WORLD HEALTH ORGANIZATION

INTERNATIONAL AGENCY FOR RESEARCH ON CANCER

IARC MONOGRAPHS

ON THE

EVALUATION OF CARCINOGENIC

RISKS TO HUMANS

Ionizing Radiation, Part 1:
X- and Gamma (γ)-Radiation, and Neutrons

VOLUME 75

This publication represents the views and expert opinions
of an IARC Working Group on the
Evaluation of Carcinogenic Risks to Humans,
which met in Lyon,

26 May–2 June 1999

2000

IARC MONOGRAPHS

In 1969, the International Agency for Research on Cancer (IARC) initiated a programme on the evaluation of the carcinogenic risk of chemicals to humans involving the production of critically evaluated monographs on individual chemicals. The programme was subsequently expanded to include evaluations of carcinogenic risks associated with exposures to complex mixtures, life-style factors and biological agents, as well as those in specific occupations.

The objective of the programme is to elaborate and publish in the form of monographs critical reviews of data on carcinogenicity for agents to which humans are known to be exposed and on specific exposure situations; to evaluate these data in terms of human risk with the help of international working groups of experts in chemical carcinogenesis and related fields; and to indicate where additional research efforts are needed.

The lists of IARC evaluations are regularly updated and are available on Internet: http://www.iarc.fr/.

This project was supported by Cooperative Agreement 5 UO1 CA33193 awarded by the United States National Cancer Institute, Department of Health and Human Services. Additional support has been provided since 1986 by the European Commission, since 1993 by the United States National Institute of Environmental Health Sciences and since 1995 by the United States Environmental Protection Agency through Cooperative Agreement Assistance CR 824264.

IARC Library Cataloguing in Publication Data

Ionizing radiation, Part 1, X- and γ-radiation and neutrons /
    IARC Working Group on the Evaluation of Carcinogenic Risks to Humans
    (1999 : Lyon, France)

    (IARC monographs on the evaluation of carcinogenic risks to humans ; 75)

    1. Carcinogens – congresses 2. Neoplasms, radiation-induced, part 1 – congresses
    3. X- and γ-radiation and neutrons – congresses I. IARC Working Group on the
    Evaluation of Carcinogenic Risks to Humans II. Series

    ISBN 92 832 1275 4   (NLM Classification: W1)
    ISSN 1017-1606

PRINTED IN FRANCE

CONTENTS

NOTE TO THE READER

The term 'carcinogenic risk' in the *IARC Monographs* series is taken to mean the probability that exposure to an agent will lead to cancer in humans.

Inclusion of an agent in the *Monographs* does not imply that it is a carcinogen, only that the published data have been examined. Equally, the fact that an agent has not yet been evaluated in a monograph does not mean that it is not carcinogenic.

The evaluations of carcinogenic risk are made by international working groups of independent scientists and are qualitative in nature. No recommendation is given for regulation or legislation.

Anyone who is aware of published data that may alter the evaluation of the carcinogenic risk of an agent to humans is encouraged to make this information available to the Unit of Carcinogen Identification and Evaluation, International Agency for Research on Cancer, 150 cours Albert Thomas, 69372 Lyon Cedex 08, France, in order that the agent may be considered for re-evaluation by a future Working Group.

Although every effort is made to prepare the monographs as accurately as possible, mistakes may occur. Readers are requested to communicate any errors to the Unit of Carcinogen Identification and Evaluation, so that corrections can be reported in future volumes.

IARC WORKING GROUP ON THE EVALUATION OF CARCINOGENIC RISKS TO HUMANS: IONIZING RADIATION, PART I, X- AND γ-RADIATION AND NEUTRONS

Lyon, 26 May–2 June 1999

LIST OF PARTICIPANTS

Members[1]

A. Auvinen, Radiation and Nuclear Safety Authority, Research and Environmental Surveillance, PO Box 14, 00881 Helsinki, Finland

J.D. Boice, Jr, International Epidemiology Institute, Ltd, 1500 Research Boulevard, Suite 210, Rockville, MD 20850-3127, United States

A. Bouville, Radiation Epidemiology Branch, National Cancer Institute, Executive Plaza South, Room 7094, Bethesda, MD 20892, United States

B.A. Bridges, MRC Cell Mutation Unit, University of Sussex, Falmer, Brighton BN1 9RR, United Kingdom

W. Burkart, Institute for Radiation Hygiene, Bundesamt für Strahlenschutz, Ingolstadter Landstrasse 1, 85764 Oberschleissheim, Germany

R.J. Fry, Life Sciences Division, Oak Ridge National Laboratory, 1060 Commerce Park, MS 6480, Oak Ridge, TN 37830-8026, United States

E. Gilbert, Radiation Epidemiology Branch, National Cancer Institute, 6120 Executive Boulevard, MS 7238, Rockville, MD 20852, United States

P. Hall, Department of Medical Epidemiology, Karolinska Institute, PO Box 218, 17177 Stockholm, Sweden

V.K. Ivanov, Medical Radiological Research Center, 4 Korolev Street, Obninsk 249020, Russian Federation

---

[1] Unable to attend: D.J. Brenner, Department of Radiation Oncology, Center for Radiobiological Research, College of Physicians and Surgeons of Columbia University, New York, NY 10032, United States; K. Mabuchi, Radiation Epidemiology Branch, National Cancer Institute, 6130 Executive Boulevard, EPN Suite 408, Bethesda, MD 20892, United States; F.A. Mettler, Department of Radiology, University of New Mexico, Health Sciences Center, Albuquerque, NM 87131-5336, United States; W.K. Sinclair, National Council on Radiation Protection and Measurements, 7910 Woodmont Avenue, Suite 800, Bethesda, MD 20814-3095, United States; C. Streffer, Institute of Medical Radiobiology, University Hospital of Essen, Hufelandstrasse 55, 45147 Essen, Germany

M. Lavin, Cancer Unit, Queensland Institute of Medical Research, Royal Brisbane Hospital, GPO Herston, Brisbane 4029, Australia

M. Lundell, Department of Hospital Physics, Karolinska Hospital, 171 76 Stockholm, Sweden

T. Nomura, Department of Radiation Biology B4, Faculty of Medicine, Osaka University, 2-2 Yamada Oka, Suita, Osaka 565-0871, Japan

C.M. Shy, School of Public Health, Department of Epidemiology, University of North Carolina, CB 7400, Chapel Hill, NC 27599, United States (*Chairman*)

H.H. Storm, Institute of Cancer Epidemiology, Department of Cancer Prevention, Danish Cancer Society, Strandboulevarden 49, 2100 Copenhagen, Denmark

R.L. Ullrich, The University of Texas Medical Branch, Department of Radiation Oncology, 3310 Gail Borden Building, 301 University Boulevard, Galveston, TX 77555-0656, United States

F. de Vathaire, INSERM Unit 351, Gustave Roussy Institute, 16 rue Paul Vaillant Couturier, 94800 Villejuif, France

J.W. Wilson, Environmental Interaction Branch, Materials Division, Building 1148, Mailstop 188B, NASA Langley Research Center, 8 West Taylor Street, Hampton, VA 23681-2199, United States

A.A. van Zeeland, Department of Radiation Genetics and Chemical Mutagenesis, Sylvius Laboratory, Leiden University, Wassenaarseweg 72, 2333 AL Leiden, The Netherlands

Representatives/Observers

United Nations Scientific Committee on the Effects of Atomic Radiation (UNSCEAR)
Represented by Dr A. Bouville

United States National Academy of Sciences, Committee on Biological Effects of Ionizing Radiation
Represented by Dr E. Gilbert

Radiation and Genome Stability Unit, Medical Research Council
D.T. Goodhead, Radiation and Genome Stability Unit, Medical Research Council, Harwell, Didcot, Oxfordshire OX11 ORD, United Kingdom

United States National Institute for Occupational Safety and Health
M. Schubauer-Berigan, Health Energy Research Branch, Division of Surveillance, Hazard Evaluations and Health, MS R-44, R.A. Taft Laboratories, 4676 Columbia Parkway, Cincinnati, OH 45226, United States

T. Taulbee, Health Energy Research Branch, Division of Surveillance, Hazard Evaluations and Health, MS R-44, Taft Laboratories, 4676 Columbia Parkway, Cincinnati, OH 45226, United States

International Social Security Association
G. Seitz, Group of Radiation Protection, Society of Mechanics and Electrotechnics, Gustav-Heinemann-Ufer 130, 50968 Cologne, Germany

IARC Secretariat
E. Amoros, Programme of Radiation and Cancer
R. Baan, Unit of Carcinogen Identification and Evaluation (*Responsible Officer*)
M. Blettner[2], Unit of Carcinogen Identification and Evaluation
I. Bray, Unit of Environmental Cancer Epidemiology
P. Brennan, Unit of Environmental Cancer Epidemiology
E. Cardis, Programme of Radiation and Cancer
Y. Grosse, Unit of Carcinogen Identification and Evaluation
J. Hall-Posner, Unit of Mechanisms of Carcinogenesis
Z. Herceg, Unit of Gene–Environment Interactions
E. Heseltine (*Editor*)
A. Kesminiene, Programme of Radiation and Cancer
D. McGregor, Unit of Carcinogen Identification and Evaluation
A.B. Miller[3], Unit of Chemoprevention
F. Nyberg, Unit of Environmental Cancer Epidemiology
H. Ohshima, Unit of Endogenous Cancer Risk Factors
C. Partensky, Unit of Carcinogen Identification and Evaluation
J. Rice, Unit of Carcinogen Identification and Evaluation (*Head of Programme*)
I. Thierry-Chef, Programme of Radiation and Cancer
E. Ward, Unit of Environmental Cancer Epidemiology
J. Wilbourn, Unit of Carcinogen Identification and Evaluation
R. Winkelmann[4], Unit of Descriptive Epidemiology

Technical assistance
M. Lézère
A. Meneghel
D. Mietton
J. Mitchell
S. Reynaud
S. Ruiz

---

[2] Present address: Department of Epidemiology and Medical Statistics, School of Public Health, PO Box 100131, 33501 Bielefeld, Germany
[3] Present address: Department of Epidemiology, German Cancer Research Center, Im Neuenheimer Feld 280, 69120 Heidelberg, Germany
[4] Present address: World Health Organization, 1211 Geneva 27, Switzerland

PREAMBLE

IARC MONOGRAPHS PROGRAMME ON THE EVALUATION OF CARCINOGENIC RISKS TO HUMANS

PREAMBLE

1. BACKGROUND

In 1969, the International Agency for Research on Cancer (IARC) initiated a programme to evaluate the carcinogenic risk of chemicals to humans and to produce monographs on individual chemicals. The *Monographs* programme has since been expanded to include consideration of exposures to complex mixtures of chemicals (which occur, for example, in some occupations and as a result of human habits) and of exposures to other agents, such as radiation and viruses. With Supplement 6 (IARC, 1987a), the title of the series was modified from *IARC Monographs on the Evaluation of the Carcinogenic Risk of Chemicals to Humans* to *IARC Monographs on the Evaluation of Carcinogenic Risks to Humans*, in order to reflect the widened scope of the programme.

The criteria established in 1971 to evaluate carcinogenic risk to humans were adopted by the working groups whose deliberations resulted in the first 16 volumes of the *IARC Monographs series*. Those criteria were subsequently updated by further ad-hoc working groups (IARC, 1977, 1978, 1979, 1982, 1983, 1987b, 1988, 1991a; Vainio *et al.*, 1992).

2. OBJECTIVE AND SCOPE

The objective of the programme is to prepare, with the help of international working groups of experts, and to publish in the form of monographs, critical reviews and evaluations of evidence on the carcinogenicity of a wide range of human exposures. The *Monographs* may also indicate where additional research efforts are needed.

The *Monographs* represent the first step in carcinogenic risk assessment, which involves examination of all relevant information in order to assess the strength of the available evidence that certain exposures could alter the incidence of cancer in humans. The second step is quantitative risk estimation. Detailed, quantitative evaluations of epidemiological data may be made in the *Monographs*, but without extrapolation beyond the range of the data available. Quantitative extrapolation from experimental data to the human situation is not undertaken.

The term 'carcinogen' is used in these monographs to denote an exposure that is capable of increasing the incidence of malignant neoplasms; the induction of benign neoplasms may in some circumstances (see p. 19) contribute to the judgement that the exposure is carcinogenic. The terms 'neoplasm' and 'tumour' are used interchangeably.

Some epidemiological and experimental studies indicate that different agents may act at different stages in the carcinogenic process, and several mechanisms may be involved. The aim of the *Monographs* has been, from their inception, to evaluate evidence of carcinogenicity at any stage in the carcinogenesis process, independently of the underlying mechanisms. Information on mechanisms may, however, be used in making the overall evaluation (IARC, 1991a; Vainio *et al.*, 1992; see also pp. 25–27).

The *Monographs* may assist national and international authorities in making risk assessments and in formulating decisions concerning any necessary preventive measures. The evaluations of IARC working groups are scientific, qualitative judgements about the evidence for or against carcinogenicity provided by the available data. These evaluations represent only one part of the body of information on which regulatory measures may be based. Other components of regulatory decisions vary from one situation to another and from country to country, responding to different socioeconomic and national priorities. **Therefore, no recommendation is given with regard to regulation or legislation, which are the responsibility of individual governments and/or other international organizations.**

The *IARC Monographs* are recognized as an authoritative source of information on the carcinogenicity of a wide range of human exposures. A survey of users in 1988 indicated that the *Monographs* are consulted by various agencies in 57 countries. About 3000 copies of each volume are printed, for distribution to governments, regulatory bodies and interested scientists. The Monographs are also available from IARC*Press* in Lyon and via the Distribution and Sales Service of the World Health Organization in Geneva.

3.   SELECTION OF TOPICS FOR MONOGRAPHS

Topics are selected on the basis of two main criteria: (a) there is evidence of human exposure, and (b) there is some evidence or suspicion of carcinogenicity. The term 'agent' is used to include individual chemical compounds, groups of related chemical compounds, physical agents (such as radiation) and biological factors (such as viruses). Exposures to mixtures of agents may occur in occupational exposures and as a result of personal and cultural habits (like smoking and dietary practices). Chemical analogues and compounds with biological or physical characteristics similar to those of suspected carcinogens may also be considered, even in the absence of data on a possible carcinogenic effect in humans or experimental animals.

The scientific literature is surveyed for published data relevant to an assessment of carcinogenicity. The IARC information bulletins on agents being tested for carcinogenicity (IARC, 1973–1996) and directories of on-going research in cancer epidemiology (IARC, 1976–1996) often indicate exposures that may be scheduled for future meetings. Ad-hoc working groups convened by IARC in 1984, 1989, 1991, 1993 and 1998 gave recommendations as to which agents should be evaluated in the IARC Monographs series (IARC, 1984, 1989, 1991b, 1993, 1998a,b).

As significant new data on subjects on which monographs have already been prepared become available, re-evaluations are made at subsequent meetings, and revised monographs are published.

4. DATA FOR MONOGRAPHS

The *Monographs* do not necessarily cite all the literature concerning the subject of an evaluation. Only those data considered by the Working Group to be relevant to making the evaluation are included.

With regard to biological and epidemiological data, only reports that have been published or accepted for publication in the openly available scientific literature are reviewed by the working groups. In certain instances, government agency reports that have undergone peer review and are widely available are considered. Exceptions may be made on an ad-hoc basis to include unpublished reports that are in their final form and publicly available, if their inclusion is considered pertinent to making a final evaluation (see pp. 25–27). In the sections on chemical and physical properties, on analysis, on production and use and on occurrence, unpublished sources of information may be used.

5. THE WORKING GROUP

Reviews and evaluations are formulated by a working group of experts. The tasks of the group are: (i) to ascertain that all appropriate data have been collected; (ii) to select the data relevant for the evaluation on the basis of scientific merit; (iii) to prepare accurate summaries of the data to enable the reader to follow the reasoning of the Working Group; (iv) to evaluate the results of epidemiological and experimental studies on cancer; (v) to evaluate data relevant to the understanding of mechanism of action; and (vi) to make an overall evaluation of the carcinogenicity of the exposure to humans.

Working Group participants who contributed to the considerations and evaluations within a particular volume are listed, with their addresses, at the beginning of each publication. Each participant who is a member of a working group serves as an individual scientist and not as a representative of any organization, government or industry. In addition, nominees of national and international agencies and industrial associations may be invited as observers.

6. WORKING PROCEDURES

Approximately one year in advance of a meeting of a working group, the topics of the monographs are announced and participants are selected by IARC staff in consultation with other experts. Subsequently, relevant biological and epidemiological data are collected by the Carcinogen Identification and Evaluation Unit of IARC from recognized sources of information on carcinogenesis, including data storage and retrieval systems such as MEDLINE and TOXLINE.

For chemicals and some complex mixtures, the major collection of data and the preparation of first drafts of the sections on chemical and physical properties, on analysis, on production and use and on occurrence are carried out under a separate contract funded by the United States National Cancer Institute. Representatives from industrial associations may assist in the preparation of sections on production and use. Information on production and trade is obtained from governmental and trade publications and, in some cases, by direct contact with industries. Separate production data on some agents may not be available because their publication could disclose confidential information. Information on uses may be obtained from published sources but is often complemented by direct contact with manufacturers. Efforts are made to supplement this information with data from other national and international sources.

Six months before the meeting, the material obtained is sent to meeting participants, or is used by IARC staff, to prepare sections for the first drafts of monographs. The first drafts are compiled by IARC staff and sent before the meeting to all participants of the Working Group for review.

The Working Group meets in Lyon for seven to eight days to discuss and finalize the texts of the monographs and to formulate the evaluations. After the meeting, the master copy of each monograph is verified by consulting the original literature, edited and prepared for publication. The aim is to publish monographs within six months of the Working Group meeting.

The available studies are summarized by the Working Group, with particular regard to the qualitative aspects discussed below. In general, numerical findings are indicated as they appear in the original report; units are converted when necessary for easier comparison. The Working Group may conduct additional analyses of the published data and use them in their assessment of the evidence; the results of such supplementary analyses are given in square brackets. When an important aspect of a study, directly impinging on its interpretation, should be brought to the attention of the reader, a comment is given in square brackets.

7.   EXPOSURE DATA

Sections that indicate the extent of past and present human exposure, the sources of exposure, the people most likely to be exposed and the factors that contribute to the exposure are included at the beginning of each monograph.

Most monographs on individual chemicals, groups of chemicals or complex mixtures include sections on chemical and physical data, on analysis, on production and use and on occurrence. In monographs on, for example, physical agents, occupational exposures and cultural habits, other sections may be included, such as: historical perspectives, description of an industry or habit, chemistry of the complex mixture or taxonomy. Monographs on biological agents have sections on structure and biology, methods of detection, epidemiology of infection and clinical disease other than cancer.

For chemical exposures, the Chemical Abstracts Services Registry Number, the latest Chemical Abstracts Primary Name and the IUPAC Systematic Name are recorded; other synonyms are given, but the list is not necessarily comprehensive. For biological agents, taxonomy and structure are described, and the degree of variability is given, when applicable.

Information on chemical and physical properties and, in particular, data relevant to identification, occurrence and biological activity are included. For biological agents, mode of replication, life cycle, target cells, persistence and latency and host response are given. A description of technical products of chemicals includes trade names, relevant specifications and available information on composition and impurities. Some of the trade names given may be those of mixtures in which the agent being evaluated is only one of the ingredients.

The purpose of the section on analysis or detection is to give the reader an overview of current methods, with emphasis on those widely used for regulatory purposes. Methods for monitoring human exposure are also given, when available. No critical evaluation or recommendation of any of the methods is meant or implied. The IARC published a series of volumes, *Environmental Carcinogens: Methods of Analysis and Exposure Measurement* (IARC, 1978–93), that describe validated methods for analysing a wide variety of chemicals and mixtures. For biological agents, methods of detection and exposure assessment are described, including their sensitivity, specificity and reproducibility.

The dates of first synthesis and of first commercial production of a chemical or mixture are provided; for agents which do not occur naturally, this information may allow a reasonable estimate to be made of the date before which no human exposure to the agent could have occurred. The dates of first reported occurrence of an exposure are also provided. In addition, methods of synthesis used in past and present commercial production and different methods of production which may give rise to different impurities are described.

Data on production, international trade and uses are obtained for representative regions, which usually include Europe, Japan and the United States of America. It should not, however, be inferred that those areas or nations are necessarily the sole or major sources or users of the agent. Some identified uses may not be current or major applications, and the coverage is not necessarily comprehensive. In the case of drugs, mention of their therapeutic uses does not necessarily represent current practice, nor does it imply judgement as to their therapeutic efficacy.

Information on the occurrence of an agent or mixture in the environment is obtained from data derived from the monitoring and surveillance of levels in occupational environments, air, water, soil, foods and animal and human tissues. When available, data on the generation, persistence and bioaccumulation of the agent are also included. In the case of mixtures, industries, occupations or processes, information is given about all agents present. For processes, industries and occupations, a historical description is also given, noting variations in chemical composition, physical properties and levels of occupational exposure with time and place. For biological agents, the epidemiology of infection is described.

Statements concerning regulations and guidelines (e.g., pesticide registrations, maximal levels permitted in foods, occupational exposure limits) are included for some countries as indications of potential exposures, but they may not reflect the most recent situation, since such limits are continuously reviewed and modified. The absence of information on regulatory status for a country should not be taken to imply that that country does not have regulations with regard to the exposure. For biological agents, legislation and control, including vaccines and therapy, are described.

8.   STUDIES OF CANCER IN HUMANS

(a)   Types of studies considered

Three types of epidemiological studies of cancer contribute to the assessment of carcinogenicity in humans—cohort studies, case–control studies and correlation (or ecological) studies. Rarely, results from randomized trials may be available. Case series and case reports of cancer in humans may also be reviewed.

Cohort and case–control studies relate the exposures under study to the occurrence of cancer in individuals and provide an estimate of relative risk (ratio of incidence or mortality in those exposed to incidence or mortality in those not exposed) as the main measure of association.

In correlation studies, the units of investigation are usually whole populations (e.g. in particular geographical areas or at particular times), and cancer frequency is related to a summary measure of the exposure of the population to the agent, mixture or exposure circumstance under study. Because individual exposure is not documented, however, a causal relationship is less easy to infer from correlation studies than from cohort and case–control studies. Case reports generally arise from a suspicion, based on clinical experience, that the concurrence of two events—that is, a particular exposure and occurrence of a cancer—has happened rather more frequently than would be expected by chance. Case reports usually lack complete ascertainment of cases in any population, definition or enumeration of the population at risk and estimation of the expected number of cases in the absence of exposure. The uncertainties surrounding interpretation of case reports and correlation studies make them inadequate, except in rare instances, to form the sole basis for inferring a causal relationship. When taken together with case–control and cohort studies, however, relevant case reports or correlation studies may add materially to the judgement that a causal relationship is present.

Epidemiological studies of benign neoplasms, presumed preneoplastic lesions and other end-points thought to be relevant to cancer are also reviewed by working groups. They may, in some instances, strengthen inferences drawn from studies of cancer itself.

(b)   Quality of studies considered

The Monographs are not intended to summarize all published studies. Those that are judged to be inadequate or irrelevant to the evaluation are generally omitted. They may be mentioned briefly, particularly when the information is considered to be a useful supplement to that in other reports or when they provide the only data available. Their inclusion does not imply acceptance of the adequacy of the study design or of the analysis and interpretation of the results, and limitations are clearly outlined in square brackets at the end of the study description.

It is necessary to take into account the possible roles of bias, confounding and chance in the interpretation of epidemiological studies. By 'bias' is meant the operation of factors in study design or execution that lead erroneously to a stronger or weaker association than in fact exists between disease and an agent, mixture or exposure circumstance. By 'confounding' is meant a situation in which the relationship with disease is made to appear stronger or weaker than it truly is as a result of an association between the apparent causal factor and another factor that is associated with either an increase or decrease in the incidence of the disease. In evaluating the extent to which these factors have been minimized in an individual study, working groups consider a number of aspects of design and analysis as described in the report of the study. Most of these considerations apply equally to case–control, cohort and correlation studies. Lack of clarity of any of these aspects in the reporting of a study can decrease its credibility and the weight given to it in the final evaluation of the exposure.

Firstly, the study population, disease (or diseases) and exposure should have been well defined by the authors. Cases of disease in the study population should have been identified in a way that was independent of the exposure of interest, and exposure should have been assessed in a way that was not related to disease status.

Secondly, the authors should have taken account in the study design and analysis of other variables that can influence the risk of disease and may have been related to the exposure of interest. Potential confounding by such variables should have been dealt with either in the design of the study, such as by matching, or in the analysis, by statistical adjustment. In cohort studies, comparisons with local rates of disease may be more appropriate than those with national rates. Internal comparisons of disease frequency among individuals at different levels of exposure should also have been made in the study.

Thirdly, the authors should have reported the basic data on which the conclusions are founded, even if sophisticated statistical analyses were employed. At the very least, they should have given the numbers of exposed and unexposed cases and controls in a case–control study and the numbers of cases observed and expected in a cohort study. Further tabulations by time since exposure began and other temporal factors are also important. In a cohort study, data on all cancer sites and all causes of death should have been given, to reveal the possibility of reporting bias. In a case–control study, the effects of investigated factors other than the exposure of interest should have been reported.

Finally, the statistical methods used to obtain estimates of relative risk, absolute rates of cancer, confidence intervals and significance tests, and to adjust for confounding should have been clearly stated by the authors. The methods used should preferably have been the generally accepted techniques that have been refined since the mid-1970s. These methods have been reviewed for case–control studies (Breslow & Day, 1980) and for cohort studies (Breslow & Day, 1987).

(c)   *Inferences about mechanism of action*

Detailed analyses of both relative and absolute risks in relation to temporal variables, such as age at first exposure, time since first exposure, duration of exposure, cumulative exposure and time since exposure ceased, are reviewed and summarized when available. The analysis of temporal relationships can be useful in formulating models of carcino-genesis. In particular, such analyses may suggest whether a carcinogen acts early or late in the process of carcinogenesis, although at best they allow only indirect inferences about the mechanism of action. Special attention is given to measurements of biological markers of carcinogen exposure or action, such as DNA or protein adducts, as well as markers of early steps in the carcinogenic process, such as proto-oncogene mutation, when these are incorporated into epidemiological studies focused on cancer incidence or mortality. Such measurements may allow inferences to be made about putative mecha-nisms of action (IARC, 1991a; Vainio *et al.*, 1992).

(d)   *Criteria for causality*

After the individual epidemiological studies of cancer have been summarized and the quality assessed, a judgement is made concerning the strength of evidence that the agent, mixture or exposure circumstance in question is carcinogenic for humans. In making its judgement, the Working Group considers several criteria for causality. A strong asso-ciation (a large relative risk) is more likely to indicate causality than a weak association, although it is recognized that relative risks of small magnitude do not imply lack of causality and may be important if the disease is common. Associations that are replicated in several studies of the same design or using different epidemiological approaches or under different circumstances of exposure are more likely to represent a causal relation-ship than isolated observations from single studies. If there are inconsistent results among investigations, possible reasons are sought (such as differences in amount of exposure), and results of studies judged to be of high quality are given more weight than those of studies judged to be methodologically less sound. When suspicion of carcino-genicity arises largely from a single study, these data are not combined with those from later studies in any subsequent reassessment of the strength of the evidence.

If the risk of the disease in question increases with the amount of exposure, this is considered to be a strong indication of causality, although absence of a graded response is not necessarily evidence against a causal relationship. Demonstration of a decline in risk after cessation of or reduction in exposure in individuals or in whole populations also supports a causal interpretation of the findings.

Although a carcinogen may act upon more than one target, the specificity of an asso-ciation (an increased occurrence of cancer at one anatomical site or of one morphological type) adds plausibility to a causal relationship, particularly when excess cancer occur-rence is limited to one morphological type within the same organ.

Although rarely available, results from randomized trials showing different rates among exposed and unexposed individuals provide particularly strong evidence for causality.

When several epidemiological studies show little or no indication of an association between an exposure and cancer, the judgement may be made that, in the aggregate, they show evidence of lack of carcinogenicity. Such a judgement requires first of all that the studies giving rise to it meet, to a sufficient degree, the standards of design and analysis described above. Specifically, the possibility that bias, confounding or misclassification of exposure or outcome could explain the observed results should be considered and excluded with reasonable certainty. In addition, all studies that are judged to be methodologically sound should be consistent with a relative risk of unity for any observed level of exposure and, when considered together, should provide a pooled estimate of relative risk which is at or near unity and has a narrow confidence interval, due to sufficient population size. Moreover, no individual study nor the pooled results of all the studies should show any consistent tendency for the relative risk of cancer to increase with increasing level of exposure. It is important to note that evidence of lack of carcinogenicity obtained in this way from several epidemiological studies can apply only to the type(s) of cancer studied and to dose levels and intervals between first exposure and observation of disease that are the same as or less than those observed in all the studies. Experience with human cancer indicates that, in some cases, the period from first exposure to the development of clinical cancer is seldom less than 20 years; latent periods substantially shorter than 30 years cannot provide evidence for lack of carcinogenicity.

9.   STUDIES OF CANCER IN EXPERIMENTAL ANIMALS

All known human carcinogens that have been studied adequately in experimental animals have produced positive results in one or more animal species (Wilbourn *et al.*, 1986; Tomatis *et al.*, 1989). For several agents (aflatoxins, 4-aminobiphenyl, azathioprine, betel quid with tobacco, bischloromethyl ether and chloromethyl methyl ether (technical grade), chlorambucil, chlornaphazine, ciclosporin, coal-tar pitches, coal-tars, combined oral contraceptives, cyclophosphamide, diethylstilboestrol, melphalan, 8-methoxypsoralen plus ultraviolet A radiation, mustard gas, myleran, 2-naphthylamine, nonsteroidal oestrogens, oestrogen replacement therapy/steroidal oestrogens, solar radiation, thiotepa and vinyl chloride), carcinogenicity in experimental animals was established or highly suspected before epidemiological studies confirmed their carcinogenicity in humans (Vainio *et al.*, 1995). Although this association cannot establish that all agents and mixtures that cause cancer in experimental animals also cause cancer in humans, nevertheless, **in the absence of adequate data on humans, it is biologically plausible and prudent to regard agents and mixtures for which there is *sufficient evidence* (see p. 24) of carcinogenicity in experimental animals as if they presented a carcinogenic risk to humans**. The possibility that a given agent may cause cancer through a species-specific mechanism which does not operate in humans (see p. 27) should also be taken into consideration.

The nature and extent of impurities or contaminants present in the chemical or mixture being evaluated are given when available. Animal strain, sex, numbers per group, age at start of treatment and survival are reported.

Other types of studies summarized include: experiments in which the agent or mixture was administered in conjunction with known carcinogens or factors that modify carcinogenic effects; studies in which the end-point was not cancer but a defined precancerous lesion; and experiments on the carcinogenicity of known metabolites and derivatives.

For experimental studies of mixtures, consideration is given to the possibility of changes in the physicochemical properties of the test substance during collection, storage, extraction, concentration and delivery. Chemical and toxicological interactions of the components of mixtures may result in nonlinear dose–response relationships.

An assessment is made as to the relevance to human exposure of samples tested in experimental animals, which may involve consideration of: (i) physical and chemical characteristics, (ii) constituent substances that indicate the presence of a class of substances, (iii) the results of tests for genetic and related effects, including studies on DNA adduct formation, proto-oncogene mutation and expression and suppressor gene inactivation. The relevance of results obtained, for example, with animal viruses analogous to the virus being evaluated in the monograph must also be considered. They may provide biological and mechanistic information relevant to the understanding of the process of carcinogenesis in humans and may strengthen the plausibility of a conclusion that the biological agent under evaluation is carcinogenic in humans.

(a)   Qualitative aspects

An assessment of carcinogenicity involves several considerations of qualitative importance, including (i) the experimental conditions under which the test was per-formed, including route and schedule of exposure, species, strain, sex, age, duration of follow-up; (ii) the consistency of the results, for example, across species and target organ(s); (iii) the spectrum of neoplastic response, from preneoplastic lesions and benign tumours to malignant neoplasms; and (iv) the possible role of modifying factors.

As mentioned earlier (p. 11), the *Monographs* are not intended to summarize all published studies. Those studies in experimental animals that are inadequate (e.g., too short a duration, too few animals, poor survival; see below) or are judged irrelevant to the evaluation are generally omitted. Guidelines for conducting adequate long-term carcinogenicity experiments have been outlined (e.g. Montesano *et al.*, 1986).

Considerations of importance to the Working Group in the interpretation and eva-luation of a particular study include: (i) how clearly the agent was defined and, in the case of mixtures, how adequately the sample characterization was reported; (ii) whether the dose was adequately monitored, particularly in inhalation experiments; (iii) whether the doses and duration of treatment were appropriate and whether the survival of treated animals was similar to that of controls; (iv) whether there were adequate numbers of animals per group; (v) whether animals of each sex were used; (vi) whether animals were allocated randomly to groups; (vii) whether the duration of observation was adequate; and (viii) whether the data were adequately reported. If available, recent data on the incidence of specific tumours in historical controls, as well as in concurrent controls, should be taken into account in the evaluation of tumour response.

When benign tumours occur together with and originate from the same cell type in an organ or tissue as malignant tumours in a particular study and appear to represent a stage in the progression to malignancy, it may be valid to combine them in assessing tumour incidence (Huff *et al.*, 1989). The occurrence of lesions presumed to be pre-neoplastic may in certain instances aid in assessing the biological plausibility of any neo-plastic response observed. If an agent or mixture induces only benign neoplasms that appear to be end-points that do not readily progress to malignancy, it should nevertheless be suspected of being a carcinogen and requires further investigation.

(*b*) *Quantitative aspects*

The probability that tumours will occur may depend on the species, sex, strain and age of the animal, the dose of the carcinogen and the route and length of exposure. Evidence of an increased incidence of neoplasms with increased level of exposure strengthens the inference of a causal association between the exposure and the develop-ment of neoplasms.

The form of the dose–response relationship can vary widely, depending on the particular agent under study and the target organ. Both DNA damage and increased cell division are important aspects of carcinogenesis, and cell proliferation is a strong deter-minant of dose–response relationships for some carcinogens (Cohen & Ellwein, 1990). Since many chemicals require metabolic activation before being converted into their reactive intermediates, both metabolic and pharmacokinetic aspects are important in determining the dose–response pattern. Saturation of steps such as absorption, activation, inactivation and elimination may produce nonlinearity in the dose–response relationship, as could saturation of processes such as DNA repair (Hoel *et al.*, 1983; Gart *et al.*, 1986).

(*c*) *Statistical analysis of long-term experiments in animals*

Factors considered by the Working Group include the adequacy of the information given for each treatment group: (i) the number of animals studied and the number examined histologically, (ii) the number of animals with a given tumour type and (iii) length of survival. The statistical methods used should be clearly stated and should be the generally accepted techniques refined for this purpose (Peto *et al.*, 1980; Gart *et al.*, 1986). When there is no difference in survival between control and treatment groups, the Working Group usually compares the proportions of animals developing each tumour type in each of the groups. Otherwise, consideration is given as to whether or not appropriate adjustments have been made for differences in survival. These adjustments can include: comparisons of the proportions of tumour-bearing animals among the effective number of animals (alive at the time the first tumour is discovered), in the case where most differences in survival occur before tumours appear; life-table methods, when tumours are visible or when they may be considered 'fatal' because mortality rapidly follows tumour development; and the Mantel-Haenszel test or logistic regression, when occult tumours do not affect the animals' risk of dying but are 'incidental' findings at autopsy.

In practice, classifying tumours as fatal or incidental may be difficult. Several survival-adjusted methods have been developed that do not require this distinction (Gart *et al.*, 1986), although they have not been fully evaluated.

10.   OTHER DATA RELEVANT TO AN EVALUATION OF CARCINOGENICITY AND ITS MECHANISMS

In coming to an overall evaluation of carcinogenicity in humans (see pp. 25–27), the Working Group also considers related data. The nature of the information selected for the summary depends on the agent being considered.

For chemicals and complex mixtures of chemicals such as those in some occupational situations or involving cultural habits (e.g. tobacco smoking), the other data considered to be relevant are divided into those on absorption, distribution, metabolism and excretion; toxic effects; reproductive and developmental effects; and genetic and related effects.

Concise information is given on absorption, distribution (including placental transfer) and excretion in both humans and experimental animals. Kinetic factors that may affect the dose–response relationship, such as saturation of uptake, protein binding, metabolic activation, detoxification and DNA repair processes, are mentioned. Studies that indicate the metabolic fate of the agent in humans and in experimental animals are summarized briefly, and comparisons of data on humans and on animals are made when possible. Comparative information on the relationship between exposure and the dose that reaches the target site may be of particular importance for extrapolation between species. Data are given on acute and chronic toxic effects (other than cancer), such as organ toxicity, increased cell proliferation, immunotoxicity and endocrine effects. The presence and toxicological significance of cellular receptors is described. Effects on reproduction, teratogenicity, fetotoxicity and embryotoxicity are also summarized briefly.

Tests of genetic and related effects are described in view of the relevance of gene mutation and chromosomal damage to carcinogenesis (Vainio *et al.*, 1992; McGregor *et al.*, 1999). The adequacy of the reporting of sample characterization is considered and, where necessary, commented upon; with regard to complex mixtures, such comments are similar to those described for animal carcinogenicity tests on p. 18. The available data are interpreted critically by phylogenetic group according to the end-points detected, which may include DNA damage, gene mutation, sister chromatid exchange, micronucleus formation, chromosomal aberrations, aneuploidy and cell transformation. The concentrations employed are given, and mention is made of whether use of an exogenous metabolic system *in vitro* affected the test result. These data are given as listings of test systems, data and references. The Genetic and Related Effects data presented in the *Monographs* are also available in the form of Graphic Activity Profiles (GAP) prepared in collaboration with the United States Environmental Protection Agency (EPA) (see also

Waters *et al.*, 1987) using software for personal computers that are Microsoft Windows®
compatible. The EPA/IARC GAP software and database may be downloaded free of
charge from *www.epa.gov/gapdb*.

Positive results in tests using prokaryotes, lower eukaryotes, plants, insects and
cultured mammalian cells suggest that genetic and related effects could occur in
mammals. Results from such tests may also give information about the types of genetic
effect produced and about the involvement of metabolic activation. Some end-points
described are clearly genetic in nature (e.g., gene mutations and chromosomal aberrations), while others are to a greater or lesser degree associated with genetic effects (e.g.
unscheduled DNA synthesis). In-vitro tests for tumour-promoting activity and for cell
transformation may be sensitive to changes that are not necessarily the result of genetic
alterations but that may have specific relevance to the process of carcinogenesis. A
critical appraisal of these tests has been published (Montesano *et al.*, 1986).

Genetic or other activity manifest in experimental mammals and humans is regarded
as being of greater relevance than that in other organisms. The demonstration that an
agent or mixture can induce gene and chromosomal mutations in whole mammals indicates that it may have carcinogenic activity, although this activity may not be detectably
expressed in any or all species. Relative potency in tests for mutagenicity and related
effects is not a reliable indicator of carcinogenic potency. Negative results in tests for
mutagenicity in selected tissues from animals treated *in vivo* provide less weight, partly
because they do not exclude the possibility of an effect in tissues other than those
examined. Moreover, negative results in short-term tests with genetic end-points cannot
be considered to provide evidence to rule out carcinogenicity of agents or mixtures that
act through other mechanisms (e.g. receptor-mediated effects, cellular toxicity with rege-
nerative proliferation, peroxisome proliferation) (Vainio *et al.*, 1992). Factors that may
lead to misleading results in short-term tests have been discussed in detail elsewhere
(Montesano *et al.*, 1986).

When available, data relevant to mechanisms of carcinogenesis that do not involve
structural changes at the level of the gene are also described.

The adequacy of epidemiological studies of reproductive outcome and genetic and
related effects in humans is evaluated by the same criteria as are applied to epidemiological studies of cancer.

Structure–activity relationships that may be relevant to an evaluation of the carcinogenicity of an agent are also described.

For biological agents—viruses, bacteria and parasites—other data relevant to
carcinogenicity include descriptions of the pathology of infection, molecular biology
(integration and expression of viruses, and any genetic alterations seen in human
tumours) and other observations, which might include cellular and tissue responses to
infection, immune response and the presence of tumour markers.

11.   SUMMARY OF DATA REPORTED

In this section, the relevant epidemiological and experimental data are summarized. Only reports, other than in abstract form, that meet the criteria outlined on p. 11 are considered for evaluating carcinogenicity. Inadequate studies are generally not summarized: such studies are usually identified by a square-bracketed comment in the preceding text.

(a)   Exposure

Human exposure to chemicals and complex mixtures is summarized on the basis of elements such as production, use, occurrence in the environment and determinations in human tissues and body fluids. Quantitative data are given when available. Exposure to biological agents is described in terms of transmission and prevalence of infection.

(b)   Carcinogenicity in humans

Results of epidemiological studies that are considered to be pertinent to an assessment of human carcinogenicity are summarized. When relevant, case reports and correlation studies are also summarized.

(c)   Carcinogenicity in experimental animals

Data relevant to an evaluation of carcinogenicity in animals are summarized. For each animal species and route of administration, it is stated whether an increased incidence of neoplasms or preneoplastic lesions was observed, and the tumour sites are indicated. If the agent or mixture produced tumours after prenatal exposure or in single-dose experiments, this is also indicated. Negative findings are also summarized. Dose–response and other quantitative data may be given when available.

(d)   Other data relevant to an evaluation of carcinogenicity and its mechanisms

Data on biological effects in humans that are of particular relevance are summarized. These may include toxicological, kinetic and metabolic considerations and evidence of DNA binding, persistence of DNA lesions or genetic damage in exposed humans. Toxicological information, such as that on cytotoxicity and regeneration, receptor binding and hormonal and immunological effects, and data on kinetics and metabolism in experimental animals are given when considered relevant to the possible mechanism of the carcinogenic action of the agent. The results of tests for genetic and related effects are summarized for whole mammals, cultured mammalian cells and nonmammalian systems.

When available, comparisons of such data for humans and for animals, and particularly animals that have developed cancer, are described.

Structure–activity relationships are mentioned when relevant.

For the agent, mixture or exposure circumstance being evaluated, the available data on end-points or other phenomena relevant to mechanisms of carcinogenesis from studies in humans, experimental animals and tissue and cell test systems are summarized within one or more of the following descriptive dimensions:

(i) Evidence of genotoxicity (structural changes at the level of the gene): for example, structure–activity considerations, adduct formation, mutagenicity (effect on specific genes), chromosomal mutation/aneuploidy

(ii) Evidence of effects on the expression of relevant genes (functional changes at the intracellular level): for example, alterations to the structure or quantity of the product of a proto-oncogene or tumour-suppressor gene, alterations to metabolic activation/inactivation/DNA repair

(iii) Evidence of relevant effects on cell behaviour (morphological or behavioural changes at the cellular or tissue level): for example, induction of mitogenesis, compensatory cell proliferation, preneoplasia and hyperplasia, survival of premalignant or malignant cells (immortalization, immunosuppression), effects on metastatic potential

(iv) Evidence from dose and time relationships of carcinogenic effects and interactions between agents: for example, early/late stage, as inferred from epidemiological studies; initiation/promotion/progression/malignant conversion, as defined in animal carcinogenicity experiments; toxicokinetics

These dimensions are not mutually exclusive, and an agent may fall within more than one of them. Thus, for example, the action of an agent on the expression of relevant genes could be summarized under both the first and second dimensions, even if it were known with reasonable certainty that those effects resulted from genotoxicity.

12.   EVALUATION

Evaluations of the strength of the evidence for carcinogenicity arising from human and experimental animal data are made, using standard terms.

It is recognized that the criteria for these evaluations, described below, cannot encompass all of the factors that may be relevant to an evaluation of carcinogenicity. In considering all of the relevant scientific data, the Working Group may assign the agent, mixture or exposure circumstance to a higher or lower category than a strict interpretation of these criteria would indicate.

(a)   Degrees of evidence for carcinogenicity in humans and in experimental animals and supporting evidence

These categories refer only to the strength of the evidence that an exposure is carcinogenic and not to the extent of its carcinogenic activity (potency) nor to the mechanisms involved. A classification may change as new information becomes available.

An evaluation of degree of evidence, whether for a single agent or a mixture, is limited to the materials tested, as defined physically, chemically or biologically. When the agents evaluated are considered by the Working Group to be sufficiently closely related, they may be grouped together for the purpose of a single evaluation of degree of evidence.

(i)   Carcinogenicity in humans

The applicability of an evaluation of the carcinogenicity of a mixture, process, occupation or industry on the basis of evidence from epidemiological studies depends on the variability over time and place of the mixtures, processes, occupations and industries. The Working Group seeks to identify the specific exposure, process or activity which is considered most likely to be responsible for any excess risk. The evaluation is focused as narrowly as the available data on exposure and other aspects permit.

The evidence relevant to carcinogenicity from studies in humans is classified into one of the following categories:

Sufficient evidence of carcinogenicity: The Working Group considers that a causal relationship has been established between exposure to the agent, mixture or exposure circumstance and human cancer. That is, a positive relationship has been observed between the exposure and cancer in studies in which chance, bias and confounding could be ruled out with reasonable confidence.

Limited evidence of carcinogenicity: A positive association has been observed between exposure to the agent, mixture or exposure circumstance and cancer for which a causal interpretation is considered by the Working Group to be credible, but chance, bias or confounding could not be ruled out with reasonable confidence.

Inadequate evidence of carcinogenicity: The available studies are of insufficient quality, consistency or statistical power to permit a conclusion regarding the presence or absence of a causal association between exposure and cancer, or no data on cancer in humans are available.

Evidence suggesting lack of carcinogenicity: There are several adequate studies covering the full range of levels of exposure that human beings are known to encounter, which are mutually consistent in not showing a positive association between exposure to the agent, mixture or exposure circumstance and any studied cancer at any observed level of exposure. A conclusion of 'evidence suggesting lack of carcinogenicity' is inevitably limited to the cancer sites, conditions and levels of exposure and length of observation covered by the available studies. In addition, the possibility of a very small risk at the levels of exposure studied can never be excluded.

In some instances, the above categories may be used to classify the degree of evidence related to carcinogenicity in specific organs or tissues.

(ii)   *Carcinogenicity in experimental animals*

The evidence relevant to carcinogenicity in experimental animals is classified into one of the following categories:

Sufficient evidence of carcinogenicity: The Working Group considers that a causal relationship has been established between the agent or mixture and an increased incidence of malignant neoplasms or of an appropriate combination of benign and malignant neoplasms in (a) two or more species of animals or (b) in two or more independent studies in one species carried out at different times or in different laboratories or under different protocols.

Exceptionally, a single study in one species might be considered to provide sufficient evidence of carcinogenicity when malignant neoplasms occur to an unusual degree with regard to incidence, site, type of tumour or age at onset.

Limited evidence of carcinogenicity: The data suggest a carcinogenic effect but are limited for making a definitive evaluation because, e.g. (a) the evidence of carcino-genicity is restricted to a single experiment; or (b) there are unresolved questions regarding the adequacy of the design, conduct or interpretation of the study; or (c) the agent or mixture increases the incidence only of benign neoplasms or lesions of uncertain neoplastic potential, or of certain neoplasms which may occur spontaneously in high incidences in certain strains.

Inadequate evidence of carcinogenicity: The studies cannot be interpreted as showing either the presence or absence of a carcinogenic effect because of major qualitative or quantitative limitations, or no data on cancer in experimental animals are available.

Evidence suggesting lack of carcinogenicity: Adequate studies involving at least two species are available which show that, within the limits of the tests used, the agent or mixture is not carcinogenic. A conclusion of evidence suggesting lack of carcinogenicity is inevitably limited to the species, tumour sites and levels of exposure studied.

(*b*)   *Other data relevant to the evaluation of carcinogenicity and its mechanisms*

Other evidence judged to be relevant to an evaluation of carcinogenicity and of sufficient importance to affect the overall evaluation is then described. This may include data on preneoplastic lesions, tumour pathology, genetic and related effects, structure–activity relationships, metabolism and pharmacokinetics, physicochemical parameters and analogous biological agents.

Data relevant to mechanisms of the carcinogenic action are also evaluated. The strength of the evidence that any carcinogenic effect observed is due to a particular mechanism is assessed, using terms such as weak, moderate or strong. Then, the Working Group assesses if that particular mechanism is likely to be operative in humans. The strongest indications that a particular mechanism operates in humans come from data on humans or biological specimens obtained from exposed humans. The data may be consi-dered to be especially relevant if they show that the agent in question has caused changes in exposed humans that are on the causal pathway to carcinogenesis. Such data may, however, never become available, because it is at least conceivable that certain com-pounds may be kept from human use solely on the basis of evidence of their toxicity and/or carcinogenicity in experimental systems.

For complex exposures, including occupational and industrial exposures, the chemical composition and the potential contribution of carcinogens known to be present are considered by the Working Group in its overall evaluation of human carcinogenicity. The Working Group also determines the extent to which the materials tested in experi-mental systems are related to those to which humans are exposed.

(*c*)   *Overall evaluation*

Finally, the body of evidence is considered as a whole, in order to reach an overall evaluation of the carcinogenicity to humans of an agent, mixture or circumstance of exposure.

An evaluation may be made for a group of chemical compounds that have been eva-luated by the Working Group. In addition, when supporting data indicate that other, related compounds for which there is no direct evidence of capacity to induce cancer in humans or in animals may also be carcinogenic, a statement describing the rationale for this conclusion is added to the evaluation narrative; an additional evaluation may be made for this broader group of compounds if the strength of the evidence warrants it.

The agent, mixture or exposure circumstance is described according to the wording of one of the following categories, and the designated group is given. The categorization of an agent, mixture or exposure circumstance is a matter of scientific judgement, reflec-ting the strength of the evidence derived from studies in humans and in experimental animals and from other relevant data.

Group 1 —The agent (mixture) is carcinogenic to humans.
The exposure circumstance entails exposures that are carcinogenic to humans.

This category is used when there is *sufficient evidence* of carcinogenicity in humans. Exceptionally, an agent (mixture) may be placed in this category when evidence of carci-nogenicity in humans is less than sufficient but there is *sufficient evidence* of carcino-genicity in experimental animals and strong evidence in exposed humans that the agent (mixture) acts through a relevant mechanism of carcinogenicity.

Group 2

This category includes agents, mixtures and exposure circumstances for which, at one extreme, the degree of evidence of carcinogenicity in humans is almost sufficient, as well as those for which, at the other extreme, there are no human data but for which there is evidence of carcinogenicity in experimental animals. Agents, mixtures and exposure circumstances are assigned to either group 2A (probably carcinogenic to humans) or group 2B (possibly carcinogenic to humans) on the basis of epidemiological and experi-mental evidence of carcinogenicity and other relevant data.

Group 2A—The agent (mixture) is probably carcinogenic to humans.
The exposure circumstance entails exposures that are probably carcinogenic to humans.

This category is used when there is *limited evidence* of carcinogenicity in humans and *sufficient evidence* of carcinogenicity in experimental animals. In some cases, an agent (mixture) may be classified in this category when there is *inadequate evidence* of carcinogenicity in humans, *sufficient evidence* of carcinogenicity in experimental animals and strong evidence that the carcinogenesis is mediated by a mechanism that also operates in humans. Exceptionally, an agent, mixture or exposure circumstance may be classified in this category solely on the basis of *limited evidence* of carcinogenicity in humans.

Group 2B—The agent (mixture) is possibly carcinogenic to humans.
The exposure circumstance entails exposures that are possibly carcinogenic to
humans.

This category is used for agents, mixtures and exposure circumstances for which there is *limited evidence* of carcinogenicity in humans and less than *sufficient evidence* of carcinogenicity in experimental animals. It may also be used when there is *inadequate evidence* of carcinogenicity in humans but there is *sufficient evidence* of carcinogenicity in experimental animals. In some instances, an agent, mixture or exposure circumstance for which there is *inadequate evidence* of carcinogenicity in humans but *limited evidence* of carcinogenicity in experimental animals together with supporting evidence from other relevant data may be placed in this group.

Group 3—The agent (mixture or exposure circumstance) is not classifiable as to its carcinogenicity to humans.

This category is used most commonly for agents, mixtures and exposure circumstances for which the *evidence of carcinogenicity* is *inadequate* in humans and *inadequate* or *limited* in experimental animals.

Exceptionally, agents (mixtures) for which the *evidence of carcinogenicity* is *inadequate* in humans but *sufficient* in experimental animals may be placed in this category when there is strong evidence that the mechanism of carcinogenicity in experimental animals does not operate in humans.

Agents, mixtures and exposure circumstances that do not fall into any other group are also placed in this category.

Group 4—The agent (mixture) is probably not carcinogenic to humans.

This category is used for agents or mixtures for which there is *evidence suggesting lack of carcinogenicity* in humans and in experimental animals. In some instances, agents or mixtures for which there is *inadequate evidence* of carcinogenicity in humans but *evidence suggesting lack of carcinogenicity* in experimental animals, consistently and strongly supported by a broad range of other relevant data, may be classified in this group.

References

Breslow, N.E. & Day, N.E. (1980) *Statistical Methods in Cancer Research*, Vol. 1, *The Analysis of Case–Control Studies* (IARC Scientific Publications No. 32), Lyon, IARC Press

Breslow, N.E. & Day, N.E. (1987) *Statistical Methods in Cancer Research*, Vol. 2, *The Design and Analysis of Cohort Studies* (IARC Scientific Publications No. 82), Lyon, IARC Press

Cohen, S.M. & Ellwein, L.B. (1990) Cell proliferation in carcinogenesis. *Science*, **249**, 1007–1011

Gart, J.J., Krewski, D., Lee, P.N., Tarone, R.E. & Wahrendorf, J. (1986) *Statistical Methods in Cancer Research*, Vol. 3, *The Design and Analysis of Long-term Animal Experiments* (IARC Scientific Publications No. 79), Lyon, IARC Press

Hoel, D.G., Kaplan, N.L. & Anderson, M.W. (1983) Implication of nonlinear kinetics on risk estimation in carcinogenesis. *Science*, **219**, 1032–1037

Huff, J.E., Eustis, S.L. & Haseman, J.K. (1989) Occurrence and relevance of chemically induced benign neoplasms in long-term carcinogenicity studies. *Cancer Metastasis Rev.*, **8**, 1–21

IARC (1973–1996) *Information Bulletin on the Survey of Chemicals Being Tested for Carcinogenicity/Directory of Agents Being Tested for Carcinogenicity*, Numbers 1–17, Lyon, IARC Press

IARC (1976–1996), Lyon, IARC Press

    Directory of On-going Research in Cancer Epidemiology 1976. Edited by C.S. Muir & G. Wagner

    Directory of On-going Research in Cancer Epidemiology 1977 (IARC Scientific Publications No. 17). Edited by C.S. Muir & G. Wagner

    Directory of On-going Research in Cancer Epidemiology 1978 (IARC Scientific Publications No. 26). Edited by C.S. Muir & G. Wagner

    Directory of On-going Research in Cancer Epidemiology 1979 (IARC Scientific Publications No. 28). Edited by C.S. Muir & G. Wagner

    Directory of On-going Research in Cancer Epidemiology 1980 (IARC Scientific Publications No. 35). Edited by C.S. Muir & G. Wagner

    Directory of On-going Research in Cancer Epidemiology 1981 (IARC Scientific Publications No. 38). Edited by C.S. Muir & G. Wagner

    Directory of On-going Research in Cancer Epidemiology 1982 (IARC Scientific Publications No. 46). Edited by C.S. Muir & G. Wagner

    Directory of On-going Research in Cancer Epidemiology 1983 (IARC Scientific Publications No. 50). Edited by C.S. Muir & G. Wagner

    Directory of On-going Research in Cancer Epidemiology 1984 (IARC Scientific Publications No. 62). Edited by C.S. Muir & G. Wagner

    Directory of On-going Research in Cancer Epidemiology 1985 (IARC Scientific Publications No. 69). Edited by C.S. Muir & G. Wagner

    Directory of On-going Research in Cancer Epidemiology 1986 (IARC Scientific Publications No. 80). Edited by C.S. Muir & G. Wagner

    Directory of On-going Research in Cancer Epidemiology 1987 (IARC Scientific Publications No. 86). Edited by D.M. Parkin & J. Wahrendorf

    Directory of On-going Research in Cancer Epidemiology 1988 (IARC Scientific Publications No. 93). Edited by M. Coleman & J. Wahrendorf

    Directory of On-going Research in Cancer Epidemiology 1989/90 (IARC Scientific Publications No. 101). Edited by M. Coleman & J. Wahrendorf

    Directory of On-going Research in Cancer Epidemiology 1991 (IARC Scientific Publications No.110). Edited by M. Coleman & J. Wahrendorf

    Directory of On-going Research in Cancer Epidemiology 1992 (IARC Scientific Publications No. 117). Edited by M. Coleman, J. Wahrendorf & E. Démaret

Directory of On-going Research in Cancer Epidemiology 1994 (IARC Scientific Publications
No. 130). Edited by R. Sankaranarayanan, J. Wahrendorf & E. Démaret

Directory of On-going Research in Cancer Epidemiology 1996 (IARC Scientific Publications
No. 137). Edited by R. Sankaranarayanan, J. Wahrendorf & E. Démaret

IARC (1977) *IARC Monographs Programme on the Evaluation of the Carcinogenic Risk of
Chemicals to Humans*. Preamble (IARC intern. tech. Rep. No. 77/002), Lyon, IARC Press

IARC (1978) *Chemicals with* Sufficient Evidence *of Carcinogenicity in Experimental Animals—*
IARC Monographs *Volumes 1–17* (IARC intern. tech. Rep. No. 78/003), Lyon, IARC Press

IARC (1978–1993) *Environmental Carcinogens. Methods of Analysis and Exposure Measurement*, Lyon, IARC Press

  Vol. 1. Analysis of Volatile Nitrosamines in Food (IARC Scientific Publications No. 18).
  Edited by R. Preussmann, M. Castegnaro, E.A. Walker & A.E. Wasserman (1978)

  *Vol. 2. Methods for the Measurement of Vinyl Chloride in Poly(vinyl chloride), Air, Water and
  Foodstuffs* (IARC Scientific Publications No. 22). Edited by D.C.M. Squirrell & W.
  Thain (1978)

  Vol. 3. Analysis of Polycyclic Aromatic Hydrocarbons in Environmental Samples (IARC
  Scientific Publications No. 29). Edited by M. Castegnaro, P. Bogovski, H. Kunte & E.A.
  Walker (1979)

  Vol. 4. Some Aromatic Amines and Azo Dyes in the General and Industrial Environment
  (IARC Scientific Publications No. 40). Edited by L. Fishbein, M. Castegnaro, I.K.
  O'Neill & H. Bartsch (1981)

  Vol. 5. Some Mycotoxins (IARC Scientific Publications No. 44). Edited by L. Stoloff,
  M. Castegnaro, P. Scott, I.K. O'Neill & H. Bartsch (1983)

  Vol. 6. N-Nitroso Compounds (IARC Scientific Publications No. 45). Edited by R. Preussmann, I.K. O'Neill, G. Eisenbrand, B. Spiegelhalder & H. Bartsch (1983)

  Vol. 7. Some Volatile Halogenated Hydrocarbons (IARC Scientific Publications No. 68).
  Edited by L. Fishbein & I.K. O'Neill (1985)

  Vol. 8. Some Metals: As, Be, Cd, Cr, Ni, Pb, Se, Zn (IARC Scientific Publications No. 71).
  Edited by I.K. O'Neill, P. Schuller & L. Fishbein (1986)

  Vol. 9. Passive Smoking (IARC Scientific Publications No. 81). Edited by I.K. O'Neill, K.D.
  Brunnemann, B. Dodet & D. Hoffmann (1987)

  *Vol. 10. Benzene and Alkylated Benzenes (*IARC Scientific Publications No. 85). Edited by L.
  Fishbein & I.K. O'Neill (1988)

  Vol. 11. Polychlorinated Dioxins and Dibenzofurans (IARC Scientific Publications No. 108).
  Edited by C. Rappe, H.R. Buser, B. Dodet & I.K. O'Neill (1991)

  Vol. 12. Indoor Air (IARC Scientific Publications No. 109). Edited by B. Seifert, H. van de
  Wiel, B. Dodet & I.K. O'Neill (1993)

IARC (1979) *Criteria to Select Chemicals for* IARC Monographs (IARC intern. tech. Rep.
No. 79/003), Lyon, IARC Press

IARC (1982) *IARC Monographs on the Evaluation of the Carcinogenic Risk of Chemicals to
Humans*, Supplement 4, *Chemicals, Industrial Processes and Industries Associated with
Cancer in Humans* (IARC Monographs, Volumes 1 to 29), Lyon, IARC Press

IARC (1983) *Approaches to Classifying Chemical Carcinogens According to Mechanism of Action* (IARC intern. tech. Rep. No. 83/001), Lyon, IARC Press

IARC (1984) *Chemicals and Exposures to Complex Mixtures Recommended for Evaluation in IARC Monographs and Chemicals and Complex Mixtures Recommended for Long-term Carcinogenicity Testing* (IARC intern. tech. Rep. No. 84/002), Lyon, IARC Press

IARC (1987a) *IARC Monographs on the Evaluation of Carcinogenic Risks to Humans*, Supplement 6, *Genetic and Related Effects: An Updating of Selected* IARC Monographs *from Volumes 1 to 42*, Lyon, IARC Press

IARC (1987b) *IARC Monographs on the Evaluation of Carcinogenic Risks to Humans*, Supplement 7, *Overall Evaluations of Carcinogenicity: An Updating of* IARC Monographs *Volumes 1 to 42*, Lyon, IARC Press

IARC (1988) *Report of an IARC Working Group to Review the Approaches and Processes Used to Evaluate the Carcinogenicity of Mixtures and Groups of Chemicals* (IARC intern. tech. Rep. No. 88/002), Lyon, IARC Press

IARC (1989) *Chemicals, Groups of Chemicals, Mixtures and Exposure Circumstances to be Evaluated in Future IARC Monographs, Report of an ad hoc Working Group* (IARC intern. tech. Rep. No. 89/004), Lyon, IARC Press

IARC (1991a) *A Consensus Report of an IARC Monographs Working Group on the Use of Mechanisms of Carcinogenesis in Risk Identification* (IARC intern. tech. Rep. No. 91/002), Lyon

IARC (1991b) *Report of an ad-hoc* IARC Monographs *Advisory Group on Viruses and Other Biological Agents Such as Parasites* (IARC intern. tech. Rep. No. 91/001), Lyon, IARC Press

IARC (1993) *Chemicals, Groups of Chemicals, Complex Mixtures, Physical and Biological Agents and Exposure Circumstances to be Evaluated in Future* IARC Monographs, *Report of an ad-hoc Working Group* (IARC intern. Rep. No. 93/005), Lyon, IARC Press

IARC (1998a) *Report of an ad-hoc* IARC Monographs *Advisory Group on Physical Agents* (IARC Internal Report No. 98/002), Lyon, IARC Press

IARC (1998b) *Report of an ad-hoc* IARC Monographs *Advisory Group on Priorities for Future Evaluations* (IARC Internal Report No. 98/004), Lyon, IARC Press

McGregor, D.B., Rice, J.M. & Venitt, S., eds (1999) *The Use of Short and Medium-term Tests for Carcinogens and Data on Genetic Effects in Carcinogenic Hazard Evaluation* (IARC Scientific Publications No. 146), Lyon, IARC Press

Montesano, R., Bartsch, H., Vainio, H., Wilbourn, J. & Yamasaki, H., eds (1986) *Long-term and Short-term Assays for Carcinogenesis—A Critical Appraisal* (IARC Scientific Publications No. 83), Lyon, IARC Press

Peto, R., Pike, M.C., Day, N.E., Gray, R.G., Lee, P.N., Parish, S., Peto, J., Richards, S. & Wahrendorf, J. (1980) Guidelines for simple, sensitive significance tests for carcinogenic effects in long-term animal experiments. In: *IARC Monographs on the Evaluation of the Carcinogenic Risk of Chemicals to Humans*, Supplement 2, *Long-term and Short-term Screening Assays for Carcinogens: A Critical Appraisal*, Lyon, IARC Press, pp. 311–426

Tomatis, L., Aitio, A., Wilbourn, J. & Shuker, L. (1989) Human carcinogens so far identified. *Jpn. J. Cancer Res.*, **80**, 795–807

Vainio, H., Magee, P.N., McGregor, D.B. & McMichael, A.J., eds (1992) *Mechanisms of Carcinogenesis in Risk Identification* (IARC Scientific Publications No. 116), Lyon, IARC Press

Vainio, H., Wilbourn, J.D., Sasco, A.J., Partensky, C., Gaudin, N., Heseltine, E. & Eragne, I. (1995) *Identification of human carcinogenic risk in* IARC Monographs. *Bull. Cancer,* **82**, 339–348 (in French)

Waters, M.D., Stack, H.F., Brady, A.L., Lohman, P.H.M., Haroun, L. & Vainio, H. (1987) Appendix 1. Activity profiles for genetic and related tests. In: *IARC Monographs on the Evaluation of Carcinogenic Risks to Humans*, Suppl. 6, *Genetic and Related Effects: An Updating of Selected IARC Monographs from Volumes 1 to 42*, Lyon, IARC Press, pp. 687–696

Wilbourn, J., Haroun, L., Heseltine, E., Kaldor, J., Partensky, C. & Vainio, H. (1986) Response of experimental animals to human carcinogens: an analysis based upon the IARC Monographs Programme. *Carcinogenesis*, **7**, 1853–1863

OVERALL INTRODUCTION
TO THE MONOGRAPHS

OVERALL INTRODUCTION

Ionizing radiation consists of particles and photons that have sufficient energy to ionize atoms in the human body, thus inducing chemical changes that may be biologically important for the functioning of cells. The greatest exposure to ionizing radiation is from natural sources.

Humans have always been exposed to ionizing radiation, since natural sources existed on earth even before life emerged. Natural γ-radiation is of two origins, extra-terrestrial and terrestrial. Extraterrestrial radiation originates in outer space as primary cosmic rays and reaches the atmosphere, with which the incoming energy and particles interact, giving rise to the secondary cosmic rays to which living beings on the earth's surface are exposed. Terrestrial radiation is emitted from primordial radioactive atoms that have been present in the earth since its formation. These radioactive atoms (called radionuclides) are present in varying amounts in all soils and rocks, in the atmosphere and in the hydrosphere. Radionuclides are characterized by the numbers of protons and neutrons in their nuclei, as ^AX, where X is the name of the element, uniquely defined by the number of protons, Z, in its nucleus, and A is the total number of protons and neutrons in the nucleus. For example, ^{137}Cs is a radionuclide of the element caesium (symbol Cs, $Z = 55$) with $A = 137$.

Until the end of the nineteenth century, human beings were exposed only to natural radiation. The discovery of X-rays by Wilhelm Röntgen in 1895 and of radioactivity by Henri Becquerel in 1896 led to the development of many applications of ionizing radiation and to the introduction of man-made radiation. The new sources of ionizing radiation consist of further kinds of radionuclides and machines that produce ionizing radiation. The most important applications of ionizing radiation which result in human exposures are in the diagnosis of diseases and the treatment of patients, in the production of nuclear weapons and in the production of electricity by means of nuclear reactors.

Members of the public can be exposed to man-made sources of radiation as a result of environmental releases of radionuclides from facilities where ionizing radiation is used and when they are subjected to medical diagnosis or treatment involving ionizing radiation. In addition, occupational exposure occurs in such facilities. An important natural source of exposure that has been enhanced by human activity is the radioactive indoor pollutant radon and its short-lived daughters. α-Emitting radon is an element of the uranium and thorium decay chains and was considered in depth in the *Monographs* series (IARC, 1988). Radon will be considered again at a later meeting of the *IARC Monographs* in 2000.

Exposure to ionizing radiation can be external or it can be internal when produced by incorporated radionuclides, usually by inhalation or ingestion. Internal exposure can also occur after absorption through intact or damaged skin and after injections for medical reasons.

The various forms of radiation are emitted with different energies and penetrating power (see Figure 1). For example, the radiation produced by radioactivity includes:

- alpha (α)-particles, consisting of helium nuclei, which can be halted by a sheet of paper and can thus hardly penetrate the dead outer layers of the skin; α-radiation is therefore primarily an internal hazard;
- beta (β)-particles, consisting of electrons, which can penetrate up to 2 cm of living tissue;
- gamma (γ)-radiation, consisting of photons, which can traverse the human body and
- neutron radiation, which is indirectly ionizing by interaction with hydrogen atoms and larger nuclei, producing proton radiation and high linear energy transfer (LET) recoil atoms.

Cosmic rays are high-energy particles which easily penetrate and traverse the human body. X-rays used in diagnostic procedures must penetrate the human body to be useful, although much of the energy is absorbed by the body tissues.

Exposure resulting from various sources of radiation is summarized approximately every five years by the United Nations Scientific Committee on the Effects of Atomic Radiation (UNSCEAR), and this introduction is based mainly on the two most recent reports (UNSCEAR, 1988, 1993). UNSCEAR also reviews studies of health effects resulting from ionizing radiation.

Figure 1. (a) Depth of penetration of α- and β-particles in tissue, for selected energy values; (b) depth of penetration of X- and γ-rays in tissue at which 50% of the radiation energy is lost

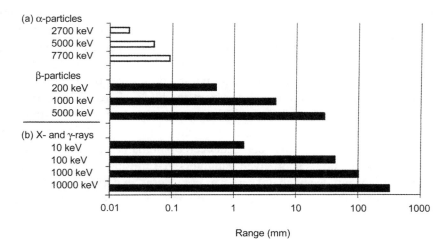

The International Commission on Radiological Protection (ICRP) is an advisory body which offers recommendations to regulatory and advisory agencies at international, national and regional levels on the fundamental principles on which appropriate radiological protection can be based (ICRP, 1999). The recommendations are usually followed at the national level.

In principle, two kinds of effects of radiation on tissues are observed. So-called 'deterministic effects' occur when a sufficiently large number of cells has been damaged, stem cells have lost their proliferative capacity, or tissue structure or function is adversely affected. At doses above this threshold, the probability of occurrence and the severity of effects increase steeply. Since organisms may compensate for the loss of cells, the harm may be temporary.

The second type of effect, called the 'stochastic effect', occurs when cells are not killed but are modified in some way. In certain cases, they produce modified daughter cells. If the cells have malignant potential and cannot be eliminated by the affected organism, they may eventually lead to cancer. The dose of radiation applied to an individual or group affects the probability of cancer but not its aggressivity. High doses and large groups of exposed individuals are generally required to study these effects accurately, as the probabilistic nature of the carcinogenic effect makes it hard to detect in groups exposed to low doses. For this reason, most of the information on the health effects of radiation has come from observations of populations exposed to high doses at high dose rates. Nevertheless, the lower doses to which significant portions of the population are exposed in some situations and those to which everyone is exposed during a lifetime are of greater interest.

The main goals of the ICRP are to prevent the occurrence of deterministic effects, by keeping doses below the relevant thresholds, and to ensure that all reasonable steps are taken to reduce the induction of stochastic effects.

1.   Nomenclature

For an assessment of the carcinogenicity of ionizing radiation, four quantities must be defined: activity, energy, exposure and dose. Various units have been used for each of these quantities: SI units of measure are used now, but in several important older studies traditional units were used. Table 1 gives the SI units and older units with the conversion factors.

1.1   Activity

Hazardous substances are usually measured in units of mass, but radionuclides are measured in activity. Mass and activity are related by the decay constant of the radionuclide. The activity of a radionuclide is defined as the number of nuclear transformations occurring per unit time. The standard unit is the becquerel (Bq); 1 Bq equals 1 nuclear transformation per second. The older unit of activity is the curie (Ci), which corresponds to 3.7×10^{10} nuclear transformations per second.

Table 1. SI and older units used in radiation dosimetry, with conversion factors

Quantity	SI unit	Older unit	Conversion factor (traditional/SI)	Conversion factor (SI/traditional)
Activity	becquerel (Bq); 1 Bq = 1 nuclear transformation s^{-1}	curie (Ci)	1 Ci = 3.7 10^{10} Bq	1 Bq = 2.7 10^{-11} Ci
Absorbed dose	gray (Gy) 1 Gy = 1 J kg^{-1}	rad	1 rad = 0.01 Gy	1 Gy = 100 rad
Equivalent dose or effective dose	sievert (Sv) 1 Sv = 1 J kg^{-1}	rem	1 rem = 0.01 Sv	1 Sv = 100 rem
Exposure	coulomb per kilogram of air (C kg^{-1})	roentgen (R)	1 R = 2.58 10^{-4} C kg^{-1}	1 C kg^{-1} = 3876 R

1.2   Energy

The energy of a particle emitted during the nuclear transformation of a radionuclide is expressed in electron-volts (eV). One electron-volt is the energy of an electron submitted to a potential difference of 1 V, and 1 eV is equal to 1.6×10^{-19} J. The energy of X-rays and γ-rays ranges between 10 and 10^{11} eV (Figure 2).

Figure 2. Bands of the electromagnetic spectrum in which X- and γ-rays fall

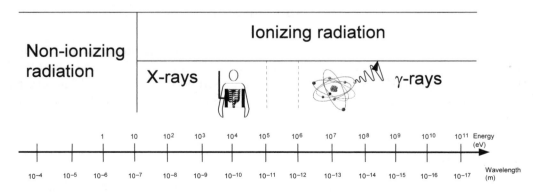

1.3   Exposure

The roentgen (R) is the unit of exposure to γ- or X-radiation and is defined as the quantity of γ- or X-radiation that will produce a charge of 2.58×10^{-4} C kg^{-1} of dry air. An exposure of 1 R is approximately equivalent to 10 milligray (mGy) of absorbed dose for γ- and X-rays in soft tissue. The roentgen is defined only for γ- and X-radiation with an energy of 10 keV to 3 MeV (Kathren & Petersen, 1989).

Another measure of radiation exposure is the 'kinetic energy released in matter' (kerma), which is the sum of the initial kinetic energies of all charged particles released in a specific volume or mass by the interaction of an uncharged particle such as a γ-ray, X-ray or neutron. The SI unit for kerma is the gray, as for absorbed dose, but the kerma differs in many circumstances from the absorbed dose in that it accounts for the initial energy released in a material but not directly for the energy absorbed per unit mass, as defined by absorbed dose. The kerma is sometimes used in epidemiological studies of the survivors of the atomic bombings in Japan (Kathren & Petersen, 1989).

1.4   Dose

The radiation dose (or dose) is related to the damage inflicted on the body and can be expressed as the absorbed dose, the equivalent dose, the effective dose or the collective dose. The dose rate is the dose per unit of time. It is a determinant of the deterministic effect and may affect the probability of occurrence of a stochastic effect.

The absorbed dose is the primary physical quantity of radiation dosimetry. It is defined as the radiation energy absorbed per unit mass of an organ or tissue and is used in studies of the damage to a particular organ or tissue. The unit is J kg^{-1}, and the special name is the gray, which is equal to 1 J kg^{-1}.

The equivalent dose (H) to an organ or tissue is the primary dosimetric quantity of radiation protection, which is concerned with inferring the biological effects associated with irradiation of tissues with rays of various characteristics (α-particles, electrons and photons). The equivalent dose is obtained by weighting the absorbed dose in an organ or tissue by a radiation weighting factor which reflects the biological effectiveness of the charged particles that produce the ionization within the tissue.

The radiation weighting factors (w_R) currently recommended by the ICRP (1991; Table 2) were selected to encompass appropriate values for the relative biological effectiveness (RBE) of the radiation but to be independent of the tissue or the biological end-point under consideration. The equivalent dose in tissue, H_T, is given as: $H_T = \sum_R w_R D_{T,R}$ where w_R is the radiation weighting factor for radiation R, $D_{T,R}$ is the absorbed dose in tissue T associated with radiation R, and the sum extends over all radiations that impart ionizing energy in tissue T. The SI unit for H_T is J kg^{-1}; the special name for the unit of equivalent dose is the sievert (Sv): 1 Sv = 1 J kg^{-1}.

The effective dose (E) is a single dosimetric quantity for the overall biological insult associated with irradiation, which takes into account variations in equivalent

Table 2. Radiation weighting factors

Type and energy range	Radiation weighting factor
Photons, all energies	1
Electrons and muons[a], all energies[b]	1
Neutrons, energy:	
< 10 keV	5
10–100 keV	10
0.1–2 MeV	20
2–20 MeV	10
> 20 MeV	5
Protons, other than recoil protons, energy	
> 2 MeV	5
α-particles, fission fragments, heavy nuclei	20

From ICRP (1991); all values relate to the radiation incident on the body or, for internal sources, emitted from the source.
[a] One of the elementary particles, a member of a category of light-weight particles called leptons which also include electrons and neutrinos
[b] Excluding Auger electrons (280–2100 eV) emitted from nuclei bound to DNA, which are ejected after excitation by an incident electron beam

dose among radiosensitive organs and tissues. The effective dose, E, is given as: $E = \sum_T w_T H_T$, where w_T is a tissue weighting factor that reflects the contribution of the tissue to the total detriment to health when the body is uniformly irradiated, and H_T is the equivalent dose in tissue *T*. The tissue weighting factors currently recommended by the ICRP (1991; Table 3) are based on the overall health detriment associated with radiation, which includes the number of fatal health effects, the non-fatal effects and the magnitude of the loss of life expectancy. For regulatory purposes, the ICRP defines the 'committed effective dose', which is the time integral of the effective dose rate with an integration time of 50 years for an adult and from the time of intake to age 70 years for children.

It is important to note that 'equivalent dose' and 'effective dose', which are derived from the estimation of 'exposure' or 'absorbed dose', are dosimetric quantities that are used for regulatory purposes. Their numerical values may change as regulatory authorities change the values for the radiation-weighting and tissue-weighting factors. 'Exposure' and 'absorbed dose', however, are physical quantities that are not subject to modification by regulatory authorities.

In order to compare the effects of several sources of radiation, data on individual doses must be supplemented by information on the number of people exposed. The simplest means of reflecting both the dose and the number of people is *the collective dose*, which is the product of the mean dose of an exposed group and the number of individuals in the group. This quantity is most useful when the individual doses are of

Table 3. Tissue weighting factors

Tissue or organ	Tissue weighting factor
Gonads	0.20
Bone marrow (active)	0.12
Colon	0.12
Lung	0.12
Stomach	0.12
Bladder	0.05
Breast	0.05
Liver	0.05
Oesophagus	0.05
Thyroid	0.05
Skin	0.01
Bone surface	0.01
Remainder[a]	0.05

From ICRP (1991). The values were derived on the basis of data for a reference population of equal numbers of males and females and a wide range of ages. In the definition of effective dose, these factors apply to workers, to the whole population and to males and females.

[a] For the purposes of calculation, the 'remainder' is composed of the following additional tissues and organs: adrenal glands, brain, upper large intestine, small intestine, kidney, muscle, pancreas, spleen, thymus and uterus. The list includes organs that are likely to be irradiated selectively and some organs which are known to be susceptible to cancer induction. If other tissues and organs are subsequently identified as being at significant risk for induced cancer, they will either be given a specific weighting factor or included in the 'remainder'. In the exceptional case in which one of the 'remainder' tissues or organs receives an equivalent dose in excess of the highest dose received by any of the 12 organs for which a weighting factor is specified, a weighting factor of 0.025 should be applied to that tissue or organ and a weighting factor of 0.025 to the average dose for the rest of the 'remainder', as defined above.

much the same magnitude and are delivered within periods that do not greatly exceed a few years. If the distribution of individual doses covers many orders of magnitude and the time distribution covers centuries, the concept of collective dose is not useful because it aggregates too much diverse information (ICRP, 1999).

It is worth noting that 'dose' is an integral quantity, corresponding to the deposition of energy over time, and the time over which a dose is calculated must be specified. This is not a problem for doses of external irradiation since the dose is, as a first approximation, proportional to the exposure and independent of the age of the person in question. In the case of internal irradiation from long-lived radionuclides with biological half-times of residence in the body of several years, however, the calculation of dose must take into account variation in metabolic parameters as a function of age. Most tabulations, such as those of the ICRP (1989, 1993, 1995a,b, 1996), provide estimates of 'committed absorbed doses' and of 'committed effective doses' per unit intake by inhalation or ingestion of the radionuclides usually encountered in occupational or environmental settings. Estimates of dose coefficients for periods shorter than a lifetime are not readily available nor easily derived from committed dose coefficients. For a large majority of the radionuclides usually considered, the dose corresponding to a single intake is delivered in a matter of weeks or months, so that the annual dose coefficient of those radionuclides is numerically equal to the committed dose coefficient.

For occupational exposure, the ICRP (1991) recommends a limit on the effective dose of 20 mSv per year averaged over five years, with the further provision that the effective dose should not exceed 50 mSv in any single year. For exposure of the general public, the ICRP (1991) recommends a limit on the effective dose of 1 mSv per year. A higher annual value could be allowed in special circumstances, provided that the average over five years does not exceed 1 mSv per year. These limits do not include the effective doses from natural background radiation or those received during medical diagnosis or treatment.

Special techniques have been developed to reconstruct doses years or decades after the event in which they were generated, for example those resulting from the release of radionuclides near the Techa River, Russian Federation, in the 1940s and 1950s, the atmospheric nuclear weapons tests conducted at the Nevada (USA) test site in the 1950s and the accident at Chernobyl, Ukraine, in 1986 (see the monograph on 'X-radiation and γ-radiation'). The techniques used for such retrospective dose assessments are described in section 2.4.

2.   Dosimetric Methods and Models

As none of the quantities of radiation such as the absorbed dose, the equivalent dose or the effective dose can be measured directly in practice, they must be estimated on the basis of other measured or assessed quantities. A distinction will be made between the occupational setting, where workers' doses of radiation are monitored systematically in order to meet regulatory requirements; the environmental setting, in which the doses received by members of the public are generally much lower and thus need not be measured accurately but are usually derived from measurements of radiation or of radionuclides in the environment or from mathematical models; and the medical setting, where the doses received by patients are determined from measurements in phantoms[1] or by calculations based on models of the human body. A further distinction is made between the doses resulting from external and internal irradiation.

---

[1] A phantom is an object made of substances with densities similar to tissue, which simulates tissues in absorbing and scattering radiation and permits determination of the dose of radiation delivered to the surface of and within the simulated tissues through measurements with ionization chambers placed within the phantom material.

2.1 Occupational setting

Monitoring practices in the workplace vary from country to country, from industry to industry and sometimes even from site to site within a given industry. Some of the differences stem from historical, technical, cost or convenience considerations. In general, more workers are monitored than is strictly necessary to meet regulatory requirements, and only a fraction of those monitored are found to have received measurable doses.

2.1.1 *Doses from external irradiation*

The choice of dosimeter used in particular circumstances is influenced by the objectives of the monitoring programme and by the nature of the radiation likely to be encountered. In most instances, workers are monitored for exposure to external radiation from β-, X- and γ-rays and are less frequently monitored for exposure to neutrons.

(*a*) *External β- and γ-rays*

Film, thermoluminescence and other personal dosimeters are used to monitor individual exposure to external β- and γ-rays. Film dosimeters are the oldest and still among the most widely used personal dosimetry systems. Modern films consist of a thin plastic base that supports a 30–50-μm gelatin layer throughout which are distributed silver bromide crystals about 1 μm in diameter; these constitute the sensitive part of the photographic emulsion. The dose to the film is measured as light transmission: the darker the film, the higher the dose. Because the sensitive portion of the film is composed of elements with relatively high Z values, namely silver and bromine, the response of the film is much more strongly dependent on the radiation energy than the response of soft tissues. Filters are used to flatten the response and to allow estimation of the dose irrespective of photon energy. A typical film badge has several filters and an open window that allows β-particles to reach the film. In the field, film dosimeters provide satisfactory accuracy and precision if properly calibrated, and the response of the film can be interpreted in terms of dose to the wearer at the point of measurement. In well-characterized radiation fields, an accuracy of 10–20% has been reported routinely at doses > 1 mGy, although an uncertainty of 50–200% is not unusual at doses below a few milligrays, particularly for mixed β-rays and low-energy photons (Kathren, 1987).

Thermoluminescence dosimetry is well suited to personal monitoring of exposure to β-particles and photons and has replaced film dosimetry in many situations. The dose is read after heating the thermoluminescent material at a uniform rate in a light-tight chamber and allowing the emitted light to fall directly on the photosensitive cathode of a photomultiplier tube. Each thermoluminescent compound has a characteristic emission as a function of temperature, known as a 'glow curve' (Kathren, 1987). The chemicals most commonly used for photon dosimetry are lithium fluoride, beryllium oxide and lithium borate. Thermoluminescent detectors containing these chemicals can be used to measure doses ranging from 0.1 mGy to 1000 Gy, and their response, like that of soft tissues, is not strongly dependent on the radiation energy, as they are made up of low-Z elements. Other compounds, like calcium fluoride and calcium sulfate, are more sensitive but give an energy-dependent response. The uncertainty in doses measured by means of lithium fluoride is less than 20% in the normal dose range, but the dosimetry of β-rays and of mixed β-ray and photon fields is considerably more difficult than that of pure photons (Deus & Watanabe, 1975; Kathren, 1987).

Optically stimulated luminescence is another method of monitoring personal exposure to β- and γ-rays. The method is similar to thermoluminescence dosimetry, except that light of a specific wavelength is used to induce luminescence, instead of heat.

Other types of personal dosimeter include electronic dosimeters, with active and passive gas-filled detectors, and glass dosimeters, which measure luminescence emitted by radiophotoluminescent materials when stimulated by ultraviolet light after irradiation (Deus & Watanabe, 1975; Kathren, 1987).

(b)   Neutrons

Personal dosimeters for use in nuclear reactors and commercial neutron sources are now well developed. When the contribution of neutrons to the effective dose is much smaller than that of photons, the neutron dose is sometimes determined by reference to the photon dose and an assumed ratio of the two components. Alternatively, measurements in the workplace and an assumed number of working hours are used.

Incident thermal and epithermal neutrons, with a low energy distribution, can be monitored relatively simply by detectors with high intrinsic sensitivity to such neutrons (for example, thermoluminescence detectors) or detectors sensitive to other types of radiation (photons and charged particles) and a converter. Neutron interactions in the converter produce secondary radiation that is detectable by the dosimeter. The commonest example of the latter technique is use of a film badge with a cadmium filter.

Personal doses from fast neutrons are assessed by means of nuclear emulsion detectors, bubble detectors or track-etch detectors. Nuclear emulsion dosimeters can measure neutrons at thermal energies and at energies above 700 keV. They have the disadvantages of being relatively insensitive to neutrons of intermediate energy and being sensitive to photons; they also suffer from fading. Bubble detectors respond to fast neutrons with energies from 100 keV upwards and have the advantages of direct reading, insensitivity to photons and being re-usable, but they have the disadvantages of being sensitive to temperature and shock. Track-etch detectors based on polyallyl diglycol carbonate respond to fast neutrons with energies from about 100 keV upwards.

Atmospheric neutrons pose a separate problem in dosimetry because of their broad energy spectrum, which extends to very high energies. The difficulty in measuring high-energy neutrons is that they are detected only after nuclear interaction, by detection of the charged interaction products; however, a neutron interaction can result in a multitude of possible products rather than a unique outcome. Sophisticated techniques are required to evaluate the spectral characteristics of the neutron environment; instruments of this type include liquid proton recoil scintillators, tissue equivalent proportional counters and tritium proportional counters. The scintillators produce a light pulse proportional to the proton recoil energy, while the proportional counters record an electrical current proportional to the energy released.

Another type of neutron detector is based on limitation of penetration through a hydrogenous material (usually polyethylene). Detectors of this kind with varying amounts of shielding, called 'Bonner sphere spectrometers', are sensitive to different neutron energies, and the range extends to very high-energy neutrons (Nakamura *et al.*, 1984).

2.1.2   *Doses from internal irradiation*

Occupations in which exposure to internal radiation is significant include uranium mining and milling (inhalation of radon decay products (IARC, 1988) and of ore dust); underground work in general and other forms of mining in particular (inhalation of radon decay products); the luminizing industry (tritium); the radiopharmaceutical industry (e.g. iodine, tritium and thallium); the operation of heavy-water reactors (tritium); fuel fabrication (uranium); fuel reprocessing (various actinides) and nuclear weapons production (tritium, uranium and plutonium) (UNSCEAR, 1993).

Three approaches are used to derive internal doses: (i) quantification of exposure to the time-integrated air concentrations of radioactive materials by means of air sampling techniques; (ii) determination of internal contamination by direct counting of γ- and X-ray emitters in the whole body, thorax, skeleton and thyroid *in vivo* and (iii) measurement of activity *in vitro*, usually in samples of urine or faeces. The choice of approach is determined by the radiation emitted by the radionuclide, its biokinetics, its retention in the body taking into account both biological clearance and radioactive decay, the required frequency of measurements, and the sensitivity, availability and convenience of the appropriate measurement facilities. The most accurate method in the case of radionuclides that emit penetrating photons (e.g. ^{137}Cs and ^{60}Co) is usually a measurement *in vivo*. Although such methods can provide information about long-term accumulation of internal contamination, they may not be sufficient for assessing the committed dose due to a single year's intake. An assessment may also require air monitoring. In many situations, therefore, a combination of methods is used. Air monitoring (individual or area) is the only available routine method for assessing doses of radon.

2.2   Environmental setting

In the environmental setting, doses are usually derived from measurements of ambient radiation and radionuclides which are then inserted in mathematical models.

The models can be complex, to account for numerous factors, such as duration of exposure, intake of certain foods and biokinetics.

2.2.1   *Environmental measurements*

Most environmental measurements can be categorized into determination of ambient radiation or of radionuclides.

(a)   *Ambient radiation*

Radiation in the environment is measured by a variety of instruments. Ambient γ- and X-radiation at a specific location can be measured with large-volume ionization chambers, which have a sensitivity in the microsievert range (Figure 3). Thermo- luminescence dosimeters can also be used, but the dosimeter reading is a measure of the environmental radiation in a particular area since these dosimeters are designed for individual monitoring. Neutron radiation can be measured with similar thermo- luminescent material enriched in ^{6}Li, in conjunction with various filters for neutron energy.

Figure 3. Structure and function of an ionization chamber

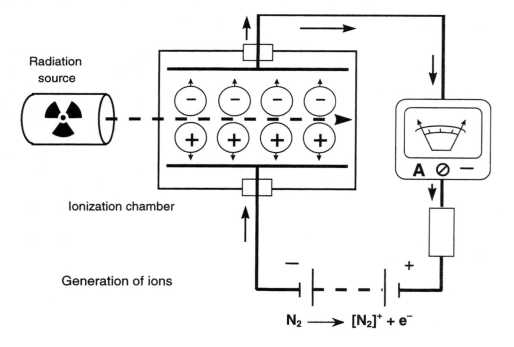

(b) Radionuclides

Radionuclides in the environment are measured either *in situ* or in samples of air, soil, sediment and water.

(i) In-situ measurements

Radionuclides in the air that emit α- or β-particles are typically measured on a filter on which matter has been collected or in a flow-through ionization chamber. α- and β-emitting radionuclides cannot be measured accurately in soil or sediment because of the strong attenuation of the particles in such samples, but γ- and X-rays can be measured in soil, sediment and water because these emissions undergo relatively little attenuation in these media. Radionuclides that emit γ- and X-rays are measured with a high-purity germanium detector or a scintillation detector. The detector is typically positioned 1 m above the surface and the emission spectrum is collected. The radionuclides are identified and the activity is quantified on the basis of the observed emission spectrum.

(ii) Sampling measurements

Radioactive particles in air can be collected on a filter and those immersed in soil, sediment or water in a standardized container. The analysis is usually conducted in two phases. The first phase is chemical reduction of the medium and the deposited radionuclides, which is done by dissolving the filter for air samples and by ashing soil, sediment and water samples to remove the water, leaving only the solid matter. The second phase is direct measurement of the prepared sample. Radionuclides that emit primarily α-particles are usually measured with a gas proportional detector or a solid-state detector. Radionuclides that emit only β-particles, such as ^{3}H, ^{14}C and ^{90}Sr/^{90}Y, are usually measured with either a gas proportional counter or a liquid scintillation counter.

2.2.2 Environmental modelling

(a) Doses from external irradiation

External irradiation usually arises from immersion in contaminated air or water containing γ-emitting radionuclides or from proximity to γ-emitting radionuclides deposited on the ground. The dose that a person receives depends on the environmental distribution of the radionuclide concentration. Because photons can travel hundreds of metres in air and tens of centimetres in water or soil, large volumes must be considered. In addition, the morphology of the person influences his or her absorption of photons. Doses from external irradiation are therefore derived from knowledge of the spatial and temporal distributions of the γ-emitting radionuclides around the person and the morphology of that person. Although simplifying assumptions and tabulated results are generally used in reconstructing doses, it has become increasingly possible to represent the irradiation conditions mathematically and to compute distributions of dose from knowledge of the interaction. Mathematical anthropometric phantoms, in which the locations of the organs in the human body are defined by geometrical coordinates, are used in that procedure. The distribution of dose within the body is usually calculated by means of Monte Carlo simulations, a type of mathematical modelling that has proved to be extremely flexible and powerful, as it can deal effectively with complex irradiation conditions. The calculations and the values of the associated interaction parameters have an inherent degree of uncertainty, however, and the anatomical parameters vary considerably.

The simplifying assumptions and tabulated results that are generally used to reconstruct doses after immersion in a radioactive cloud or from radionuclides deposited on the ground are summarized below.

(i)   *Immersion dose*

External exposure due to immersion in contaminated air or water or to radiation from an overhead plume usually makes only a small contribution to the total dose received by members of the public. It is therefore usually warranted to use simplifying assumptions to estimate immersion doses.

The external dose from cloud immersion is generally calculated on the assumption that: (1) the person considered is outdoors at all times during the passage of the radioactive cloud; (2) the radioactive cloud is 'semi-infinite' with uniform radionuclide concentrations (this is called the 'semi-infinite' assumption because only the half-space above the ground is considered); and (3) results calculated for reference adults apply to individuals of all ages. Tables giving values of dose per unit air concentration for many radionuclides are available in the literature, notably in the *United States Federal Radiation Guide* No. 12 (Eckerman & Ryman, 1993).

Persons who are indoors receive much lower doses than those who are outdoors because of the shielding effect of buildings. The indoor:outdoor dose ratio, called the 'shielding factor', varies according to the γ-energy spectrum of the radionuclide considered, the distribution of activity in the radioactive cloud and the characteristics of the building. According to Le Grand *et al.* (1990), the shielding factor can range from 0.5 on the first floor of a semi-detached house to less than 0.001 in the basement of a multistorey building. Within a building, the effective shielding factor varies by 30% depending on where the measurement is made, as shown by Fujitaka and Abe (1984a). These authors also showed that the dose rate does not depend on the details of the building interior (Fujitaka & Abe, 1984b); the location of other buildings can affect exposure on the lower floors, but all such parameters have only a 30% effect on exposure. The most important parameters are floor thickness and building size (Fujitaka & Abe, 1986). A radioactive cloud is never really semi-infinite, with uniform concentrations of radionuclides. Typically, the doses received outdoors in an urban area are about half those received in a flat, open area because of the presence of building materials between the individual considered and some part of the radioactive cloud.

For a given air kerma, the organ and effective doses received by individuals of various sizes (or ages) vary to some extent. Within the energy range of interest in most dose reconstructions (0.2–2 MeV), the effective doses per air kerma are estimated to be higher for infants than for children, which are in turn higher than those for adults. The differences are not, however, very large: the infant:adult dose ratios vary for most energies within a factor of 2 (Saito *et al.*, 1990).

(ii)   *Ground deposition dose*

The ground deposition dose can be relatively important. It is usually calculated on the basis of simplifying assumptions that are less crude than those used to calculate the immersion doses. In the absence of information on the lifestyle of a person, it is typically assumed that: (1) the contaminated area can be represented by an infinite plane source at the air–ground interface; (2) the fractions of time that the person spent indoors and outdoors correspond to population averages; (3) average indoor shielding factors can be applied to the person; and (4) the morphology of the person corresponds to that of ICRP 'reference man' (ICRP, 1975), the organ masses and body size of which were determined on the basis of an extensive literature review.

The assumption of an infinite plane source is conservative, as radionuclides migrate into the soil and are removed from surfaces by erosion and cleaning. These effects are dependent on the chemical properties and radioactive half-lives of the radionuclides. The most extensive data are available for ^{137}Cs.

The fractions of time spent indoors and outdoors are usually taken to be 80% and 20%, respectively (UNSCEAR, 1993). Being indoors provides a degree of protection from shielding that depends on factors such as the thickness and composition of walls. The indoor shielding factor is usually taken to be 0.2 (UNSCEAR, 1993). Shielding effects were reviewed by Burson and Profio (1977), who concluded that the shielding factors were highest for wood-frame houses without a cellar (average, 0.4; representative range, 0.2–0.5) and lowest for the cellars of multistorey stone structures (average, 0.005; representative range, 0.001–0.015).

The organ and effective doses received by individuals of various sizes from radiation of a given activity superficially deposited on the ground over an infinite area vary to some extent. Calculations made by Jacob *et al.* (1990) and by Saito *et al.* (1990), using four anthropomorphic phantoms representing an adult male, an adult female, a child and an infant, showed that the effective doses received by an infant are usually about 20% higher than those received by an adult.

(b)   *Doses from internal irradiation*

Doses may be incurred from internal irradiation by inhalation of radionuclide-contaminated air or by ingestion of radionuclides in water and food. Doses from internal irradiation are usually derived from knowledge of the radionuclide concentrations relevant to the pathway under consideration, data on human intake of the radionuclides (breathing rates or food consumption rates) and biokinetic modelling of the radionuclides taken in.

In some cases in which large doses were delivered, for example during radiation accidents, measurements were made to establish the radionuclide content of excreta, the thyroid or the whole body. Even in such cases, however, data on lifestyle and dietary habits are necessary to determine the magnitude of the exposure to radionuclides from internal irradiation. When the doses are very low, radionuclides cannot be detected, and the doses are determined from models based on the source of exposure (for example, the amounts of radioactive materials released into the environment). Most biokinetic models of human intake of radionuclides are based on information in recent ICRP publications (ICRP, 1989, 1993, 1994, 1995a,b, 1996), in which the absorbed doses in various organs and tissues, as well as the effective doses, are calculated for unit intakes of radionuclides and for typical infants, children and adults on the basis of reviews of biokinetics in man and animals.

Calculation of the doses received by inhalation requires not only knowledge of the outdoor and indoor air concentrations and the physical and chemical characteristics of the aerosol inhaled but also information on the breathing characteristics of the person involved, a model of the respiratory tract that allows determination of the amount of airborne particles deposited in the airways, and models simulating the uptake of radionuclides by blood and their subsequent absorption and retention in the organs and tissues of the body. The models used to estimate the deposition and retention of airborne contaminants in the respiratory tract have been revised (ICRP, 1994; National Council on Radiation Protection and Measurements, 1997). Committed dose coefficients for inhalation are generally extracted from ICRP publications. Annual dose coefficients, when numerically different from the committed dose coefficients, can be calculated from the models developed by the ICRP (1995b, 1996).

The procedure for calculating doses from ingested radionuclides is similar to that for calculating the doses from inhalation. Calculation of the doses received by ingestion requires not only knowledge of the radionuclide concentrations in various foodstuffs but also information on the amounts of food consumed by the person in question and models of the behaviour of radionuclides in the gastrointestinal tract and the subsequent absorption and retention of radionuclides in the various organs and tissues of the body. The dietary information is usually obtained from national food surveys, food surveys applicable to the population considered or personal interviews. The dosimetric models are generally extracted from ICRP publications.

2.3   Medical setting

The doses received by patients during external irradiation (diagnostic radiography or radiotherapy) or internal irradiation (nuclear diagnosis and therapy) are usually determined from measurements in phantoms or by Monte Carlo calculations with computer models of the human body (Drexler *et al.*, 1990; Hart *et al.*, 1996). Detailed tables of average doses from various kinds of examinations were compiled by UNSCEAR (1993).

External irradiation results in a dose to the part of the body within the primary radiation beam and a dose in adjacent tissues. The dose from the primary beam for diagnostic X-rays ('soft' X-rays) and computed tomography is measured with thermoluminescence dosimeters or ionization chambers in a phantom. The dose from the secondary or scattered radiation is determined with computer software shown by Monte Carlo calculations to model the absorbed dose in adjacent tissue. Modelling is important since the absorbed dose from the soft X-rays in surrounding tissue changes radically with density (i.e. bone versus soft tissue). The absorbed dose to the breast from mammography is estimated in a standard phantom that simulates breast tissue, in combination with a photographic film. The darkening of the film reflects the absorbed dose.

In radiotherapy, the dose in the primary beam from an accelerator or ^{60}Co unit is determined in a water phantom, with an ionization chamber to measure the energy of the radiation and the dose rate directly. The phantom may be less precise than in other applications since in this case the primary beam consists of high-energy photons which can penetrate the body easily and deliver a fairly uniform absorbed dose throughout the region of interest. The dose outside the primary beam is determined by use of computer software.

In brachytherapy, sealed radioactive sources are inserted into a body cavity, placed on the surface of a tumour or on the skin, or implanted throughout a tumour. A phantom is used in conjunction with a thermoluminescence dosimeter or an ionization chamber to determine the dose at specific points. For a complete evaluation of the distribution, software is used which takes into consideration absorption in the applicator, scattering and absorption in surrounding tissues.

The doses from internal irradiation in therapeutic uses of nuclear medicine are due mainly to β-rays (which will be considered in a future IARC monograph), but when nuclear medicine is used in diagnosis, it is mostly γ-rays from the various radio-isotopes that are detected. The absorbed doses of radiation from radiopharmaceuticals have been assessed from the literature, and the complicated calculation of the doses to various organs has been addressed primarily by the ICRP (1987) and the Medical International Radiation Dose committees (Loevinger *et al.*, 1988).

2.4   Retrospective dose assessment

Doses may be assessed retrospectively when they were not estimated at the time of exposure but are needed for epidemiological or other reasons. The methods that can be used to assess individual doses retrospectively are analysis of teeth by electron paramagnetic resonance, analysis of chromosomal aberrations in peripheral blood lymphocytes by biological techniques such as fluorescence in-situ hybridization, and measurement of γ-radiation emitted from the body by radionuclides such as ^{90}Sr and ^{239}Pu.

Doses to unspecified representative individuals in a group (group doses) can also be measured, and the doses to specified individuals can then be derived. The methods used to assess group doses include analysis of ceramic materials such as bricks by thermoluminescence, to determine the total dose from external irradiation in a given location; analysis of the ratio of ^{239}Pu and ^{240}Pu concentrations in soil to determine the contribution of fall-out from a specific test site; and measurement of ^{129}I in soil to derive the ^{131}I fall-out at that location.

3.   Transmission and Absorption in Biological Tissues

Ionizing radiation such as photon and neutron radiation interacts with matter in a way that is qualitatively different from that of most other mutagens or carcinogens. Specifically, the energy imparted and the consequent chemical changes are not distributed in uniform, random patterns. Instead, the radiation track is structured, with energy depositions occurring in clusters along the trajectories of charged particles. Depending on the absorbed dose and on the type and energy of the radiation, the resulting non-homogeneity of the microdistribution can be substantial. Measurements in randomly selected microscopic volumes yield concentrations of energy or of subsequent radiation products that deviate considerably from their average values, and these variations depend in intricate ways on the size of the reference volume, the magnitude of the dose and the type of ionizing radiation (ICRU, 1983; Goodhead, 1988).

The amount of radiation that produces an effect is specified as the energy deposited per unit mass in the irradiated system, the absorbed dose. Although defined at a point, the absorbed dose can be considered to be a macroscopic quantity because its value is unaffected by microscopic fluctuations in energy deposition. These fluctuations are important, however, if only because they are the reason why equal doses of different types of radiation have effects of different magnitude. While the absorbed dose determines the average number of energy deposition events, each cell reacts to the actual energy deposited in it, the actual spatial distribution of the energy within the cell and its relationship to critical cellular structures or molecules. The average response of a system of cells should therefore depend on the energy distribution on a scale that is at least as small as the dimensions of the cell, although events on a larger multicell or tissue dimension can also influence the response. The characterization of microscopic energy depositions and radiation track structure is the field of micro-dosimetry (Goodhead, 1987).

3.1   Track structure of radiation with low and high linear energy transfer

All ionizing radiation deposits energy primarily through ionization or excitation of the atoms and molecules in the material through which it travels. Generally speaking, most of the energy deposition is produced by secondary or higher-order electrons that are set in motion by the primary radiation, be it a photon, a neutron or a charged particle. It is likely that the biologically significant energy deposition events involve ionization, where an electron is actually removed from an atom or molecule, and particularly local clusters of ionizations (Hutchinson, 1985; Goodhead, 1994; Prise, 1994). Such ionizations can occur directly in a critical molecule, such as DNA, or in nearby molecules such as water (Nikjoo *et al.*, 1997). In either case, or in combination, they can result in single or multiple damage to critical molecules, such as strand breaks and base damage in DNA (Ward, 1994).

Because the probabilities of all the relevant interactions between the different types of radiation and the atoms and molecules of the medium can be estimated (with various degrees of accuracy), it is possible to simulate on a computer the passage of a particle (and its secondaries) as it travels through a medium (Brenner & Zaider, 1984). Figure 4 is a schematic illustration of radiation tracks in a cell irradiated with γ-rays (low-LET) or slow α-particles (high-LET). The energy deposition of the γ-rays is spread throughout the cell, although there is considerable non-uniformity at the submicrometer scale. The energy of α-particles is deposited along a much smaller number of narrow tracks, while large parts of the cell do not receive any energy at all. It is important to realize that radiation energy deposition is a stochastic process, and no two radiation tracks are the same.

3.2   Quantitative characterization of energy deposition at cellular and subcellular sites

A fundamental quantity of the radiation deposited in tissue is the specific energy, z, defined as the energy imparted to finite volumes per unit mass (ICRU, 1983); it is measured in the same units as absorbed dose, and was introduced in order to quantify the stochastic nature of energy deposition in cellular and subcellular objects (Rossi, 1967). The variation of specific energy across identical targets is characterized by the distribution function $f(z;D)dz$, representing the probability of deposition of a specific energy between z and $z+dz$. This distribution depends, among other things, on the dimensions of the volume under consideration and the dose D (i.e. the average value of z). The statistical fluctuations of z about its mean value are larger for smaller volumes, smaller doses and higher LET.

The unit of LET is keV μm^{-1}. This is far from a perfect descriptor, because energy is not deposited uniformly along the path of the particle. An alternative approach is based on lineal energy, y, the energy deposited in an event divided by the mean chord length of the volume in which it occurs, and z, the energy deposited by one or more events, divided by the mass of the volume in which it occurs (ICRU, 1983). This approach became possible with the introduction of proportional counters filled with tissue-equivalent gas for the measurement of the spectra of y and z (see Rossi, 1979). Despite its deficiencies, LET has remained the term of choice among radiotherapists and radiologists.

Figure 4. Schematic representation of a cell nucleus irradiated with two electron tracks from radiation with low linear energy transfer (LET; γ-rays; panel A) or two high-LET α-particle tracks (panel B)

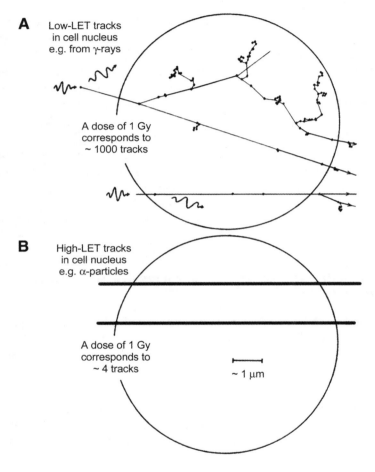

A Low-LET tracks
in cell nucleus
e.g. from γ-rays

A dose of 1 Gy
corresponds to
~ 1000 tracks

B High-LET tracks
in cell nucleus
e.g. α-particles

A dose of 1 Gy
corresponds to
~ 4 tracks

~ 1 μm

Adapted from Goodhead (1988)

Energy can be deposited in the volume of interest by the passage of one or more tracks of radiation. Because of the relevance of single tracks to the low-dose situation, it is useful to consider the corresponding spectrum of energy depositions, which is the single-event spectrum, $f_1(z)$, due to single tracks only. The frequency average of $f_1(z)$, i.e. $\bar{z}_F = \int z\, f_1(z)\; dz$, is then simply the average specific energy deposition produced by a single track of that radiation through or in the sensitive site. Thus, for a given dose, D, the mean number of radiation tracks through or in a given target volume, is $n = D/z_F$.

Typical values of $\bar{z}_F$ are shown in Figure 5. Note that $\bar{z}_F$ increases with both LET and decreasing target site size. Thus, a given dose of high-LET radiation, such as neutrons or α-particles, will result from a much lower average number of tracks than would be the case for the same dose of low-LET radiation, such as γ-rays (see Figure 4). The significance of the average number of tracks is in the objective deposition of a 'low dose' of a given type of radiation and the argument for the dose-dependence of independent cellular effects at low doses on the basis of microdosimetric considerations.

The average number of events (n), however, and the average specific energy (z_F) do not tell the entire story. A group of identical cells exposed to the same dose of radiation will be subject to a range of specific energy depositions, characterized by the distributions $f(z;D)$ or $f_i(z)$, because of a variety of effects such as geometric path, energy loss fluctuation (straggling), track length distribution and energy dissipation by δ-rays (Kellerer & Chmelevsky, 1975). Such distribution can often be broad. Furthermore, even for identical specific energy, the biological consequences depend on the spatial distribution of the energy deposition within each cell.

Figure 5. Frequency-averaged specific energy per event, $\bar{z}_F$, in unit density spheres of diameter d for γ-rays and neutrons of different energies

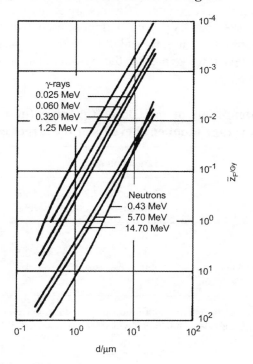

Adapted from ICRP (1983)

3.3   'Low dose'

On the basis of these considerations, a measure of what constitutes 'low dose' can be established by estimating the dose at which the average number of events (tracks) in a given cell is 1. Below this dose, effects due to the interactions between different tracks will be rare, and the number of cells subject to one single-track insult will simply decrease in proportion to the dose. As shown by Poisson statistics, even when the average number of tracks in a given target is 1, 26% of the targets will be hit more than once. A slightly more conservative definition of 'low dose', used by Goodhead (1988), corresponds to a mean number of 0.2 tracks per cell (or per cell nucleus). In this case, less than 2% of the cells will be subject to traversals by more than one radiation track, and less than 10% of all the hit cells will have been hit by more than one radiation track. This and other operational definitions of 'low dose' have been considered by UNSCEAR (1993).

Appropriately sized targets for consideration may include those of typical human cell nuclei (100–1000 μm^3) or whole cells (Altman & Katz, 1976). Table 4 shows representative estimates of 'low dose' derived from the measured specific energy spectra for spherical target volumes of 240 μm^3 (average nucleus) and for a larger target (5500 μm^3). The latter is meant to simulate a small cluster of cells, each of which is potentially able to communicate the effect of the radiation to other cells in the cluster, thus comprising a larger effective target. Results are given for γ-rays (here, 1.25 MeV from ^{60}Co), for X-rays (here, 25 kVp, typical of those used in mammography), for intermediate energy neutrons (0.44 MeV, typical of those from a reactor) and for α-particles with an energy of 100 keV μm^{-1} (typical of those from radon progeny incident on target lung cells).

Table 4. Definition of low dose: the dose (in mGy) below which the average number of events in the target is less than 1

Radiation	Target volume	
	240 μm^3 (d=7.7 μm) (nucleus)	5500 μm^3 (d=22 μm) (cluster of cells)
γ-rays (1.25 MeV)	0.9	0.1
X-rays (25 kVp)	4.5	0.5
Neutrons (0.44 MeV)	50	4
α-particles (100 keV μm^{-1})	300	30

To derive a more conservative definition of low dose, corresponding to < 0.2 tracks per target, the doses should be divided by 5 (Goodhead, 1988).

3.4 Clusters of energy deposition events and correlations with biological lesions

The detailed spatial and temporal properties of the initial physical features of radiation energy deposition influence the final biological consequences, despite the physical, chemical and biological processes that eliminate the vast majority of the initial damage (Goodhead & Brenner, 1983; Brenner & Ward, 1992; Goodhead, 1994). Ionizing radiation produces many different possible clusters of spatially adjacent damage, and analysis of track structures from different types of radiation has shown that clustered DNA damage of complexity greater than double-strand breaks can occur at biologically relevant frequencies with all types of ionizing radiation, at any dose (Brenner & Ward, 1992; Goodhead, 1994). In other words, such clustered damage can be produced by a single track of ionizing radiation, with a probability that increases with ionization density but is not zero even for sparsely ionizing radiation such as X- and γ-rays.

3.5 Biological effects of low doses

A general conclusion that follows from the stochastics of ionizing radiation energy deposition in small sites is that the average effect of small absorbed doses (average number of tracks in the cell, < 1) on independent cells is always proportional to dose (Goodhead, 1988). Such a linear relation between observed cellular effect and dose must be expected regardless of the dependence of cellular effect on specific energy; it is due to the fact that, even at very low doses, finite amounts of energy are deposited in a cell when the cell is traversed by a charged particle. As the energy deposited during such single events does not depend on the dose, the effect in those cells that are traversed by a charged particle does not change with decreasing dose. The only change that occurs with decreasing dose is the decrease in the proportion of cells which are subject to a single energy deposition. This can be treated quantitatively (Kellerer & Rossi, 1975; Goodhead, 1988), and microdosimetry can supply information about the range of doses to which the statement applies for different radiation qualities. A schematic illustration of these concepts is given in Figure 6.

A possible objection to this conclusion is that a single track might have no effect at the appropriate target, although an effect might be produced after more than one hit. This hypothesis is inconsistent with both microdosimetric and biological evidence, however. First, the spectrum of specific energy produced in single events is distributed widely, both for sparsely and densely ionizing radiation. Consequently, there is a finite probability, although it may be small, that the same amount of energy deposited during two events could be deposited during one event. Second, there is much experimental evidence to suggest that DNA damage and chromosomal and other cellular damage can be induced by individual radiation tracks. The evidence is based largely on the observation of a linear component to the dose–response relationship at doses for

Figure 6. Schematic dose–response curves for radiation of low and high linear energy transfer

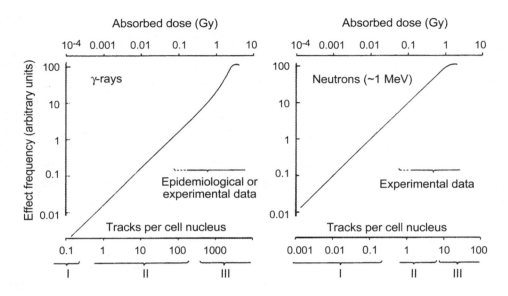

Adapted from Goodhead (1988)
The mean number of tracks was evaluated for 8-μm diameter spherical nuclei. Region I corresponds to 'definite' single-track action on individual cells, corresponding to ~0.2 tracks per cell nucleus. Region II corresponds to intermediate doses, at which single-track action on individual cells will still dominate. Region III corresponds to regions in which multi-track action will dominate. Note the difference in number of tracks per cell nucleus at equal absorbed doses of γ-rays and neutrons.

which track overlap in DNA and other cellular components is highly improbable (ICRP, 1991) and on theoretical simulations of the clustered ionizations within a track and the ensuing clustered DNA damage (Goodhead, 1994; Nikjoo *et al.*, 1997). Experiments with the new generation of single-particle microbeams have confirmed that, at least for high-LET radiation, traversals of cell nuclei by single tracks do produce observable biological effects (Hei *et al.*, 1997). These arguments imply that single tracks of ionizing radiation can induce damage to individual cells, however low the macroscopic dose. Of course, the probability of a cellular effect resulting from a single track of low-LET radiation is extremely small.

4. Occurrence and Exposure

4.1 Military uses

Military uses of ionizing radiation include the production of materials for nuclear weapons and the testing and use of nuclear weapons.

4.1.1 *Detonation of atomic bombs over Hiroshima and Nagasaki*

The initial nuclear radiation from an exploding nuclear device consists mainly of neutrons and primary γ-rays, and secondary γ-rays are produced by neutron inter-actions in the environment. These components must be considered in establishing the relationship between tissue kerma and distance, which determines the decrease in initial nuclear radiation with distance from the hypocentre.

After the atomic bombings in 1945 in Hiroshima and Nagasaki, Japan, a com-mission (the Atomic Bomb Casualty Commission, currently known as the Radiation Effects Research Foundation) was established to investigate the long-term health effects among the survivors in the two cities.

The first estimates of the doses received by the survivors were based on distance from the hypocentre. In the late 1950s, a dosimetric system was developed on the basis of responses to a detailed questionnaire on the location and position of the survivors at the time of the bombings. These tentative doses were later replaced by a more extensive, refined set of tentative doses (T65D), which was used for risk assessment throughout the 1970s. In the late 1970s, scientists from the USA noted differences between the T65 dose and newer theoretical estimates, and a joint Japan–USA study was initiated to reassess various factors related to the atomic bomb explosions that determined the actual doses of ionizing radiation. As a result, Dosi-metry System 1986 (DS86) was established (Roesch, 1987) which permits calculation of the exposures of various organs (referred to as organ doses) from estimates of individual exposures to γ-rays and neutrons. These shielded kerma doses were determined by analysis of information on each survivor's location and shielding at the time of the bombings. Most of the exposure was to γ-rays, but there was a small neutron component. The magnitude of this component is unknown, but it would have contributed no more than a few per cent. The neutron dose in Hiroshima is considered to have been larger than that in Nagasaki, which is believed to have been negligible.

Data on the survivors of the atomic bombings are the main source of information on the risks for cancer associated with exposure to low-LET γ-radiation. As neutrons are considered to have a greater biological effect per unit dose than γ-rays, a weighted total dose (in Sv) based on a radiation weighting factor (w_R) for neutrons was used in many recent studies. A typical value for the weighting factor is 10, although there is still no agreement.

DS86 estimates of dose are available for a majority of the participants in the so-called Life Span Study (see section 2.2.1), which consists of about 120 000 persons who were in one of the two cities at the time of the bombings. The latest version of the DS86 system (version 3) was used to estimate the doses received by a subcohort of 86 572 persons. Recent analyses of the data from this study have been limited to members of the cohort for whom such estimates were available (Thompson *et al.*, 1994; Pierce *et al.*, 1996). The weighted dose to the colon, considered to be a typical dose for deep organs, was < 0.1 Sv for most of the cohort. The distribution of doses to the colon for this cohort is summarized by city in Table 5. DS86 provides estimates of γ-ray and neutron doses to 15 organs. The doses account for shielding of the organs by the body and the survivors' orientation, position and shielding at the time of the bombings. The analyses for specific cancer sites are based on these organ doses. The collective dose to the colon for the 86 572 survivors was about 24 000 person–Sv (Burkart, 1996).

4.1.2   *Nuclear weapons testing*

Nuclear weapons are of two types: fission devices (so-called 'atomic bombs'), in which the energy released is due to fission of uranium or plutonium nuclei, and fusion devices (so-called 'hydrogen bombs' or 'thermonuclear bombs'), in which the atomic bomb serves as a trigger to cause fusion of tritium and deuterium nuclei, thus producing a more powerful explosion.

Fission produces a wide spectrum of radionuclides (fission products); fusion in principle creates only tritium, but a fusion explosion leads to reactions of neutrons with surrounding materials, producing ^{14}C and other neutron activation products. Furthermore, since a thermonuclear bomb needs a fission device as a trigger, fission products are also found after a thermonuclear explosion.

An atmospheric nuclear explosion creates a fireball and a very large cloud that contains all the radioactive materials that have been formed. The top of the cloud rises high into the atmosphere and often reaches the stratosphere. If the cloud enters into contact with the ground, large radioactive particles settle rapidly in the vicinity of the test site (local fall-out). Smaller particles descend gradually to the earth's surface in the latitude band where the explosion took place (tropospheric fall-out) over days or weeks, during which time the radioactive cloud may have circled the globe. Finally, the radioactive particles that are contained in the portion of the cloud that reaches the stratosphere remain there for much longer, and may take several years to descend to the surface of the earth (stratospheric or global fall-out). During that time, the radio-nuclides with short half-lives will have decayed.

The series of large tests of nuclear weapons in the atmosphere conducted between 1945 and 1980 involved unrestrained releases of radioactive materials into the environment and caused the largest collective dose thus far from man-made environmental sources of radiation. Only a small fraction of that collective dose came from the bombs

Table 5. Numbers of survivors of the atomic bombings in Japan, by weighted dose to the colon and city, in the Life Span Study

City	Total	DS86 weighted colon dose (Sv)[a]								
		<0.005	0.005–0.02	0.02–0.05	0.05–0.1	0.1–0.2	0.2–0.5	0.5–1.0	1.0–2.0	≥2.0
Hiroshima	58 459	21 370	11 300	6 847	5 617	4 504	5 078	2 177	1 070	496
Nagasaki	28 113	15 089	5 621	2 543	921	963	1 230	1 025	538	183
Total	86 572	36 459	16 921	9 390	6 538	5 467	6 308	3 202	1 608	679

From Pierce *et al.* (1996)
[a] Categories defined with a weighting factor of 10 for neutrons

detonated over Hiroshima and Nagasaki in 1945, and most was due to the tests conducted in 1961 and 1962.

Atmospheric nuclear explosions were carried out at several locations by China, France, the United Kingdom, the USA and the former USSR. The first such test was conducted in the USA in 1945; subsequent periods of intensive testing were 1952–54, 1957–58 and 1961–62. Much less frequent testing in the atmosphere occurred after a limited nuclear test ban treaty was signed in August 1963. It is estimated that 520 atmospheric nuclear explosions occurred at a number of locations, mainly in the Northern Hemisphere, between 1945 and 1980. The total explosive yield amounts to 545 megatonnes (Mt) of TNT equivalent, consisting of 217 Mt from fission and 328 Mt from fusion (UNSCEAR, 1993).

Nuclear weapons have also been tested underground, most recently in 1998, but the resulting doses to humans are insignificant in comparison with those from atmospheric weapons tests, as the radioactive materials produced during underground testing usually remain under the earth's surface.

(a)   Doses from local fall-out

Local fall-out affects areas within a few hundred kilometres surrounding the test site, where the highest individual doses are found. The doses resulting from the atmospheric explosions conducted in Nevada (USA), mainly between 1952 and 1957, have been relatively well investigated. The highest effective doses from external irradiation are estimated to have been in the range 60–90 mSv, with an average of 2.8 mSv to the population of 180 000 living < 300 km from the site (Anspaugh et al., 1990). The internal doses to most organs and tissues were found to be much smaller than the external doses, with the exception of the thyroid, in which ^{131}I from ingestion of milk contributed relatively higher doses. The doses absorbed in the thyroid of 3545 locally exposed individuals were estimated to range from 0 to 4600 mGy, with an average of about 100 mGy (Till et al., 1995). In comparison, the estimated mean dose to the thyroid for the entire population of the 48 contiguous states of the USA (approximately 160 million people) was about 20 mGy (National Cancer Institute, 1997).

The nuclear explosions carried out by the USA at locations in the Pacific Ocean were usually conducted under conditions that limited local fall-out. An exception was the 'Bravo shot' in 1954 at Bikini atoll in the Marshall Islands. Unexpected wind conditions resulted in heavy fall-out eastwards on inhabited atolls rather than over open seas to the north, resulting in the exposure of 82 persons (and four in utero) on Rongelap and Ailinginae atolls, 23 fishermen aboard a fishing vessel, 28 servicemen on Rongerik atoll and 159 residents (and eight in utero) of Utrik atoll. These persons were evacuated within a few days of their exposure. The average external doses were estimated to be 1.9 Sv on Rongelap, 1.1 Sv on Ailinginae, 1.7–6 Sv for the fishermen, 0.8 Sv on Rongerik and 0.1 Sv on Utrik. The doses to the skin of the most heavily exposed fishermen were several grays. The average doses to the thyroid for the atoll residents, due mainly to ingestion of contaminated food, were estimated to be 12 Gy to adults, 22 Gy to children and 52 Gy to infants (UNSCEAR, 1993). The doses to the thyroid for the fishermen were due mainly to inhalation and were estimated to range from 0.8 to 4.5 Gy (Conard *et al.*, 1980).

The heaviest near-field exposure from nuclear weapons testing occurred around a test site near Semipalatinsk in north-eastern Kazakhstan. Five of the nuclear explosions conducted at the test site, in 1949, 1951, 1953, 1956 and 1962, account for most of the exposure of the populations to local fall-out. Relatively high effective doses, 2–4 Sv, were estimated at several locations. The absorbed doses to the thyroid after the tests of 1949 were estimated to be 1.3 Gy for adults and 6.5–13 Gy for children in three nearby villages (Gusev *et al.*, 1997). A provisional estimate of the combined collective dose of two cohorts presently under study near the test site and in the region of the Altai Range at the borders of Kazakhstan, Mongolia and China is 50 000 person–Sv (Burkart, 1996).

(b)   Doses from tropospheric and global fall-out

The doses from tropospheric and global fall-out were studied extensively (UNSCEAR, 1993) on the basis of data from environmental measurement networks complemented with mathematical models. One way of expressing the doses from this source is as the integral over time of the average collective effective dose rate of the world population: the 'collective effective dose commitment'. In this calculation, the variation of the world's population with time is taken into account. The effective dose commitment to the year 2200 from atmospheric testing is about 1.4 mSv; over 'all time'—until the radioactivity has decreased to negligible values—it is 3.7 mSv. The two figures are of the same order of magnitude as the effective dose from one year of exposure to natural sources. The estimated collective effective dose commitments of the world's population for individual radionuclides from atmospheric nuclear testing are presented in Table 6. The total collective effective dose commitment from weapons testing is about 30 million person–Sv, of which about 7 million person–Sv will have been delivered by the year 2200; the rest, due to long-lived ^{14}C, will be delivered over the next 10 000 years or so. The next most important radionuclides, in terms of collective effective dose commitments, are ^{137}Cs and ^{90}Sr, both of which have radioactive half-lives of about 30 years. Most of the doses from ^{137}Cs and ^{90}Sr have already been delivered, ^{137}Cs through both external and internal irradiation and ^{90}Sr through internal irradiation. The collective effective dose commitment from ^{131}I is much lower than those from ^{14}C, ^{137}Cs and ^{90}Sr because most of the ^{131}I released decayed in the stratosphere before contaminating the biosphere and because the thyroid has a low weighting factor in calculations of effective dose.

4.1.3   Production of materials for nuclear weapons

The production of nuclear weapons involves use of enriched uranium or plutonium for fission devices and tritium and deuterium for fusion devices. The fuel cycle for

Table 6. Collective effective dose commitments of the world population from atmospheric nuclear testing

Radionuclide	Half-life	Activity produced ($\times 10^{18}$ Bq)	Collective effective dose commitment (1000 person–Sv)			
			External	Ingestion	Inhalation	Total
^{14}C	5730 years	0.220		25 800	2.6	25 800
^{137}Cs	30.1 years	0.910	1 210	677	1.1	1 890
^{90}Sr	28.6 years	0.600		406	29	435
^{95}Zr	64.0 days	143	272		6.1	278
^{106}Ru	372 days	11.8	140		82	222
^{3}H	12.3 years	240		176	13	189
^{54}Mn	312 days	5.20	181		0.4	181
^{144}Ce	285 days	29.6	44		122	165
^{131}I	8.02 days	651	4.4	154	6.3	164
^{95}Nb	35.2 days	–	129		2.6	132
^{125}Sb	2.73 years	0.524	88		0.2	88
^{239}Pu	24 100 years	0.00652		1.8	56	58
^{241}Am	432 years	–		8.7	44	53
^{140}Ba	12.8 days	732	49	0.81	0.66	51
^{103}Ru	39.3 days	238	39		1.8	41
^{240}Pu	6560 years	0.00435		1.3	38	39
^{55}Fe	2.74 years	2.00		26	0.06	26
^{241}Pu	14.4 years	0.142		0.01	17	17
^{89}Sr	50.6 days	91.4		4.5	6.0	11
^{91}Y	58.5 days	116			8.9	8.9
^{141}Ce	32.5 days	254	3.3		1.4	4.7
^{238}Pu	87.7 years	–		0.003	2.4	2.3
Total (rounded)			2 160	27 200	440	30 000

From UNSCEAR (1993)

military purposes is similar to that for generation of nuclear electric energy: uranium mining and milling, enrichment, fuel fabrication, reactor operation and fuel reprocessing. Environmental releases of radioactive materials from military facilities were greatest during the earliest years of the nuclear arsenals, in the 1940s and 1950s, although the scale of such activities is not disclosed and must be assessed indirectly. According to UNSCEAR (1993), the global collective effective dose committed by these operations is at most 0.1 million person–Sv, which is small when compared with the collective effective dose of 30 million person–Sv committed by the test programmes (Table 6).

As in the case of nuclear weapons testing, substantial doses have been received locally. The doses to the thyroid near a plutonium production plant at Hanford, Washington, USA, as a result of atmospheric releases of ^{131}I between 1944 and 1956 were ≤ 2 Gy (UNSCEAR, 1993). The release into the Techa River of radioactive wastes from the processing of irradiated fuel at the Mayak facility, a military plant in Ozersk, in the Ural Mountains in the Russian Federation, resulted in widescale environmental contamination (Trapeznikov *et al.*, 1993; Bougrov *et al.*, 1998). These activities peaked shortly after the onset of operations in 1948 and in the early 1950s. Between 1949 and 1956, the activity in liquid releases into the Techa river amounted to 10^{17} Bq, consisting mainly of $^{89/90}$Sr (20.4%), ^{137}Cs (12.2%), ^{95}Zr/^{95}Nb (13.6%), $^{103/106}$Ru (25.9%) and rare earth elements (26.9%) (UNSCEAR, 1993). The cumulative dose from external radiation fields in river sediments and contaminated flood plains was up to 4 Gy, as determined by environmental thermoluminescence dosimetry on bricks from a mill in the nearest village downstream from the Mayak plant (Bougrov *et al.*, 1998). Internal exposure from drinking-water and irrigation with contaminated water added to the external exposure, resulting in effective doses > 1 Gy. The total exposure of the population was about 15 000 person–Sv. Exposure of workers in nuclear weapons production facilities is discussed in section 4.3.

The two most important nuclear accidents in military installations took place in Kyshtym, a village near the Mayak facility, and in Windscale in the United Kingdom in 1957.

(a)   The Kyshtym accident

In September 1957, a large concrete vessel containing highly radioactive waste (10^{18} Bq) in a chemically reactive mixture of acetate and nitrate exploded due to failure of both the cooling and the surveillance equipment. About 10^{17} Bq of radioactive material, mainly ^{144}Ce (66%), ^{95}Zr/^{95}Nb (24.9%), ^{106}Ru (3.7%) and ^{90}Sr (5.4%), were dispersed over 300 km. The collective dose over 30 years was estimated to be about 2500 person–Sv; it was shared about equally between people who were evacuated from the area of high contamination (about 10 000) and those who remained in the less contaminated areas (about 260 000). The highest individual doses were those of people who were evacuated within a few days of the accident. The average effective dose for this group of 1150 people was about 0.5 Sv. The cumulative exposure of the population living along the Techa River was even higher, as highly radioactive waste was released into the Techa–Iset–Tobol river system (UNSCEAR, 1993; Burkart, 1996).

(b)   The Windscale accident

The accident at the Windscale I reactor (United Kingdom) in October 1957 attracted little public attention, because it occurred during a decade when there was high fall-out from weapons testing and the impact of the accident on the environment was comparatively small. The reactor was a graphite-moderated nuclear reactor of approximately 30 MW power, cooled by forced draught air, which was used to produce plutonium for military purposes. The accident occurred when the safe operating temperature in the core was exceeded during a controlled heating process on 8 October

1957. The fuel elements were damaged, and the uranium started to burn. This was not detected until 11 October when the operators removed a fuel channel plug and saw that 150 fuel elements were burning. When an attempt to extinguish the fire by injecting carbon dioxide failed, the core was flooded with water. The release of fission products started on 10 October and lasted 18 h, during which period about 1.5×10^{16} Bq of radioactive material left the stack and were distributed in the environment. The material included 1.4×10^{16} Bq of ^{133}Xe and 0.7×10^{15} Bq of ^{131}I. Other nuclides such as ^{137}Cs and ^{89}Sr/^{90}Sr were retained in the fuel elements or filters, but about 0.04×10^{15} Bq of ^{137}Cs was released. The radioactive cloud spread over the southern part of Great Britain and other parts of Europe (Stewart & Crooks, 1958; UNSCEAR, 1993).

The British Medical Research Council decided to conduct extensive measurements of ^{131}I in milk in an area of 500 km^2 around the reactor and to allow a maximum level of radioactivity in milk of 3700 Bq/L. The aim of this action was to limit individual doses to the thyroid to < 200 mSv. The countermeasure was justified because up to 300 000 Bq/L were actually measured (Spiers, 1959). The highest doses were to the thyroids of children living near the site, which were up to 100 mGy (Burch, 1959). The total collective effective dose from the release is estimated to have been 2000 person–Sv, while that received from external irradiation in northern Europe was 300 person–Sv (Crick & Linsley, 1984). The route of exposure that contributed the most to the collective dose was inhalation. ^{131}I was the predominant radionuclide (UNSCEAR, 1993).

4.2   Medical uses

The amount of radiation received from medical uses is second only to that from natural background radiation and is the largest source of man-made radiation. In terms of collective worldwide effective dose, medical diagnostic sources account for about 2–5 million person–Sv annually, whereas natural background accounts for 14 million person–Sv. All other sources are relatively small in comparison (UNSCEAR, 1993).

Medical use of ionizing radiation began within months of the discovery of X-rays by Röntgen in 1895. By 1900, X-rays were being used for a wide variety of medical applications in both diagnosis and therapy. Similarly, radioactive sources—particularly radium—have been in use for medical purposes since 1898. During the twentieth century, the medical use of radiation spread to most parts of the world, and is becoming more frequent. A number of new techniques, such as computed tomography and interventional radiation, result in particularly high doses.

The medical use of neutrons is limited, as no therapeutic benefit has been noted when compared with conventional radiotherapy; however, neutrons are used to a limited extent in external beam therapy and boron neutron capture therapy.

Exposure to radiation during medical use involves exposure not only of patients but also of technical staff and physicians and some of the general public, such as that from radiation emitted by patients treated by nuclear medicine. In this section, the discussion is limited to the exposure of patients; occupational exposure is discussed in section 4.3.

Medical radiation differs from most other such exposures in that the radiation is purposefully administered in a controlled fashion to individuals who are expected to receive a direct benefit. Furthermore, the age, sex and health status of medically exposed populations differ from those of the general population: the age distribution tends to be centred in older age groups (which would reduce the potential carcinogenic risk) and in younger age groups (who may have a higher risk for cancer than the general population). The approximate distribution by age and sex of recipients of medical radiation in developed countries is shown in Table 7.

Table 7. Approximate percentage distribution of medical procedures by age and sex in developed countries

Procedure	Age 0–15	Age 16–40	Age > 40	Male	Female
Diagnostic radiology, except dental X-rays	8	29	64	47	53
Diagnostic nuclear medicine	3	26	71	47	53
Teletherapy	15	20	65	47	53
Brachytherapy	0	28	72	36	64

From UNSCEAR (1993)

The exposure of the world's population to medical radiation has been estimated by UNSCEAR in its periodic reports (UNSCEAR, 1988, 1993). While exposure from natural background radiation varies somewhat between countries, the variation in medical exposure is much greater, as both exposure and the incidence of procedures can vary by as much as a factor of 100. As might be expected, the more developed a country, the greater the use of medical radiation, and the number of medical radiation procedures correlates quite well with the level of health care. Global practice is usually assessed from surveys in many countries, which may be divided into four levels of health care on the basis of the number of physicians per 1000 population: level I, one physician per 1000 population; level II, one physician per 1000–3000; level III, one physician per 3000–10 000; and level IV, fewer than one physician per 10 000 persons. In 1993, countries with level I health care had about 26% of the world's population, those with level II had 53%, those with level III had 11% and those with level IV had 10%. The approximate numbers of medical radiation procedures performed in countries in each of these categories are shown in Table 8.

The global or national average dose from medical radiation can be quite misleading, as a minority of persons are ill but receive most X-ray exposure, while the majority of healthy persons receive little or no medical radiation exposure. The fact that ill persons receive the most medical exposure has a number of implications: as

Table 8. Approximate annual frequency of various radiation procedures for medical purposes per 1000 population

Health care level	I	II	III	IV
Estimated population in millions	1350 (26%)	2630 (53%)	850 (11%)	460 (10%)
Diagnostic radiology	890	120	67	9
Dental radiology	350	2.5	1.7	–
Diagnostic nuclear medicine	16	0.5	0.3	–
Teletherapy	1.2	0.2	0.1	–
Brachytherapy	0.24	0.06	0.02	–
Nuclear medicine therapy	0.1	0.02	0.02	–

From UNSCEAR (1993)

they are ill, their potential lifespan is likely to be shorter than that of the general population, and the incidence of cancer as a result of the exposure is likely to be lower in this group than that which would be predicted for the general population.

A wide range of doses is applied to patients, spanning a range of at least five orders of magnitude. Doses from chest X-rays are < 1 mGy, whereas the absorbed doses from series of fluoroscopies in the past or from interventional radiology can be 100–1000 mGy, and those from radiation therapy are even higher (in the range of 50 Gy) to ensure cell killing (UNSCEAR, 1993).

4.2.1   *Diagnostic radiology*

Diagnostic radiology typically involves the use of a standard X-ray beam to make an image on film, for example a chest radiograph. The absorbed dose from such a procedure can vary by up to a factor of 10 depending on the X-ray equipment and the film or intensifying screen used. In highly developed countries, the use of rare-earth screens and fast film has significantly reduced the dose. Most plain film examinations of the chest and extremities involve relatively low doses (effective doses of about 0.05–0.2 mSv), whereas the abdomen and lower back are examined at higher doses (effective doses of about 1–3 mSv) in order to penetrate more, critical tissues. The approximate doses to the skin and the effective doses from a number of diagnostic radiology procedures in developed countries are shown in Table 9 (UNSCEAR, 1993). The direction of the beam in relation to the patient is important in determining the distribution of the dose, as only about 1–5% of the entrance dose actually leaves the other side of the patients's body to make the image; the rest of the radiation is either absorbed in the patient or scattered. For example, the dose to the breast during a chest X-ray examination is 50-fold higher if the X-ray beam passes from anterior to posterior than if it passes from posterior to anterior; conversely, a posterior–anterior projection exposes relatively more active bone marrow.

Table 9. Approximate mean effective doses from diagnostic radiological procedures in highly developed countries

Procedure	Average effective dose (mSv) per examination	Average number of examinations per 1000 population per year
Chest radiograph	0.14	197
Lumbar spine radiograph	1.7	61
Abdominal radiograph	1.1	36
Urography	3.1	26
Gastrointestinal tract radiograph	5.6	72
Mammography	1.0	14
Radiograph of extremity	0.06	137
Computed tomography, head	0.8	44
Computed tomography, body	5.7	44
Angiography	6.8	7.1
Dental X-ray	0.07	350
Overall	1.05	988

From UNSCEAR (1993). Doses may vary from these values by as much as an order of magnitude depending on the technique, equipment, film type and processing.

Use of fluoroscopy allows physicians to see images in real time. It is typically used in combination with barium meals, barium enemas, during orthopaedic operations and for interventional procedures such as angiography, biopsy and drainage-tube placement. Higher doses are used than in plain-film examinations, the typical dose rate to the skin in the primary beam being about 30–50 mGy min^{-1} and the effective dose from most procedures about 1–10 mSv. The regulatory maximum in some countries is as high as 180 mGy min^{-1}. Long interventional procedures (such as coronary angioplasty with widening of obstructed blood vessels) often result in absorbed doses to the skin of 0.5–5 Gy and effective doses of about 10–50 mSv. Particularly difficult or long procedures can result in skin doses that are high enough to cause deterministic effects such as epilation and necrosis.

Use of imaging procedures that do not involve ionizing radiation (ultrasound and magnetic resonance imaging) has increased over the past two decades in the hope that they would reduce the overall use of ionizing radiation. While this has occurred for selected applications such as obstetrical imaging, the overall number of procedures in which ionizing radiation is used has continued to increase. In level I countries, the total frequency of diagnostic radiology examinations per 1000 population increased approximately 10% over the last two decades. The growth in the number of examinations in less-developed countries is even more pronounced (UNSCEAR, 1993).

Computed tomography scanning has become widely available in many developed countries. In contrast to most plain-film radiography, it provides excellent visualization of soft tissue as well as good spatial resolution. The scans require, however, a significantly higher dose of radiation (an effective dose of about 2.5–15 mSv) than plain film-based diagnoses. The rapid growth of use of computed tomography has meant that in many countries both the total and the average absorbed dose from medical diagnosis is increasing. In the USA, even though computed tomography accounts for less than 10% of procedures, it accounts for over 30% of the absorbed dose (UNSCEAR, 1993).

4.2.2   *Diagnostic nuclear medicine*

Nuclear medicine involves the deliberate introduction of radioactive materials into the body. These radionuclides can be presented in various chemical or radiopharmaceutical forms so that they reach different organs of the body. In contrast to diagnostic radiology, which is used predominantly to evaluate anatomy, diagnostic nuclear medicine procedures are usually used to evaluate the perfusion or function of various organs. Images are obtained from the γ-rays, or less commonly from positrons, emitted from the radionuclide inside the body. Radionuclides such as ^{125}I, ^{131}I and ^{201}Tl are used in diagnostic procedures.

In developed countries, about 25% of such procedures are used to scan bone, 20% each to scan the cardiovascular system and the thyroid and 10% to scan the liver and spleen and lung. As can be seen from Table 7, about 70% of diagnostic nuclear medicine scans are performed on patients over 40 years of age (UNSCEAR, 1993).

The distribution of doses from diagnostic nuclear medicine is not uniform, as the majority of the dose is to the target organ that is being imaged and to the organs involved in excretion. For example, with bone-seeking agents, about 50% of the radiotracer reaches the bone, while the other 50% is cleared by urinary excretion. Examples of the effective doses received by various organs are shown in Table 10.

4.2.3   *Radiation therapy*

In radiation therapy, high doses of radiation are used to kill neoplastic cells in an area of the body that is often referred to as the 'target volume'. The cell killing reduces the chance that cells in the target volume will subsequently become malignant as a result of the exposure to radiation, but attenuated and scattered radiation from the primary beam goes outside the target volume. Thus, the doses to normal tissues near the target volume can be quite high, and individuals who survive the tumour for which they were being treated may have a measurable increase in the risk for cancer as a result of the radiation therapy. Many patients who receive radiation therapy are not treated with curative intent but rather for palliative purposes, and, because of their limited survival, have essentially no risk for a secondary, radiation-induced malignancy. No firm data exist on the percentage of patients treated for cure and for

Table 10. Typical administered activities and effective doses during common diagnostic nuclear medicine procedures

Scan	Radiopharmaceutical	Administered activity (MBq)	Effective dose (mSv)
Brain	^{99m}Tc-HMPAO	500	6.5
Thyroid	^{99m}Tc-Pertechnetate	100	1.3
Heart	^{201}Tl-chloride	100	23
Lung perfusion	^{99m}Tc-microaggregated albumin	100	1.5
Liver and gall-bladder	^{99m}Tc-HIDA	100	2.4
Bone	^{99m}Tc-phosphate	550	4.4

From ICRP (1987). HMPAO, hexamethyl propyleneamine oxime; HIDA, *N*-substituted-2,6-dimethyl phenyl carbamoylethyl iminodiacetic acid (hepatic iminodiacetic acid)

palliation, but it is probable that at least 50% of treatments are palliative, particularly in patients with cancers of the lung, brain, pancreas, stomach, liver and ovary and with sarcomas. The cancers for which long-term treatment is likely to be more successful include leukaemia, lymphoma and cancers of the thyroid, cervix uteri and breast. Radiation therapy has been used occasionally to treat benign lesions, such as presumed thymic enlargement in children and ankylosing spondylitis in adults, but that use has decreased significantly.

Radiation therapy usually involves high-energy X-rays (4–50 MeV) and ^{60}Co γ-rays. For superficial lesions, electron beams are used (UNSCEAR, 1993). Radiation therapy is typically divided into teletherapy, brachytherapy and nuclear therapy. Teletherapy is performed with an external beam of radiation. The beam may consist of poorly penetrating electrons for superficial lesions, but more energetic beams from cobalt sources or particle accelerators may be used. Brachytherapy is the placement in a tumour of a sealed radioactive source, which may be ^{192}Ir wire, encapsulated ^{125}I or another radionuclide. Relatively short-lived sources may be left inside patients, while longer-lived radionuclides must be removed. Nuclear medicine therapy involves oral or intravenous administration of radionuclides in solutions which then travel to a target organ, where decay may occur (UNSCEAR, 1993).

Teletherapy is used for a wide variety of tumours. As seen in Table 7, about two-thirds of all teletherapy patients are over the age of 40; only 15% are children, and most of these have leukaemia or lymphoma. The target doses for most teletherapy regimens are 20–60 Gy, usually delivered in daily fractions of 2–4 Gy over five weeks. Treatment for leukaemia usually involves total bone-marrow irradiation, and the total doses are about 10–20 Gy delivered in one to four fractions (UNSCEAR, 1993).

Radioactive implants in brachytherapy are used predominantly for the treatment of tumours of the head and neck, breast, cervix uteri and prostate. The typical doses to the target volume are 20–50 Gy. Often, patients receive teletherapy in addition to local brachytherapy.

The doses of radiation used in therapeutic nuclear medicine are much larger than those used in diagnosis. Radiopharmaceuticals are administered to accumulate in specific tissues, to deliver high absorbed doses and to kill cells. Most therapeutic radio-pharmaceuticals emit β-particles, which travel only a few millimetres in tissue. The commonest procedure is use of radioactive ^{131}I for treatment of hyperthyroidism and thyroid cancer. As in diagnosis, thyroid therapy is given predominantly to women (male:female ratio, 1:3). The activities of ^{131}I given orally for hyperthyroidism are 200–1000 MBq, and those for thyroid cancer are 3500–6800 MBq (UNSCEAR, 1993). Other therapeutic uses of unsealed radionuclides include administration of bone-seeking agents (such as [89]SrCl) for palliative treatment of osseous metastases, at a typical intravenously administered activity of 150 MBq.

Less common procedures include the use of labelled monoclonal antibodies for the treatment of metastases at other sites. Occasionally, patients are treated with intra-venous ^{32}P for polycythaemia vera or synovitis (UNSCEAR, 1993).

4.3 Occupational exposure

Many categories of workers use radioactive materials or are exposed at work to man-made or natural sources of radiation. Many of these workers are individually monitored. The main sources of exposure for most workers involved with radiation sources or radioactive materials are external to the body. Occupational exposures during 1985–89 were compiled and analysed by UNSCEAR (1993). The annual average effective doses to individually monitored workers vary according to their occupation, and range from 0.1 to 6 mSv, with an estimated annual collective effective dose of 4300 person–Sv.

4.3.1 Natural sources (excluding uranium mining)

Approximately 5 million workers are estimated to be exposed to natural sources of radiation at levels in excess of the average background. About 75% are coal miners, about 13% are underground miners in non-coal mines and about 5% are aircrew (UNSCEAR, 1993). Workers in occupations involving exposure to natural sources are not usually individually monitored. The numbers of monitored workers and the average annual effective doses in various occupational categories during 1985–89 are summarized in Table 11.

The typical annual effective doses of workers are 1–2 mSv in coal mines and 1–10 mSv in other mines. In the mineral extraction industry, the main exposure is to radon, although there is some exposure to γ-radiation. The annual collective effective

Table 11. Worldwide occupational exposures to radiation, 1985–89

Occupational category	Annual average number of monitored workers (thousands)	Annual average collective effective dose (person–Sv)	Annual average effective dose to monitored workers (mSv)
Natural sources (excluding uranium mining)			
Coal mining	3 900	3 400	0.9
Other mining	700	4 100	6
Air crew	250	800	3
Other	300	< 300	< 1
Total	5 200	8 600	1.7
Medical profession	2 200	1 000	0.5
Commercial fuel cycle			
Uranium mining	260	1 100	4.4
Uranium milling	18	120	6.3
Fuel enrichment	5	0.4	0.08
Fuel fabrication	28	22	0.78
Reactor operation	430	1 100	2.5
Fuel reprocessing	12	36	3.0
Research	130	100	0.82
Total	880	2 500	2.9
Industrial sources	560	510	0.9
Military activities	380	250	0.7
Total	9 200	13 000	1.4

From UNSCEAR (1993)

dose of these workers is estimated to be 8600 person–Sv (UNSCEAR, 1993). Detailed information on exposure to radon is given in volume 43 of the *IARC Monographs* (IARC, 1988), which is to be updated in 2000.

Aircraft pilots and cabin crews are exposed to both γ-radiation and neutrons. The North Atlantic flight corridor is one of the busiest in the world and also involves heavy exposure, whereas many European flights are within a geomagnetically protected region, and somewhat lower exposures are expected. Flights over Canada result in the heaviest exposure. If an annual effective dose to aircrews of 3 mSv is assumed, the worldwide total collective effective dose in 1985–89 was about 800 person–Sv (UNSCEAR, 1993). There is some uncertainty about the neutron energy spectrum to which aircrews are exposed, but the effective dose equivalent for a transatlantic flight has been estimated to be up to 0.1 mSv (Schalch & Scharmann, 1993; see also the monograph on neutrons).

4.3.2   *Man-made sources*

About 4 million monitored workers worldwide were potentially exposed to man-made radiation in 1985–89, about 55% to medical sources of radiation, about 22% in the commercial nuclear fuel cycle, 14% in industrial uses of radiation and 10% in military activities. Table 12 shows the time trend between 1975 and 1989 in occupational exposures from man-made sources and indicates that the total average annual dose decreased from 1.9 mSv in 1975–79 to 1.1 mSv in 1985–89.

Table 12. Trends in worldwide occupational exposure to man-made sources of radiation

Source	Annual average number of monitored workers (thousands)			Annual average effective dose to monitored workers (mSv)		
	1975–79	1980–84	1985–89	1975–79	1980–84	1985–89
Medical uses	1280	1890	2220	0.78	0.60	0.47
Commercial nuclear fuel cycle	560	800	880	4.1	3.7	2.9
Industrial uses	530	690	560	1.6	1.4	0.9
Military activities	310	350	380	1.3	0.71	0.66
Total	2680	3730	4040	1.9	1.4	1.1

From UNSCEAR (1993)

(*a*)   *Medical profession*

Workers in the medical industry are exposed to a wide range of radiations and radionuclides. Workers in the medical industry who were monitored for exposure to radiation had an average annual effective dose of 0.5 mSv and an average annual collective dose of approximately 1000 person–Sv between 1985 and 1989 (UNSCEAR, 1993). Their exposures, like those of patients, can be categorized into irradiation from diagnostic and therapeutic procedures.

When X-irradiation was first used, in the early twentieth century, radiologists were exposed to high doses of X-rays, but these doses are now usually low because of improved shielding and a greater distance of the worker from the radiation source. X-ray technicians exposed to radiation in the USA in 1983 had an average effective dose of 0.96 mSv (National Council on Radiation Protection and Measurements, 1989).

Exposure to γ- and β-rays may occur during teletherapy and brachytherapy, although technicians are less exposed than patients because of shielding of the sources and the limited duration of exposure. Some therapeutic procedures such as boron neutron capture therapy involve exposure to neutrons, but the occupational dose equivalents are typically low, 1–4 mSv over four months (Finch & Bonnett, 1992).

(b) Commercial fuel cycle

Workers in commercial nuclear power plants are typically exposed to γ-radiation. The main routes of exposures are from fission products and activation products. The activation product of greatest concern is ^{60}Co, which emits energetic γ-rays of 1.17 and 1.33 MeV per nuclear transformation. The average annual effective dose of monitored workers in the commercial fuel cycle between 1985 and 1989 was 2.9 mSv, and the annual average collective dose was 2500 person–Sv (UNSCEAR, 1993). A small proportion of workers in the nuclear industry are also exposed to neutrons; less than 3% of the total annual effective dose of nuclear industry workers during the period 1946–88 in the United Kingdom was from neutrons (Carpenter et al., 1994). In the USA, the average equivalent doses at selected nuclear power plants in 1984 were 4.9 mSv of γ-radiation and 5.6 mSv of neutrons, and the total collective doses were 4.69 person–Sv for γ-radiation and 0.038 person–Sv for neutrons, since few workers were exposed to neutrons. Thus, the collective dose of neutrons comprises approximately 1% of the total collective dose in the commercial fuel cycle (National Council on Radiation Protection and Measurements, 1989).

High doses may be received in remedial situations. The external doses of the workers involved in clean-up operations after the accident at the Chernobyl nuclear power plant in the Ukraine (see section 4.4.2) and registered in Belarus, the Russian Federation and the Ukraine were for the most part in excess of 50 mSv (Table 13).

(c) Industrial sources

Radioactive materials have numerous applications in industrial processes. One of the main uses is radiography of welded joints with large sources of γ-radiation. The average annual effective dose of workers exposed in this way in the USA in 1985 was

Table 13. Distribution of external doses of clean-up workers after the accident at the Chernobyl nuclear power plant, Ukraine

Country of origin of workers	Year of arrival	Reference	External dose (mGy)			
			0–49	50–99	100–249	≥ 250
Belarus	1986–87	Okeanov et al. (1996)	15%	30%	48%	7%
Russian	1986	Ivanov et al. (1997)	18%	10%	67%	5%
Federation	1987		24%	52%	24%	< 1%
	1988–90		87%	10%	3%	< 1%
Ukraine	1986–87	Buzunov et al. (1996)	11%	30%	48%	11%
	1988–90		81%	17%	2%	< 1%

2.8 mSv (National Council on Radiation Protection and Measurements, 1989). Industrial irradiators are used to sterilize products or to irradiate foods in order to destroy harmful bacteria. The annual average effective dose from industrial uses of radiation between 1985 and 1989 was 0.9 mSv, and the annual average collective effective dose was 510 person–Sv (UNSCEAR, 1993).

Oil-field workers are exposed to low doses of neutron radiation during 'well logging', in which γ-ray or neutron sources are used to assess the geological structures in a bore hole. The typical annual dose equivalents from exposure to neutrons are 1–2 mSv (Fujimoto et al., 1985).

(d)   Military activities

Workers involved in the production of nuclear weapons are exposed to a wide range of radiation types and radionuclides. Those involved in fuel fabrication are primarily exposed to uranium, which is chemically toxic, and have some exposure to γ- and β-radiation. The primary exposure of workers in reactor operations is to γ-radiation and neutrons from the fission process and to γ- and β-radiation from fission products and neutron activation products. During fuel reprocessing and separation of weapon material, workers are exposed first to γ-radiation from the fission products and then during fuel reprocessing to α-radiation from plutonium, uranium and americium. During the later stages of weapons production, they are also exposed to neutrons from α-particle reactions with light materials, although such exposure is low. In 1979, of the 24 787 workers in the USA who were monitored for exposure to neutrons, only 326 (1.4%) had received neutron dose equivalents greater than 5 mSv. Almost 80% of these workers were involved in military activities (National Council on Radiation Protection and Measurements, 1989).

In the early days of operation of the first plutonium production facility in the former USSR, the Mayak facility in Ozersk in the Ural Mountains, reactor operators (about 1800 persons) and workers involved in the separation of plutonium from irradiated fuel (about 3300 persons) received annual effective doses in the range of 1 Sv. The percentage of women in the radiochemistry processing plant was about 38% (Akleyev & Lyubchansky, 1994; Koshurnikova et al., 1994). External γ-irradiation was the major route of exposure for workers operating and repairing reactors or transporting radioactive materials, leading to an average dose of 940 mSv in 1949, the first full year of operation. Table 14 gives estimates based on film badge dosimetry for the first 15 years of operation. The doses from external exposure in the radiochemistry processing plant reached a maximum of 1130 mSv. The doses to the lung due to inhalation of ^{239}Pu aerosol were considerable.

Several epidemiological studies of workers in military activities involving exposure to radiation have reported collective dose equivalents. A study of 28 347 male workers employed between 1943 and 1985 at the X-10 and Y-12 plants in Oak Ridge, Tennessee (USA), and monitored for exposure to external radiation, showed a collective dose of 376 Sv (Frome et al., 1997). A combined international study of 95 673 monitored

Table 14. External γ-radiation doses from the production of plutonium at the Mayak facility in Ozersk, Russian Federation, during the first 15 years of operation

Period of employment	Average annual dose (mGy)		Per cent exposed to > 1 Gy	
	Reactor	Processing plant	Reactor	Processing plant
1948–53	326	704	6.5	22.5
1954–58	64	172	0.15	0.1
1959–63	25	105	0	0

From Koshurnikova *et al.* (1994)

nuclear workers from the Sellafield nuclear fuel processing plant, the Atomic Energy Authority and the Atomic Weapons Establishment in the United Kingdom; the Hanford and Rocky Flats facilities and Oak Ridge National Laboratory in the USA; and Atomic Energy of Canada (a non-military facility) found a total collective dose of 3843.2 Sv (Cardis *et al.*, 1995). Table 15 shows the sizes of the respective cohorts, their collective doses and their average cumulative effective doses.

Table 15. Collective doses received by monitored workers in nuclear facilities involving exposure to radiation

Facility	No. of workers	Cumulative	
		Collective dose (Sv)	Average dose (mSv)
Sellafield, United Kingdom	9 494	1 310	138
Atomic Energy Authority and Atomic Weapons Establishment, United Kingdom	29 000	960	33
Atomic Energy of Canada	11 355	310	28
Hanford, Washington, USA	32 595	880	27
Rocky Flats, Colorado, USA	6 638	240	36
Oak Ridge National Laboratory, Tennessee, USA	6 591	140	21
Total	95 673	3 840	40

Adapted from Cardis *et al.* (1995)

4.4   Environmental exposure

4.4.1   *Natural sources*

Natural radiation comprises external sources of extraterrestrial origin, i.e. cosmic radiation, and sources of terrestrial origin. The worldwide average annual effective dose from natural sources is estimated to be 2.4 mSv, of which about 1.1 mSv is due to basic background radiation (cosmic rays, terrestrial radiation and ingested radionuclides excluding radon) and 1.3 mSv is due to exposure to radon. Estimates of the average annual effective doses from the various sources of natural radiation are given in Table 16. The annual collective effective dose to the world population of 5.3 thousand million people is about 13 million person–Sv.

Table 16. Annual effective doses to adults from natural sources of radiation

Source of exposure	Annual effective dose (mSv)	
	Typical	Elevated[a]
Cosmic rays	0.39	2.0
Terrestrial γ-rays	0.46	4.3
Radionuclides in the body (except radon)	0.23	0.6
Radon and its decay products	1.3	10
Total (rounded)	2.4	–

From UNSCEAR (1993)
[a] The elevated values are representative of large regions; higher values may be observed locally.

(*a*)   *Cosmic radiation*

It has long been known that ions are present in the atmosphere. V.F. Hess developed an electrometer capable of operating at the temperature and pressure extremes of the altitudes to which balloons rise and derived conclusive evidence that radiation arrives at the outer layers of the earth's atmosphere. The components of natural radiation and the extent of human exposure are outlined below, with indications of the quality of the radiation involved and levels of exposure.

(i)   *Sources*

Galactic sources: When cosmic rays originating in the galaxy by processes not entirely understood enter the solar system, they interact with the outwards propagating solar wind in which the solar magnetic field is embedded. Most particles are found in the broad energy range 100–1000 MeV per nucleon. Although these radiations penetrate deep into the atmosphere, only the most energetic particles produce effects at ground level. The mechanism by which they interact with the atmosphere is still being investigated, as are the biological risks of exposure (Schimmerling *et al.*, 1998).

Solar sources: Solar cosmic radiation, or solar particle events, were first observed as sudden, short-term increases in the rate of ionization at ground level. The close correlation with solar flare events first indicated that they originated in the solar surface plasma and were eventually released into the solar system. Thus, it was assumed that observation of solar surface phenomena would allow forecasting of such events.

The only solar particle events of interest for radiation protection are those in which high-energy particles are produced that can increase ground-level radiation. The rate of occurrence of such events between 1955 and 1990 (Shea & Smart, 1993) is shown in Figure 7. These high-energy events vary greatly in intensity, and only the most intense events affect high-altitude aircraft. The largest event yet observed occurred on 23 February 1956, during which the rates of neutron counts at ground level rose to 3600% above normal background levels. No other events of this scale have since been observed. The next largest event (370% over background) was that of 29 September 1989. Events of this magnitude are also rare, occurring about once per decade.

Figure 7. Temporal distribution of ground-level solar particle events, 1955–90

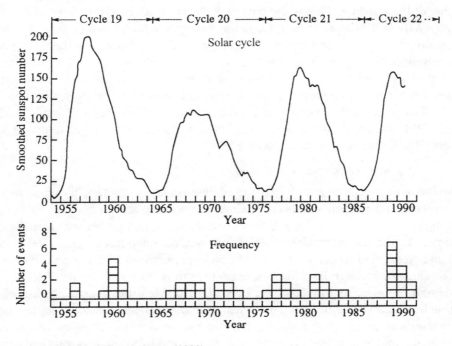

Adapted from Shea & Smart (1993)

(ii)   *Interactions*

Geomagnetic effects: Charged particles arriving at some location within the geomagnetosphere are deflected by the geomagnetic field, which prevents penetration of particles with lower energies near the equator. Studies of such phenomena showed the existence of a dipolar magnetic field, which provides the basis for classifying the orbital trajectories of charged particles arriving at some location within the field.

Atmospheric interactions: The number of galactic cosmic rays incident on the earth's atmosphere is modified first by the modulating effects of the solar wind and second by the deflections in the earth's magnetic field. Upon entering the earth's atmosphere, cosmic rays collide through coulomb interaction with air molecules, but the cosmic ions lose only a small fraction of their energy in these collisions and must undergo many collisions before slowing down significantly. On rare occasions, cosmic ions collide with the nuclei of air atoms and large energies are exchanged. More complex ions may also lose particles through direct knockout with subsequent cooling, adding decay products to the high-energy radiation field. As a result of nuclear reactions with air nuclei, the complexity of cosmic radiations increases further as the atmosphere is penetrated. When these collisional events occur in tissues of living organisms, they become biologically important (Wilson *et al.*, 1991; Cucinotta *et al.*, 1996). For example, the release of energy in biological systems due to ion or neutron collisions has a high probability of causing cell injury with a low probability of repair of the damage. This is the basis for the large RBE of this type of radiation (Shinn & Wilson, 1991; see section 1.2 in the monograph on neutrons). Figure 8 shows estimates of the flux of charged particles and nucleonic components in the atmosphere.

Atmospheric radiation: The ionizing radiation within the earth's atmosphere has been studied by many groups with various instruments. Observations made over many decades with a common instrument give a consistent picture of changes with time and latitude. Two detectors have played important roles: high-pressure ion chambers (Neher, 1961; Neher & Anderson, 1962; Neher, 1967, 1971) and Geiger-Mueller counters (Bazilevskaya & Svirzhevskaya, 1998).

(iii)   *External irradiation*

Background: Foelsche *et al.* (1974) used neutron spectrometers, tissue equivalent ion chambers and nuclear emulsion dosimeters to study atmospheric radiation at a wide range of altitudes, latitudes and times to construct a comprehensive global model over time. The data on atmospheric ionization were obtained from Neher (1961, 1967, 1971) and Neher and Anderson (1962). As most populations of the world live on the coastal plains of the large land masses, exposures to cosmic rays from sea level to an altitude of a few thousand meters have been studied. Measurements of the associated radiation levels can be confounded by terrestrial radionuclide emissions, depending on local geological factors; in addition, cosmic radiation itself changes character at ground level since interaction with the local terrain modifies the neutron fields above the surface.

Figure 8. Particle flux at 50° geomagnetic latitude

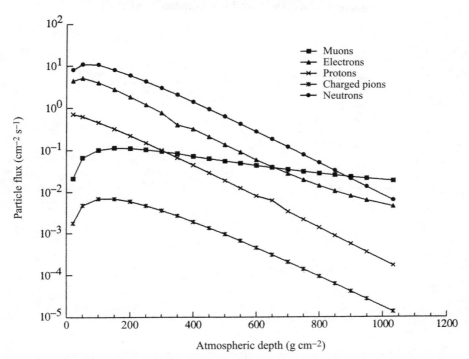

From National Council on Radiation Protection and Measurements (1987a)

As the rate of ionization due to cosmic rays at sea level at intermediate to high latitudes was found to be consistently in the range of 1.9–2.6 ion pairs cm^{-3} s^{-1}, an average value of 2.1 has been adopted (UNSCEAR, 1982). If it is assumed that the formation of an ion pair in moist air requires 33.7 eV, the absorbed dose rate is 32 nGy h^{-1}. The absorbed doses at high and low latitudes are shown in Figure 9.

The neutron flux at sea level at 50° geomagnetic North is estimated to be 0.008 neutrons cm^{-2} s^{-1}, but as the energy spectrum is very broad and difficult to measure estimates of dose equivalents are still uncertain. The average effective dose equivalent was estimated to be 2.4 nSv h^{-1} (UNSCEAR, 1988). With application of the quality factor recommended by the ICRP in 1991, the dose equivalent would increase by about 50%, to a value of 3.6 nSv h^{-1} (UNSCEAR, 1993). The dependence of the neutron dose equivalent rate (with the older quality factors) on latitude is shown in Figure 10; application of the 1991 quality factors would increase the values by about 50%. Figure 11 shows that the dose equivalent of neutrons is small for altitudes < 3 km and increases rapidly to half of the total dose equivalent near 6 km.

Figure 9. Absorbed dose rates in air as a function of altitude and geomagnetic latitude

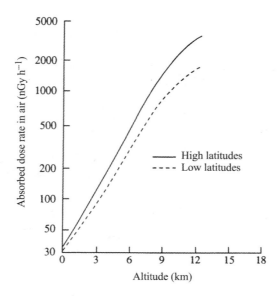

From Hewitt *et al.* (1980)

Figure 10. Measured neutron dose equivalent rate at latitudes in the Northern Hemisphere

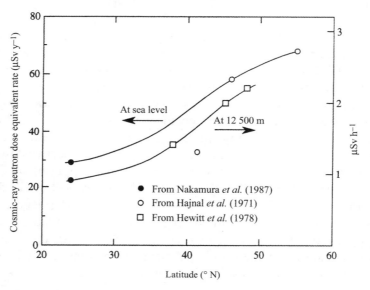

From Nakamura *et al.* (1987)

Figure 11. Annual effective dose equivalents of ionizing radiation and neutrons as a function of altitude

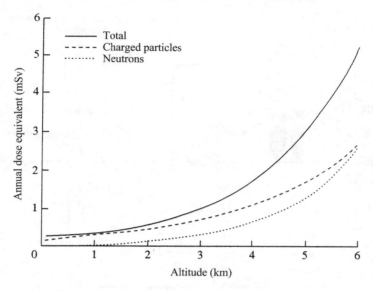

From Bouville and Lowder (1988)

Atmospheric solar particle events: Bazilevskaya and Svirzhevskaya (1998) showed that even a modest ground-level solar particle event such as that which occurred in October 1989 could dominate the particle flux at aircraft altitudes, but their importance to human exposure can be determined only by measurements with instruments capable of distinguishing the biologically important components. Foelsche *et al.* (1974) conducted two balloon flights with such instruments during the solar particle event of March 1969, which was modest at ground level but provided important information on the exposure in high-altitude aircraft (Figure 12). The high-energy fluence relevant to exposure in aircraft is nearly proportional to the ground-level response, and this relationship has been assumed to provide an estimate of the dose equivalent rate of other, larger ground-level events (dose equivalent was used in studies in which the LET-dependent quality factor was used). Of particular importance are the high dose rates over the North Atlantic air routes. The accumulated dose equivalent on such flights during the event of March 1969 was high (5 mSv) even at subsonic flight altitudes (Foelsche *et al.*, 1974).

Radiation doses at high altitudes: The distribution of effective dose equivalent was modelled by Bouville and Lowder (1988) and used to estimate the exposure of the world population on the basis of terrain height (Figure 13) and population distribution. About one-half of the effective dose equivalent is received by people living at altitudes below 0.5 km, and about 10% of those exposed live above 3 km. Thus, in 90% of all exposures, less than 25% of the dose equivalent is contributed by

Figure 12. Energetic solar events measured on the ground and at supersonic travel (SST) altitude

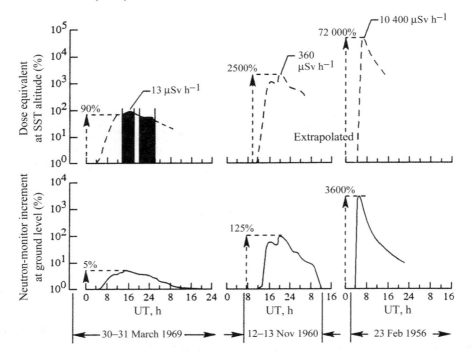

Adapted from Foelsche *et al.* (1974). UT, universal time

neutrons (see Figure 11). A small fraction of people living at high altitudes receive exposures of which 40–50% is from neutrons. Some countries, such as the USA, have large coastal regions where the population effective dose is similar to that at sea level; countries with large cities on elevated plateaux, such as Ethiopia, the Islamic Republic of Iran, Kenya and Mexico, have relatively heavy exposure (Table 17). For example, the cities of Bogota, Lhasa and Quito receive annual effective dose equivalents from cosmic radiation in excess of 1 mSv, of which 40–50% is from neutrons (UNSCEAR, 1988).

The passengers and crew of commercial aircraft experience even higher dose equivalent rates, of which 60% are from neutrons. The exposure depends on altitude, latitude and time in the solar cycle. Most aircraft have optimal operating altitudes of 13 km, but short flights operate at altitudes of 7–8 km at speeds of 600 km h^{-1}, and longer flights at 11–12 km. Human exposure was estimated by UNSCEAR (1993). Assuming 3×10^9 passenger–hours aloft annually and an effective dose rate of 2.8 μSv h^{-1} at 8 km, the collective dose equivalent was found to be 10 000 person–Sv. The worldwide annual average effective dose would thus be 2 μSv, although that in North

America is about 10 µSv. Nevertheless, the dose from air travel makes only a small contribution to the annual worldwide effective dose from cosmic rays, which is about 380 µSv.

Figure 13. Collective effective dose equivalent from cosmic radiation as a function of altitude

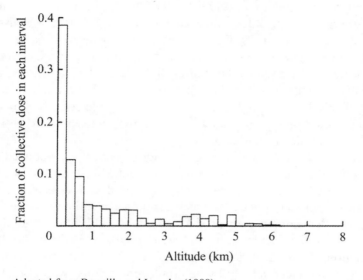

Adapted from Bouville and Lowder (1988)

Table 17. Worldwide average annual exposure to cosmic rays according to altitude

Location	Population (millions)	Altitude (m)	Annual effective dose (µSv)		
			Ionizing	Neutron	Total
High-altitude cities					
La Paz, Bolivia	1.0	3900	1120	900	2020
Lhasa, Tibet, China	0.3	3600	970	740	1710
Quito, Ecuador	11.0	2840	690	440	1130
Mexico City, Mexico	17.3	2240	530	290	820
Nairobi, Kenya	1.2	1660	410	170	580
Denver, USA	1.6	1610	400	170	570
Teheran, Iran	7.5	1180	330	110	440
Sea level			240	30	270
World average			300	80	380

From UNSCEAR (1993)

The supersonic Concorde airplanes operated by France and the United Kingdom fly at cruise altitudes of 15–17 km. The average dose equivalent rate on the six French planes during the two years after July 1987, from solar minimum through near solar maximum, was 12 $\mu Sv\ h^{-1}$, with monthly values up to 18 $\mu Sv\ h^{-1}$. During 1990, the average for the French planes was 11 $\mu Sv\ h^{-1}$, and the annual dose equivalent to the crew was about 3 mSv, while the average for 2000 flights of the British planes was 9 $\mu Sv\ h^{-1}$, with a maximum of 44 $\mu Sv\ h^{-1}$. All of the dose equivalent estimates for the Concorde were made with older values of the quality factor; the revised estimates would be about 30% higher (UNSCEAR, 1993). The exposure of passengers on these aircraft is about the same as that on equivalent subsonic flights, since the higher rate of exposure is nearly matched by the shorter flight time. The exposure of the crew can be substantially higher, since the time they spend at altitude is about the same and independent of speed. These flights make only a negligible contribution to the collective dose, since supersonic plane travellers and crews represent a small fraction of all people involved with the airline industry.

Cosmogenic radionuclides: Cosmogenic radionuclides are produced in the many nuclear reactions of cosmic particles with atomic nuclei in the air and to a lesser extent with ground materials. The dominant isotopes are produced in reactions with oxygen and nitrogen and with other trace gases such as argon and carbon dioxide. Their importance to humans depends on their production rate, their lifetime, the chemistry and physics of the atmosphere and terrain, and their processing in the body after ingestion and/or inhalation. Only four such isotopes are important for human exposure (Table 18). ^{14}C is produced mainly by neutron events in ^{14}N, whereas ^{3}H and ^{7}Be are produced in high-energy interactions with nitrogen and oxygen nuclei; ^{22}Na is produced in interactions with argon. All of these radionuclides are produced mainly in the atmosphere, where their residence time can be one year in the stratosphere before mixing with the troposphere. The residence time of non-gaseous products in the troposphere is only 30 days. ^{14}C undergoes oxidation soon after production to form $^{14}CO_2$. Not all of these radionuclides contribute to human exposure. For example, about 90% of the ^{14}C is dissolved in deep ocean reservoirs or remains as ocean sediment; the remainder is found on the land surface (4%), in the upper mixed layers of the ocean (2.2%) and in the troposphere (1.6%). ^{14}C enters the biosphere mainly through photosynthesis. ^{3}H oxidizes and precipitates as rainwater. The concentrations of ^{7}Be are distributed unevenly over the earth's surface as they are strongly affected by global precipitation patterns (National Council on Radiation Protection and Measurements, 1987a,b). The bioprocessing of ^{22}Na is affected by the tree canopy, which serves as a filter to ground vegetation and is one of the main factors responsible for the large variation in ^{22}Na concentrations observed in plants. Hence, in studies in animals, it was found that deer and elk from wooded areas of Washington State (USA) contained two to three times less ^{22}Na than Arctic caribou (Jenkins *et al.*, 1972).

Table 18. Cosmogenic radionuclides that contribute to human exposure

Radionuclide	Half-life	Main decay modes	Global inventory (Bq)
^{3}H	12.33 years	β	1.8×10^{18}
^{7}Be	53.3 days	γ	6.0×10^{16}
^{14}C	5730 years	β	1.6×10^{22}
^{22}Na	2.62 years	β, γ	6.1×10^{17}

From Lal & Peters (1967)

(iv)　*Internal irradiation*

Of the radionuclides produced by cosmic rays, ^{14}C results in the greatest internal exposures. UNSCEAR (1977) assessed exposure from the known specific activity of ^{14}C, 230 Bq kg^{-1} of carbon resulting in an annual effective dose of 12 µSv. Internal exposure to the other abundant radionuclides (^{3}H, ^{7}Be and ^{22}Na) is negligible.

(b)　*Terrestrial radiation*

The radioactive elements remaining from the formation of the earth are sustained by their unusually long lifetimes. ^{238}U, ^{232}Th, ^{87}Rb and ^{40}K are chemically bound and found in various mineral formations in various quantities. The lifetime of ^{235}U is so short that it plays a lesser role in exposure. The decay of ^{238}U and ^{232}Th consists of complex sequences of events that terminate with stable nuclei (Figure 14). ^{87}Rb and ^{40}K decay by simple β-emission directly into stable isotopes. The decay sequences are determined by nuclear instability, which is characterized by an excess of either protons or neutrons as is required for a stable configuration. α- and β-particles are emitted in order to reach this configuration, but excited states may result from such emissions, which are subsequently resolved by emission of γ-radiation.

The radioactive nuclei are chemically bound and reside as minerals in the earth's crust. As such, they are generally immobile and contribute little to human exposure except as an external source. Indeed, only the upper 25 cm of the crust provide escaping γ-radiation that results in exposure, except for the radioisotopes of radon. Radon has a closed electronic shell structure and is therefore chemically inert and normally in a gaseous state. Although all of the ^{238}U and ^{232}Th decay sequences pass through this noble gas, radon is trapped within the mineral matrix; its chance of escape depends on the porosity of the material. Generally, diffusion within minerals occurs along the grain, from which the radionuclides can escape to the atmosphere or to groundwater. The decay of radium by α-emission results in nuclear recoil of the radon atom, which may then escape from the mineral matrix. The lifetimes of ^{219}Rn and ^{220}Rn are short, allowing little time for escape before they decay into chemically reactive polonium. Consequently, exposure to α-particles is due mainly to the decay of the single isotope, ^{222}Rn.

Figure 14. Principal nuclear decay sequences of the uranium and thorium series

Uranium series

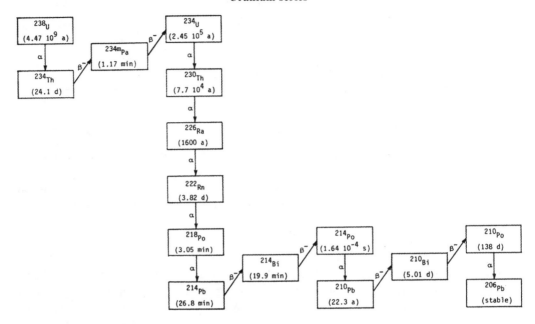

Thorium series

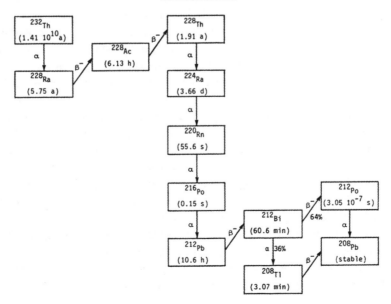

From UNSCEAR (1988)

(i)   *Distribution of terrestrial radioactive nuclei*

The earth's mantle is a relatively uniform mixture of molten minerals, but the mineral content depends on how the crust was formed during cooling. The early rock formations of silicate crystals are rich in iron and magnesium (dark mafic rocks), whereas later cooling resulted in silicates rich in silicon and aluminium (light salic rocks), and the final cooling provided silicates rich in potassium and rubidium. Thorium and uranium are incompatible with the silicate crystal structure and appear only as trace elements within silicate rocks; in contrast, they are the main components of minor minerals.

Physical and chemical processes collectively known as 'weathering' further separate mineral types. Erosion by water, wind and ice breaks down the grain sizes mechanically and separates them into those that are resistant and those that are susceptible to weather. Although the minerals are only slightly soluble in water, leaching by dissolution into unsaturated running water transports minerals to sedimentation points where they are mixed with other sedimented products. Weather-resistant minerals such as zircon and monazite break down into small grains rich in thorium and uranium, which ultimately appear as small, dense grains in coarse sand and gravel in alluvium. Dissolved thorium and uranium minerals add to clay deposits. Thus, weathering of igneous rock results in sands depleted in radioactivity, fine clays rich in radioactivity and dense grains rich in thorium and uranium. Decomposing organic materials produce organic acids which form complexes with uranium minerals to increase their mobility.

Water carries dissolved minerals and mechanically eroded particulates to places with a downward thrust, where sedimentation occurs. The build-up of successive layers of sedimentation forms an insulating layer against the outward transport of heat from the mantle and increases the pressure in the lower layers, and the heat and pressure cause phase transitions, resulting in new segregation of mineral types. The same general process applies to the formation of coal, crude oil and natural gas. Uranium has a particular affinity for these organic products. The radionuclide content is fairly closely correlated to sedimentary rock type (Table 19), and the majority of the population of most countries lives over sedimentary bedrock (van Dongen & Stoute, 1985; Ibrahiem *et al.*, 1993).

The radioactivity of the soil is related to the rock from which it originates but is altered by leaching, dilution by organic root systems and the associated changes in water content and is augmented by sorption and precipitation (National Council on Radiation Protection and Measurements, 1987a; Weng *et al.*, 1991). Soil is transported laterally by water and wind and modified by human activities such as erosion, topsoil transport and the use of fertilizers. Biochemical processes modify the activity in several ways: root systems increase the porosity and water content; humic acids decompose rock into smaller fragments, increasing their water content and resulting in leaching; and the lower soil is changed from an oxidizing to a reducing medium. The overall effect of natural soil development is to reduce activity. The radioactivity of a specific soil type depends on the region and the active processes, as can be seen by comparing the data for similar soil types in Tables 20 and 21. Although geological maps based on the uppermost bedrock are useful for general characterization of activity, they are not a reliable guide to quantitative evaluation.

Table 19. Concentrations (Bq kg⁻¹) of radioactivity in major rock types and soils

Rock type	^{40}K	^{87}Rb	^{232}Th	^{238}U
Igneous rocks				
Basalt (average)	300	30	10–15	7–10
Sedimentary rocks				
Shale sandstones	800	110	50	40
Beach sands (unconsolidated)	< 300	< 40	25	40
Carbonate rocks	70	8	8	25
Continental upper crust				
Average	850	100	44	36
Soils	400	50	37	66

From National Council on Radiation Protection and Measurements (1987a)

Table 20. Concentrations (Bq kg⁻¹) of radioactivity in soil in the Nordic countries

Soil type	^{40}K	^{232}Th
Sand and silt	600–1200	4–30
Clay	600–1300	25–80
Moraine	900–1300	20–80
Soils with alum shale	600–1000	20–80

From Christensen *et al.* (1990)

Table 21. Mean concentrations (Bq kg⁻¹) of radioactivity in the Nile Delta and middle Egypt

Soil type	^{40}K	^{232}Th
Coastal sand (monazite, zirconium)	223.6	47.7
Sand	186.4	9.8
Sandy loam and sandy clay	288.6	15.5
Clay loam and silty loam	317.0	17.9
Loam	377.5	19.1
Clay	340.7	17.9

From Ibrahiem *et al.* (1993)

(ii)   *External irradiation*

The natural cover of the larger fraction of the earth's surface, where people live, is soil resulting from weathering processes. As noted, external exposures are due mainly to γ-radiation emitted from the top 25 cm of the surface layer of the earth and the construction materials of buildings. Buildings reduce exposure from the surface but may themselves be constructed from radioactive material, which may add to exposure to radiation rather than act as a shield. The concentrations of activity of soil in China and the USA (UNSCEAR, 1993) and the associated dose rates in air are given in Table 22. The range of dose rates is broad. The concentrations of activity and associated dose rates for various building materials have been compiled by UNSCEAR (1993) and are shown in Table 23 in relation to the fraction of the materials in specific buildings. Conversion factors for air kerma to effective dose depend on the geometry of the individual and range from about 0.72 for adults to 0.93 for infants.

The results of national surveys of outdoor dose rates, covering 60% of the world population, have been compiled by UNSCEAR (1993). The national average outdoor dose rates vary from 24 nGy h^{-1} in Canada to 120 nGy h^{-1} in Namibia. The world population average is approximately 57 nGy h^{-1}. Many of the surveys included indoor dose rates, which depend on the construction materials used. The average indoor:outdoor dose rate ratio was 1.44 and varied from 0.80 (USA) to 2.02 (Netherlands).

Table 22. Activity concentrations of natural radionuclides in soil and absorbed dose rates in air in China and the USA

Radionuclide	Concentration (Bq kg^{-1})		Dose coefficient (nGy h^{-1} per Bq kg^{-1})	Dose rate (nGy h^{-1})	
	Mean[a]	Range		Mean	Range
China					
^{40}K	580 ± 200	12–2190	0.0414	24	0.5–90
^{232}Th series	49 ± 28	1.5–440	0.623	31	0.9–270
^{238}U series	40 ± 34	1.8–520	–	b	
^{226}Ra subseries	37 ± 22	2.4–430	0.461	17	1.1–200
Total				72	2–560
USA					
^{40}K	370	100–700	0.0414	15	4–29
^{232}Th series	35	4–130	0.623	22	2–81
^{238}U series	35	4–140	–	b	
^{226}Ra subseries	40	8–160	0.461	18	4–74
Total				55	10–200

From UNSCEAR (1993)

[a] Area-weighted mean for China; arithmetic mean for the USA

[b] Dose from ^{226}Ra subseries

Table 23. Estimated absorbed dose rates in air in masonry dwellings

Material	Concentration (Bq kg⁻¹)			Activity utilization index[a]	Absorbed dose rate in air for indicated fractional mass of building material (nGy h⁻¹)			
	C_K	C_{Ra}	C_{Th}		1.0	0.75	0.5	0.25
Typical masonry	500	50	50	1.0	80	60	40	20
Granite blocks	1200	90	80	1.9	140	105	70	35
Coal-ash aggregate	400	150	150	2.4	180	135	90	45
Alum–shale concrete	770	1300	67	9.0	670	500	390	170
Phosphogypsum	60	600	20	3.9	290	220	145	70
Natural gypsum	150	20	5	0.25	20	15	10	5

From UNSCEAR (1993)

[a] Assuming full use of the materials

UNSCEAR (1988) listed several areas in which unusually high dose rates are associated with the presence of ^{232}Th and ^{238}U. These sites include Kerala and Tamil Nadu, India, where the rates were 150–6000 nGy h⁻¹; and Guarapari, Meaipe and Poços de Caldas, Brazil, with 100-4000 nGy h⁻¹. Exceptionally high dose rates have been reported in Kenya (12 000 nGy h⁻¹) and Ramsar, Islamic Republic of Iran (≤ 30 000 nGy h⁻¹).

(iii) *Internal irradiation*

Inhalation and ingestion of naturally occurring radionuclides give rise to internal irradiation. The absorbed and effective doses can be derived from measured tissue concentrations (UNSCEAR, 1982, 1988) or from measured concentrations in air, water and food (UNSCEAR, 1993). The two methods yield similar results (UNSCEAR, 1993). ^{40}K and the radionuclides in the uranium and thorium series are considered separately. Radon was considered in a previous monograph (IARC, 1988).

The data for ^{40}K are well established, being based mainly on direct measurements in persons of various ages but also on analysis of post-mortem specimens. Because the concentration of potassium is under homeostatic control in the body, the concentrations of ^{40}K in soft tissues do not depend on those in food, air or water and are relatively constant. For an average ^{40}K concentration of 55 Bq kg⁻¹ bw and a rounded conversion coefficient of 3 µSv per Bq kg⁻¹, the annual effective dose is 165 µSv for adults, most of the dose being delivered by β-particles (UNSCEAR, 1993).

In contrast, the internal doses from radionuclides in the uranium and thorium series reflect intake with the diet and air. The intakes of the various radionuclides can be estimated from reference activity concentrations in food and air, reference food consumption profiles and breathing rates (UNSCEAR, 1993). The effective doses are then calculated with ICRP dose coefficients. Table 24 presents the reference activity

Table 24. Reference activity concentrations of natural radionuclides in food and air

Intake	Activity concentration (mBq kg^{-1})								
	^{238}U+^{234}U	^{230}Th	^{226}Ra	^{210}Pb	^{210}Po	^{232}Th	^{228}Ra	^{228}Th	^{235}U
Milk products	1	0.5	5	40	60	0.3	5	0.3	0.05
Meat products	2	2	15	80	60	1	10	1	0.05
Grain products	20	10	80	100	100	3	60	3	1.0
Leafy vegetables	20	20	50	30	30	15	40	15	1.0
Roots and fruits	3	0.5	30	25	30	0.5	20	0.5	0.1
Fish products	30	–	100	200	2000	–	–	–	–
Water supplies	1	0.1	0.5	10	5	0.05	0.5	0.05	0.04
Air[a]	1	0.5	0.5	500	50	1	1	1	0.05

From UNSCEAR (1993). All values for food are for wet weight.
[a] Activity concentration in μBq m^{-3}, assumed to apply both indoors and outdoors

concentrations of natural radionuclides in food and air, based mainly on data for northern, temperate latitudes (UNSCEAR, 1993).

Table 25 presents the food consumption profiles and breathing rates of adults, children and infants. The food consumption profiles are based on the normalized average consumption rates adopted by WHO, which are derived from food balance sheets compiled by FAO. The food consumption rates for children and infants are taken to be two-thirds and one-third of the adult values, except for milk products, for which the rates are taken to be higher. Intake of water, both directly and in beverages, is based on reference water balance data (ICRP, 1975).

The resulting age-weighted annual intakes and effective doses are shown in Table 26 in which it has been assumed that the fractional distribution of adults,

Table 25. Reference annual intakes of food and air

Intake	Food consumption (kg year^{-1})		
	Adults	Children	Infants
Milk products	105	110	120
Meat products	50	35	15
Grain products	140	90	45
Leafy vegetables	60	40	20
Roots and fruits	170	110	60
Fish products	15	10	5
Water and beverages	500	350	150
Air[a]	8000	5500	1400

From UNSCEAR (1993)
[a] Breathing rate (m^3 year^{-1}); from ICRP (1975)

Table 26. Average age-weighted annual intakes of natural radionuclides and associated effective doses

Radionuclide	Ingestion		Inhalation	
	Intake (Bq)	Dose (μSv)	Intake (mBq)	Dose (μSv)
^{238}U	4.9	0.12	6.9	0.21
^{234}U	4.9	0.15	6.9	0.21
^{230}Th	2.5	0.18	3.5	0.18
^{226}Ra	19	3.8	3.5	0.01
^{210}Pb	32	32	3500	7.0
^{210}Po	55	11	350	0.35
^{232}Th	1.3	0.52	6.9	1.4
^{228}Ra	13	3.9	6.9	0.01
^{228}Th	1.3	0.09	6.9	0.69
^{235}U	0.21	0.01	0.4	0.01
Total		52		10

From UNSCEAR (1993)

children and infants is 0.65, 0.3 and 0.05, respectively. The total effective doses resulting from the intake of the radionuclides considered are 52 μSv for ingestion and 10 μSv for inhalation. Most of the effective dose is due to the intake of ^{210}Pb, both by inhalation and by ingestion. These dose estimates are nominal and uncertain, and variation in individual doses must be expected owing to the variability of food consumption rates and of the radionuclide concentrations of foods. As shown in Table 27, the reference radionuclide concentrations in foodstuffs can be exceeded by orders of magnitude. For example, in the volcanic areas of Minas Gerais, Brazil, and in the mineral sands of Kerala, India, excess activity is found in milk, meat, grains, leafy vegetables, roots and fruit. The most pronounced increases over reference levels are found, however, in Arctic and sub-Arctic regions, where ^{210}Pb and ^{210}Po accumulate in the flesh of reindeer and caribou, an important part of the diet of the inhabitants of those regions. Reindeer and caribou feed on lichens, which accumulate these radionuclides from the atmosphere. The overall effective dose from ingestion of these meats is about 300 μSv per year for adults (UNSCEAR, 1993).

As in foods, high concentrations of natural radionuclides can be found in water. For example, in Finland, remarkably high concentrations (≤ 74 000 mBq/L of ^{238}U, ≤ 5300 mBq/L of ^{226}Ra and ≤ 10 200 mBq/L of ^{210}Pb) were found in wells drilled in bed rock throughout the south of the country near Helsinki. When the dose received from these waters is added to reference intakes, the overall annual committed effective dose of adults becomes 550 μSv (UNSCEAR, 1993).

Exposure to radon, which is the most significant source of human exposure to radiation from natural sources, occurs mainly by inhalation of short-lived decay

Table 27. Foods in which high activity concentrations of natural radionuclides are found

Food	Country	Radionuclide	Activity concentration in fresh food ($mBq\ kg^{-1}$)	
			Range	Arithmetic mean
Cows' milk	Brazil	^{226}Ra	29–210	108
		^{210}Pb	5–60	45
Chicken meat	Brazil	^{226}Ra	37–163	86
		^{228}Ra	141–355	262
Beef	Brazil	^{226}Ra	30–59	44
		^{228}Ra	78–111	96
Pork	Brazil	^{226}Ra	7–22	13
		^{228}Ra	93–137	121
Reindeer meat	Sweden	^{210}Pb	400–700	550
		^{210}Po	–	11 000
Cereals	India	^{226}Ra	≤ 510	174
		^{228}Th	≤ 5590	536
Corn	Brazil	^{226}Ra	70–229	118
		^{210}Pb	100–222	144
Rice	China	^{226}Ra		250
		^{210}Pb		570
Green vegetables	India	^{226}Ra	325–2120	1 110
		^{228}Th	348–5180	1 670
Carrots	Brazil	^{226}Ra	329–485	411
		^{210}Pb	218–318	255
Roots and tubers	India	^{226}Ra	477–4780	1 490
		^{228}Th	70–32 400	21 700
Fruits	India	^{226}Ra	137–688	296
		^{228}Th	59–21 900	2 590

From UNSCEAR (1993)

products of the principal isotope, ^{222}Rn, with indoor air. The average annual effective dose resulting from inhalation of radon and its short-lived decay products is estimated to be 1200 μSv (UNSCEAR, 1993).

4.4.2 *Man-made sources*

(*a*) *Routine releases from facilities*

The generation of electrical energy in nuclear power stations has continued to increase since its beginning in the 1950s, although the rate of increase slowed to an average of just over 2% per year during 1990–96. According to the International Atomic Energy Agency (IAEA, 1997), at the end of 1997, there were 437 nuclear reactors operating in 37 countries with a total installed capacity of 352 GW and generating 254 GW–years, about 17% of the world's electrical energy generated in that year, a GW–year being the energy produced in a year by a 1-GW (10^6 kW) power plant.

As described above, the nuclear fuel cycle includes the mining and milling of uranium ore and its conversion to nuclear fuel material, the fabrication of fuel elements, the production of energy in the nuclear reactor, the storage of irradiated fuel or its reprocessing with the recycling of the fissile and fertile materials recovered and the storage and disposal of radioactive wastes. In some types of reactors, enrichment of the isotopic content of ^{235}U in the fuel material is an additional step. The nuclear fuel cycle also includes the transport of radioactive materials between various installations.

The doses of individuals from the generation of electrical energy by nuclear power vary widely, even for people near similar plants. Generally, the individual doses decrease rapidly with distance from the point of discharge. Some estimates of the maximum effective doses have been made for realistic model sites: for the principal types of power plants, these doses range from 1 to 20 μSv. UNSCEAR (1993) reported corresponding annual figures for large fuel reprocessing plants of 200–500 μSv.

Detailed information was obtained by UNSCEAR (1993) on the release of radionuclides to the environment during routine operation of most of the major nuclear power installations in the world. From this information, UNSCEAR assessed the collective effective doses committed per unit energy generated (called 'normalized collective effective doses'), making separate estimates for the normalized components resulting from local and regional exposures and from exposure to globally dispersed radionuclides (truncated at 10 000 years). Values of 3 and 200 person–Sv per GW–year were obtained for those two components, respectively. The main contributors to the normalized local and regional collective doses are radon, which is released during operation of uranium mines and mills, and ^{14}C and ^{3}H, which are released from nuclear reactors. The global component of the normalized collective effective dose is dominated by radon released from abandoned mill tailings and ^{14}C released from nuclear reactors. The main contributions to the total normalized collective dose of 200 person–Sv per GW–year are shown in Table 28. The total nuclear power generated up to 1990 (about 2000 GW–years) is therefore estimated to have committed a collective effective dose of approximately 0.4 million person–Sv.

(b)   Accidents

(i)   Accidents other than from nuclear reactors

A historical review of radiological accidents shows that industrial accidents account for most of the immediate fatalities. A total of 178 fatal and non-fatal accidents occurred between 1945 and 1985, of which 153 were radiological accidents in industrial radiography, X-ray crystallography, industrial and research X-radiography, research accelerators, radiotherapy and irradiation or sterilization.

Table 28. Normalized collective effective dose commitments to the public from nuclear power production

Source	Collective effective dose commitment per unit energy generated (person–Sv per GW–year)
Local and regional	
Mining, milling and tailings	1.5
Fuel fabrication	0.003
Reactor operation	1.3
Fuel reprocessing	0.25
Transport	0.1
Total (rounded)	3
Global (including solid-waste disposal)	
Mine and mill tailings (releases over 10 000 years)	150
Reactor operation waste disposal	0.5
Globally dispersed radionuclides	50
Total (rounded)	200

From UNSCEAR (1993)

Many non-nuclear accidents occur when strong γ-radiation sources used for radiotherapy or industrial radiography are abandoned by their first users and removed from their shielding by unqualified persons, such as scrap dealers (Stephan *et al.*, 1983). With increased use of linear accelerators for industrial purposes, the number of accidents in this area has also increased (Lanzl *et al.*, 1967). One of the most severe non-nuclear accidents occurred in Goiânia, near Brasilia, Brazil, in 1987 and accounted for four deaths, 28 cases of severe radiation burns and 249 cases of internal or external contamination (IAEA, 1988). The cytogenetic effects of this exposure are described in the monograph on X- and γ-radiation (section 4.4.1). Another accident, with a ^{60}Co source, occurred in Ciudad Juárez, Mexico, in 1983: seven persons received doses of 3–7 Sv, and 700 persons received 0.005–0.25 Sv (Marshall, 1984).

(ii) *Nuclear reactor accidents*

The two largest nuclear accidents in civilian installations took place at the Three-Mile Island facility, Harrisburg, Pennsylvania, USA, in 1979 and in Chernobyl, Ukraine, in 1986.

Three-Mile Island accident: The Three-Mile Island pressurized water reactor unit 2 was a commercial reactor with 2800 MW thermal power. At the time of the accident on 28 March 1979, it had been in operation for one year. Owing to several technical problems, the reactor core was not covered with coolant for 2 h and started to melt, partially as a result of overheating. As the operator was unaware of this critical situation, considerable amounts of radioactive gases entered an auxiliary building from which mainly inert gas escaped to the environment. About 3.7×10^{17} Bq of ^{133}Xe were released with other xenon and krypton fission products. Iodine was successfully retained in the auxiliary building and only 6×10^{11} Bq were released to the environment (Lakey, 1993). The individual doses were low, and the total dose to the population within a 80-km radius of the reactor was estimated to have been about 20 person–Sv (Gernsky, 1981). The individual doses to thyroids of one-year-old children resulting from inhalation and ingestion of iodine were ≤ 0.07 mGy.

Chernobyl accident: Reactors of the channelized large power reactor (RBMK) type which are moderated by graphite and cooled by water generate 1000 MW of electrical power. Four of them were operating at Chernobyl, about 100 km north of Kiev. During a poorly implemented test on 26 April 1986, a critical excursion occurred, which was followed by a steam explosion that destroyed unit 4. About 3.5–4% of the reactor fuel was blown out with this explosion, and the entire content of radioactive noble gases, about 50% of the iodine, 30% of the caesium and 4% of the strontium content were released to the environment between 26 April and 6 May 1986. The total amount of radioactive material released apart from the noble gases was several times 10^{18} Bq (Buzulukov & Dobrynin, 1993; Nuclear Energy Agency, 1995). Several hundred people exposed to doses > 2 Gy had acute radiation sickness, and 29 of them died.

Fall-out of radioiodine was one of the most important factors in human irradiation in the contaminated areas. Radioiodine from food and inhalation accumulates in the thyroid gland, where it may produce large doses. Almost all of the dose is due to β-particles. ^{131}I was the predominant source of exposure during the first weeks after the accident, but its contribution was negligible thereafter when compared with long-lived nuclides like ^{137}Cs and ^{90}Sr, owing to its half-life of eight days. A detailed analysis of the relative contributions of different sources to the total exposure of the thyroid to iodine isotopes was made for the citizens of Kiev (Likhtarev *et al.*, 1994a,b). The measured doses correspond well to calculations based on the ingestion of contaminated milk and water, although individual doses can be considerably underestimated by this method.

By October 1986, about 116 000 persons had been evacuated. Those first eva-cuated were the residents of the town of Pripyat (49 360 persons) and of villages near the reactor site. The average whole-body dose from external radiation for these people was estimated to be 0.2 Gy, with individual values ranging from 0.0001 to 0.4 Gy (Likhtarev *et al.*, 1994c). In comparison, the average dose to the thyroid of the evacuees from Pripyat, which was delivered mainly by inhalation of radioiodine, was estimated to be 0.2 Gy and to be highest for 0–3-year-old children (about 1.4 Gy). A collective dose of about 2×10^6 person–Sv is expected over the next 50 years (Goulko *et al.*, 1996). About 150 000 individual measurements of the dose to the thyroid were carried out in the Ukraine, one-third of them with energy-selective equipment. The collective dose can be estimated to be 64 000 person–Gy (Likhtarev et al., 1993).

Twenty per cent of the Belarussian territory containing 27 cities and 2736 villages with 2 million inhabitants was contaminated with ^{137}Cs at levels over 37 kBq m^{-2} (Henrich & Steinhäusler, 1993; Hoshi et al., 1994). In this area, the ground deposition density of ^{131}I was $> 2.6 \times 10^5$ Bq m^{-2}. The individual exposure of about 200 000 people was derived from a survey of the ^{131}I activity in thyroids, carried out within five weeks of the accident by measuring γ-radiation near the thyroid gland. The exposure of other inhabitants of the region was estimated by adjusting for age and milk consumption, and the contamination pattern of the whole country was used to estimate exposure of the thyroid. The collective thyroid dose for the population of Belarus was thus estimated to about 500 000 person–Gy as a result of the intake of ^{131}I (Gavrilin et al., 1999).

(c)   Miscellaneous releases

For the sake of completeness, miscellaneous sources which contribute little to the exposure of the general public are described briefly. These sources include consumer products such as smoke alarms, clocks and watches, compasses, tritium light sources and gas mantles (Schmitt-Hannig et al., 1995). Various national and international bodies stipulate the criteria for inclusion of radioactive materials in consumer and household goods (Nuclear Energy Agency, 1985; National Radiological Protection Board, 1992).

(i)   Smoke alarms

Ionizing-chamber smoke alarms contain a source of ^{241}Am incorporated in metal foil. Current smoke alarms contain less than 40 kBq of ^{241}Am, although alarms with activities of up to 3.7 MBq were used in the past in industrial and commercial premises (National Radiological Protection Board, 1985; Nuclear Energy Agency, 1985). The annual individual effective dose from current smoke alarms has been estimated to be about 0.1 μSv, on the basis of the assumption that an individual spends 8 h daily at a distance of 2 m from the alarm.

(ii)   Radioluminous clocks and watches

Clocks and watches have been luminized since the 1920s, initially with ^{226}Ra and later with ^{147}Pm and ^{3}H. The maximum radioactivity in modern timepieces is restricted, and the average annual dose for wearers of these timepieces is estimated to be around 1 μSv (IAEA, 1967; International Association for Standardization, 1975).

(iii)   Gaseous tritium light devices

Gaseous tritium light devices are glass containers filled with gaseous tritium and coated internally with phosphor. They are frequently used to illuminate exit signs, telephone dials, clocks and watches, instrument panels and compasses. During normal use, tritium escapes from the devices by diffusion or leakage from inadequately sealed tubes. The average annual doses of individuals wearing watches with a gaseous tritium light device are likely to be < 1 μSv (Nuclear Energy Agency, 1973; National Radiological Protection Board, 1992).

(iv)   *Thoriated gas mantles*

Thoriated gas mantles consist of a mesh impregnated with thorium and cerium compounds and are used in gas burners to provide illumination. They are bought mainly for camping and caravanning and are used for only short periods of the year. Radioactive decay products are released from the mantle as it burns, and the doses of regular users can be higher than those from other consumer products. If five gas mantles were used by a camper each year, each gas mantle being burnt for 4 h, the annual dose would be 100 μSv for children and 50 μSv for adults (National Radiological Protection Board, 1992).

(v)   *Other miscellaneous sources*

Other sources of radiation in consumer products include the use of radioactive attachments to lightning conductors, static elimination devices, fluorescent lamp starters, porcelain teeth, gemstones activated by neutrons, thoriated tungsten welding rods and television sets. A recent concern is use of depleted uranium in ammunition and in airplane balancing weights, although chemotoxicity may be of greater importance in this instance. Uranium was formerly used as a glaze colourant in pottery, and other past exposures include cardiac pacemakers (^{238}Pu) and radioactive tiles. Individual exposure from these sources is likely to be low (Nuclear Energy Agency, 1973, 1985; Schmitt-Hannig *et al.*, 1995).

Coal-fired plants release naturally occurring radioactive materials during the combustion of coal. The collective effective dose based on global annual energy production is approximately 20 person–Sv per GW–year (UNSCEAR, 1993).

4.5   Summary

In order to compare the effect of radiation from the main sources, UNSCEAR (1993) estimated the collective effective doses to the world's population committed by 50 years of practice for each of the significant sources of exposure and by discrete events since 1945. The results are shown in Table 29. By far the largest source of exposure is natural background radiation; the next most significant source is the medical use of X-rays and radiopharmaceuticals in diagnostic examination and treatment. Exposure from atmospheric testing of nuclear weapons comes next. The collective doses from other sources of radiation are much less important.

Variation in individual doses from man-made sources over time and place make it difficult to summarize individual doses coherently, although some indications can be given. The average annual effective dose from natural sources is 2.4 mSv, with elevated values commonly up to 10–20 mSv. Medical procedures in developed

Table 29. Collective effective dose committed to the world's population between 1945 and 1992

Source	Basis of commitment	Collective effective dose (million person–Sv)
Natural sources	Cumulative dose for 1945–92	650
Medical exposures	Cumulative dose for 1945–92	
Diagnosis		90
Treatment		75
Atmospheric nuclear weapons tests	Completed practice	30
Nuclear power	Events to date	0.4
	Cumulative dose for 1945–92	2
Severe accidents	Events to date	0.6
Occupational exposures	Cumulative dose for 1945–92	
Military activities		0.01
Nuclear power generation		0.12
Medical uses		0.05
Industrial uses		0.03
Non-uranium mining		0.4

From UNSCEAR (1993)

countries result in an average annual effective dose of 1–2 mSv, with local skin doses of several grays in interventional radiology and values up to 100 mSv in diagnostic radiology. The annual effective dose due to atmospheric nuclear weapons testing peaked at about 0.2 mSv in the Northern Hemisphere in the early 1960s and is currently about 0.005 mSv. The annual effective doses to people living near nuclear power installations are currently 0.001–0.2 mSv. The annual effective doses of monitored workers are commonly 1–10 mSv (UNSCEAR, 1993).

5.   Deterministic effects of exposure to ionizing radiation

The effects of exposure to radiation other than cancer are classified as deterministic, and are distinguished from stochastic effects (cancer and genetic effects) by the following features: Both the incidence and the severity increase above a threshold dose with increasing dose (Figure 15). The threshold dose is usually defined as the dose above which signs and symptoms of the effect on a specific organ or tissue can be detected. Thus, in some cases, the sensitivity of the method of detection is fundamental; for example, clinical methods are available to detect small radiation-induced lesions in the lens of the eye which do not affect vision significantly. The time at which deterministic effects can be detected after irradiation varies among tissues, which are classified as early-responding and late-responding.

Figure 15. Schematic representation of dose–response relationship of the incidence and the severity of deterministic effects as a function of the dose of radiation

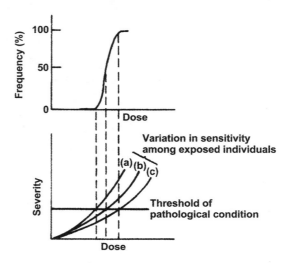

Adapted from ICRP (1984)

Only a short time after the discovery of X-rays in 1895, workers exposed to this type of radiation suffered damage to the skin. The lesions observed led to the conclusion that localized exposure to low-energy photons could cause both early and late effects (Upton, 1977). Knowledge of the deterministic effects of radiation stems from studies of patients undergoing radiotherapy, patients who receive whole-body irradiation before bone-marrow transplantation, the persons exposed during or after nuclear accidents, for example the firemen at Chernobyl, and the atomic bomb survivors. Informative reviews are available that are of a general nature (ICRP, 1984; UNSCEAR, 1988; National Radiation Protection Board, 1996) or deal specifically with effects on the skin (ICRP, 1991) or in exposed children (UNSCEAR, 1993).

5.1   Dose–survival relationships

Cell killing is crucial to the development of deterministic effects, except in radiation-induced cataract (see section 4.2.9 in the monograph on X-radiation and γ-radiation). The response of tissues to radiation reflects not only the killing of cells but also the cell kinetics and the architecture of the organ or tissue. In addition, the severity of the damage and the time between the exposure and the effect are influenced by the dose rate, dose fractionation and radiation quality. As the early effects of radiation are due to cell killing or inactivation, an understanding of the loss of reproductive integrity is essential for interpretation of dose–response curves (Figure 15).

The first curve of radiation dose–survival for single mammalian cells was determined by Puck and Marcus (1956), who used a human cancer cell line derived from a malignant tumour, which has become widely known as HeLa. The survival curve had an initial shoulder and then became steeper and straight on a semilogarithmic plot. It was the shoulder that attracted attention, and various interpretations of the curve and the role of repair in determining the shoulder have been mooted. It has been claimed that neoplastic transformation does not alter the survival curve for a specific cell type, but the difference between the curves for primary human cells and neoplastically transformed cells appears to negate such a sweeping claim. In fact, the complex roles of many genes in the response of cells to radiation are being revealed. The initial part of the survival curve for cells *in vivo* is difficult to determine directly, except for some blood cell progenitors. As survival curves for more types of normal and tumour cells were obtained, it became clear that radiosensitivity and repair capability vary between individuals and between animal strains. Such variations also occur among cells and tissues within an individual and between individuals, and cell survival in tissues irradiated *in vivo* appeared to be influenced by more factors than can be reproduced *in vitro*. A number of models have been proposed to explain the shape of the survival curve. One commonly used is the multi-target model (Figure 16A), in which the initial slope D_1 represents cell killing from a single event, and the final slope D_0 represents cell killing from multiple events. The values for D_1 and D_0 are the reciprocals of the initial and final slopes. The width of the shoulder is measured from the extrapolation number n, or D_q.

The model that predominates the interpretation of survival curves is the linear–quadratic model which stems from the early work and analysis of radiation-induced chromosomal aberrations (Figure 16B). The model implies that there are two components of radiation-induced loss of proliferative capacity: the first (αD) represents a single-track non-repairable event that is proportional to dose, and the second component (βD^2) represents the interaction of two events that can occur if spatially close and before either event is repaired. It is the βD^2 component that is reduced or eliminated when the dose rate is lowered:

$$S = \exp\left[-(\alpha D + \beta D^2)\right]$$

From this relationship, it follows that the contributions of the linear and quadratic components to cell inactivation are equal at a dose that is equal to α/β. When the β coefficient is large and the $\alpha{:}\beta$ ratio is small, it suggests a higher proportion of repairable damage. The $\alpha{:}\beta$ ratio has been useful for comparing both the early and late responses of tissues. Early or acute effects in normal tissues have $\alpha{:}\beta$ ratios of about 10, whereas the range of values for late responses is broad, many ratios being about 2–5. For accounts of the models that are based on the use of the $\alpha{:}\beta$ ratio and have had an impact on radiobiology and radiotherapy, see Fowler *et al.* (1963) and Withers *et al.* (1983).

Figure 16. Survival as a function of dose

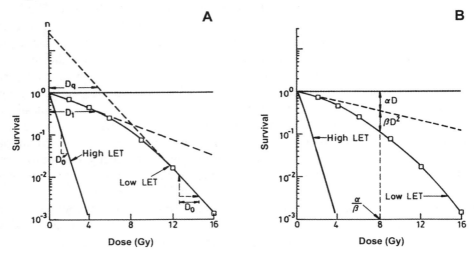

Adapted from Hall (1994). LET, linear energy transfer
A, data fitted to a multi-target model; B, data fitted to a linear–quadratic model

A meticulous examination of the initial slope of radiation survival curves by Marples and Joiner (1993) demonstrated that cell survival at doses below 1 Gy was actually lower than that predicted by the linear–quadratic model on the basis of higher doses. It was suggested that the higher dose points reflect the induction of repair, which is absent, or less effective, at the lower doses.

For primary human fibroblasts, the survival curves are essentially exponential and different from those of most established cell lines. Mutations in several genes, including *p53*, may influence the shape of the survival curve in response to radiation, and especially the shoulder. These findings emphasize the importance of dose–survival curves *in vivo* for interpreting the response of tissues. The methods used to determine survival curves for clonogenic cells within specific tissues are discussed in the monograph on X-radiation and γ-radiation.

The shape of the population and tissue dose–response curve is sigmoid (Figure 15) and shows considerable individual variation. Various functions have been used to describe the responses, including cumulative normal, log normal and Weibull distributions. The response based on the Weibull distribution is described by:

$$R = 1 - e^{-H},$$

where H is the hazard function given by:

$$H = \ln_2 (D/D_{50}),$$

where D is the dose and D_{50} is the dose that causes a specific effect in 50% of the irradiated population (LD_{50} is commonly used to describe lethality for whole organisms and ED_{50} for specific effects on tissues or the function of organs).

5.2   Time–dose relationships

5.2.1   *Dose rate*

The effectiveness of low-LET radiation to inactivate cells is reduced when the dose rate is lowered because of repair of sublethal damage and, at very low dose rates, by the ability of cell renewal systems to restore or maintain the integrity of the tissue by increasing cell proliferation to offset the increased cell loss.

The term 'low dose rate' is used loosely and defined differently by various committees. UNSCEAR (1993) defined it as 0.1 mGy min^{-1}. As the dose rate is reduced, so is the effect, until further reduction in dose rate results in no further reduction in effect. The effect is then no longer dependent on the dose rate but only on the total dose. The dose rate at which independence from dose rate is reached differs among tissues and end-points; Bedford and Mitchell (1973) reported a maximal reduction of the effect on cell killing *in vitro* at a rate of about 5.2 Gy d^{-1}, whereas Sacher and Grahn (1964) found that the dose rate at which life-shortening in mice became independent of dose rate was about 0.2 Gy d^{-1}. The dose-rate effect has been quantified by use of the dose-rate factor, which is the ratio of the effect at a given dose rate and the same effect at the reference dose rate.

5.2.2   *Dose fractionation*

Dividing a radiation dose into two or more fractions reduces the effect because, it is thought, it allows time for the repair of sublethal damage and, if the fractions are separated by sufficient time, for repopulation. Other factors may be altered by fractionation that affect the damage and its repair. The differential in the effect of fractionation on normal and cancerous tissues is the basis of radiotherapy (Thames & Hendry, 1987).

Dose fractionation affects both early and late deterministic effects, and the reduction in effect is tissue-dependent. Tissues respond to radiation at different times after exposure: early-responding tissues, such as gut and skin, and late-responding tissues, such as brain and spinal cord, differ in their responses to fractionation regimens. One explanation is that resting cells or cells that progress slowly through the cell cycle are more resistant to radiation than dividing cells; late-responding tissues contain many more resting cells than early-responding tissues, which have many proliferating cells.

Administration of small fractions twice or more frequently per day is known clinically as 'hyperfractionation'. Under these conditions, the late effects of radiation are less severe than those seen with a small number of larger fractions. Withers (1994) showed that if each of a series of multiple fractions caused the same proportionate decrease in cell survival, the effective survival curve for the multiple fraction regimen would be linear (Figure 17).

In summary, time–dose relationships are complex. In the case of dose fractionation, the total dose, the dose per fraction, the duration of the interval between fractions and

Figure 17. Single and multi-fraction dose–survival curves based on experiments with intestinal crypt cells

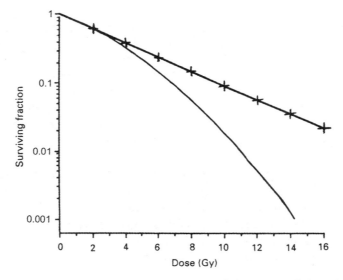

The parameters for the curves are $\alpha = 0.2$ Gy^{-1}, $\beta = 0.02$ Gy^{-2}, the $\alpha{:}\beta$ ratio being 10 Gy. At low doses the α, single-hit non-repairable component predominates. At higher doses the β, repairable injury component predominates. The response to 2-Gy fractions, if there is an equal effect per fraction and there is no repopulation, is linear, with a D_0 of 4.15 Gy.
Adapted from Withers (1994)

the overall time of exposure all influence the response. The occurrence of late effects is largely determined by the dose per fraction and not by the overall time of the exposures, whereas the effects on early-responding tissues are influenced not only by the dose per fraction but also by the overall exposure time. An important mechanism by which tissues tolerate radiation is repopulation. The ability to repopulate is very different in early- and late-responding tissues, being greater in the former.

The response of cell renewal systems such as the bone marrow and gut depends on the inherent radiosensitivity of the stem cells, the life span of the differentiated functional cells, the sensitivity of the feed-back mechanisms and the ability of stem cells in unirradiated areas to repopulate distant areas, which occurs, for example, by migration of haematopoietic stem cells from one site in the bone marrow to another. The replacement of stem cells involves an increase in the proportion of the progeny of stem cells retained in the stem-cell pool. A decrease in the cycle time of the stem cells and an increase in the number of amplification divisions in the committed but still proliferative cells can maintain a functional cell population even with a temporarily reduced stem-cell population. Cell kinetics differs among tissues. These principles and the response of squamous epithelia to fractionated irradiation have been reviewed (Dörr, 1997).

6. References

Akleyev, A.V. & Lyubchansky, E.R. (1994) Environmental and medical effects of nuclear weapon production in the southern Urals. *Sci. total Environ.*, **142**, 1–8

Altman, P.L. & Katz, D.D. (1976) *Cell Biology*, Bethesda, MD, Federal American Society Experimental Biology

Anspaugh, L.R., Ricker, Y.E., Black, S.C., Grossman, R.F., Wheeler, D.L., Church, B.W. & Quinn, V.E. (1990) Historical estimates of external gamma exposure and collective external gamma exposure from testing at the Nevada test site. II. Test series after Hardtack II, 1958, and summary. *Health Phys.*, **59**, 525–532

Bazilevskaya, G.A. & Svirzhevskaya, A.K. (1998) On the stratospheric measurements of cosmic rays. *Space Sci. Rev.*, **85**, 431–521

Bougrov, N.G., Göksu, H. Y., Haskell, E., Degteva, M.O., Meckbach, R. & Jacob, P. (1998) Issues in the reconstruction of environmental doses on the basis of thermoluminescence measurements in the Techa riverside. *Health Phys.*, **75**, 574–583

Bouville, A. & Lowder, W.M. (1988) Human population exposure to cosmic radiation. *Radiat. Prot. Dosim.*, **24**, 293–299

Brenner, D.J. & Ward, J.F. (1992) Constraints on energy deposition and target size of multiply damaged sites associated with DNA double-strand breaks. *Int. J. Radiat. Biol.*, **61**, 737–748

Brenner, D.J. & Zaider, M. (1984) The application of track calculations to radiobiology. II. Calculations of microdosimetric quantities. *Radiat. Res.*, **98**, 14–25

Burch, P.J.R. (1959) Iodine-131 in human thyroids and iodine-131 and cesium-137 in milk. *Nature*, **183**, 515–517

Burkart, W. (1996) Radioepidemiology in the aftermath of the nuclear program of the former Soviet Union: Unique lessons to be learnt. *Radiat. Environ. Biophys.*, **35**, 65–73

Burson, Z.G. & Profio, A.E. (1977) Structure shielding in reactor accidents. *Health Phys.*, **33**, 287–299

Buzulukov, Y.P. & Dobrynin, Y.L. (1993) Releases of radionuclides during the Chernobyl accident. In: Merwin, S.E. & Banonar, M.J., eds, *The Chernobyl Papers. Doses to the Soviet Population and Early Health Effect Studies*, Vol. 1, Richland, WA, Research Enterprises, pp. 3–21

Buzunov, V., Omelyanetz, N., Strapko, N., Ledoschuk, B., Krasnikova, L. & Kartushin, G. (1996) Chernobyl NPP accident consequences cleaning up participants in Ukraine— Health status epidemiologic study—main results. In: Karaoglou, A., Desmet, G., Kelly, G.N. & Menzel, H.G., eds, *The Radiological Consequences of the Chernobyl Accident* (Proceedings of the First International Conference, Minsk, Belarus, 18–22 March 1996), Luxembourg, Office for Official Publications of the European Communities, pp. 871–878

Cardis, E., Gilbert, E.S., Carpenter, L., Howe, G., Kato, I., Armstrong, B.K., Beral, V., Cowper, G., Douglas, A., Fix, J., Fry, S.A., Kaldor, J., Lavé, C., Salmon, L., Smith, P.G., Voelz, G.L. & Wiggs, L.D. (1995) Effects of low doses and low dose rates of external ionizing radiation: Cancer mortality among nuclear industry workers in three countries. *Radiat. Res.*, **142**, 117–132

Carpenter, L., Higgins, C., Doublas, A., Fraser, P., Beral, V. & Smith, P. (1994) Combined analysis of mortality in three United Kingdom nuclear industry workforces, 1946–1988. *Radiat. Res.*, **138**, 224–238

Christensen, T., Ehdwall, H. & Stranden, E., eds (1990) *Natural Radiation, Nuclear Wastes and Chemical Pollutants*, Stockholm, Nordic Liaison Committee for Atomic Energy, pp. 1–51

Conard, R.A., Paglia, D.E., Larsen, R.P., Sutow, W.W., Dobyns, B.M., Robbins, J., Krotosky, W.A., Field, J.B., Rall, J.E. & Wolff, J. (1980) *Review of Medical Findings in a Marshallese Population Twenty-six Years after Accidental Exposure to Radioactive Fallout* (Brookhaven National Laboratory Report BNL 51261), Springfield, VA, National Technical Information Service

Crick, M.J. & Linsley, G.S. (1984) An assessment of the radiological impact of the Windscale reactor fire. October 1957. *Int. J. Radiat. Biol.*, **46**, 479–506

Cucinotta, F.A., Katz, R., Wilson, J.W. & Dubey, R.D., (1996) Radial dose distributions in the delta-ray theory of track structures. In: Gay, T.J. & Starace, A.F., eds, *Two Center Effects in Ion–Atom Collisions* (AIP Conference Proceedings 362), College Park, MD, American Institute of Physics, pp. 245–265

Deus, S.F. & Watanabe, S. (1975) Intercomparison between photographic, thermoluminescent and radiophotoluminescent dosimeters. *Health Phys.*, **28**, 793–799

van Dongen, R., Stoute, J. R. D. (1985) Outdoor natural background radiation in the Netherlands. *Sci. total Environ.*, **45**, 381–388

Dörr, W. (1997) Three A's of repopulation during fractionated irradiation of squamous epithelia: Asymmetry loss, acceleration of stem cell division and abortive divisions. *Int. J. Radiat. Biol.*, **72**, 635–643

Drexler, G., Panzer, W., Widenmann L., Williams, G. & Zankl, M. (1990) *The Calculation of Dose from External Photon Exposures Using Reference Human Phantoms and Monte Carlo Methods. Part III: Organ Doses in X-ray Diagnostics* (GSF Report 11/90), Neuherberg, Forschungszentrum für Umwelt und Gesundheit

Eckerman, K.F. & Ryman, J.C. (1993) *External Exposure to Radionuclides in Air, Water and Soil* (Federal Guidance Report 12; EPA 402-R-93-081), Washington DC, US Environmental Protection Agency

Finch, J. & Bonnett, D.E. (1992) An investigation of the dose equivalent to radiographers from a high-energy neutron therapy facility. *Br. J. Radiol.*, **65**, 327–333

Foelsche, T., Mendell, R.B., Wilson, J.W. & Adams, R.R. (1974). *Measured and Calculated Neutron Spectra and Dose Equivalent Rates at High Altitudes: Relevance to SST Operations and Space Research* (NASA TN D-7715), Washington DC, National Aeronautics and Space Administration

Fowler, J.F., Morgan, R.L., Silvester, J.A., Bewley, D.K. & Turner, B.A. (1963) Experiments with fractionated X-ray treatment of the skin of pigs. 1. Fractionation up to 28 days. *Br. J. Radiol.*, **36**, 188–196

Frome, E.L., Cragle, D.L., Watkins, J.P., Wing, S., Shy, C.M., Tankersley, W.G. & West, C.M. (1997) A mortality study of employees of the nuclear industry in Oak Ridge, Tennessee. *Radiat. Res.*, **148**, 64–80

Fujimoto, K., Wilson, J.A. & Ashmore, J.P. (1985) Radiation exposure risks to nuclear well loggers. *Health Phys.*, **48**, 437–445

Fujitaka, K. & Abe, S. (1984a) Calculation on cosmic-ray muon exposure rate in non-walled concrete buildings. *Radioisotopes*, **33**, 350–356

Fujitaka, K. & Abe, S. (1984b) Modelling of cosmic-ray muon exposure in building's interior. *Radioisotopes*, **33**, 343–349

Fujitaka, K. & Abe, S. (1986) Effects of partition walls and neighboring buildings on the indoor exposure rate due to cosmic-ray muons. *Health Phys.*, **51**, 647–659

Gavrilin, Y.I., Krouch, V.T., Shinkarev, S.M., Krysenko, N.A., Skryabin, A.M., Bouville, A. & Anspaugh, L.R. (1999) Chernobyl accident: Reconstruction of thyroid dose for inhabitants of the Republic of Belarus. *Health Phys.*, **76**, 105–119

Gernsky T.M. (1981) Three Mile Island: Assessment of radiation exposures and environmental contamination. *Ann. N.Y. Acad. Sci.*, **365**, 54–62

Goodhead, D.T. (1987) Relationship of microdosimetric techniques to applications in biological systems. In: Kase, K.R., Bjarngaard, B.E. & Attix, F.H., eds, *The Dosimetry of Ionizing Radiation*, Vol. II, Orlando, FL, Academic Press, pp. 1–89

Goodhead, D.T. (1988) Spatial and temporal distribution of energy. *Health Phys.*, **55**, 231–240

Goodhead, D.T. (1994) Initial events in the cellular effects of ionizing radiations: Clustered damage in DNA. *Int. J. Radiat. Biol.*, **65**, 7–17

Goodhead, D.T. & Brenner, D.J. (1983) Estimation of a single property of low LET radiations which correlates with biological effectiveness. *Phys. Med. Biol.*, **28**, 485–492

Goulko, G.M., Chumak, V.V., Chepurny, N.I., Henrichs, K., Jacobs, P., Kairo, I.A., Likhtarev, I..A., Repin, V.S., Sobolev, B.G. & Voigt, G. (1996) Estimation of ^{131}I doses for the evacuees from Pripyat. *Radiat. environ. Biophys.*, **35**, 81–87

Gusev, B.I., Abylkassimova, Z.N. & Apsalikov, K.N. (1997) The Semipalatinsk nuclear test site: A first assessment of the radiological situation and the test-related radiation doses in the surrounding territories. *Radiat. Environ. Biophys.*, **36**, 201–204

Hajnal, F., McLaughlin, J.E., Weinstein, M.S. & O'Brien, K. (1971) *1970 Sea-level Cosmic-ray Neutron Measurements (USAEC Report HASL-241)*, New York, NY, Environmental Measurements Laboratory

Hall, E.J. (1994) *Radiobiology for the Radiologist*, Philadelphia, PA, J.B. Lippincott Co.

Hart, D., Jones D.G. & Wall, B.F. (1996) *Coefficients for Estimating Effective Doses from Pediatric X-ray Examinations (NRPB-R279)*, Chilton, Berkshire, National Radiological Protection Board

Hei, T.K., Wu, L.J., Liu, S.X., Vannais, D., Waldren, C.A. & Randers-Pehrson, G. (1997) Mutagenic effects of a single and an exact number of alpha particles in mammalian cells. *Proc. natl Acad. Sci. USA*, **94**, 3765–3770

Henrich, E. & Steinhäusler, F. (1993) Dose assessment for recent inhabitants living adjacent to zones heavily contaminated from the Chernobyl fallout. *Health Phys.*, **64**, 473–478

Hewitt, J.E., Hughes, L., Baum, J.W., Kuehner, A.V., McCaslin, J.B., Rindi, A., Smith, A.B., Stephens, L.D., Thomas, R.H., Griffith, R.V. & Wells, C.G. (1978) AMES collaborative study of cosmic ray neutrons: Mid-latitude flights. *Health Phys.*, **34**, 375–384

Hewitt, J.E., Hughes, L., McCaslin, J.B., Smith, A.R., Stephens, L.D., Syvertson, C.A., Thomas, R.H. & Tucker, A.B. (1980) Exposure to cosmic-ray neutrons at commercial jet aircraft altitudes. In: Gessell, T.F. & Lowder, W.M., eds, *Natural Radiation Environment III* (US Department of Energy Report Conf-780422), Springfield, VA, National Technical Information Service, pp. 855–881

Hoshi, M., Shibata, Y., Okajima, S., Takatsuji, T., Yamashita, S., Namba, H., Yokoyama, N., Izumi, M., Nagataki, S., Fujimura, K., Kuramoto, A., Krupnik, T.A., Dolbeshkin, N.K., Danilchik, S.A., Derzhitsky, V.E., Wafa, K.A., Kiikuni, K. & Shigematsu, I. (1994) ^{137}Cs concentration among children in areas contaminated with radioactive fallout from the Chernobyl accident: Mogilev and Gomel oblasts, Belarus. *Health Phys.*, **67**, 272–275

Hutchinson, F. (1985) Chemical changes induced in DNA by ionizing radiation. *Prog. nucl. Acid Res. mol. Biol.*, **32**, 115–154

IAEA (International Atomic Energy Agency) (1967) *Radiation Protection Standards for Radioluminous Timepieces*, Vienna

IAEA (International Atomic Energy Agency) (1988) *The Radiological Accident in Goiânia* (STI/PUB/815), Vienna

IAEA (International Atomic Energy Agency) (1997) *IAEA Yearbook 1997* (STI/PUB/1034), Vienna

IARC (1988) *IARC Monographs on the Evaluation of Carcinogenic Risks to Humans*, Vol. 43, *Man-made Mineral Fibres and Radon*, Lyon, IARC Press

Ibrahiem, N.M., Abd el Ghani, A.H., Shawky, S.M., Ashraf, E.M. & Farouk, M.A. (1993) Measurement of radioactivity levels in soil in the Nile Delta and middle Egypt. *Health Phys.*, **64**, 620–627

ICRP (International Commission on Radiological Protection) (1975) *Report of the Task Group on Reference Man* (ICRP Publication 23), Oxford, Pergamon Press

ICRP (International Commission on Radiological Protection) (1984) *Nonstochastic Effects of Ionising Radiation* (ICRP Report 41; Annals of the ICRP Vol. 14, No. 3), Oxford, Pergamon Press

ICRP (International Commission on Radiological Protection) (1987) *Radiation Dose to Patients from Radiopharmaceuticals* (ICRP Publication 53), Oxford, Pergamon Press

ICRP (International Commission on Radiological Protection) (1989) *Age-dependent Doses to Members of the Public from Intake of Radionuclides*, Part 1 (ICRP Publication 56), Oxford, Pergamon Press

ICRP (International Commission on Radiological Protection) (1991) *1990 Recommendations of the International Commission on Radiological Protection* (ICRP Report 60), Oxford, Pergamon Press

ICRP (International Commission on Radiological Protection) (1993) *Age-dependent Doses to Members of the Public from Intake of Radionuclides*, Part 2, *Ingestion Dose Coefficients* (ICRP Publication 67), Oxford, Pergamon Press

ICRP (International Commission on Radiological Protection) (1994) *Human Respiratory Tract Model for Radiological Protection* (ICRP Publication 66), Oxford, Pergamon Press

ICRP (International Commission on Radiological Protection) (1995a) *Age-dependent Doses to Members of the Public from Intake of Radionuclides*, Part 3, *Ingestion Dose Coefficients* (ICRP Publication 69), Oxford, Pergamon Press

ICRP (International Commission on Radiological Protection) (1995b) *Age-dependent Doses to Members of the Public from Intake of Radionuclides*, Part 4, *Inhalation Dose Coefficients* (ICRP Publication 71), Oxford, Pergamon Press

ICRP (International Commission on Radiological Protection) (1996) *Age-dependent Doses to Members of the Public from Intake of Radionuclides*, Part 5, *Compilation of Ingestion and Inhalation Dose Coefficients* (ICRP Publication 72), Oxford, Pergamon Press

ICRP (International Commission on Radiological Protection) (1999) *History, Policies, Procedures*, Amsterdam, Elsevier

ICRU (International Commission on Radiation Quantities and Units) (1983) *Microdosimetry* (Report 36), Bethesda, MD

International Association for Standardization (1975) *Radioluminescence for Time Measurement Instruments—Specifications* (ISO 3157), Geneva

Ivanov, V.K., Tsyb, A.F., Gorsky, A.I., Maksyutov, M.A., Rastopchin, E.M., Konogorov, A.P., Korelo, A.M., Biryukov, A.P. & Matyash, V.A. (1997) Leukaemia and thyroid cancer in emergency workers of the Chernobyl accident: Estimation of radiation risks (1986–1995). *Radiat. environ. Biophys.*, **36**, 9–16

Jacob, P., Rosenbaum, H., Petoussi, N. & Zankl, M. (1990) *Calculation of Organ Doses from Environmental Gamma Rays using Human Phantoms and Monte Carlo Phantoms*, Part II, *Radionuclides Distributed in the Air or Deposited on the Ground* (GSF Report 12/90), Forschungszentrum für Umwelt und Gesundheit, Neuherberg

Jenkins, C.E., Wogman, N.A. & Rieck, H.G. (1972) Radionuclide distributions in Olympic National Park, WA. *Water Air Soil Pollut.*, **1**, 181–204

Kathren, R.L. (1987) *External Beta-photon Dosimetry for Radiation Protection.* In: Kase, K.R., Bjarngard, B.E. & Attix, F.H., eds, *The Dosimetry of Ionizing Radiation*, Vol. II, New York, Academic Press, pp. 321–370

Kathren, R.L. & Petersen, G.R. (1989) Reviews and commentary. Units and terminology of radiation measurement: A primer for the epidemiologist. *Am. J. Epidemiol.*, **130**, 1076–1087

Kellerer, A.M. & Chmelevsky, D. (1975) Criteria for the applicability of LET. *Radiat. Res.*, **63**, 226–234

Kellerer, A.M. & Rossi, H.H. (1975) Biophysical aspects of radiation carcinogenesis. In: Becker, F.F., ed., *Cancer, A Comprehensive Treatise*, Vol. I, New York, Plenum Press, pp. 405–439

Koshurnikova, N.A., Buldakov, L.A., Bysogolov, G.D., Bolotnikova, M.G., Komleva, N.S. & Pesternikova V.S. (1994) Mortality from malignancies of the hematopoietic and lymphatic tissues among personnel of the first nuclear plant in the USSR. *Sci. total Environ.*, **142**, 19–23

Lakey, J.R.A. (1993) Review of radiation accidents. In: *Off-site Emergency Response to Nuclear Accidents*, Luxembourg, Commission of the European Communities, pp. 41–53

Lal, D. & Peters, B. (1967) Cosmic ray produced radioactivity on the earth. In: Fluegge, S. & Sitte, K., eds, *Encyclopedia of Physics*, Vol. XLVI/2, *Cosmic Rays*, Berlin, Springer-Verlag, p. 551

Lanzl, L.H., Rozenfeld, M.L. & Tarlov, A.R. (1967) Injury due to accidental high-dose exposure to 10 MeV electrons. *Health Phys.*, **13**, 241–251

Le Grand, J., Roux, Y., Meckbach, R., Jacob, P., Hedeman Jensen, P. & Thikier-Nielsen, S. (1990) External exposure from airborne radionuclides. In: *Proceedings of the Seminar on Methods and Codes for Assessing the Off-site Consequences of Radiation Accidents* (Report EUR-13013), Luxembourg, Commission of the European Communities, pp. 407–422

Likhtarev, I.A., Skandala, N.K., Gulko, G.M., Kairo, I.A. & Chepurny, N.I. (1993) Ukrainian thyroid doses after the Chernobyl accident. *Health Phys.*, **64**, 594–599

Likhtarev, I.A., Gulko, G.M., Kairo, I.A., Los, I.P., Henrichs, K. & Paretzke, H.G. (1994a) Thyroid doses resulting from the Ukraine Chernobyl accident—Part I: Dose estimates for the population of Kiev. *Health Phys.*, **66**, 137–146

Likhtarev, I.A., Chumack, V.V. & Repin, V.S. (1994b) Analysis of the effectiveness of emergency countermeasures in the 30-km zone during the early phase of the Chernobyl accident, *Health Phys.*, **67**, 541–544

Likhtarev, I., Chumak, V.V. & Repin, V.S. (1994c) Retrospective construction of individual and collective external gamma doses of population evacuated after the Chernobyl accident. *Health Phys.*, **66**, 643–652

Loevinger R., Budinger T. & Watson E. (1988) *Primer for Absorbed Dose Calculations*, New York, The Society of Nuclear Medicine

Marshall, E. (1984) Juarez: An unpredicted radiation accident. *Science*, **223**, 1152–1154

Nakamura, T., Kosako, T. & Iwai, S. (1984) Environmental neutron measurement around nuclear facilities with moderated-type neutron detector. *Health Phys.*, **47**, 729–743

Nakamura, T., Uwamino, Y., Ohkubo, T. & Hara, A. (1987) Altitude variation of cosmic-ray neutrons. *Health Phys.*, **53**, 509–517

National Cancer Institute (1997) *NCI Releases Results of Nationwide Study of Radioactive Fallout from Nuclear Tests*, Bethesda, MD, Office of Cancer Communications

National Council on Radiation Protection and Measurements (1987a) *Exposure of the US Population from Natural Background Radiation* (Report of Scientific Committee 43), Bethesda, MD

National Council on Radiation Protection and Measurements (1987b) *Exposure of the Population in the United States and Canada from Natural Background Radiation* (NCRP Report No. 94), Bethesda, MD

National Council on Radiation Protection and Measurements (1989) *Exposure of the US Population from Occupational Radiation* (NCRP Report No 101), Bethesda, MD

National Council on Radiation Protection and Measurements (1997) *Deposition, Retention and Dosimetry of Inhaled Radioactive Substances* (NCRP Report No. 125), Bethesda, MD

National Radiological Protection Board (1985) *Criteria of Acceptability Relating to the Approval of Consumer Goods Containing Radioactive Substances* (NRPB-GS2), Chilton, Oxfordshire

National Radiological Protection Board (1992) *Board Statement on Approval of Consumer Goods Containing Radioactive Substances* (NRPB 3, No. 2), Chilton, Oxfordshire

National Radiological Protection Board (1996) *Risk from Deterministic Effects of Ionizing Radiation* (Documents of the NRPB Vol & No. 3), Chilton, Oxfordshire

Neher, H.V. (1961) Cosmic-ray knee in 1958. *J. geophys. Res.*, **66**, 4007–4012

Neher, H.V. (1967) Cosmic-ray particles that changed from 1954 to 1958 to 1965. *J. geophys. Res.*, **72**, 1527–1539

Neher, H.V. (1971) Cosmic rays at high latitudes and altitudes covering four solar maxima. *J. geophys. Res.*, **76**, 1637–1851

Neher, H.V. & Anderson, H.R. (1962) Cosmic rays at balloon altitudes and the solar cycle. *J. geophys. Res.*, **67**, 1309–1315

Nikjoo, H., O'Neill, P., Goodhead, D.T. & Terrissol, M. (1997) Computational modelling of low-energy electron-induced DNA damage by early physical and chemical events. *Int. J. Radiat. Biol.*, **71**, 467–483

Nuclear Energy Agency (1973) *Radiation Protection Standards for Gaseous Tritium Light Devices*, Paris, Organisation for Economic Co-operation and Development

Nuclear Energy Agency (1985) *A Guide for Controlling Consumer Products Containing Radioactive Substances*, Paris, Organisation for Economic Co-operation and Development

Nuclear Energy Agency (1995) *Chernobyl: Ten Years on Radiological and Health Impact*, Paris, Organisation for Economic Co-operation and Development

Okeanov, A.E., Cardis, E., Antipova, S.I., Polyakov, S.M., Sobolev, A.V. & Bazulko, N.V. (1996) Health status and follow-up of the liquidators in Belarus. In: Karaoglou, A., Desmet, G., Kelly, G.N. & Menzel, H.G., eds, *The Radiological Consequences of the Chernobyl Accident* (Proceedings of the First International Conference, Minsk, Belarus, 18–22 March 1996), Luxembourg, Office for Official Publications of the European Communities, pp. 851–859

Pierce, D.A., Shimizu, Y., Preston, D.L., Vaeth, M. & Mabuchi, K. (1996) Studies of the mortality of atomic bomb survivors. Report 12, Part I. Cancer: 1950–1990. *Radiat. Res.*, **146**, 1–27

Prise, K.M. (1994) Use of radiation quality as a probe for DNA lesion complexity. *Int. J. Radiat. Biol.*, **65**, 43–48

Puck, T.T. & Marcus, P.I. (1956) Action of X-rays on mammalian cells. *J. exp. Med.*, **103**, 653–666

Roesch, W.D. (1987) *US–Japan Joint Reassessment of Atomic Bomb Radiation Dosimetry in Hiroshima and Nagasaki, Final Report*. Hiroshima, Radiation Effects Research Foundation

Rossi, H.H. (1967) Energy distribution in the absorption of radiation. *Adv. biol. Med. Phys.*, **11**, 27–85

Rossi, H.H. (1979) The role of microdosimetry in radiobiology. *Radiat. environ. Biophys.*, **17**, 29–40

Sacher, G.A. & Grahn, D. (1964) Survival of mice under duration-of-life exposure to gamma rays: I. The dosage–survival relation and the lethality function. *J. natl Cancer Inst.*, **32**, 277–321

Saito, K., Petoussi, N., Zankl, M., Veit, R., Jacob, P. & Drexler, G. (1990) *Calculation of Organ Doses from Environmental Gamma Rays using Human Phantoms and Monte Carlo Phantoms*, Part I, *Monoenergetic Sources and Natural Radionuclides Distributed in the Ground* (GSF Report 12/90), Neuherberg, Forschungszentrum für Umwelt und Gesundheit

Schalch, D. & Scharmann, A. (1993) In-flight measurements at high latitudes: Fast neutron doses to aircrew. *Radiat. Prot. Dosim.*, **48**, 85–91

Schimmerling, W., Wilson, J.W., Cucinotta, F.A. & Kim, M.Y. (1998). Evaluation of risks from space radiation with high-energy heavy ion beams. *Phys. med.*, **14** (Suppl. 1), 29–38

Schmitt-Hannig, A., Drenkard, S. & Wheatley, J. (1995) *Study on Consumer Products Containing Radioactive Substances in the EU Member States*, Luxembourg, Office for Official Publications of the European Communities

Shea, M.A. & Smart, D.F. (1993) History of energetic solar protons for the past three solar cycles including cycle 22 update. In: Swenberg, C.E., Horneck, G. & Stassinopoulos, G., eds, *Biological Effects and Physics of Solar and Galactic Cosmic Radiation*, New York, NY, Plenum Press, pp. 37–71

Shinn, J.L. & Wilson, J.W. (1991) Nuclear reaction effects in use of newly recommended quality factor. *Health Phys.*, **61**, 415–419

Spiers, F.W. (1959) Increase in background gamma-radiation and its correlation with iodine-131 in milk. *Nature*, **183**, 517–519

Stephan, G., Hadnagy, W., Hammermaier, C. & Imhof, U. (1983) Biologically and physically recorded doses after an accidental exposure to ^{60}Co-γ-rays. *Health Phys.*, **44**, 409–411

Stewart, N.G. & Crooks, R.N. (1958) Long-range travel of the radioactive cloud from the accident at Windscale. *Nature*, **182**, 627–628

Thames, H.D. & Hendry, J.H. (1987) *Fractionation Radiotherapy*, London, Taylor & Francis

Thompson, D.E., Mabuchi, K., Ron, E., Soda, M., Tokunaga, M., Ochikubo, S., Sugomoto, S., Ikeda, T., Terasaki, M., Izumi, S. & Preston, D.L. (1994) Cancer incidence in atomic bomb survivors. Part II: Solid tumours, 1958–1987. *Radiat. Res.*, **137** (Suppl. 2), S17–S67

Till, J.E., Simon, S.L., Kerber, R., Lloyd, R.D., Stevens, W., Thomas, D.C., Lyon, J.L. & Preston-Martin, S. (1995) The Utah Thyroid Cohort Study: Analysis of the dosimetry results. *Health Phys.*, **68**, 472–483

Trapeznikov, A.V., Pozolotina, V.N., Chebotina, M.Y., Chukanov, V.N., Trapeznikova, V.N., Kulikov, N.V., Nielsen, S.P. & Aarkrog, A. (1993) Radioactive contamination of the Techa river; the Urals. *Health Phys.*, **65**, 481–488

UNSCEAR (United Nations Scientific Committee on the Effects of Atomic Radiation) (1977) *Sources and Effects of Ionizing Radiation* (United Nations Publication Sales E.77.IX.1), New York

UNSCEAR (United Nations Scientific Committee on the Effects of Atomic Radiation) (1982) *Ionizing Radiation: Sources and Biological Effects* (United Nations Publication Sales E.82.IX.8), New York

UNSCEAR (United Nations Scientific Committee on the Effects of Atomic Radiation) (1988) *Sources, Effects and Risks of Ionizing Radiation* (United Nations Publication Sales E.88.IX.7), New York

UNSCEAR (United Nations Scientific Committee on the Effects of Atomic Radiation) (1993) *Sources, Effects and Risks of Ionizing Radiation* (United Nations Publication Sales E.94.IX.2), New York

Upton, A.C. (1977) Radiobiological effects of low doses. Implications for radiological protection. *Radiat. Res.*, **71**, 51–74

Ward, J.F. (1994) The complexity of DNA damage: Relevance to biological consequences. *Int. J. Radiat. Biol.*, **66**, 427–432

Weng, P.-S., Chu, T.-C. & Chen, C.-F. (1991) Natural radiation background in metropolitan Taipei. *J. Radiat. Res.*, **32**, 165–174

Wilson, J.W., Cucinotta, F.A. & Hajnal, F. (1991) Analytical relationships of nuclear fields and microdosimetric quantities for target fragmentation in tissue systems. *Health Phys.*, **60**, 559–565

Withers, H.R. (1994) Biology of radiation oncology. In: Tobias J.S. & Thomas, P.R.M., eds, *Current Radiation Oncology*, Vol. 1, London, Edward Arnold, pp. 5–23

Withers, H.R. Thames, H.D., Jr & Peters, L.J. (1983) A new isoeffect curve for change in dose per fraction. *Radiother. Oncol.*, **1**, 187–191

THE MONOGRAPHS

X-RADIATION AND γ-RADIATION

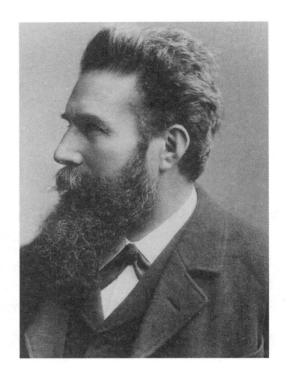

Wilhelm Conrad Röntgen (1845–1923)
Munich University, Munich, Germany

Röntgen received the Nobel Prize in Physics in 1901,
for the discovery of X-rays.

Photo © The Nobel Foundation

X-RADIATION AND γ-RADIATION

1. Exposure data

1.1 Occurrence

1.1.1 *X-radiation*

X-rays are electromagnetic waves in the spectral range between the shortest ultraviolet (down to a few tens of electron volts) and γ-radiation (up to a few tens of mega electron volts) (see Figure 2, Overall introduction). The term γ-radiation is usually restricted to radiation originating from the atomic nucleus and from particle annihilation, while the term X-radiation covers photon emissions from electron shells. X-rays are emitted when charged particles are accelerated or decelerated, during transitions of electrons from the outer regions of the atomic shell to regions closer to the nucleus, and as *bremsstrahlung*, i.e. radiation produced when an electron collides with, or is deflected by, a positively charged nucleus. The resulting line spectra are characteristic for the corresponding element, whereas *bremsstrahlung* shows a continuous spectrum with a steep border at the shortest wavelengths.

Interaction of X-rays with matter is described by the Compton scattering and photoelectric effect and their resulting ionizing potentials, which lead to significant chemical and biological effects. Ions and radicals are produced in tissues from single photons and cause degradation and changes in covalent binding in macromolecules such as DNA. In other parts of the electromagnetic spectrum, below the spectra of ultraviolet and visible light, the single photon energies are too low to cause genotoxic effects. The intensity (I) of X-rays inside matter decreases according to $I = I_0 \times 10^{-\mu \cdot d}$, where d is the depth and μ a coefficient specific to the interacting material and the corresponding wavelength. The ability to penetrate matter increases with increasing energy and decreases with increasing atomic number of the absorbing material. When X-rays penetrate the human body, they are absorbed more effectively in the bones than in the adjacent tissue because of the greater density of bone and the larger proportion in bone of elements with higher atomic numbers, such as calcium.

X-rays are usually generated with X-ray tubes in which electrons emitted from a cathode are accelerated by a high electric potential and hit a target which emits *bremsstrahlung* and a line spectrum characteristic for the material of the target. The expression 'kVp' refers to the applied voltage (kV) of an X-ray machine and is given as the maximum (p for peak) voltage that the machine can produce. According to the applied voltage, ultrasoft (5–20 kVp), soft (20–60 kVp), medium hard (60–120 kVp), hard (120–250 kVp) and very hard (> 250 kVp) X-rays can be distinguished. Extremely hard X-rays are generated with betatrons, synchrotrons and linear accelerators and are in the mega electron volt range.

X-rays are used in many medical and technical applications. The most common are X-ray examinations of the human body and analysis of technical materials. In X-ray therapy, the biological effect of X-rays is used to destroy malignant tissue. It is applied mainly to treat cancer patients, when high doses are delivered to a limited area of the body, with restricted irradiation of adjacent tissue.

1.1.2   γ-radiation

Ernest Rutherford in 1899 found that the radiation from radioactive sources consisted of several components, which he called α-, β- and γ-rays. In 1914, he proved by interference experiments that γ-rays were electromagnetic waves. They are emitted by γ-transitions in atomic nuclei. The corresponding photons, called γ-quants, have widely different energies, ranging from 0.01 to 17.6 MeV, which reflect the fact that the energy of the transitions in the atomic nucleus is higher than that of the transitions of the orbiting electrons. The emission of γ-rays usually follows nuclear trans-formations, which place an atomic nucleus in a state of enhanced energy during processes of radioactivity and during capture of particles. Unlike α- and β-radiation, γ-rays cannot be deflected by electric and magnetic fields. The γ-transition, also called γ-decay, is not radioactive decay in the usual sense, because neither the charge nor the mass number of the nucleus changes.

Electromagnetic radiation in the same energy range can also be produced by the decay of elementary particles, annihilation of electron–positron pairs and acceleration and deceleration of high-energy electrons in cosmic magnetic fields or in elementary particle accelerators. γ-rays, especially those with high energy, can penetrate matter easily, and their absorption and deflection follow an exponential law, as in the case of X-rays. Their physiological effect is also similar to that of X-rays.

Interaction of γ-rays with matter is described by the Compton scattering and photoelectric effect. At energies above 1.02 MeV, pair production occurs, resulting in emission of electron and positron radiation. At even higher energies, in the range of several mega electron volts, absorption of γ-quants results in neutron emission.

1.2   Exposure

Electromagnetic waves in the ionizing range are ubiquitous in the human environ-ment and are responsible with α- and β-rays and to a lesser extent with particle radiation, such as neutrons or muons, for the total radiation dose to which the average person is exposed.

Exposure to X-rays and γ-rays can be external or internal, depending on the location of the source with respect to the human body. External exposure occurs, for example, during X-ray examinations or during natural irradiation from building materials containing γ-ray emitters. Most of the dose from external irradiation is due to X- or γ-rays, because α- and β-particles are readily absorbed by the clothes covering the body or by the superficial layer of skin, whereas X- and γ-rays can penetrate the body and even traverse it if their energy is sufficiently high (see Figure 1, Overall introduction). Internal irradiation occurs during the decay of radionuclides absorbed in the body, usually after ingestion or inhalation. In this case, α- and β-particles are more important than X- or γ-rays, because α- and β-emitters lose most or all of their energy in the tissues or organs in which they decay, while the energy of X- and γ-rays, which is usually lower than those of α- and β-rays, is diffused throughout the body or even leaves the body without creating any damage.

Doses of all types of radiation from external and internal exposure are summarized in the Overall introduction. In this chapter, only external exposure to X and γ-rays is discussed.

Although it is difficult to evaluate the relative contribution of electromagnetic radiation in mixed radiation fields, it can be estimated to be about 50% (Figure 1). There are major natural and man-made sources of exposure, some of which are increasing. Estimates of the average doses received by the general population are reviewed regularly by the United Nations Scientific Committee on the Effects of Atomic Radiation (UNSCEAR) and by many national bodies, such as the Bundesministerium für Umwelt, Naturschutz und Reaktorsicherheit in Germany, the National Council on Radiation Protection and Measurements in the USA and the National Radiological Protection Board in the United Kingdom. Medical exposure and natural terrestrial exposure are due mainly to X- and γ-rays. Other important components of these estimates are mixed radiation fields, such as internal β-emitters with a considerable γ-ray component, whereas the important man-enhanced exposure from indoor radon and its short-lived daughter products is mainly internal exposure to α-radiation. Cosmic radiation at ground level consists of particle radiation (mainly muons), with increasing contributions from neutrons at higher altitudes (see section 4.4.1, Overall introduction).

1.2.1   *Natural sources*

Most natural exposure to X- and γ-rays is from terrestrial sources, with a small part from extraterrestrial sources. Exposure from terrestrial sources depends on the geological properties of the soil, which vary significantly. The average annual external exposure to γ-rays worldwide from terrestrial sources is 0.46 mSv (UNSCEAR, 1993). This value is derived from the average indoor (80 nGy h^{-1}) and outdoor (57 nGy h^{-1}) absorbed dose rates in air, assuming an indoor occupancy factor of 0.8 and a conversion factor from the absorbed dose in air to the effective dose of 0.7 Sv Gy^{-1}.

Figure 1. Estimated average exposure to ionizing radiation from various sources in Germany

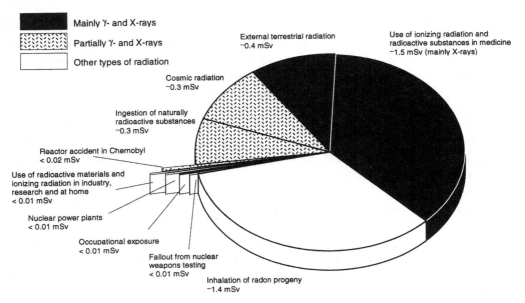

From Bundesamt für Strahlenschutz (1998)

UNSCEAR (1993) also gives detailed data for exposure in various regions of the world. The lowest outdoor dose rates in air are reported for Canada (24 nGy h⁻¹) and the lowest indoor rates for Iceland and New Zealand (20 nGy h⁻¹). The maximum average values are found in Namibia (outdoors, 120 nGy h⁻¹; indoors, 140 nGy h⁻¹). In a survey of terrestrial γ-radiation in the USA, 1074 measurements were made in and around 247 dwellings (Miller, 1992). The absorbed dose rate in outdoor air was 14–118 nGy h⁻¹ with an average of 46.6 nGy h⁻¹, whereas the average indoor rate was 12–160 nGy h⁻¹ with an average of 37.6 nGy h⁻¹. The last value is considerably lower than the worldwide average reported by UNSCEAR (1993) and apparently results from the predominant use of wood-frame construction and other building materials with a low content of radionuclides in the USA. The average exposures in eight countries of Europe ranged from 50 to 110 nGy h⁻¹ in buildings and from 30 to 100 nGy h⁻¹ in the open air (Green *et al.*, 1992; Commission of the European Communities, 1993).

Little exposure is derived from X- and γ-rays in extraterrestrial natural sources (i.e. cosmic rays), as muons and electrons are the most important contributors to the average annual effective dose at ground level of about 0.4 mSv (UNSCEAR, 1993).

1.2.2 Medical uses

The medical uses of radiation include diagnostic examinations and treatment. The dose to individual patients undergoing radiotherapy is much higher than that experienced during diagnosis, although the number of patients is much smaller. As treatment with radiotherapy is intended to deliver high doses to target organs, mostly in elderly patients, attempts to transform collateral doses to non-target organs into effective doses are open to criticism. For this reason, data on exposure during radiotherapy are not described, although UNSCEAR (1993) made the crude estimate that the effective collective dose of the world population due to radiotherapy is comparable to that due to diagnostic applications (see section 4.2, Overall introduction).

Medical diagnosis involving ionizing radiation is based mainly on X-rays. Although the dose per examination is generally low, the extent of the practice makes diagnostic radiography the main source of radiation from medical use. The use of X-rays and γ-rays for medical purposes is distributed very unevenly throughout the world, being closely associated with general health care level (see section 4.2, Overall introduction). A survey undertaken by UNSCEAR in 1990–91, in which responses to a questionnaire were received from 50 countries, indicated that at that time there were 210 000 radiologists worldwide, 720 000 diagnostic X-ray units, 1.6 thousand million X-ray examinations performed in 1990 and 6 million patients undergoing some form of radiotherapy. Seventy per cent of these services were available in countries with a well-developed health-care system. In highly developed countries, most plain-film examinations of the chest and extremities involve relatively low doses (effective doses of about 0.05–0.2 mSv), whereas the doses used to examine the abdomen and lower back are higher (about 1–3 mSv). The approximate doses to the skin and the effective doses from a number of diagnostic procedures in developed countries are shown in Table 1. Computed tomography scanning has become widely available in many developed countries. In the USA, even though it accounts for less than 10% of procedures, it provides more than 30% of the absorbed dose since the effective dose is about 2.5–15 mSv, which is higher than that from most procedures in which plain-film X-rays are used for diagnosis (UNSCEAR, 1993). The estimated annual effective dose from all diagnostic uses of radiation in those countries was estimated to be 1.0 mSv per person, while that averaged over the whole world was about 0.3 mSv per person (UNSCEAR, 1993).

A source of uncertainty in these estimates is the use of fluoroscopy, which results in much higher doses than radiography; furthermore, its prevalence is not fully known and is changing with time. The doses may vary widely: modern equipment with image amplifiers results in lower doses than older equipment with fluorescent screens, but high doses may still be received when fluoroscopy is used in interventional radiology as a means of guidance during surgical procedures, although this practice is infrequent. The effective dose from most procedures is about 1–10 mSv. The collective dose is due mainly to the more frequent fluoroscopic examinations of the gastrointestinal tract. In the USA, the average effective doses are 2.4 mSv during examination of the upper

Table 1. Approximate mean effective doses from diagnostic radiology procedures in highly developed countries

Procedure	Average effective dose (mSv) per examination	Average number of examinations per 1000 population per year
Chest radiograph	0.14	197
Lumbar spine radiograph	1.7	61
Abdominal radiograph	1.1	36
Urography	3.1	26
Gastrointestinal tract radiograph	5.6	72
Mammography	1.0	14
Radiograph of extremity	0.06	137
Computed tomography, head	0.8	44
Computed tomography, body	5.7	44
Angiography	6.8	7.1
Dental X-ray	0.07	350
Average	1.05	887

From UNSCEAR (1993). Doses may vary from these values by as much as an order of magnitude depending on the technique, equipment, film type and processing.

gastrointestinal tract and 4.1 mSv during a barium enema. These two types of examination are the source of about 40% of the annual collective dose due to diagnostic X-ray application, whereas chest examinations account for over 5% of the *per caput* effective dose equivalent from medical X-rays in the USA (National Council on Radiation Protection and Measurements, 1989). The dose from chest examinations in a Canadian study was 0.07 mSv (Huda & Sourkes, 1989).

1.2.3   *Nuclear explosions and production of nuclear weapons*

The atomic bombings of Hiroshima and Nagasaki, Japan, in 1945 exposed hundreds of thousands of people to substantial doses of external radiation from γ-rays. Estimates of the doses are available for 86 572 persons in the Life Span Study out of about 120 000 persons who were in one of the cities at the time of the explosions. The collective dose to the colon for the 86 472 persons for whom dosimetry is available was 24 000 person–Sv (Burkart, 1996; see section 4.1, Overall introduction), to give an average of about 300 mSv. The doses decreased with distance from the epicentres, but the highest doses to the colon were > 2000 mSv.

Atmospheric nuclear explosions were carried out at several locations, mostly in the Northern Hemisphere, between 1945 and 1980. The most intense period of testing was between 1952 and 1962. In all, approximately 520 tests were carried out, with a total yield of 545 Mt. Since 1963, nuclear tests have been conducted mainly underground, and the principal source of worldwide exposure due to weapons testing is the earlier atmospheric tests. The total collective effective dose of X- and γ-rays committed by weapons testing to date is about 2.2×10^6 person–Sv. The radionuclides that contribute the most to this dose are listed in Table 2. With the exception of ^{137}Cs and [125]Sb, all of these radionuclides have radioactive half-lives of less than one year, and therefore delivered their doses soon after the explosions. [137]Ce, with a radioactive half-life of about 30 years, is still present in the environment and continues to deliver its dose at a low rate. For the world population of 3.2×10^9 in the 1960s, the average effective dose from global fall-out resulting from external irradiation was about 0.7 mSv (UNSCEAR, 1993).

Table 2. Collective effective doses of the world population from external radiation committed by atmospheric nuclear testing

Radionuclide	Radioactive half-life	Collective effective dose (1000 person–Sv)
[137]Cs	30 years	1210
[95]Zr	64 days	270
[54]Mn	310 days	180
[106]Ru	370 days	140
[95]Nb	35 days	130
[125]Sb	2.7 years	88
[140]Ba	13 days	49
[144]Ce	280 days	44
[103]Ru	39 days	39
[131]I	8.0 days	4.4
[141]Ce	33 days	3.3
Total (rounded)		2200

From UNSCEAR (1993)

People living near the sites where nuclear weapons were tested received higher doses than the average, but the magnitude of the local dose varies according to the conditions under which the tests were conducted. In the USA, about 100 surface or near-surface tests were conducted at a test site in Nevada between 1951 and 1962. The collective dose to the local population of about 180 000 persons has been estimated to be approximately 500 person–Sv (Anspaugh *et al.*, 1990), corresponding to an average dose of about 3 mSv.

After a US test in 1954 at Bikini atoll in the Marshall Islands, the residents of Rongelap and Utirik atolls, located 210 and 570 km, respectively, east of Bikini, received high external exposures, mainly from short-lived radionuclides, with doses of 1900 mSv on Rongelap (67 persons, including three *in utero*), 1100 mSv on nearby Ailinginae atoll (19 persons, including one *in utero*) and 100 mSv on Utirik (167 persons, including eight *in utero*) (Conard *et al.*, 1980).

At the Semipalatinsk test site in the Kazakh region of the former USSR, atmospheric tests were conducted from 1949 through 1962, exposing 10 000 people in settlements bordering the test site. The collective dose from external irradiation was estimated to be 2600 person–Sv, corresponding to an average dose of 260 mSv (Tsyb *et al.*, 1990).

γ-ray fields resulting from production of weapons material and chemical separation can be considerable, and, as in the case of testing, some local exposures have been substantial. For example, the release of nuclear wastes into the Techa River from a military plant of the former USSR near Kyshtym, in the Ural Mountains, resulted in a cumulative effective dose in the early 1950s of up to 1 Sv (Trapeznikov *et al.*, 1993; Bougrov *et al.*, 1998).

1.2.4   *Generation of nuclear power*

The generation of electrical energy in nuclear power stations has also contributed to exposure to radiation. The collective effective dose committed by the generation of 1 GW–year of electrical energy has been estimated by UNSCEAR (1993) for the entire fuel cycle, from mining and milling, through enrichment and fuel fabrication, reactor operation, to fuel processing and waste disposal, including transport of radioactive materials from one site to another. The doses of X- and γ-rays have not been estimated explicitly as most of the exposure is due to internal irradiation. The local collective effective dose from X- and γ-rays from external irradiation can be crudely estimated to be about 0.2 person–Sv per GW–year. If it is assumed that about 2000 GW–year of electricity have been generated by nuclear reactors throughout the world, the local collective effective dose from external irradiation is about 400 person–Sv, corresponding to an average dose for the world's population of about 0.1 μSv. An additional component of the exposure is the long-lived radionuclides that are distributed worldwide; the only one that contributes significantly to external irradiation, however, is ^{85}Kr, which has a radioactive half-life of about 10 years. UNSCEAR (1993) indicated that the global component of the collective effective dose due to environmental releases of ^{85}Kr is 0.1 person–Sv per GW–year, corresponding to an average dose for the world's population of about 0.05 μSv.

1.2.5   *Accidents*

The production and transport of nuclear weapons have resulted in several accidents. The two most serious accidents in nuclear weapons production were at Kyshtym and at the Windscale plant at Sellafield in the United Kingdom, both occurring in 1957 (see section 4.1.3, Overall introduction). A major accident in a nuclear power plant occurred in Chernobyl, Ukraine, in 1986 (see section 4.4.2, Overall introduction).

The Kyshtym accident was a chemical explosion that followed failure of the cooling system in a storage tank of highly radioactive fission wastes. The highest doses were received by 1150 people who received an estimated effective dose from external irradiation of about 170 mSv (UNSCEAR, 1993; Burkart & Kellerer, 1994; Burkart, 1996).

The Windscale accident was caused by a fire in the uranium and graphite core of an air-cooled reactor primarily intended for the production of plutonium for military use. An important route of intake was through milk consumption, which was controlled near the accident, although it was a significant source of exposure further away. The total collective effective dose from external irradiation received in northern Europe was 300 person–Sv (Crick & Linsley, 1984). The total collective effective dose from the release is estimated to have been 2000 person–Sv (UNSCEAR, 1993).

The Chernobyl accident consisted of a steam explosion in one of the four reactors and a subsequent fire, which resulted in the release of a substantial fraction of the core inventory of the reactor. The collective effective dose from the accident is estimated to have been about 600 000 person–Sv, approximately half of which was due to external irradiation (UNSCEAR, 1988). The main contributor to the dose from external irradiation was [137]Cs. The doses to individuals throughout the Northern Hemisphere varied widely, some staff and rescue workers on duty during the accident receiving fatal doses > 4 Sv and the most affected people in the evacuated zone receiving effective doses approaching 0.5 Sv (Savkin et al., 1996).

Sealed sources used for industrial and medical purposes have occasionally been lost or damaged, resulting in exposure of members of the public. Examples include the sale of a ^{60}Co source as scrap metal in the city of Juarez, Mexico, in 1983 (Marshall, 1984); the theft and breaking up of a ^{137}Cs source in Goiânia, Brazil, in 1987 (IAEA, 1988); and the retrieval of a lost ^{60}Co source in Shanxi Province, China, in 1992 (UNSCEAR, 1993). While these incidents resulted in significant individual doses to a small number of people, the collective effective doses were not large. Tables 3 and 4 are based on recently published data and summarize radiation accidents and resulting early fatalities. Table 4 shows that the steady increase in the use of sources of ionizing radiation has led to an increase in the number of fatalities, despite progress in radiation protection.

1.2.6   *Occupational groups*

Occupational exposure to radiation occurs during nuclear fuel recycling, military activities and medical applications. The doses, including those from internal exposure, are given in Table 5.

Table 3. Major radiation accidents (1945–97) and early fatalities in nuclear and non-nuclear industries

Year	Place	Source	Dose (or activity intake)	No. of persons with significant exposure[a]	No. of deaths
1945–46	Los Alamos, USA	Criticality	≤ 13 Gy	10	2
1958	Vinča, Yugoslavia	Experimental reactor	2.1–4.4 Gy	8	1
1958	Los Alamos, USA	Criticality	0.35–45 Gy	3	1
1960	USSR	^{137}Cs (suicide)	~15 Gy	1	1
1960	USSR	Radium bromide (ingestion)	74 mBq	1	1 (after 4 years)
1961	USSR	Submarine accident	10–50 Gy	> 30	8
1961	Switzerland	^{3}H	3 Gy	3	1
1961	Idaho Falls, USA	Explosion in reactor	≤ 3.5 Gy	7	3
1962	Mexico City, Mexico	^{60}Co capsule	9.9–52 Sv	5	4
1963	China	^{60}Co	0.2–80 Gy	6	2
1964	Federal Republic of Germany	^{3}H	10 Gy	4	1
1964	Rhode Island, USA	Criticality	0.3–46 Gy	4	1
1966	Pennsylvania, USA	^{198}Au	Unknown	1	1
1967	USSR	X-radiation medical diagnostic facility	50 Gy	1	1 (after 7 years)
1968	Wisconsin, USA	^{198}Au	Unknown	1	1
1968	Chicago, USA	^{198}Au	4–5 Gy (bone marrow)	1	1
1972	Bulgaria	^{137}Cs (suicide)	> 200 Gy (local, chest)	1	1
1975	Brescia, Italy	^{60}Co	10 Gy	1	1
1978	Algeria	^{192}Ir	≤ 13 Gy	7	1
1982	Norway	^{60}Co	22 Gy	1	1
1983	Constitu, Argentina	Criticality	43 Gy	1	1
1984	Morocco	^{192}Ir	Unknown	11	8
1985	China	^{198}Au (mistake in treatment)	Unknown, internal	2	1

Table 3 (contd)

Year	Place	Source	Dose (or activity intake)	No. of persons with significant exposure[a]	No. of deaths
1985–86	USA	Accelerator	Unknown	3	2
1986	Chernobyl, USSR	Nuclear power plant	1–16 Gy	134	28
1987	Goiânia, Brazil	^{137}Cs	≤ 7 Gy	50[b]	4
1989	El Salvador	^{60}Co irradiation facility	3–8 Gy	3	1
1990	Israel	^{60}Co irradiation facility	> 12 Gy	1	1
1990	Spain	Radiotherapy accelerator	Unknown	27	≤ 11
1991	Nesvizh, Belarus	^{60}Co irradiation facility	10 Gy	1	1
1992	China	^{60}Co	> 0.25–10 Gy	8	3
1992	USA	^{192}Ir brachytherapy	> 1000 Gy (local)	1	1
1994	Tammiku, Estonia	^{137}Cs	1830 Gy (thigh) + 4 Gy (whole body)	3	1
1996	Costa Rica	Radiotherapy	Unknown	110	≤ 40
1997	Kremlev, Sarov, Russian Federation	Criticality experiment	5–10 Gy	1	1

From IAEA (1998)

[a] 0.25 Sv to the whole body, haematopoietic or other critical organs: < 6 Gy to the skin locally; < 0.75 Gy to other tissues or organs from an external source, or exceeding half the annual limit on intake

[b] The number of persons who received significant overexposure is probably lower, as some of the 50 contaminated persons received doses < 0.25 Sv.

Table 4. Time trends in numbers of major radiation accidents and early fatalities, 1945–97

Years	Nuclear or military installations		Other installations	
	Accidents	Fatalities	Accidents	Fatalities
1945–54	3	2	0	0
1955–64	12	14	15	10
1965–74	9	0	38	6
1975–84	1	0	35	12
1985–97	3	29[a]	20	66[b]

From IAEA (1998)
[a] Including 28 fatalities after the reactor accident in Chernobyl, 1986
[b] Including 40 fatalities after a radiotherapy accident in Costa Rica, 1996

Table 5. Annual occupational exposures of monitored workers to radiation, 1985–89

Occupational category	Annual collective effective dose (person–Sv)	Annual average effective dose per monitored worker (mSv)
Mining	1100	4.4
Milling	120	6.3
Enrichment	0.4	0.08
Fuel fabrication	22	0.8
Reactor operation	1100	2.5
Reprocessing	36	3.0
Research	100	0.8
Total	2500	2.9
Other occupations		
Industrial applications	510	0.9
Military activities	250	0.7
Medical applications	1030	0.5
Total	1800	0.6
All applications	4300	1.1

From UNSCEAR (1993). Radiological, terrestrial and most occupational exposures are dominated by X- and γ-radiation.

1.2.7   *Summary of collective effective doses*

Typical collective effective doses from all significant sources of exposure over the period 1945–92 are presented in Table 6, which indicates that the two largest sources of X- and γ-rays are natural radiation and the use of X-rays in medicine. Exposures from atmospheric testing have diminished, and only small contributions to the collective dose are made by the generation of electrical energy from nuclear reactors, from accidents and from occupational exposure. These contributions can, however, result in significant exposure of small groups of individuals.

Table 6. Collective doses from X- and γ-radiation committed to the world population by continuing practices or by single events, 1945–92

Source	Basis of commitment	Collective effect dose from X- and γ-rays (million person–Sv)
Natural	Current rate for 50 years	120
Medical use	Current rate for 50 years	
Diagnosis		80
Treatment		75
Atmospheric nuclear weapons tests	Completed practice	2.5
Nuclear power generation	Total practice to date	0.2
	Current rate for 50 years	2
Severe accidents	Events to date	0.3
Occupational exposure	Current rate for 50 years	
Medical		0.05
Nuclear power		0.12
Industrial uses		0.03
Military activities		0.01
Non-uranium mining		0.4
Total		0.6

From UNSCEAR (1993)

Variations in individual doses over time and place make it difficult to summarize individual doses accurately, although some indications can be given. The average annual effective dose from γ-rays from natural sources is about 0.5 mSv, with excursions up to about 5 mSv. Medical procedures in developed countries result in an annual effective dose of about 1–2 mSv, of which about two-thirds results from diagnostic radiology. The annual effective doses of monitored workers are commonly 1–10 mSv (UNSCEAR, 1993).

1.2.8   *Variations in exposure to X- and γ-radiation*

Figure 1 shows the estimated average exposures to ionizing radiation in a developed country. As described in the Overall introduction, some of the components may vary by a factor of up to 10, and the distribution is almost log-normal. The distribution of doses from X- and γ-irradiation in medical diagnosis is extremely skewed, as the majority of the population receives no exposure in a given year, while the effective dose may be up to 100 mSv for a small number of people receiving computed tomography scans of the abdomen. Table 7 lists the exposure of the general population that includes considerable X- or γ-ray components.

1.3   Human populations studied in the epidemiology of cancer due to X- and γ-radiation

In view of the large, often poorly understood fluctuations in natural and non-occupational artificial radiation, studies of the carcinogenic potential of ionizing radiation should concentrate on populations with known exposures well above the background load of 2–4 mSv per year from all qualities of radiation from internal and external sources. Many such populations were exposed in the past either routinely or during accidents. A number of persons are still irradiated at high doses in the course of radiation therapy to eradicate tumour tissue. Figure 2 shows those organs and systems in which significant health effects have occurred in such population groups. Although these cohorts are often well characterized with respect to the dose and dose rate they received, possible confounders such as increased susceptibility to toxicants and accompanying chemical treatment must be considered. In addition, patients undergoing cancer therapy are usually in an age distribution that excludes the early years of life, which are of special importance in view of the assumed greater sensitivity of children to radiation. Unselected populations of all ages are therefore of particular interest. In view of the many instances of high exposure to radiation at the workplace in the past, occupational exposure is another important facet of risk (Schneider & Burkart, 1998).

1.3.1   *Unselected populations*

Entire communities received heavy exposure through military action, accidents and poorly controlled releases from weapon material production facilities. Table 8 lists the doses received by the cohorts that have been studied in order to quantify the carcinogenic potential of X- and γ-rays, the study of radiation effects in the survivors of the atomic bombs contributing a major element. Several populations exposed during the nuclear programme of the former USSR are now potentially accessible for epidemiological study, although it is unclear whether reliable retrospective dosimetry will be feasible. Nevertheless, except for partially unconfirmed high collective doses, the dose rates to which these populations were exposed are closer to those that

Table 7. Lifetime exposure of the general public to X- and γ-radiation, with doses and variations

Population	Route of exposure	Individual lifetime (75 years) dose (mSv)		Collective dose (person–Sv per year)	Variation
		Average	Maximum		
World (5800 million)	All	180	750	13 920 000	
Medical diagnosis, health-care level I (1500 million)	Diagnostic radiology	75	500	1 500 000	Highly skewed distribution
Medical diagnosis, health-care levels III and IV (1200 million)	Diagnostic radiology	3	380	48 000	Highly skewed distribution

From UNSCEAR (1993). For a description of health-care levels, see the Overall introduction, section 4.2.

Figure 2. Populations who received heavy exposure to ionizing radiation and were followed for cancer and other long-term effects on health

Site of cancer	Type of exposure																		
	Atomic bombs, Chernobyl				Radiotherapy and diagnosis										Occupation				
	Atomic bomb survivors	Inhabitants of Marshall islands	Participants in weapons tests	Chernobyl	Ankylosing spondylitis (X-rays)	Ankylosing spondylitis (radium)	Benign gynaecological disorders	Benign breast disease	Fluoroscopy of the chest	Tinea capitis	Thymus	Thorotrast	Thyroid (^{131}I)	X-rays *in utero*	Radium-dial painters	Radiologists	Underground miners	Nuclear workers	Aircraft personnel
Leukaemia	■		○	□	■		□	○		□	○	■	○	■		■		○	
Thyroid	■	□		■						■	■			○					
Breast	■					□		■	■		□				○				○
Lung	■				■							○					■		
Bone						■						○			■				
Stomach	■				□												○		
Oesophagus	□				□				□										
Bladder	■						□												
Lymphoma	□				□		○					○		□		□			
Central nervous system	○				■					□			○	□		□			○
Uterus	○						□												
Liver	■											■					○		
Skin										■	□					■	○		
Salivary gland	□									□	□								
Kidney					○	○													
Colon	■				■		○												
Small intestine															○				

■ Statistically significant correlation □ Strongly suspected but in some studies no significant correlation ○ Some correlation found but not significant

From Schneider and Burkart (1998)

Table 8. Major human populations exposed to considerable doses of X- and γ-rays

Population	Main exposure	Individual lifetime dose (mSv)		Collective dose (person–Sv)
		Average	Maximum	
Survivors of atomic bombs, Japan (86 000)	Acute γ-rays, neutron component for subcohort with low exposure	280	4000	24 000
Chernobyl: population in 'contaminated areas' (7 million in Belarus, Ukraine and Russian Federation)	External from ^{137}Cs (deposition density of ^{137}Cs, 37 Bq/m^2)	6–17	> 100	45 000–120 000
Population along the Techa River, Russian Federation (80 000)	External and internal ^{90}Sr	200	3000	15 000
Population in area near Semipalatinsk, Kazakhstan	External and internal ^{131}I, ^{137}Cs, ^{103}Ru			
Near Polygon test field (10 000)		(1000)	3000	(20 000)
Altair area (northeast of test field) (90 000)		(300)	1500	(30 000)

From UNSCEAR (1993); Burkart (1996); Cardis *et al.* (1996). Values in parentheses are highly uncertain estimates.

contribute to current exposure to radiation than to those experienced during the atomic bombings in Hiroshima and Nagasaki (UNSCEAR, 1993).

1.3.2   *Workers*

Large work forces experienced considerable individual exposures during the first few decades of the nuclear age. Whereas uranium mining results in internal exposure to α-particles from radon daughter products, reactor operation and reprocessing result mostly in external exposure to X- and γ-rays. In the past, radiologists and other medical personnel were exposed to considerable doses of radiation. In the clean-up operations near Chernobyl, a workforce of several hundred thousand persons was exposed to a cumulative effective dose of up to 250 mSv, and even higher doses were received immediately after the accident. Several tens of thousands of military personnel were exposed primarily to external γ-radiation when they participated in the atomic bomb tests conducted by the United Kingdom and the USA in the 1950s and 1960s, but the individual doses were typically a few millisieverts. Table 9 lists the doses received by cohorts used to assess the effects of radiation among workers.

1.3.3   *Patients*

Even optimized tumour therapy results in high doses of X- and γ-rays to healthy tissue adjacent to or overlying the target volume. Whole-body irradiation before bone-marrow transplantation in leukaemia patients is an example of treatment used in younger patients with potentially long survival and a concomitant risk for a second cancer. Ionizing radiation was also used in the past against fungal infections by inducing epilation of the scalp, to reduce inflammatory processes and against enlarged thymuses. Patients with tuberculosis who underwent multiple fluoroscopies also received high doses (UNSCEAR, 1993). Table 10 gives an overview of the doses received by some of the cohorts used in studies to assess cancer risks in patients exposed to X- and γ-rays.

2.   Studies of Cancer in Humans

2.1   Introduction

A wealth of information exists about the health consequences of human exposure to ionizing radiation (Committee on the Biological Effects of Ionizing Radiations, 1990 (BEIR V), 1998 (BEIR VIII); ICRP, 1991a; UNSCEAR, 1994; Boice, 1996, 1997; Upton, 1999). Important epidemiological studies of humans exposed to radiation are listed in Table 11. It is from these epidemiological studies that radiation risks are identified and quantified in humans.

Table 9. Main occupational populations exposed to X- and γ-radiation

Population	Major exposure	Individual lifetime dose (mSv)		Collective dose (person–Sv)
		Average	Maximum	
Mayak workers (8800)	External from short-lived fission products, ^{239}Pu inhalation	1300	> 5500	12 000 000
Nuclear workers (86 000, three countries)	External γ-radiation	40	> 500	3800
Chernobyl liquidators, 1986–87 (200 000)	External from fission products	100	Several Sv	20 000
Early radiologists (5000)		–	10 000	–
Bomb testing personnel (70 000)		1–4	–	100–200

From Seltser & Sartwell (1965); Smith & Doll (1981); Robinette et al. (1985); Darby et al. (1993); UNSCEAR (1993)

Table 10. Main populations of patients exposed to X- and γ-radiation

Disease	Major exposure	Individual dose to critical tissue (Gy)		Collective dose (person–Sv)
		Average	Maximum	
Ankylosing spondylitis	X-radiation to bone marrow	4.4		61 000
Bone-marrow eradication in leukaemia	X-radiation	2	14	–
Haemangioma	Soft X-radiation + ^{226}Ra γ-radiation	0.2	47	2800
Tinea capitis	X-radiation to head and neck	6.8	24	73 000
Mastitis	X-radiation to breast	3.8	14	2 300
Tuberculosis treated by fluoroscopy	X-radiation to chest, breast	0.8	6.4	2 000

From UNSCEAR (1993)

Table 11. Epidemiological studies that provide quantitative estimates of doses of radiation to specific organs and cancer risks

Outcome	Type of exposure	Study population
Cancer mortality	Atomic bombs	Japanese bomb survivors (Pierce *et al.*, 1996)
	Radiotherapy for benign disease	Patients with ankylosing spondylitis (Weiss *et al.*, 1994, 1995)
		Patients with benign gynaecological disorders (Inskip *et al.*, 1990a, 1993; Darby *et al.*, 1994)
		Patients with peptic ulcer (Griem *et al.*, 1994)
	Occupation	Nuclear workers (Cardis *et al.*, 1995)
	Diagnostic procedures	Patients with tuberculosis examined by fluoroscopy (Davis *et al.*, 1989; Howe, 1995; Howe & McLaughlin, 1996)
Cancer incidence	Atomic bombs	Japanese bomb survivors (Preston *et al.*, 1994; Thompson *et al.*, 1994)
	Radiotherapy for malignant disease	Patients with cervical cancer (Boice *et al.*, 1987, 1988)
		Patients with childhood cancer (Tucker *et al.*, 1987a,b, 1991; Hawkins *et al.*, 1992, 1996; Wong *et al.*, 1997; de Vathaire *et al.*, 1999a)
		Patients with breast cancer (Boice *et al.*, 1992; Curtis *et al.*, 1992; Storm *et al.*, 1992)
		Patients with endometrial cancer (Curtis *et al.*, 1994)
		Patients with Hodgkin disease (Hancock *et al.*, 1993; Bhatia *et al.*, 1996)
	Radiotherapy for benign disease	Patients undergoing bone-marrow transplantation (Curtis *et al.*, 1997)
		Patients with breast disease (Shore *et al.*, 1986; Mattson *et al.*, 1993, 1997)
		Patients with tinea capitis (Ron *et al.*, 1988a,b, 1989, 1991)
		Patients with an enlarged thymus (Shore *et al.*, 1993)
		Patients with enlarged tonsils (Schneider *et al.*, 1993)
		Patients with haemangioma (Lundell *et al.*, 1994; Lundell & Holm, 1995; Lundell *et al.*, 1996, 1999)
	Diagnostic procedures	Patients with tuberculosis examined by fluoroscopy (Boice *et al.*, 1991a,b)

From UNSCEAR (1994); Boice (1996); Upton (1999)

The epidemiological studies that provided evidence that ionizing radiation, and X-rays and γ-rays in particular, are associated with cancer in humans are summarized below. The studies are divided into four categories of exposure: that due to military use, to medical use, to occupational exposure and environmental exposure. Not all studies are discussed: the Working Group emphasized those with large numbers, documented exposure and minimum influences of bias or confounding factors. Case reports are not included.

Radiation is unique among other known or suspected carcinogenic exposures in that standing committees have existed for over 50 years that periodically review the human and experimental evidence linking radiation to cancer. Table 11 indicates the wide range of studies, practically all of cohort design, that have provided quantitative estimates of cancer risk in human populations. Studies of both mortality and incidence have been conducted in populations around the world. The single most important investigation, that of the atomic bomb survivors, has been under way for over 45 years and provides quantitative risk estimates for use by committees in setting standards. Most information on the effects of radiation comes from studies of patients treated for malignant or benign conditions, and the most informative study of the medical use of radiotherapy is the International Cervical Cancer Patient Study (Day & Boice, 1984), which involved nearly 200 000 women who were followed for over 40 years. Studies of patients treated for benign conditions, such as ankylosing spondylitis, also provided data on the carcinogenicity of radiation. Studies of diagnostic examinations such as frequent chest fluoroscopies to monitor lung collapse, used in the treatment of tuberculosis, are important sources of information on the effects of fractionation, when a dose is spread over long periods as opposed to a brief period as occurred during the atomic bombings. The doses observed in studies of occupational exposure are much lower than those in studies of medical uses, except those of pioneering radiologists who must have received very high doses, although they were not recorded. As the doses to which most people are exposed occupationally and in the environment are very low, studies of such populations are uninformative for establishing a causal relationship with cancer. The final sections cover issues in quantitative risk assessment and a discussion of the many factors that affect the development of radiation-induced cancer, such as age at exposure.

2.2   Military uses

2.2.1   *Detonation of atomic bombs over Hiroshima and Nagasaki*

The Life Span Study is an on-going study conducted by the Radiation Effects Research Foundation (and its predecessor, the Atomic Bomb Casualty Commission (Shimizu *et al.*, 1990)) to investigate the long-term health effects of exposure to radiation during the atomic bombings of Hiroshima and Nagasaki, Japan, in 1945. A number of features make this study a singularly important source of information for assessing the risks associated with exposure to radiation. These include the large size of the exposed population, consisting of both men and women of a wide range of ages who received various doses, long-term follow-up for mortality from and incidence of cancer, well-characterized estimates of the doses received by individual study subjects and the availability of clinical, biological and other information relevant for epidemiological studies. This study has resulted in hundreds of publications which are relevant to understanding various aspects of the effects of exposure to radiation on human health and has served as the primary source of data for quantitative assessments of the risk due to exposure to ionizing radiation (see also sections 2.6 and 2.7).

The study has a number of limitations which must be considered in interpreting its results. The subjects were all Japanese exposed during wartime, and host and environmental factors may have modified their risk for cancer. In addition, the study sample includes only those still alive five years after the bombings. The effect of this initial selection on the estimated cancer risk is a subject of debate. Although it is known that the dose was predominantly from exposure to γ-radiation, the contribution of neutrons and the yield of the bomb dropped on Hiroshima are uncertain. Although these limitations may affect the estimated magnitude of the risk for radiation-induced cancers and their generalizability to other populations, they do not affect the overall conclusion of an association between exposure to radiation and cancer.

The Life Span Study cohort consists of approximately 120 000 people (UNSCEAR, 1994) who were identified at the time of the 1950 census, and individual doses have been reconstructed. Several versions of the dose estimates have been published (see Overall introduction). The current version, DS86, is available for 86 572 survivors who were in the cities at the time of the bombings, and most of the recent analyses (and all of the results presented here) were limited to this subcohort. Table 12 summarizes the distribution of doses among these subjects. Sieverts are used to express weighted organ doses, while grays are used for exposure (shielded kerma) unadjusted for attenuation by the body. Doses to organs, such as 'marrow dose', are given as weighted doses unless reference is made specifically to γ-rays or neutrons. When no specific type of cancer is mentioned, dose refers to weighted dose to the colon, chosen as representative of a more general dose.

A major strength of the Life Span Study is the virtually complete ascertainment of deaths ensured by use of the Japanese family registration system, known as *koseki*. Follow-up of the cohort began in 1950 and was updated at three-year cycles. The latest published data on mortality from cancer cover the period 1950–90 (Pierce *et al.*, 1996). An additional source of information on leukaemia and related haematological disease is the Leukemia Registry (Brill *et al.*, 1962; Ichimaru *et al.*, 1978). It later became possible to analyse cancer incidence by linkage to the Hiroshima and Nagasaki tumour registries (Mabuchi *et al.*, 1994; Thompson *et al.*, 1994), which allows ascertainment of persons who remained in the two cities. A limitation of these data is that they do not include diagnoses of cancers before 1958 or for persons who migrated from the two cities. The incidences of haematological malignancies and of other cancers (referred to below as 'solid tumours') in 1958–87 have been published (Preston *et al.*, 1994; Thompson *et al.*, 1994). The main results of the latest analyses of cancer mortality and incidence are summarized below. The modifying effects of age at exposure, sex and time since exposure are addressed in section 2.7.

Figure 3 shows the excess relative risk (ERR; relative risk −1) per sievert for each of several cancers and for all solid tumours combined. Slightly more recent results for mortality (1950–90) were reported by Pierce *et al.* (1996); the only change is that the

Table 12. Numbers of subjects by radiation dose and city in the Life Span Study of survivors of the atomic bombings

City	Total no.	DS86 weighted dose to the colon (Sv)								
		< 0.005	0.005–0.02	0.02–0.05	0.05–0.1	0.1–0.2	0.2–0.5	0.5–1.0	1.0–2.0	> 2.0
Hiroshima	58 459	21 370	11 300	6 847	5 617	4 504	5 078	2 177	1 070	496
Nagasaki	28 113	15 089	5 621	2 543	921	963	1 230	1 025	538	183
Total	86 572	36 459	16 921	9 390	6 538	5 467	6 308	3 202	1 608	679

From Pierce et al. (1996)

Figure 3. Excess relative risks per sievert and 90% confidence intervals for the incidence of solid tumours (1958–87) and mortality from solid tumours (1950–87) among survivors of the atomic bombings

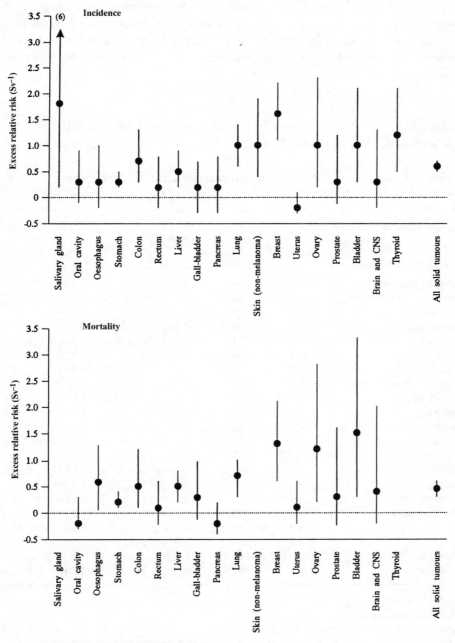

From UNSCEAR (1994). CNS, central nervous system

ERR for cancer of the gall-bladder is closer to the level of statistical significance in the new data ($p = 0.06$) than in the older data ($p = 0.13$; Shimizu *et al.*, 1990). The most recent published estimates of the ERR and excess absolute risk (EAR; number of excess cases or deaths per 10 000 person-years Sv) for cancer incidence are shown in Table 13 for several sites of cancer. The findings for leukaemia, all solid tumours and cancers of the female breast and thyroid are presented below, followed by an indication of the extent to which cancers at other specific sites have been linked with radiation in the Life Span Study cohort.

(a)   Leukaemia

Leukaemia was the first cancer to be linked with exposure to radiation after the atomic bombings (Folley *et al.*, 1952), and the ERR for this malignancy is by far the

Table 13. Estimates of risk for increased incidence of cancer by site, 1958–87, in the Life Span Study of survivors of the atomic bombings

Cancer site/organ system	No. of cases		ERR_{1Sv} (95% CI)	EAR per 10 000 person–years Sv (95% CI)
	Exposed[a]	Unexposed		
All solid tumours	4327	4286	0.63 (0.52, 0.74)	29.7 (24.7, 34.8)
Oral cavity and pharynx	64	68	0.29 (−0.09, 0.93)	0.23 (−0.08, 0.65)
Salivary gland	13	9	1.8 (0.15, 6.0)	NR
Oesophagus	84	101	0.28 (−0.21, 1.0)	0.30 (−0.23, 1.0)
Stomach	1305	1353	0.32 (0.16, 0.50)	4.8 (2.5, 7.4)
Colon	223	234	0.72 (0.29, 1.3)	1.8 (0.74, 3.0)
Rectum	179	172	0.21 (−0.17, 0.75)	0.43 (−0.35, 1.5)
Liver	283	302	0.49 (0.16, 0.92)	1.6 (0.54, 2.9)
Gall-bladder	143	152	0.12 (−0.27, 0.72)	0.18 (−0.41, 1.1)
Pancreas	122	118	0.18 (−0.25, 0.82)	0.24 (−0.36, 1.1)
Trachea, bronchus and lung	449	423	0.95 (0.60, 1.4)	4.4 (2.9, 6.0)
Non-melanoma skin	91	77	1.0 (0.41, 1.9)	0.84 (0.40, 1.4)
Female breast	289	240	1.6 (1.1, 2.2)	6.7 (4.9, 8.7)
Uterus	349	375	−0.15 (−0.29, 0.10)	−1.1 (−2.1, 0.68)
Ovary	66	67	0.99 (0.12, 2.3)	1.1 (0.15, 2.3)
Prostate	61	79	0.29 (−0.21, 1.2)	0.61 (−0.46, 2.2)
Urinary bladder	115	95	1.0 (0.27, 2.1)	1.2 (0.34, 2.1)
Kidney	34	39	0.71 (−0.11, 2.2)	0.29 (−0.50, 0.79)
Nervous system	69	56	0.26 (−0.23, 1.3)	0.19 (−0.17, 0.81)
Thyroid	129	96	1.2 (0.48, 2.1)	1.6 (0.78, 2.5)
Leukaemia[b]	141	67	4.4 (3.2, 5.6)	2.7 (2.0, 3.5)

From Thompson *et al.* (1994). ERR_{1Sv}, excess relative risk at 1 Sv; EAR, excess absolute risk; CI, confidence interval

[a] Defined as a dose to the colon ≥ 0.01 Sv

[b] Based on data for 1950–87 and bone-marrow dose, from UNSCEAR (1994); 90% CI

highest (Table 13). Figure 4 shows the EARs for leukaemia plotted as a function of dose to the bone marrow, based on the most recent mortality analyses (Pierce *et al.*, 1996). This Figure demonstrates a clear increase in risk with increasing dose over the range 0–2.5 Sv.

Figure 4. Excess absolute risks for death from leukaemia per person in the Life Span Study, 1950–90, of survivors of the atomic bombings

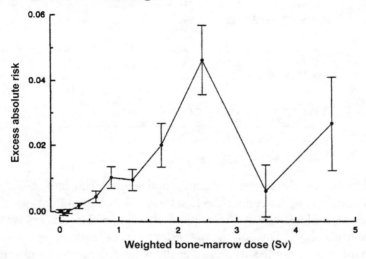

From Pierce *et al.* (1996); bars = standard error

Table 14, also based on the analysis of Pierce *et al.* (1996), presents the observed numbers of leukaemia deaths, the estimated expected background numbers and their differences, by dose category. The excess deaths are those estimated to be attributable to radiation. Because these values are estimates, they are subject to statistical variation, and thus negative values are possible; the negative excesses in the first dose category are well within sampling variation of a true value of zero. The excess of deaths among people whose dose was greater than zero, i.e. (87–9)/(249–73) = 44%, may be considered to correspond to the percentage of tumours due to exposure to radiation, or the attributable risk among exposed persons.

Although the temporal patterns of leukaemia risk are more complex than those of solid tumours (see below), the largest excess risks were generally seen in the early years of follow-up. For people exposed as children, essentially all of the excess deaths appear to have occurred early in the follow-up. For people exposed as adults, the excess risk was lower than that of people exposed as children and appears to have persisted throughout the follow-up. Detailed investigations (Preston *et al.*, 1994) have been made of the patterns of risk by time since exposure, age at exposure and sex for four major subtypes of leukaemia—acute lymphocytic leukaemia, acute myelogenous

Table 14. Observed and expected numbers of deaths from leukaemia in the Life Span Study, 1950–90, of survivors of the atomic bombings

Dose (Sv)[a]	No. of subjects	No. of deaths observed	No. of deaths expected	Excess no. of deaths
< 0.005	35 458	73	64	9
0.005–0.1	32 915	59	62	−3
0.1–0.2	5 613	11	11	0
0.2–0.5	6 342	27	12	15
0.5–1.0	3 425	23	7	16
1.0–2.0	1 914	26	4	22
> 2.0	905	30	2	28
Total	86 572	249	162	87

From Pierce *et al.* (1996)
[a] Dose to red bone marrow

leukaemia, chronic myelogenous leukaemia and adult T-cell leukaemia—and dose–response relationships were seen for the first three. The other major type of leukaemia, chronic lymphocytic leukaemia, is infrequent in Japan, and no excess was seen in the Life Span Study cohort. One of the important recent developments in studies of leukaemia in the atomic bomb survivors was the reclassification of leukaemia cases by new systems and criteria, including the French–American–British classification after 1975 (Matsuo *et al.*, 1988; Tomonaga *et al.*, 1991), which made it possible to analyse the data on leukaemia in the Life Span Study by subtype.

(*b*)   *All solid tumours*

Figure 5 shows the ERRs for all solid tumours by dose to the colon. As for leukaemia, an increase in risk with increasing dose over the range 0–2.5 Sv is seen.

Excess deaths from solid tumours are shown in Table 15. The attributable risk for solid tumours is estimated to be 8%—much smaller than the estimate of 44% for leukaemia. The temporal pattern of solid tumours differs from that of leukaemia as it includes a longer minimal latent period. The ERR for solid tumours remained remarkably constant from about 5–9 years after exposure to the end of the follow-up period, but the number of excess deaths increases monotonically with each successive five-year period of follow-up, and the EAR is roughly proportional to the rapid age-specific increase in background risk. For people who were exposed when they were under the age of 30, nearly half of the excess deaths during the entire 40 years of follow-up have occurred in the last five years.

Figure 5. Excess relative risks for solid tumours, adjusted to men aged 30 at the time of exposure, in the Life Span Study of survivors of the atomic bombings

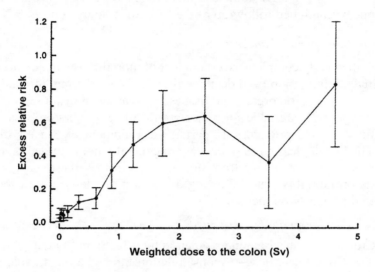

From Pierce *et al.* (1996); bars = standard error

Table 15. Observed and expected numbers of deaths from solid tumours in the Life Span Study, 1950–90, of survivors of the atomic bombings

Dose (Sv)[a]	No. of subjects	No. of deaths observed	No. of deaths expected	Excess no. of deaths
< 0.005	36 459	3 013	3 055	–42
0.005–0.1	32 849	2 795	2 710	85
0.1–0.2	5 467	504	486	18
0.2–0.5	6 308	632	555	77
0.5–1.0	3 202	336	263	73
1.0–2.0	1 608	215	131	84
> 2.0	679	83	44	39
Total	86 572	7 578	7 244	334

From Pierce *et al.* (1996)
[a] Weighted dose to the colon used to represent all solid tumours

Of the 86 572 subjects for whom DS86 dose estimates are available, 56% were still alive at the end of 1990, the end of the period for which mortality has been reported. Of the 46 263 subjects who were under the age of 30 at the time of the bombings, 87% were still alive at the end of 1990 (Pierce *et al.*, 1996). This indicates the importance of continued follow-up of the Life Span Study cohort.

(c)   *Site-specific cancer risks*

Although the nearly complete ascertainment of mortality is a major strength of the Life Span Study, information from death certificates is not optimal for analyses of the risks for cancers in specific organs and tissues. The causes of death reported on death certificates are generally reliable for major groups of cancer but are less reliable for some specific sites, and provide only partial ascertainment of cancers that are less often fatal. The histological types of cancer are generally not recorded on death certificates. Data on cancer incidence from tumour registries fill these gaps and complement the data on mortality. The following discussion of site-specific cancer risks is therefore based primarily on incidence.

(i)   *Female breast cancer*

The risk for breast cancer among women in the Life Span Study (Tokunaga *et al.*, 1994) shows a strong linear dose–response relationship and a remarkable age dependence (Figure 6). The ERR for this cancer is one of the largest of those for solid tumours (see Table 13), but it decreases smoothly and significantly with increasing age at the time of exposure. Figures on incidence from the tumour registries showed, for example, that the ERR of women who were under 10 years of age at the time of exposure was five times that of women who were over 40 years of age at that time. Land *et al.* (1994a,b) investigated the interaction between exposure to radiation and known risk factors for breast cancer in a case–control study nested in the Life Span Study and found a multiplicative relationship between exposure and age at the time of a first full-term pregnancy, the number of children and cumulative period of breast-feeding.

(ii)   *Thyroid cancer*

After early reports of increased risks for thyroid cancer among atomic bomb survivors, a dose-related increase in the incidence of thyroid cancer was demonstrated in the early 1960s (Socolow *et al.*, 1963) from the results of periodic clinical examinations of a subcohort of approximately 20 000 persons (the 'Adult Health Study'). More detailed analyses based on incidence in the Life Span Study cohort showed a strong dependence of risk with age at exposure, the risk being higher among people who had been less than 19 years old at the time of the bombings (Thompson *et al.*, 1994). In fact, no association was found for subjects who had been over the age of 14 when exposed (ERR/Gy, 0.4; 95% CI, –0.1, 0.2; $n = 169$), while the risk of people exposed as children (< 15 years) was significantly elevated (ERR/Gy, 4.7; 95% CI,

Figure 6. Estimated excess relative risks (ERRs) per sievert for breast cancer among women in the Life Span Study, according to age at the time of the atomic bombings

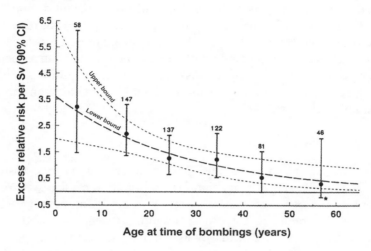

From Tokunaga *et al.* (1994). Derived from the model ERR $(D;E) = \alpha D \exp(\beta_1 E)$, where D is the equivalent dose in sieverts (relative biological effectiveness of neutrons = 10) and E is age at the time of the bombings. The estimates and 90% confidence intervals (CIs) are stratified on city, age at the time of the bombings, attained age and period of follow-up. The numbers above the CIs are the numbers of cases for each age interval.

*Minimum value feasible for lower confidence limit

1.7–11; $n = 56$) (Ron *et al.*, 1995). Among children who were under 15 at the time of the bombings, a steep decrease in risk with age at exposure was found, and children who were exposed between the ages of 10 and 14 had one-fifth the risk of those exposed when they were under 5.

(iii) *Other sites*

Cancers at other sites that are clearly linked with exposure to radiation in the Life Span Study include those of the salivary glands, stomach, colon, lung, liver, ovary and urinary bladder, and nonmelanoma skin cancer. For most of these sites, statistically significant associations were found for both mortality and incidence. A study of cancers of the salivary glands involving reviews of slides strengthened the evidence for an association (Land *et al.*, 1996). A similar study of nonmelanoma skin cancer showed a significant dose–response relationship for all nonmelanoma skin cancer as a group, for basal-cell carcinoma and for non-basal-, non-squamous-cell epithelial skin carcinoma, but not for squamous-cell carcinoma (Ron *et al.*, 1998a).

The evidence for an association with exposure to radiation is equivocal for cancers of the oesophagus, gall-bladder, kidney and nervous system and for non-Hodgkin lymphoma and multiple myeloma, as the results are either of borderline statistical significance or those for incidence and mortality conflict (UNSCEAR, 1994).

Cancers for which there is little evidence of an association with exposure to radiation include those of the oral cavity (except salivary glands), rectum, pancreas, uterus and prostate and Hodgkin disease. Small numbers of cases and diagnostic mis-classification may have contributed to the failure to demonstrate an association, as all of the upper confidence limits of the risk estimates were positive. Therefore, the possibility of associations with these cancers cannot be excluded on the basis of the Life Span Study alone (UNSCEAR, 1994).

2.2.2   Nuclear weapons testing

A number of epidemiological studies have been carried out to assess the risks for cancer associated with exposure to radiation resulting from nuclear weapons tests. The populations that have been studied are those who were living near the tests sites and were thus exposed to radioactive fall-out, and military personnel who participated in the tests and were thus exposed primarily to external γ-radiation with possible internal exposure by ingestion or inhalation of radionuclides. Many of the results are incon-clusive, largely because of the lack of individual doses and in some cases because the approaches used, such as population-based ecological (correlation) studies, are not adequate for assessing risk.

(a)   People living near weapons test sites

(i)   Nevada test site

Between 1951 and 1958, the US Atomic Energy Commission carried out more than 100 atmospheric tests of nuclear weapons at a test site in Nevada, resulting in the deposition of radioactive fall-out in regions surrounding the site. The heaviest expo-sure was in southwestern Utah and in adjacent areas of Nevada and Arizona. The cancer risks of residents of areas downwind of the test site have been the subject of studies of varying kind and quality. Studies of leukaemia clusters and risks and of the risks for thyroid disease led to a population-based case–control study in Utah of 1177 persons who had died of leukaemia (cases) and 5330 who had died of other causes (controls) (Stevens et al., 1990). The median dose of cases and controls was estimated to be 3.2 mGy. A weak, nonsignificant association was found between dose to the bone marrow and acute leukaemias (excluding chronic lymphocytic leukaemia) when all ages and all periods after exposure were considered (odds ratio, 1.7; 95% CI, 0.94–3.1 for those exposed to ≥ 6 mGy; n = 17). [The Working Group noted that the dose estimates were largely determined by the doses assigned to the place of residence.]

(ii)   *Semipalatinsk test site*

In 1949, the Semipalatinsk test site was created in northeastern Kazakhstan, then part of the USSR, and 118 atmospheric nuclear and thermonuclear devices were exploded before 1962, 26 of which were near the ground; between 1965 and 1989, 370 underground nuclear explosions were carried out, and two additional atmospheric tests were conducted in 1965. Most of the contamination and exposure resulted from the early atmospheric testing. The estimated effective doses from external and internal exposure attributable to the 1949 and 1953 tests (the two largest atmospheric tests) in villages near the test site range from 70 to 4470 mSv (Gusev *et al.*, 1997), most local residents being exposed to an effective dose of 100 mSv. The incidence of cancer among children under the age of 15 during 1981–90 in four administrative zones of Khazakhstan in relation to distance from the test site was studied by Zaridze *et al.* (1994): the risk for acute leukaemia rose significantly with increasing proximity of residence to the testing areas, although the absolute value of the risk gradient was relatively small. [The Working Group noted that potential confounders, notably urban–rural and ethnic differences, were not considered in the analyses.]

(*b*)   *Military personnel participating in weapons tests*

Follow-up of more than 20 000 participants in the 21 atmospheric nuclear tests conducted by the United Kingdom in 1952–58 in Australia and islands in the Pacific Ocean (Darby *et al.*, 1988) and of an equally large control group of military personnel through 1991 showed that the rate of death from leukaemia among participants was similar to that of the general population (SMR, 1.0 [95% CI, 0.7–1.4]) but was higher than that of the control group (RR, 1.8; 95% CI, 1.0–3.1) (Darby *et al.*, 1993).

A small study, with follow-up for the period 1957–87, of approximately 500 personnel of the Royal New Zealand Navy involved in the test programme of the United Kingdom in the Pacific Ocean in 1957–58, showed that mortality from all cancers was similar (RR, 1.2; 95% CI, 0.8–1.7) to that of 1504 Navy personnel who were not involved in the tests (Pearce *et al.*, 1997); however, mortality from leukaemia was greater among participants than controls (RR, 5.6; 95% CI, 1.0–42; four cases).

In a cohort study of participants in five US nuclear bomb test series between 1953 and 1957 (Robinette *et al.*, 1985), more than 46 000 subjects were followed-up by linkage to Veterans' Administration records, which showed 5113 deaths. No increase in mortality from leukaemia was observed (SMR, 0.9; 95% CI, 0.6–1.2), suggesting that the findings of a previous smaller study of 3217 participants in a single test (Caldwell *et al.*, 1983), which showed a relative risk of 2.6 (95% CI, 1.1–5.1), were probably not due to exposure to radiation.

Approximately 8500 Navy veterans who had participated in the US 'Hard tack I' operation in 1958, which included 35 tests in the Pacific Ocean, were found to have had a median dose of 4 mSv (Watanabe *et al.*, 1995). The mortality rates from all cancers (RR, 1.1; 95% CI, 1.0–1.3) and leukaemia (RR, 0.7; 95% CI, 0.3–1.8) were comparable to those for an unexposed group of veterans. In a study of 40 000 military veterans who had participated in a test in the Bikini atoll, Marshall Islands, in 1946, the mortality rates from all cancers (RR, 1.0; 95% CI, 0.96–1.1) and from leukaemia (RR, 1.0; 95% CI, 0.75–1.4) were similar to those for nonparticipants (Johnson *et al.*, 1997).

[The Working Group noted that the weaknesses of these studies include low doses and insufficient dosimetry, which obviate a quantitative risk estimation.]

2.2.3   *Production of materials for nuclear weapons*

Plutonium production for nuclear weapons in the former USSR started in 1949 in the closed city of Ozersk (the Mayak facility) situated 1200 km east of Moscow in the southern Ural Mountains. During the early 1950s, the Techa River was severely contaminated with radioactive wastes discharged directly into the water (Kossenko *et al.*, 1997). Approximately 28 000 inhabitants of the river-bank villages were exposed, and 7500 were resettled. In 1957, a container of highly radioactive wastes exploded, resulting in a contaminated area known as the East Urals Radioactive Trace; this incident is referred to as the 'Kyshtym accident', after the name of a nearby village. About 11 000 individuals, including approximately 1700 who had previously lived in exposed areas along the River, were resettled. Systematic follow up of a cohort of almost 30 000 individuals who received significant exposure from the releases was begun in 1967.

The inhabitants of the riverside villages were exposed to both internal and external radiation (river water, sediments and soils). Doses are available at the village level (Degteva *et al.*, 1994), but individual doses are being constructed (Degteva *et al.*, 1996). ^{90}Sr, which accumulates in bone, was the largest component of the internal dose (Kozheurov & Degteva, 1994). The individuals living along the River thus received doses of external γ-radiation and of internal γ- and β-rays over several years. The preliminary results of follow-up from 1950 through 1989, which were analysed in linear dose–response models for excess relative risk, indicate an increased rate of mortality from leukaemia and solid tumours related to internal and external doses of ionizing radiation (Tables 16 and 17; Kossenko *et al.*, 1997).

The authors emphasize that with continuing improvement of the quality of follow-up and dosimetry, the study of the Techa River cohort could provide important information on the effects of protracted exposure to low doses of ionizing radiation in an unselected population, and that this study supplements and complements the findings of the studies of atomic bomb survivors in Japan.

Table 16. Estimated excess numbers of cases of leukaemia[a] in the Techa River cohort and person–years of risk in relation to dose to red bone marrow

Dose category (Sv)	Person–years[b]	Observed	Excess
0.005–0.1	103 031	3	−1
0.1–0.2	194 858	13	4
0.2–0.5	200 144	16	6
0.5–1	93 873	9	5
> 1	49 398	9	7
Total	641 304	50	21

From Kossenko et al. (1997)
[a] Computed as the difference between the observed number of cases and an estimate of the number expected in the absence of exposure
[b] Computed through date of death, loss to follow-up or 31 December 1989

Table 17. Estimated excess numbers of deaths from solid tumours[a] in the Techa River cohort and person–years of risk in relation to dose to soft tissue

Dose category (Sv)	Person–years[b]	Observed	Excess
0.005–0.1	459 576	716	5
0.1–0.2	96 297	126	1
0.2–0.5	19 582	34	10
0.5–1	32 204	52	6
> 1	33 645	41	8
Total	641 304	969	30

From Kossenko et al. (1997)
[a] Computed as the difference between the observed number of cases and an estimate of the number expected in the absence of exposure
[b] Computed through date of death, loss to follow-up or 31 December 1989

2.3   Medical uses

Studies of patients irradiated for the treatment or diagnosis of diseases have contributed substantial evidence about the carcinogenic effects of X-rays and γ-rays. The often detailed radiotherapy records for cancer patients and those treated for benign conditions allow precise quantification of the doses to the organs of individuals, and dose–response relationships can be studied. Further, patients with the same initial disease treated by means other than radiation are often available for comparison. Large cohorts of patients who have been followed-up for long periods are available, allowing evaluation of late effects and cancer in particular. Population-based cancer registries around the world have been used to identify these patients; for example, the risks for a second cancer after individual primary cancers in Denmark and in Connecticut, USA, have been evaluated comprehensively (Boice *et al.*, 1985a).

Studies of patients undergoing radiotherapy have provided information on the risks for cancer in relatively insensitive organs, such as the rectum, that appear to be associated with exposure to radiation only at therapeutic doses of the order of ≥ 10 Gy. Studies of organs outside the radiation treatment fields which received lower doses provide information on risks for cancer that are not influenced by the cytotoxic effects of radiation. Studies of long-term survivors of radiotherapy for benign conditions, such as past use for enlarged tonsils, have indicated that cancers such as those of the thyroid and breast can be induced, in the absence of confounding effects of the disease being treated or concomitant therapy. Studies of diagnostic procedures that involve much lower doses provide limited evidence for the carcinogenicity of radiation except when the cumulative exposure reaches a substantial level. Well over 100 studies of patients have linked exposure to radiation to increased risks for cancer (Boice *et al.*, 1985a, 1996; UNSCEAR, 1994; Curtis, 1997). Only the most informative ones, which include assessments of radiation dose, are reviewed in this section and summarized in Table 11; more detailed listings are given in Tables 18–20.

2.3.1   *Radiotherapy for malignant disease*

Chemotherapy and/or hormonal therapy used in the treatment of cancers are potential confounding factors in investigations of the risk for a second cancer. Furthermore, patients with a malignant disease may develop a second primary cancer because of common risk factors for the two cancers or genetic predisposition for the second. Increased medical surveillance may contribute to the detection and reporting of new cancers. These studies are summarized in Table 18.

(*a*)   *Cervical cancer*

External beam radiotherapy and radium and caesium applicators are used for the treatment of cervical cancer to deliver high local doses of X-rays and γ-rays to the cervix uteri and adjacent organs in the abdomen and pelvic area—notably the urinary

Table 18. Study characteristics and second cancers in patients receiving radiotherapy for a malignant disease

Reference	Index cancer (period of diagnosis)	Sex, no. of exposed and total no. of individuals (exposed + unexposed) or, for case–control studies, nos of cases and controls	Mean follow-up (years)	Organ dose (Gy, except as noted)	Second cancers studied	Results
Cohort studies						
Zippin et al. (1971)	Cervix (1932–51)	Women, 497/497	17–36	Bone marrow, 20	Leukaemia	No increase
Fehr & Prem (1973)	Cervix, squamous-cell carcinoma (1939–60)	Women, 627/627	> 9	NR	Pelvic girdle sarcoma	Pelvis: SIR = 650; n = 4
Clarke et al. (1984)	Cervix, invasive carcinoma (1960–75)	Women, 7083/7535	7.5	Cervix, 40	All	No increase
Boice et al. (1985b)*	Cervix (1920–78)	Women, 82 616/182 040	7.60; < 1–> 30	Stomach, 2 Colon, 5 Pancreas, 1.5 Lung, 0.35 Breast, 0.35 Kidney, 2.0 Bladder, 30 Thyroid, 0.15 Red bone marrow, 7.5	All, excluding cervical cancer	Oesophagus: SIR = 1.5; n = 40 Small intestine: SIR = 2.2; n = 21 Rectum: SIR = 1.3; n = 198 Pancreas: SIR = 1.3; n = 121 Lung: SIR = 3.7; n = 493 Bladder: SIR = 2.7; n = 196 Connective tissue: SIR = 1.9; n = 27 ANLL: SIR = 1.3; n = 52
Pettersson et al. (1985)	Cervix, carcinoma (1914–65)	Women, 5000[a]/13 041	>10–45	NR	Colon, rectum, corpus uteri, ovary, bladder	Rectum: O/E = 1.7; n = 118 Bladder: O/E = 3.4; n = 112

Table 18 (contd)

Reference	Index cancer (period of diagnosis)	Sex, no. of exposed and total no. of individuals (exposed + unexposed) or, for case–control studies, nos of cases and controls	Mean follow-up (years)	Organ dose (Gy, except as noted)	Second cancers studied	Results
Cohort studies (contd)						
Pettersson et al. (1990)	Cervix, invasive carcinoma (1958–80)	Women, 16 704/16 704	8	Pelvic wall, 35–50	All	Bladder: O/E 3.5; $n = 55$ Rectum: O/E = 1.8; $n = 47$ Uterus (not corpus): O/E = 1.9; $n = 11$
Arai et al. (1991)	Cervix (1961–81)	Women, 7694/11 855	8	Pelvis, 50	All	Leukaemia: SIR = 2.6; $n = 9$ Rectum: SIR = 1.9; $n = 25$ Bladder: SIR = 2.1; $n = 9$
Hancock et al. (1991)*	Hodgkin disease (1961–89)	Both sexes, 1677/1787	10	Cervical lymph node area, 44	Thyroid	Thyroid: SIR = 16; $n = 6$
Hancock et al. (1993)	Hodgkin disease (1961–90)	Women, 383/885	10	Radiotherapy alone, 7.5–≥ 40	Breast	Breast: SIR = 3.5; $n = 12$
Khoo et al. (1998)	Hodgkin disease (1970–89)	Both sexes, 320/320	9; 1–23	Thyroid, 40	Thyroid	Thyroid: RR = 6.7; $n = 4$
Harvey & Brinton (1985)	Breast (1935–82)	Women, 11 691/41 109	> 20	NR	All	Second breast cancer: RR = 3.9; $n = 544$
Yoshimoto et al. (1985)	Breast (1960–70)	Women, 733/1359	11	NR	All	Second primary cancer: SIR = 8.7; $n = 61$
Andersson et al. (1991)	Breast (1977–82)	Women, 846/3538	8	NR	All	Second breast cancer: SIR = 4.2; $n = 47$
Taghian et al. (1991)	Breast (1954–83)	Women, 6919/7620 > 1 year follow-up	7	Sarcoma, 45	Soft-tissue sarcoma	Soft tissue: SIR = 1.8; $n = 11$

Table 18 (contd)

Reference	Index cancer (period of diagnosis)	Sex, no. of exposed and total no. of individuals (exposed + unexposed) or, for case–control studies, nos of cases and controls	Mean follow-up (years)	Organ dose (Gy, except as noted)	Second cancers studied	Results
Cohort studies (contd)						
Neugut et al. (1997a)	Breast (1973–93)	Women, 62 453/251 750	<20	NR	Pleural mesothelioma	No significant increase
Pride & Buchler (1976)	Gynaecological malignancies (1956–74)	Women, 4238/4238	>10	NR	Vaginal, cervical carcinoma	No increase
Ahsan & Neugut (1998)	Breast (1973–93)	Women, 47 915/220 806	6	NR	Oesophagus	Oesophageal squamous-cell carcinoma: RR = 5.4; n = 20 (≥ 10 years after radiotherapy)
Maier et al. (1997)	Gynaecological carcinomas (1972–93)	Women, 10 709/10 709	22	Pelvis, 67.5	Urinary tract	Bladder: RR = 4.7; n = 6
Jacobsen et al. (1993); Møller et al. (1993)	Testis[b] (1943–87)	Men, 6187/6187	9.5	Lymph nodes, 20–45	All	Sarcoma: SIR = 4; n = 13; Stomach: SIR = 2.1; n = 34; Colon: SIR = 1.5; n = 28; Pancreas: SIR = 2.3; n = 21; Kidney: SIR = 2.3; n = 21; Bladder: SIR = 2.1; n = 47; Non-melanoma skin: SIR = 2.0; n = 68; Leukaemia: SIR = 2.4; n = 18
Horwich & Bell (1994)	Testicular seminoma (1961–85)	Men, 859/859	10	NR	All	Leukaemia: SIR = 6.2; n = 4

Table 18 (contd)

Reference	Index cancer (period of diagnosis)	Sex, no. of exposed and total no. of individuals (exposed + unexposed) or, for case–control studies, nos of cases and controls	Mean follow-up (years)	Organ dose (Gy, except as noted)	Second cancers studied	Results
Cohort studies (contd)						
Travis et al. (1997)*	Testis (1935–93)	Men, 8841/28 843	10	NR	All	Stomach: SIR = 1.95; n = 93; Bladder: SIR = 2.0; n = 154; Pancreas: SIR = 2.2; n = 66
Neugut et al. (1997b)	Prostate (1973–93)	Men, 34 889/141 761	0.5–> 8	NR	Bladder, rectal carcinoma, ANLL, CLL	Bladder: RR = 1.5; n = 38 (> 8 years after radiotherapy)
Maxon et al. (1981)	Head and neck (1963–67)	Both sexes, 554/1 266	21.5	Salivary gland, 5 ± 2	Salivary gland	Salivary gland: p = 0.049; n = 3
Potish et al. (1985)	Childhood cancer (1953–75)	Both sexes, 330/330	14 (5–30)	NR	All	None
Hawkins et al. (1987)*	Childhood CNS cancer[c] (1962–79)	Both sexes, 1101/9279	19	NR	All	All: RR = 6.2; n = 10
Eng et al. (1993)*	Retinoblastoma (1914–84) Bilateral	Both sexes, 965/1603 835/919	17	NR	All (results for bilateral retinoblastoma)	Bone: SMR = 630; n = 34; Soft tissue: SMR = 880; n = 15; Skin melanoma: SMR =180; n = 7; Brain: SMR = 45; n = 8
Bhatia et al. (1996)*	Childhood Hodgkin disease (1955–86)	Both sexes, 1270/1380 (897 girls)	11 (median); 0.1–37	Breast, < 20–> 40	All	Breast: 20–40 Gy; RR = 5.9; n, NR
de Vathaire et al. (1999a)*	Childhood cancer (1942–85)	Both sexes, 2827/4096	15; 3–45	Thyroid, 7.0	Thyroid	Thyroid carcinoma: SIR = 80; n = 14

Table 18 (contd)

Reference	Index cancer (period of diagnosis)	Sex, no. of exposed and total no. of individuals (exposed + unexposed) or, for case–control studies, nos of cases and controls	Mean follow-up (years)	Organ dose (Gy, except as noted)	Second cancers studied	Results
Cohort studies (contd)						
de Vathaire et al. (1999b)*	Childhood cancer (1942–85)	Both sexes, 3013/4400	15; 3–48	Brain, 8.6 Breast, 5.1 Colon, 8.1	All	Brain: O/E = 44; $n = 8$ Breast: O/E = 5.1; $n = 4$
Curtis et al. (1997)*	Bone-marrow transplantation for cancer (1964–92)	Both sexes, 14 656/19 229	5; 1–25	Whole body Single, ≥ 10 Total fractionated, ≥ 13	All	Melanoma: RR = 8.2; $n = 7$ Brain: RR = 4.3; $n = 8$ Thyroid: RR = 5.8; $n = 6$
Case–control studies						
Boivin et al. (1986)	All (1933–72)	Both sexes, 398/781	6; 1–28	NR	Leukaemia	Leukaemia excluding CLL (232 cases): RR = 1.6; $n = 82$
Nandakumar et al. (1991)	All (1974–86)	Both sexes, 97/194	NR	NR	Myeloid leukaemia	No increase
Zaridze et al. (1993)	All (1975–90)	Both sexes, 165/294	NR	NR	All	None

Table 18 (contd)

Reference	Index cancer (period of diagnosis)	Sex, no. of exposed and total no. of individuals (exposed + unexposed) or, for case–control studies, nos of cases and controls	Mean follow-up (years)	Organ dose (Gy, except as noted)	Second cancers studied	Results
Case–control studies (contd)						
Boice et al. (1988)*	Cervix (1920–78)	Women, 4188/6880	7.6; <1–>30	Stomach, 2 Small intestine, 10–20 Colon, 24 Rectum, 30–60 Uterus, 165 Ovary, 32 Vagina, 66 Bladder, 30–60 Bone, 22 Connective tissue, 7 Stomach, 2 Pancreas, 2 Kidney, 2 Breast, 0.3 Thyroid, 0.1 Red bone marrow, 7	All, excluding cervical cancer	Stomach: RR = 2.1; n = 338 Vagina: RR = 2.65; n = 100 Bladder: RR = 4.05; n = 267 Leukaemia excluding CLL: RR, 2.0; n = 133 Rectum: RR = 1.8; n = 465
Curtis et al. (1994)*	Corpus uteri (1935–85)	Women, 218/775	1–50	Bone marrow, 5.2	Leukaemia	Leukaemia excluding CLL (57 cases); RR = 1.9; n = 118
Kaldor et al. (1990a)*	Hodgkin disease (1960–87)	Both sexes, 163/455	1–≥10	Red bone marrow, <10–>20	Leukaemia	Risk increased with dose ≥ 20 Gy: RR = 8.2; n, NR
Kaldor et al. (1992)*	Hodgkin disease (1960–87)	Both sexes, 98/259	1–≥10	Lung, <1–>2.5	Lung	No significant increase

Table 18 (contd)

Case–control studies (contd)

Reference	Index cancer (period of diagnosis)	Sex, no. of exposed and total no. of individuals (exposed + unexposed) or, for case–control studies, nos of cases and controls	Mean follow-up (years)	Organ dose (Gy, except as noted)	Second cancers studied	Results
van Leeuwen et al. (1995)	Hodgkin disease (1966–86)	Both sexes, 30/82	1–23	Lung, 7.2	Lung	No significant increase, but significant trend
Travis et al. (1994)	Non-Hodgkin lymphoma (1965–89)	Both sexes, 35/140	8; 2–18	Red bone marrow, 9.3	ANLL	No significant increase
Travis et al. (1995)	Non-Hodgkin lymphoma (1965–80)	Both sexes, 48/136	9; 2–21	Bladder, 12.0 Kidney, 12.8	Bladder and kidney	No increase
Basco et al. (1985)*	Breast (1946–82)	Women, 194/194	≥ 5–≥ 10	Contralateral breast, 2.0–3.3	Contralateral breast	No significant increase
Curtis et al. (1989)*	Breast (1935–84)	Women, 48/97	12; 1.6–27	Red bone marrow, 5.3	Leukaemia	No increase
Boice et al. (1992)*	Breast (1935–82)	Women, 655/1189	5–> 10	Contralateral breast, 2.8	Contralateral breast	For < 45 years old, RR = 1.6; n = 78
Curtis et al. (1992)*	Breast (1973–85)	Women, 90/264	5; 2–12	Red bone marrow, 7.5	All leukaemia & myelodysplasia	ANLL: RR, 2.4; n = 12
Storm et al. (1992)*	Breast (1943–78)	Women, 529/529	8–> 25	Contralateral breast, 2.5	Contralateral breast	No significant increase
Inskip et al. (1994)*	Breast (1935–71)	Women, 61/120	10–46	Lung, 9.8	Lung	For ≥ 15 years after treatment, RR = 2.8; n, NR

Table 18 (contd)

Reference	Index cancer (period of diagnosis)	Sex, no. of exposed and total no. of individuals (exposed + unexposed) or, for case–control studies, nos of cases and controls	Mean follow-up (years)	Organ dose (Gy, except as noted)	Second cancers studied	Results
Case–control studies (contd)						
Neugut et al (1994)	Breast (1986–89)	Women, 121/1043	> 10	NR	Lung	Lung: OR = 2.8; n, NR
Karlsson et al. (1996)*	Breast (1960–80)	Women, 18/54	1–26	Breast (integral dose), 152 J	Soft-tissue sarcoma	Soft-tissue sarcoma: p = 0.008 with integral dose; n = 16
Kaldor et al. (1990b)*	Ovary (1960–85)	Women, 114/342	1–> 10	Red bone marrow, < 10–> 20	Leukaemia	No significant increase
Kaldor et al. (1995)*	Ovary (1960–87)	Women, 63/188	0–> 15	Bladder, 35	Bladder	No significant increase
Travis et al. (1999)*	Ovary (1980–93)	Women, 96/272	4 (max., 14)	Red bone marrow, 18.4	Leukaemia	No increased risk
Tucker et al. (1987a)*	Childhood cancer (1936–79)	Both sexes, 64/209	2–≥ 20	Bone, 27	Bone sarcoma	Bone: OR = 2.7; n = 54
Tucker et al. (1987b)*	Childhood cancer (1945–79)	Both sexes, 25/90	> 2	Red bone marrow, 10 (0–38)	Leukaemia	No increase
Tucker et al. (1991)*	Childhood cancer (1945–79)	Both sexes, 23/89	5.5; 2–48	Thyroid, 12.5 (0–76)	Thyroid	Thyroid: 2–< 10 Gy, RR = 13; n = 7; 10–< 30 Gy, RR = 12; n = 7; > 30 Gy, RR = 18; n = 5
Hawkins et al. (1992)*	Childhood cancer (1940–83)	Both sexes, 26/96	7.7	Red bone marrow, 0.01–> 15	Leukaemia	No significant increase
Hawkins et al. (1996)*	Childhood cancer (1940–83)	Both sexes, 59/220	10	Red bone marrow, 0.01–≥ 50	Bone	No significant dose–response relationship

Table 18 (contd)

Reference	Index cancer (period of diagnosis)	Sex, no. of exposed and total no. of individuals (exposed + unexposed) or, for case–control studies, nos of cases and controls	Mean follow-up (years)	Organ dose (Gy, except as noted)	Second cancers studied	Results
Case–control studies (contd)						
Wong *et al.* (1997)*	Retinoblastoma (1914–84)	Both sexes, 83/89	20	Bone, 32.8 Soft tissues, 20.4	Bone and soft-tissue sarcoma	Bone and soft-tissue sarcoma combined: RR (dose–response) = 1.9–10.7; $n = 55$
Le Vu *et al.* (1998)*	Childhood cancer (1960–86)	Both sexes, 32/160	9; 2–25	Red bone marrow, 6	Osteosarcoma	Osteosarcoma: linear increase with dose (ERR/Gy = 1.8)

ANLL, acute non-lymphocytic leukaemia; CLL, chronic lymphocytic leukaemia; CNS, central nervous system; ERR, excess relative risk; NR, not reported; O/E, observed/expected; OR, odds ratio; RR, relative risk; SIR, standardized incidence ratio; SMR, standardized mortality ratio
* Study cited in text
[a] Only patients who survived the treatment for > 10 years were taken into account.
[b] 53% seminomas
[c] Excluding second primary tumours for which there is a genetic predisposition

bladder, the rectum, the ovaries, the corpus uteri, and portions of the colon and bone marrow in the pelvis. The treatment is successful, and patients survive for many years after radiotherapy.

An international study of nearly 200 000 women treated for cervical cancer in 15 countries has provided information on dose-related risks of second cancers associated with radiotherapy (Day & Boice, 1984; Boice *et al.*, 1985b, 1987, 1988, 1989). This study is one of those that provides quantitative information on the risk for cancer (UNSCEAR, 1988, 1994): it is a study of incidence, as opposed to mortality, with long and complete follow-up; the numbers of exposed and unexposed patients were large, and chemotherapy was rarely used; the existence of radiotherapy records allowed the development of a comprehensive programme for dose reconstruction to simulate actual individual doses. Estimates of the doses to specific organs were computed for selected cases and controls (Boice *et al.*, 1987, 1988).

In the initial part of the study (Day & Boice, 1984; Boice *et al.*, 1985b), 5146 second cancers were identified in cancer registries, whereas 4736 were expected from the rates for the general population. Radiotherapy with large doses in 82 616 women was associated with increased risks for cancers close to or within the field of radiation, but the authors concluded that these doses had not significantly altered the risk for developing a second cancer at a distant site, and at most only 162 (5%) of the 3324 second cancers in these women could be attributed to radiation.

The relative risks for developing a second primary cancer after radiotherapy for cervical cancer are shown in Figure 7 (Boice *et al.*, 1985b). Some of the differences seen may be due to dose: those to organs in the pelvic area were of the order of tens of grays, those to the corpus uteri were > 200 Gy, those just outside the pelvic region were of the order of grays and those to organs at some distance from the pelvis were fractions of grays. Significantly increased risks were seen for cancers of the bladder, rectum, lung, pancreas, oesophagus, small intestine and connective tissue, and significantly decreased risks were seen for cancers of the corpus uteri and ovary. No excess risk was found within 10 years of radiotherapy for cancers at sites that received > 1 Gy. The risk rose after 10 years and remained elevated for up to 40 years of follow-up. A slight but significant excess risk for acute and nonlymphocytic leukaemia was found (RR, 1.3; $p < 0.05$); however, the radiation regimens used to treat cervical cancer were not as effective in inducing leukaemia as other regimens that have been studied, possibly because the bone marrow in the pelvis is destroyed by the very high doses of radiation used. There was little evidence that radiation affected the incidences of cancers of the colon, liver or gall-bladder or those of melanoma or chronic lymphocytic leukaemia, despite substantial exposure. The incidences of second cancers at other sites that received relatively low doses were either not increased over that expected or were increased due to other strong risk factors, such as cigarette smoking or alcohol drinking.

The expanded case–control study of this cohort involved 19 cancer registries and 20 oncology clinics, and 4188 women with second cancers were matched to 6880

Figure 7. Relative risks for developing a second primary cancer at selected sites one year or more after radiotherapy for cervical cancer, with 95% confidence intervals

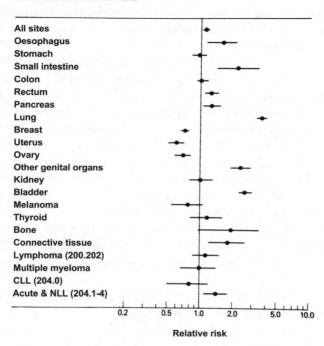

Relative risk

From Boice *et al.* (1985b). CLL, chronic and unspecified lymphocytic leukaemia; NLL, non-lymphocytic leukaemia

controls. Doses of the order of several hundred grays significantly increased the risks for cancers of the bladder (RR, 4.0), rectum (RR, 1.8) and vagina (RR, 2.7), and doses of several grays increased the risks for stomach cancer (RR, 2.1) and for leukaemia (RR, 2.0). There was no evidence of a dose-dependent increase in risk for pancreatic cancer (Boice *et al.*, 1988). The incidence of breast cancer was not increased overall, even though the average dose to this site was 0.3 Gy and 953 cases were available for evaluation; however, ovarian ablation during radiotherapy was a complicating factor (Boice *et al.*, 1989). Radiation was not found to increase the overall risks for cancers of the colon, ovary or connective tissue or for Hodgkin disease, multiple myeloma or chronic lymphocytic leukaemia (Boice *et al.*, 1988).

(b)   Hodgkin disease

The large radiation therapy fields used in the treatment of Hodgkin disease by external beam radiotherapy, the young age of patients and their long survival provide opportunities for investigating the risk for second cancer as a consequence of exposure to ionizing radiation. Most patients, however, are treated with a mixture of radiotherapy and chemotherapy (Henry-Amar, 1983; Blayney *et al*., 1987; Kaldor *et al*., 1987; Morales *et al*., 1992; Glanzmann *et al*., 1994; Beaty *et al*., 1995; Boivin *et al*., 1995), and many studies have convincingly linked exposure to alkylating agents to a high risk for leukaemia (see also IARC, 1987). A few have addressed the risks for solid tumours and the role of radiotherapy alone.

In a case–control study of 163 cases of leukaemia and 455 controls nested in an international cohort of 29 552 patients with Hodgkin disease in Canada and Europe, Kaldor *et al*. (1990a) found a ninefold increase in the relative risk for leukaemia associated with chemotherapy, whereas a dose–response relationship was suggested for patients treated with radiotherapy, the risk of leukaemia increasing with estimated dose to the red bone marrow: relative risk, 1 for < 10 Gy; 1.6 (95% CI, 0.26–10) for 10–20 Gy and 8.2 (95% CI, 1.7–39) for > 20 Gy.

Another case–control study nested in the same international cohort (Kaldor *et al*., 1992) involved 98 cases of lung cancer occurring after Hodgkin disease which were compared with 259 matched controls without lung cancer. Patients treated with chemotherapy had a higher risk than patients given radiotherapy only. Although the results indicated an increasing risk with dose of radiation to the lungs for those treated with radiation alone, neither the trend nor any of the relative risks by dose category was statistically significant.

In a cohort of 1677 patients in the USA who were treated for Hodgkin disease and received an average dose to the cervical lymph node area of 44 Gy, a significant excess risk for thyroid cancer was shown, based, however, on only six cases (standardized incidence ratio (SIR), 15.6; 95% CI, 6.3–32.5) (Hancock *et al*., 1991).

(c)   *Breast cancer*

A case–control study of leukaemia was conducted within a cohort of 82 700 women with breast cancer in the USA (Curtis *et al*., 1992). Detailed information on therapy with alkylating agents and radiotherapy was obtained for 90 patients with leukaemia and for 264 matched controls. The mean dose of radiation to red bone marrow was 7.5 Gy. The risk for acute non-lymphocytic leukaemia was significantly increased after radiotherapy alone (RR, 2.4; 95% CI, 1.0–5.8; 12 cases), and a dose–response relationship was demonstrated after adjustment for the amount of chemotherapy. It was suggested that chemotherapy might interact with radiotherapy to enhance the development of leukaemia.

In a case–control study of 655 women in whom a second breast cancer developed ≥ 5 years after a primary breast cancer and 1189 controls nested in a cohort of 41 109 women in whom breast cancer was diagnosed between 1935 and 1982 in Connecticut, USA, an increased risk for contralateral breast cancer was found in association with radiotherapy (mean dose, 2.8 Gy) only among women who were under 45 years of age at the time of treatment (RR, 1.6; 95% CI, 1.1–2.4; $n = 78$) (Boice *et al.*, 1992). No excess risk was found among older women.

A similar study performed in Denmark comprised 529 cases of contralateral breast cancer and 529 controls with unilateral breast cancer nested in a cohort of 56 540 women with breast cancer diagnosed between 1943 and 1978; 82% of each group had received radiotherapy at a mean dose of 2.5 Gy. Radiation did not increase the risk for contralateral breast cancer (RR, 1.0; 95% CI, 0.7–1.5) (Storm *et al.*, 1992). The dose to the contralateral breast of each case and each control was known from individual radiotherapy records in both the Danish and the US studies.

A case–control study nested in a cohort of 14 000 Canadian women with breast cancer diagnosed between 1946 and 1982 included 194 cases of contralateral breast cancer and 194 controls. The mean dose to the contralateral breast was 2.0–3.3 Gy, depending on the radiation source. This study showed no excess risk for contralateral breast cancer in association with radiotherapy (RR, 0.99; 95% CI, 0.76–1.3) (Basco *et al.*, 1985).

In one study, an attempt was made to reconstruct the doses of radiation to the lung and to evaluate risk in a case–control fashion within a large cohort of breast cancer patients reported to the Connecticut Tumor Registry (USA; Inskip *et al.*, 1994). The risk appeared to increase with estimated dose, but the dosimetry was complex and the location of the initial lung tumour was often unknown (RR for ≥ 15 years after radiotherapy, 2.8; 95% CI, 1.0–8.2).

In a cohort of 13 490 women with breast cancer in Sweden (Karlsson *et al.*, 1996), 19 cases of soft-tissue sarcoma (SIR, 2.2; 95% CI, 1.3–3.4) were found, one of which had been misclassified and was in fact a melanoma. A matched case–control study was conducted with respect to radiation dose and the occurrence of sarcoma inside the radiation field. A significant correlation ($p = 0.008$) with the integral dose was observed. When the analysis was restricted to sarcomas that occurred inside the radiation field, the odds ratio was no longer significant.

(d)   Ovarian cancer

A case–control study comprising 114 cases of leukaemia and 342 controls within an international cohort of 99 113 survivors of ovarian cancer showed no significant excess risk for leukaemia associated with radiotherapy alone (RR, 1.6; 95% CI, 0.51–4.8) (Kaldor *et al.*, 1990b), and no significant risk for bladder cancer was observed (RR, 1.9; 95% CI, 0.77–4.9; $n = 63$) (Kaldor *et al.*, 1995).

In a more recent international study in Europe and North America of 28 971 patients in whom ovarian cancer was diagnosed between 1980 and 1993, a case–control study of 96 cases of secondary leukaemia and 272 controls found no risk associated with exposure to radiotherapy at a median dose to the bone marrow of 18.4 Gy (RR, 0.4; 95% CI, 0.04–3.5) (Travis *et al.*, 1999).

(e)   *Testicular cancer*

In a study of 28 843 men with testicular cancer who survived for one year or more, identified in 16 population-based tumour registries in Europe and North America, 1406 patients developed a second primary malignancy (Travis *et al.*, 1997). The overall SIR was 1.43 (95% CI, 1.36–1.51), and a significantly increased risk was seen for acute leukaemia ([SIR, 3.4; 95% CI, 2.4–4.7]; $n = 36$) in relation to both chemotherapy and radiotherapy. Significantly increased risks seen for cancers of the stomach (SIR, 1.95; 95% CI, 1.6–2.4; $n = 93$), bladder (SIR, 2.0; 95% CI, 1.7–2.4; $n = 154$) and pancreas (SIR, 2.2; 95% CI, 1.7–2.8; $n = 66$) were mainly associated with radiotherapy. The dose of radiation was not estimated, and excess risks for cancer were noted among patients who did not receive radiotherapy.

(f)   *Malignant disorders during childhood*

One of the great successes in the treatment of cancer is the increased survival of patients treated in childhood for malignancies. Radiotherapy, often in combination with chemotherapy, has prolonged the life expectancy of children with cancer, leaving open the possibility for the development of late effects and particularly second cancers. Because childhood cancer is rare, national and international groups have combined their data to evaluate the risks. The most informative studies were conducted by the Late Effects Study Group (Tucker *et al.*, 1984, 1987a,b, 1991) and several groups in the United Kingdom (Hawkins *et al.*, 1987, 1992, 1996) and France (de Vathaire *et al.*, 1989, 1999b). The cohort studies of children with cancer who survived for at least two years indicate that the risk for developing a second cancer 25 years after the diagnosis of the first cancer was as high as 12% (Tucker *et al.*, 1984); that for a second cancer 50 years after diagnosis of hereditary retinoblastoma was as high as 51% (Wong *et al.*, 1997).

High doses of radiotherapy have been associated with increased risks for brain cancer, thyroid cancer and bone and soft-tissue sarcomas, with dose–response relationships. The effect of radiation on the risk for leukaemia is less clear because it is difficult to control for the effect of concomitant chemotherapy (see IARC, 1987), which is associated with a much higher risk for leukaemia than radiation and is cytotoxic at therapeutic doses.

An international cohort study of 9170 children who developed a second malignant tumour at least two years after diagnosis of a first tumour, conducted by the Late Effects Study Group (Tucker *et al.*, 1984), provided information on risks associated with radiotherapy in three nested case–control studies involving 64 cases of bone cancer and 209 controls (Tucker *et al.*, 1987a), 23 cases of thyroid cancer and 89 controls (Tucker *et al.*, 1991) and 25 cases of leukaemia and 90 controls (Tucker *et al.*, 1987b). Although the doses to red bone marrow were accurately quantified, there was no evidence of a dose–response relationship for leukaemia, and the authors concluded that high doses to small volumes of tissue probably result in killing of stem cells rather than carcinogenic transformation. When the doses to the site of secondary bone cancers were reconstructed, a dose–response relationship was demonstrated, but no increase in the risk for bone cancer was observed at doses < 10 Gy, consistent with the hypothesis that radiation-induced bone cancer occurs only after very high doses. The relationship between dose and the relative risk for bone cancer was similar among patients treated for bilateral retinoblastoma, who have a high risk for developing sarcoma, and among children treated with radiation for other malignancies. The dose–response curve for thyroid cancer (average dose, 13 Gy) was also relatively flat, suggesting to the authors that cancer induction and cell killing have competing roles at high therapeutic doses. In comparison with the general population, the SIR for thyroid cancer was 53 (95% CI, 36–80).

A British cohort study of 10 106 three-year survivors of childhood cancer (Hawkins et al., 1987) showed an SIR of 5.6 (95% CI, 3.8–8.1; $n = 40$) for second tumours among 2668 children with cancer (except retinoblastoma) who received radiotherapy, in comparison with the general population. For children with hereditary retinoblastoma, the RR for second tumours was 26 (95% CI, 14–45). Two case–control studies were nested in this study, involving 59 cases of second bone cancer and 220 controls (Hawkins et al., 1996) and 26 cases of second leukaemia and 96 controls (Hawkins et al., 1992). A dose–response relationship was reported for bone cancer, but it was not statistically significant ($p = 0.065$). The risk for leukaemia increased with dose of radiation to the red bone marrow, but the confidence interval around the overall estimate of risk was wide (RR, 8.4; 95% CI, 0.9–81). [The Working Group underlined the difficulty in controlling for the effects of chemotherapy, which is associated with very high risks for leukaemia, in analyses of the effects of radiotherapy.]

A French–British cohort study comprised 4400 three-year survivors of childhood cancer (de Vathaire et al., 1999b). As this cohort overlapped somewhat with those of the Late Effects Study and the British studies described above, it is not completely independent. The SIR for the development of any second cancer among the 1045 children who received radiotherapy alone was 5.6 (95% CI, 3.8–7.8) when compared with the general population. Brain cancer developed as a second cancer only in children who had received doses > 5 Gy (Little et al., 1998a). Brain cancer had previously been linked to cranial radiotherapy for acute lymphoblastic leukaemia in children in the USA (Neglia et al., 1991). Several case–control studies were nested in the French–British study: e.g. 32 cases of osteosarcoma and 160 controls (Le Vu et al., 1998), and 25 cases of any second cancer and 96 controls, 23 and 74 of whom had received radiotherapy, respectively (Kony et al., 1997). Thyroid carcinoma developed at a high rate (SIR, 80) among the 2827 children who received radiotherapy at a dose of 7 Gy (de Vathaire et al., 1999a), and associations with radiation dose were reported for all types of second cancer together and for osteosarcoma, leukaemia and thyroid cancer.

In a cohort study of 1380 children (483 girls) treated for Hodgkin disease, the average dose to the chest region was 40 Gy for the girls who eventually developed breast cancer; 17 cases of breast cancer were observed after radiotherapy alone or combined, giving an SIR of 75 (95% CI, 45–118) in comparison with the general population. In seven of these cases, only radiotherapy was used, but the SIR was not reported (Bhatia *et al.*, 1996). The cumulative incidence of breast cancer at 40 years of age was 35% (95% CI, 18–52). [The Working Group noted that the incompleteness of the follow-up of persons with no medical problems could have biased the risk esti- mates upwards.]

Radiotherapy for retinoblastoma is associated with an increased risk for osteo- sarcoma (Jensen & Miller, 1971). In a cohort study of cancer mortality involving 1458 patients in the USA who were followed-up for retinoblastoma for an average of 17 years, 534 of whom received only radiotherapy, the SMR of children with bilateral disease who received radiotherapy was 2.9 (95% CI, 2.2–3.7; $n = 79$) (Eng *et al.*, 1993).

In order to determine the long-term risk for new primary cancers among survivors of childhood retinoblastoma and to quantify the role of radiotherapy in the deve- lopment of sarcomas, the incidence of cancer was studied in the same cohort, involving 1604 patients who had survived for at least one year after diagnosis (Wong *et al.*, 1997). The children were treated at hospitals in Massachusetts and New York (USA) during 1914–84, and detailed records were available, allowing reconstruction of doses. The incidence of subsequent cancers was significantly increased only among the 961 patients with hereditary retinoblastoma, in whom 190 cancers were diagnosed, whereas 6.3 were expected in the general population (RR, 30). The cumulative inci- dence of a second cancer 50 years after diagnosis was $51 \pm 6.2\%$ for hereditary retino- blastoma and $5 \pm 3\%$ for non-hereditary retinoblastoma. All of the 114 sarcomas of diverse histological types occurred in patients with hereditary retinoblastoma, and the risk was associated with exposure to radiation at doses > 5 Gy, rising to 10.7-fold at doses > 60 Gy ($p < 0.05$). A dose–response relationship was demonstrated for all sarcomas and, for the first time in humans, for soft-tissue sarcomas; however, despite the role of genetic predisposition in the development of sarcomas, therapeutic doses < 5 Gy did not increase the risk for cancer.

(g)   *Bone-marrow transplant*

Studies of patients given radiotherapy to the whole body or to part of the body at doses of about 10 Gy in conjunction with bone-marrow transplants show an increased risk for second cancers with evidence of a dose–response relationship (Curtis *et al.*, 1997). The effect of prior radiotherapy and chemotherapy could not be discounted, however.

2.3.2   *Radiotherapy for benign disease*

The studies of patients treated with X- and γ-rays for benign disease (Table 19) have provided valuable information about the role of radiotherapy in the risk for cancer. The doses used are not nearly as high as those used to treat malignant disease,

Table 19. Study characteristics and second cancers in patients receiving radiotherapy for a benign disease

Reference	Disease treated (period of treatment)	Sex, no. of exposed and total no. of individuals or, for the case–control study, nos of cases and controls	Mean follow-up (years)	Organ dose (Gy)	Second cancers studied	Results
Cohort studies						
Shore et al. (1986)*	Post-partum acute mastitis (1940–57)	Women, 601/1840	29; 20–45	Breast, 3.8	Breast	Breast: RR = 3.2; n = 56
Mattsson et al. (1993, 1997)*	Benign breast disease (1925–61)	Women, 1216/3090	27; 0–61	Breast, 5.84 Lung, 0.75 Liver, 0.66 Stomach, 0.66 Pancreas, 0.37 Oesophagus, 0.28 Kidney, 0.13 Rectum, 0.008	All	Colon: RR = 1.8; n = 25 Breast: RR = 3.6; n = 183
Griem et al. (1994)*	Peptic ulcer (1973–65)	Both sexes, 1831/3609	21.5; 20–51	Stomach, 14.8 Colon, 0.1–12.3 Liver, 4.6 Lung, 1.8 Red bone marrow, 1.55	All	Stomach: RR = 2.8; n = 40 Pancreas: RR = 1.9; n = 28 Lung: RR = 1.7; n = 99 Leukaemia: RR = 3.3; n = 11
Alderson & Jackson (1971)	Uterine bleeding (1946–60)	Women, 2049/2049	15	NR	All	None
Inskip et al. (1990a,b)*	Uterine bleeding (1925–65)	Women, 4153/4153	27; < 60	Stomach, 0.2 Colon, 1.3 Liver, 0.2 Bladder, 6.0 Red bone marrow, 0.5 Uterus, 32 Vagina, 14	All	Colon: SMR = 1.3; n = 86 Pancreas: SMR = 1.5; n = 37 Uterus: SMR = 1.8; n = 105 Other genital sites: SMR = 1.5; n = 44 Leukaemia, excluding CLL: [SMR = 1.8]; n = 25

Table 19 (contd)

Cohort studies (contd)

Reference	Disease treated (period of treatment)	Sex, no. of exposed and total no. of individuals or, for the case–control study, nos of cases and controls	Mean follow-up (years)	Organ dose (Gy)	Second cancers studied	Results
Ryberg et al. (1990)*	Uterine bleeding (1912–77)	Women, 788/2007	28; 0–56	Pelvis, 6.5	All	Ovary, corpus uteri, cervix uteri, rectum and bladder combined: SIR = 1.6; n = 30
Inskip et al. (1993)*	Benign gynaecological disorders (1925–65)	Women, 9770/12 955	25	Red bone marrow, 1.2	All haematological malignancies	Leukaemia, excluding CLL: [RR = 4.7]; n = 47
Darby et al. (1994)*	Uterine bleeding (1940–60)	Women, 2067/2067	28; 5–30	Stomach, 0.23 Colon, 3.20 Liver, 0.27 Bladder, 5.20 Red bone marrow, 1.30	All	Colon: SMR = 1.4; n = 47 Bladder: SMR = 3.0; n = 20 Multiple myeloma: SMR, 2.6; n = 9 Leukaemia: SMR = 2.05; n = 12
Ron et al. (1994)*	Refractory hormonal infertility and amenorrhoea (1925–61)	Women, 816/816	35	Ovary, 0.88 Pelvis, 0.62 Uterus, 0.54 Sigmoid colon, 1.02 Red bone marrow, 0.29	All	Colon: SMR = 1.9; n = 15 Non-Hodgkin lymphoma: SMR = 2.8; n = 6

Table 19 (contd)

Cohort studies (contd)

Reference	Disease treated (period of treatment)	Sex, no. of exposed and total no. of individuals or, for the case–control study, nos of cases and controls	Mean follow-up (years)	Organ dose (Gy)	Second cancers studied	Results
Weiss et al. (1994, 1995)*	Ankylosing spondylitis (1935–57)	Both sexes, 14 556/15 577	25 (1–57)	Oesophagus, 5.55; Colon, 4.10; Stomach, 3.21; Liver, 2.13; Lung, 2.54; Bone, 4.54; Breast, 0.59; Bladder, 2.18; Kidney, 6.08; Thyroid, 1.41; Brain, 0.20; Red bone marrow, 5.10	All; ≥ 5 years since first treatment	Oesophagus: RR = 1.9; n = 74; Colon: RR = 1.3; n = 113; Pancreas: RR = 1.6; n = 84; Lung: RR = 1.2; n = 563; Bone: RR = 3.3; n = 9; Prostate: RR = 1.4; n = 88; Kidney: RR = 1.6; n = 35; Non-Hodgkin lymphoma : RR = 1.7; n = 37; Hodgkin disease: RR = 1.65; n = 13; Multiple myeloma: RR = 1.6; n = 22; Leukaemia, excluding CLL: RR = 3.1; n = 53
Damber et al. (1995)*	Benign lesions of the locomotor system or scoliosis (1950–64)	Both sexes, 20 024/20 024	1–38	Red bone marrow, 0.39	Haematological malignancies	Leukaemia: SIR = 1.2; n = 116; SMR = 1.2; n = 115
Shore et al. (1976, 1984)*	Tinea capitis (1940–59)	Both sexes, 2226/3613	26 (13–35)	Skin, 4.5; Thyroid, 0.1; Brain, 1.4	Thyroid, skin, brain, leukaemia, salivary glands, bone	Skin: RR = 3.8; n = 31

Table 19 (contd)

Reference	Disease treated (period of treatment)	Sex, no. of exposed and total no. of individuals or, for the case–control study, nos of cases and controls	Mean follow-up (years)	Organ dose (Gy)	Second cancers studied	Results
Cohort studies (contd)						
Ron & Modan (1980); Ron et al. (1988a,b, 1989, 1991)*	Tinea capitis during childhood (1948–60)	Both sexes, 10 834/27 060	30; 26–39	Thyroid, 0.09; Brain, 1.5; Breast, 0.016; Skin, 6.8; Red bone marrow, 0.3	Thyroid, brain, skin, breast, leukaemia	Non-melanoma skin: RR = 4.2; n = 44; Brain: RR = 6.9; n = 60; Thyroid: RR = 4.0; n = 43; Leukaemia: RR = 2.3; n = 14
Janower & Miettinen (1971)	Thymus enlargement during childhood (1924–46)	Both sexes, 466/972	30	Thyroid, 4	Thyroid, breast	Thyroid: [SIR = 34]; n = 2
Hildreth et al. (1985, 1989); Shore et al. (1993)*	Thymus enlargement during childhood (1926–57)	Both sexes, 2657/7490	37; 29–60	Skin, 2.3; Breast, 0.69; Thyroid, 1.4	Thyroid, breast, skin, bone, nervous system, salivary gland	Skin: RR = 2.3; n = 11; Breast: RR = 3.6; n = 22; Thyroid: SIR = 24; n = 37
Li et al. (1974)	Skin haemangioma during childhood (1946–1968)	Both sexes, 4746/4746	7	NR	All	None
Fürst et al. (1988); Lundell & Holm (1995, 1996); Lundell et al. (1996)*	Skin haemangioma during childhood (1920–59)	Both sexes, 14 351/14 351	39; 1–67	Bone, 0.40; Thyroid, 0.26; Red bone marrow, 0.13; Breast, 0.39; Brain, 0.08; Stomach, 0.09; Lung, 0.12; Gonads, 0.05	All	Pancreas: SIR = 3.3; n = 9; Breast: SIR, 1.2; n = 75; Thyroid: SIR = 2.3; n = 17; Endocrine glands: SIR = 2.0; n = 16

Table 19 (contd)

Reference	Disease treated (period of treatment)	Sex, no. of exposed and total no. of individuals or, for the case–control study, nos of cases and controls	Mean follow-up (years)	Organ dose (Gy)	Second cancers studied	Results
Cohort studies (contd)						
Lindberg et al. (1995); Karlsson et al. (1997)*	Skin haemangioma during childhood (1930–65)	Both sexes, 12 055/12 055	33; 1–59	Thyroid, 0.116; Breast, 0.155; Lung, 0.121; Brain, 0.07	All	Brain: SIR = 1.8; n = 47; Thyroid: SIR = 1.9; n = 15; Other endocrine glands: SIR, 2.6; n = 23
Maxon et al. (1980)	Various benign diseases of the head and neck (1963–67)	Both sexes, 1266/12 089	36.5	Thyroid, 2.9	Thyroid	Thyroid: [RR = 15.5]; n = 16
DeGroot et al. (1983)	Tonsil, thymus, acne (NR)	Both sexes, 263/416	26	Thyroid, 4.5	Thyroid	Thyroid: [SIR = 55]; n = 11 (results from physical examination)
van Daal et al. (1983)	Various benign diseases of the head and neck (1933–63)	Both sexes, 605/2400	38–43	Thyroid, 10.4–20.7; Skin, 10–19.5	Thyroid, skin	Skin: SIR, NR; n = 20
Fjälling et al. (1986)*	Tuberculous cervical adenitis (1975–82)	Both sexes, 444/444	43	Thyroid, 0.4–51	Thyroid	Thyroid: [SIR = 23]; n = 25
Schneider et al. (1993)	Infections and inflammatory diseases of the upper respiratory tract during childhood (1939–62)	Both sexes, 2634/2634	33; 12–51	Thyroid, 0.6	Thyroid	Thyroid: [SMR = 1.4]; n = 309

Table 19 (contd)

Reference	Disease treated (period of treatment)	Sex, no. of exposed and total no. of individuals or, for the case–control study, nos of cases and controls	Mean follow-up (years)	Organ dose (Gy)	Second cancers studied	Results
Cohort studies (contd)						
Royce et al. (1979)	Various diseases of the head and neck (1937–70)	Both sexes, 214/457	28	Thyroid, 7.1	Thyroid	No increase
Refetoff et al. (1975)	Tonsils, adenoids, enlarged thymus (NR)	Both sexes, 100/100	24	Head and neck, 8	Thyroid	Thyroid: RR, NR; n = 7
Straub et al. (1982)	Lymphoid hyperplasia, acne, enlarged thymus (1940–60)	Both sexes, 553/553	23	Thyroid, 1	Thyroid	Thyroid: no significant increase (relatively late age at irradiation)
Pottern et al. (1990)	Lymphoid hyperplasia (1938–69)	Both sexes, 1195/2258	29	Thyroid, 0.24	Thyroid	Thyroid: [SIR = 2.4]; n = 13
Brada et al. (1992)	Pituitary adenoma (1962–86)	Both sexes, 334/334	11	Brain, 45	Brain	Brain: SIR = 9.4; n = 5
Bliss et al. (1994)	Pituitary adenoma (1962–90)	Both sexes, 296/296	8; 0.1–28	Brain, 45	All	Non-central nervous system tumours: SIR = 17.5; n = 30
Hanford et al. (1962)	Tuberculous adenitis (1920–50)	Both sexes, 162[a]/296	17	Thyroid, 8.2 (no standard dose)	Thyroid	Thyroid: [RR = 80]; n = 8

Table 19 (contd)

Reference	Disease treated (period of treatment)	Sex, no. of exposed and total no. of individuals or, for the case–control study, nos of cases and controls	Mean follow-up (years)	Organ dose (Gy)	Second cancers studied	Results
Case–control study						
Fürst *et al.* (1990)	Skin haemangioma in childhood (1920–59)	Both sexes, 94/359	35 (0–59) (time since first treatment)	Thyroid, 0.3–0.8 Bone, 0.07–3 Breast, 0.2 Brain, 0.003–0.1	Breast, thyroid, brain, bone, soft tissue	Thyroid: linear trend *p* < 0.05; *n* = 14 Bone and soft tissue: OR = 19.5; *n* = 3 (≥ 0.5 Gy)

CLL, chronic lymphocytic leukaemia; NR, not reported; RR, relative risk; SIR, standardized incidence ratio; SMR, standardized mortality ratio
* Studies cited in text
[a] Examined ≥ 10 years after irradiation

so that cell-killing effects do not predominate, survival after treatment is good and there is minimal confounding from concomitant treatment.

(a)   During adulthood

(i)   Benign breast disease

A cohort of 1216 women treated for benign breast disease with radiotherapy and 1874 women treated by other means in Sweden in 1925–54 were studied for subsequent cancer development (Baral *et al.*, 1977; Mattsson *et al.*, 1993, 1995, 1997). The mean age of the women at the time of radiotherapy was 40 years. The mean estimated dose of radiation to the breast was 5.8 Gy, and that to 14 other organs ranged from 0.01 to the rectum to 0.75 Gy to the lung. The mean follow-up time was 27 years. In an internal analysis, the incidence of breast cancers was increased (RR, 3.6; 95% CI, 2.8–4.6; $n = 183$) (Mattsson *et al.*, 1993), with a linear dose–response relationship at low-to-medium doses. The risk for radiation-induced breast cancer was inversely related to age at exposure, the lowest risk being seen for women who were exposed at or after the menopause. The relative risk for all cancers together (excluding breast) was 1.2 (95% CI, 0.97–1.4; $n = 189$). In an analysis by site, the incidence of colon cancer was increased to a degree that approached statistical significance (RR, 1.8; 95% CI, 0.96–3.4; $n = 25$). The relative risk was 1.8 (95% CI, 0.75–4.5) for stomach cancer, at an average dose of 0.66 Gy, and 1.8 (95% CI, 0.65–5.0; $n = 10$) for lung cancer, at an average dose of 0.75 Gy. Deficits were noted for leukaemia (RR, 0.67; 0.18–2.1; $n = 5$) and several other cancers (Mattsson *et al.*, 1997). [The Working Group noted that some benign diseases of the breast are independent risk factors for breast cancer, and this might have contributed to the excess risk if bias was present in the selection of those who received radiotherapy. The inconsistent patterns of cancer excesses for some sites, e.g. the colon, which received little exposure, were noted.]

A cohort of 601 women in the USA treated with radiotherapy for acute post-partum mastitis and 1239 treated by other means between 1940 and 1957 were followed-up for an average of 29 years. The average dose to the breast was 3.8 Gy, and a dose–response relationship was demonstrated. In an internal analysis, an increased risk for breast cancer was shown (RR, 3.2; 90% CI, 2.3–4.3; $n = 56$) (Mettler *et al.*, 1969; Shore *et al.*, 1986). In a combined analysis of this study with those of atomic bomb survivors and of tuberculosis patients who received repeated chest fluoroscopies, the risk was similar in the three populations, at least for people aged 10–40 years at the time of exposure (Boice *et al.*, 1979; Land *et al.*, 1980).

(ii)   Peptic ulcer

A cohort of 1831 patients in the USA who received X-rays between 1937 and 1965 for the treatment of peptic ulcer and 1778 who did not were followed for an average of 22 years before 1985 (Griem *et al.*, 1994). The dose to the stomach was about 15 Gy. In an internal analysis of cancer mortality, this treatment was associated with a significantly increased relative risk for death from cancers at all sites (RR, 1.5; 95% CI,

1.3–1.8; $n = 341$) and from stomach cancer (RR, 2.8; 95% CI, 1.6–4.8; $n = 40$). Cancers at the other sites studied were not convincingly linked to radiotherapy.

(iii) *Benign gynaecological diseases*

A cohort of 4153 women in the USA who received radiotherapy between 1925 and 1965 for uterine bleeding disorders were followed-up for an average of 27 years before 1984 (Inskip *et al.*, 1990a,b). The median dose to red bone marrow was estimated to be 0.5 Gy, and the median dose to the uterus was 32 Gy. By comparison with mortality rates for the general population of the USA, this treatment was associated with a significantly increased SMR for death from all cancers (SMR, 1.3; 95% CI, 1.2–1.4; $n = 632$). A significant increase was observed in deaths from cancer of the colon (SMR, 1.3 [95% CI, 1.0–1.6]; $n = 86$), cancers of the uterus (SMR, 1.8; 95% CI, 1.5–2.2; $n = 105$), cancers of other female genital organs (SMR, 1.5; 95% CI, 1.1–2.0; $n = 44$) and leukaemia (SMR, 2.0; 95% CI, 1.4–2.8; $n = 34$).

This cohort was expanded to 9770 women, for whom the average dose to red bone marrow was estimated to be 1.2 Gy (Inskip *et al.*, 1993). In comparison with 3185 women treated by other methods, radiotherapy was associated with a significantly increased relative risk for death from leukaemia (2.5; 95% CI, 1.4–5.2; $n = 64$ after exclusion of two cases of leukaemia diagnosed before radiotherapy), but no increase in mortality from non-Hodgkin lymphoma, Hodgkin disease or multiple myeloma was observed.

A cohort of 2067 women in the United Kingdom who received radiotherapy for uterine bleeding disorders between 1940 and 1960 was followed-up for an average of 28 years before 1990 (Darby *et al.*, 1994). The average doses ranged from 0.002 Gy to the brain to 5.3 Gy to the ovary and 5.2 Gy to the uterus. In all, 331 deaths from cancer were observed (SMR, 1.1; 95% CI, 1.0–1.2), and significant excesses of deaths were observed from cancers at heavily irradiated sites in the pelvic area (SMR, 1.5; 95% CI, 1.2–1.7; $n = 129$), urinary bladder cancer (SMR, 3.0; 95% CI, 1.8–4.6; $n = 20$), colon cancer (SMR, 1.4; 95% CI, 1.05–1.9; $n = 47$), leukaemia (SMR, 2.05; 95% CI, 1.1–3.6; $n = 12$) and multiple myeloma (SMR, 2.6; 95% CI, 1.2–4.9; $n = 9$); whereas fewer deaths from breast cancer were observed than expected among women who received more than 5 Gy to the ovaries (SMR, 0.53; 95% CI, 0.34–0.78; $n = 24$).

A cohort of 788 Swedish women who received radiotherapy between 1912 and 1977 for uterine bleeding was followed-up for an average of 28 years before 1982 (Ryberg *et al.*, 1990). By comparison with cancer incidence rates for the general population, those for women who underwent radiotherapy were slightly increased (SIR, 1.2; 95% CI, 1.0–1.5; $n = 107$); however, the SIR of an unexposed group of 1219 women with the same condition was similar (1.1; 95% CI, 0.94–1.3). The exposed group had a significantly increased SIR for cancers at heavily irradiated sites in the pelvic area (ovary, corpus uteri, cervix, rectum and bladder; SIR, 1.6; 95% CI, 1.1–2.3; $n = 30$) but not for cancers at other sites.

(iv)   *Hormonal infertility*

A cohort of 816 women in the USA who received X-rays to the ovaries and/or pituitary gland for refractory hormonal infertility and amenorrhoea between 1925 and 1961 was followed-up for an average of 35 years before 1990 (Ron *et al.*, 1994). The average doses were 0.011 Gy to the breast, 0.88 Gy to the ovary and 1.02 Gy to the sigmoid colon. In an external analysis of cancer mortality, 78 deaths from cancer were observed (SMR, 1.1; 95% CI, 0.9–1.4). No increase in mortality rates was found for leukaemia or cancers of the ovary or brain, sites directly exposed to radiation.

(v)   *Ankylosing spondylitis*

A cohort of 14 556 patients in the United Kingdom who received X-rays for the treatment of ankylosing spondylitis between 1935 and 1957 and 1021 patients who received other treatments were followed-up for an average of 25 years. This study, first reported in 1957 (Court Brown & Doll, 1957), provides strong evidence that radiation can cause leukaemia and other cancers in humans. Estimates were made of the doses received by persons who developed leukaemia and by a sample of the entire cohort, irrespective of mortality outcome. The average dose to red bone marrow was estimated to be 4.4 Gy, while those to other organs ranged from 0.2 to the brain to 5.55 Gy to the oesophagus; the doses were not uniform, and the lower spine received the highest dose. In a study of mortality (Darby *et al.*, 1987; Weiss *et al.*, 1994, 1995), the irradiated patients had a significantly greater mortality rate from cancer than expected from the national rates for England and Wales (SMR, 1.30; 95% CI: 1.2–1.35), and a significant increase was noted for leukaemia other than chronic lymphocytic leukaemia (SMR, 3.1; 95% CI, 2.4–4.1; $n = 53$), although a clear dose–response relationship was not evident. The excess cancers occurred predominantly in the tissues that were likely to have been exposed during radiotherapy, such as the oesophagus, lung, bladder, kidney, bone and connective and soft tissue. The relative risks of men were significantly increased for leukaemia (RR, 2.9; $p < 0.001$; $n = 55$), colorectal cancers (RR, 1.25; $p < 0.01$; $n = 148$) and other neoplasms (RR, 1.3; $p < 0.001$; $n = 1225$). The risks for prostate cancer, non-Hodgkin lymphoma and multiple myeloma were also increased. For lung cancer, the SMR associated with radiotherapy (average dose to the lung, 2.54 Gy) was 1.2 (95% CI, 1.1–1.3; $n = 563$), but the risk declined to near the expected level after 25 years. No excess risk for death from stomach cancer was found on the basis of 127 deaths and an average estimated dose of 3.2 Gy. No significant excess of deaths from breast cancer (average dose, 0.59 Gy) was found among the 2394 treated women (SMR, 1.1; 95% CI, 0.77–1.45). The treatment for ankylosing spondylitis involved various radiation fields, some covering only the neck region and others covering the entire spine. The dose–response relationship could be evaluated only for leukaemia and was found to be relatively flat over various categories of dose to the bone marrow, possibly because of cell killing effects. The condition being treated, ankylosing spondylitis, is known to be associated with increased rates of colon cancer, independently of exposure to radiation, and perhaps with other conditions as well. It is unclear whether these factors influenced the time–response relationship and contributed to the return to levels of risk near those expected after 25 years.

A cohort of 20 024 Swedish patients who received X-rays between 1950 and 1964 for painful arthritic conditions such as spondylosis was followed-up for an average of 25 years before 1988 (Damber *et al.*, 1995; Johansson *et al.*, 1995). The average dose to red bone marrow was estimated to have been 0.39 Gy. In analyses of both cancer incidence and cancer mortality, radiotherapy was associated with increased risks for leukaemia (SIR, 1.2; 95% CI, 0.98–1.42; *n* = 116 and SMR, 1.2; 95% CI, 0.99–1.45; *n* = 115). The reported dose–response relationship for leukaemia is not easily interpreted because chronic lymphocytic leukaemia was included and contributed 50 of the 116 cases, although this disease has not been associated with exposure to radiation. The numbers of cases of non-Hodgkin lymphoma (81 cases), Hodgkin disease (17 cases) and multiple myeloma (65 cases) were no greater than expected.

(b)   During childhood

(i)   Tinea capitis

The risk for cancer of children treated for tinea capitis (ringworm of the scalp) was studied in Israel among 10 834 patients (Ron *et al.*, 1989) and in New York (USA) among 2200 children (Shore *et al.*, 1976, 1984). In the Israeli cohort, the mean dose to the skin of the scalp was estimated to be several grays, and the scatter dose to the thyroid was estimated to be about 0.10 Gy. Significantly increased risks for thyroid cancer were seen in Israel (Ron *et al.*, 1989), and an association with non-melanoma skin cancer was seen in both Israel and New York (Shore *et al.*, 1984; Ron *et al.*, 1991). An interaction between sunlight and radiotherapy was suggested in the New York study. The Israeli study also revealed a significant relation between dose of radiation and tumours of the central nervous system (Ron *et al.*, 1988a). [The Working Group noted that although an increased risk for breast cancer after radiotherapy for tinea capitis was reported (Modan *et al.*, 1989), the increase was related to a deficit of breast cancer cases among the control subjects rather than to an increase among the exposed women.]

(ii)   Enlarged thymus gland

A cohort of 2657 patients treated with radiotherapy for an enlarged thymus gland between 1926 and 1957 in Rochester, New York (USA), has been studied extensively (Shore *et al.*, 1993). Ninety per cent were treated before six months of age (Hildreth *et al.*, 1985). The individual doses, estimated from radiotherapy records (Hempelmann *et al.*, 1967), were 0.69 Gy to the breast (Hildreth *et al.*, 1989) and 1.4 Gy to the thyroid (Shore *et al.*, 1993). A significantly increased risk was found for cancer of the thyroid, with a dose–response relationship (Shore *et al.*, 1980, 1985, 1993). Of the 1201 women who received radiotherapy, 22 developed breast cancer after a mean follow-up of 36 years, and the relative risk, in comparison with sibling controls, was 3.6 (95% CI, 1.8–7.3); none of the cases occurred before 28 years after irradiation (Hildreth *et al.*, 1989). The relative risk for cancer of the skin was 2.3 (95% CI, 1.0–5.6), but no excess was found for cancers of the nervous system or salivary glands (Hildreth *et al.*, 1985).

(iii)   *Skin haemangiomas*

Various techniques, most based on X-rays or applicators of ^{226}Ra, have been used to treat skin haemangiomas, usually in children under the age of two. Two cohort studies were performed in Sweden, which comprised 12 055 patients treated between 1930 and 1965 (11 807 followed-up) (Lindberg *et al.*, 1995; Karlsson *et al.*, 1997, 1998) and 14 351 treated between 1920 and 1959 (Fürst *et al.*, 1988, 1989; Lundell & Holm, 1995; Lundell *et al.*, 1996, 1999). Lundell *et al.* (1999) combined the data for women in the two cohorts (Lindberg *et al.*, 1995; Lundell *et al.*, 1996), for a pooled analysis of 17 202 women who had received a mean dose to the breast of 0.29 Gy (range, < 0.01–36 Gy). Between 1958 and 1993, 245 breast cancers were diagnosed in this cohort, yielding a SIR of 1.2 (95% CI, 1.1–1.4). The excess relative risk per gray was estimated to be 0.35 (95% CI, 0.18–0.59), which is somewhat lower than that reported in other studies. The risk for leukaemia was not associated with the dose of radiation to bone marrow (average, 0.13 Gy; range, < 0.01–4.6 Gy). During 1920–86, there were only 20 deaths from leukaemia, and the low dose to bone marrow implied a limited possibility of detecting an effect even among 14 624 irradiated infants (Lundell & Holm, 1996). The risk for cancer of the thyroid was evaluated for 14 351 irradiated infants (Lundell *et al.*, 1994; Lundell & Holm, 1995), among whom 17 cases were found (SIR, 2.3; 95% CI, 1.3–3.65) after a mean follow-up of 39 years. The mean dose to the thyroid of the patients with cancer was 1.1 Gy (range, < 0.01–4.3 Gy). The excess risk for thyroid cancer began to be seen 19 years after irradiation. The SIRs were similar for women (SIR, 2.2) and men (SIR, 2.9), but 15 of the 17 cancers occurred in women, such that the incidence rate in this cohort was nearly 10 times higher in women than in men.

In a study of intracranial tumours in 12 055 infants who were treated for skin haemangiomas (Karlsson *et al.*, 1997), 47 tumours developed in 46 persons (SIR, 1.8; 95% CI, 1.3–2.4). No dose–response relationship was observed, and the mean dose to the brain was low (0.07 Gy), although some children received > 1 Gy. In a pooled analysis of this cohort and that of Lundell and Holm (1995), for a total of 28 008 patients, 88 brain tumours were identified in 86 persons (SIR = 1.4; 95% CI, 1.1–1.8), to give an ERR of 2.7 per Gy (95% CI, 1.0–5.6). These results strongly indicate that a dose–response relationship exists (Karlsson *et al.*, 1998).

(iv)   *Enlarged tonsils and other benign conditions*

A cohort of 2634 patients in the USA who received X-rays between 1939 and 1962 primarily for enlarged tonsils during childhood was followed-up for 33 years. The average dose to the thyroid was estimated to be 0.6 Gy. During screening of the thyroid, 309 thyroid cancers were diagnosed. Successive follow-up of this cohort confirmed a strong dose–response relationship between the dose to the thyroid and the risk for thyroid cancer (Favus *et al.*, 1976; Schneider *et al.*, 1985, 1993).

A cohort of 444 patients in Sweden treated for cervical tuberculous adenitis received an average dose to the thyroid of 0.4–51 Gy. A significant excess of thyroid carcinoma was observed ([SIR, 23] *n* = 25) (Fjälling *et al.*, 1986).

(v)   *Combined analysis of studies of thyroid cancer*

Most of the available information on radiation-induced thyroid cancer comes from studies of cohorts of children who received radiotherapy for benign diseases. In 1995, a pooled analysis of seven studies was published (Ron *et al.*, 1995), comprising the studies of atomic bomb survivors and six studies of patients who received radio-therapy: two case–control studies (Boice *et al.*, 1988; Tucker *et al.*, 1991) and four cohort studies (Ron *et al.*, 1989; Pottern *et al.*, 1990; Schneider *et al.*, 1993; Shore *et al.*, 1993). Five of the six studies concerned children who were ≤ 15 years old at the time of radiotherapy. The excess relative risk per gray after radiotherapy with X- or γ-rays during childhood was estimated to be 7.7 (95% CI, 2.1–28.7), and the excess absolute risk for thyroid carcinoma per 10^4 person–years Gy to be 4.4 (95% CI, 1.9–10.1), on the basis of 458 atomic bomb survivors and 448 exposed patients. The risk was strongly dependent on the age at exposure, being highest for people exposed when they were under the age of five years. No significant risk was found for exposure in adult life. A dose–response relationship was seen for persons exposed as children. The pooled study of irradiated children did not include several studies that had not been published at the time the analysis began (Lundell *et al.*, 1994; Lindberg *et al.*, 1995; de Vathaire *et al.*, 1999a).

2.3.3   *Diagnostic X-radiation*

These studies are summarized in Table 20.

(*a*)   *During adulthood*

(i)   *Repeated chest fluoroscopies for pulmonary tuberculosis*

In a cohort study in Canada of 64 172 patients (32 255 men and 31 917 women) who had been treated for tuberculosis, 25 007 patients had been treated by lung collapse, which requires frequent monitoring by X-ray fluoroscopy. The number of such examinations ranged from one to several hundreds; the mean dose to the lung was 1.02 Sv, and the mean dose to the breast was 0.89 Sv. In 1987, the mean follow-up time was 37 years. Two main studies of cancer mortality in this cohort have been published: one on lung cancer (Howe, 1995) and one on breast cancer (Miller *et al.*, 1989; Howe & McLaughlin, 1996). No increase in the risk for death from lung cancer was observed (RR, 1.0; 95% CI, 0.94–1.1; *n* = 1178). In contrast, an excess of breast cancer and a dose–response relationship were found (SMR, 1.5; 95% CI, 1.3–1.6;

Table 20. Study characteristics and second cancers in patients undergoing diagnostic X-ray procedures

Reference	Reason for examination (period)	Sex, no. of exposed individuals and total no. of individuals or, for case–control studies, nos of cases and controls	Mean follow-up (years)	Organ dose (Gy except as noted)	Second cancers studied	Results
Cohort studies						
Howe (1995); Howe & McLaughlin (1996)*	Tuberculosis; multiple chest fluoroscopies (1930–52)	Both sexes, 25 007/64 172	37; 0–57	Lung, 1.02 (0–24.2 Sv); Breast, 0.89 (0–18.4 Sv)	Lung, breast	Breast: SMR, 1.5; n = 349
Davis et al. (1989); Boice et al. (1991b)*	Tuberculosis; multiple chest fluoroscopies (1925–54)	Both sexes, 6285/13 385	30; 0–50	Oesophagus, 0.80; Lung, 0.84; Breast, 0.79; Red bone marrow, 0.09; Pancreas, 0.06; Stomach, 0.06	All	Oesophagus: SMR = 2.1; n = 14; Breast: SIR = 1.3; n = 147
Levy et al. (1994)	Scoliosis; multiple full spinal radiographies (1960–79)	Both sexes, 18 471/2181	NR	Breast, 0.03; Thyroid, 0.03	All	Excess risk, 2%
Hoffman et al. (1989)*	Scoliosis; multiple full spinal radiographies (1935–65)	Women, 973/1030	26; 3 –> 30	Breast, 0.13	Breast	Breast: SIR = 1.8; n = 11

Table 20 (contd)

Reference	Reason for examination (period)	Sex, no. of exposed and total no. of individuals or, for case–control studies, nos of cases and controls	Mean follow-up (years)	Organ dose (Gy except as noted)	Second cancers studied	Results
Cohort studies (contd)						
Spengler et al. (1983)	Childhood; cardiac catheterization; fluoroscopy (1946–68)	Both sexes, 4891	13	NR	All	None
McLaughlin et al. (1993a)	Cardiac catheterization; fluoroscopy (1950–65)	Both sexes, 3915	22; 0–36	NR	All	None
Case–control studies						
Storm et al. (1986)	Tuberculosis; multiple chest fluoroscopies (1937–54)	Women, 89/390	< 10–≥ 40	Breast, 0.27	Breast	No increase
Ron et al. (1987)*	All X-ray, including dental and radiotherapy (1978–80)	Both sexes, 159/285	< 20–≥ 40	NR	Thyroid	No significant increase

Table 20 (contd)

Reference	Reason for examination (period)	Sex, no. of exposed and total no. of individuals or, for case–control studies, nos of cases and controls	Mean follow-up (years)	Organ dose (Gy except as noted)	Second cancers studied	Results
Case–control studies (contd)						
Hallquist et al. (1994)*	All X-ray, including dental and radiotherapy (1980–89)	Both sexes, 171/325	> 5	Thyroid, 0–> 0.6 mGy	Thyroid	Papillary thyroid cancer: OR = 2.3; $n = 56$ (for > 0.6 mGy)
Inskip et al. (1995)*	All X-ray (1980–92)	Both sexes, 484/484	54	6 mGy	Thyroid	No increase
Wingren et al. (1997)*	All X-ray, including dental (1977–89)	Women, 186/426	1–14	Thyroid, 0–> 1 mGy	Thyroid	Thyroid: OR = 2.6; $n = 60$ (for > 1 mGy)
Preston-Martin et al. (1980)	All X-ray, including dental and radiotherapy (1972–75)	Women, 185/185	< 7	NR	Intracranial meningiomas	No increase
Preston-Martin et al. (1989)*	All X-ray (1979–85)	Both sexes, 136/136	3–20	Red bone marrow, 0–≥ 2 mGy	Chronic myeloid and monocytic leukaemia	Leukaemia: OR = 2.4 (for ≥ 2 mGy)

Table 20 (contd)

Reference	Reason for examination (period)	Sex, no. of exposed and total no. of individuals or, for case–control studies, nos of cases and controls	Mean follow-up (years)	Organ dose (Gy except as noted)	Second cancers studied	Results
Case–control studies (contd)						
Boice et al. (1991a)*	All X-ray (1956–82)	Both sexes, 1091/1390	15–> 50	Red bone marrow, 0.00001–0.23	Non-Hodgkin lymphoma, leukaemia, multiple myeloma	No increase; dose–response relationship for multiple myeloma
Ryan et al. (1992)	Dental X-ray (1987–90)	Both sexes, 170/417	< 25	NR	Brain gliomas and meningiomas	No significant increase
Linos et al. (1980)	All X-ray (1955–74)	Both sexes, 138/276	> 10	Red bone marrow, < 3	Leukaemia	No increase
Thomas et al. (1994)	All X-ray (1983–86)	Men, 227/300	1–> 36	Estimate to breast, 0.18	Breast	Breast: RR = 3; n = 12, 10 and 10 when treated in 1940–54, for 20–35 years since first or last treatment, respectively

NR, not reported; OR, odds ratio; RR, relative risk; SIR, standardized incidence ratio; SMR, standardized mortality ratio

* Cited in text

$n = 349$). The excess relative risk per sievert decreased sharply with age at irradiation (Howe & McLaughlin, 1996).

In a cohort study in Massachusetts (USA) of 6285 patients (4940 women) who received repeated fluoroscopic examinations for tuberculosis in 1925–54 and 7100 who did not, the mean dose to the breast was 0.79 Gy. In a study of cancer incidence, an excess risk for breast cancer was observed (SIR, 1.3; 95% CI, 1.1–1.5; $n = 147$), which showed a linear dose–response relationship. The risk for radiation-induced breast cancer was inversely related to age at exposure, and no risk was seen for patients who had been over the age of 40 when first exposed (Hrubec et al., 1989; Boice et al., 1991b; Little & Boice, 1999). Significantly increased risks were found for death from cancer of the breast (SMR, 1.4; 95% CI, 1.1–1.8; $n = 62$) and oesophagus (SMR, 2.1; 95% CI, 1.2–3.6; $n = 14$), but not from lung cancer or, in an internal comparison of exposed and unexposed patients, from non-chronic lymphocytic leukaemia (RR, 0.9; 95% CI, 0.5–1.8; $n = 17$) (Davis et al., 1989). The average dose to red bone marrow was 0.09 Gy.

(ii)   *Other uses of diagnostic X-rays in adults*

Other studies of the use of diagnostic X-rays have provided limited information on the effects of radiation, largely because of the low doses involved, the lack of dosimetry and problems of bias in studies involving interviews. In a case–control study of 136 pairs in Los Angeles, California (USA), the number of X-ray examinations and the associated dose to the bone marrow were associated with increased risks for chronic myeloid and monocytic leukaemia (Preston-Martin et al., 1989). [The Working Group noted that exposure was ascertained by telephone interview and not directly validated. The possibility of reporting bias and the uncertainty in the dosimetry make the results difficult to interpret.]

A case–control study of 565 patients with leukaemia, 318 patients with non-Hodgkin lymphoma, 208 patients with multiple myeloma and 1390 matched controls was conducted in the USA, in which information on exposure was extracted from medical records held by two prepaid health plans. When the first two years before diagnosis were excluded, no relation was found between the dose of radiation from diagnostic X-rays and the risks for leukaemia or non-Hodgkin lymphoma, whereas a dose–response relationship was found for multiple myeloma (Boice et al., 1991a). Exposure to diagnostic X-rays was not linked to multiple myeloma in a larger study of 399 patients and 399 controls who were interviewed in the United Kingdom (Cuzick & De Stavola, 1988).

In five case–control studies of the role of diagnostic radiation in the risk for thyroid cancer, all but one of which were performed in Sweden, exposure was assessed by interview in four studies, without validation. Of these, three found an association between the cumulative thyroid dose delivered by the diagnostic procedure and the risk for thyroid cancer (Wingren et al., 1993; Hallquist et al., 1994; Wingren et al., 1997), and one did not (Ron et al., 1987). The largest case–control study was based on data from radiological records in hospitals and comprised 484 cases and 484 controls. No association was found with the estimated dose from diagnostic X-rays to the thyroid (Inskip *et al.*, 1995). [The Working Group noted that studies based on interviews have potential recall bias, as persons with disease are more likely to recall past exposure than controls who do not have cancer.]

(*b*)   During childhood

(i)   Multiple diagnostic X-rays for scoliosis

A cohort study was conducted of 973 women in the USA who had received multiple diagnostic X-rays during follow-up for scoliosis between 1935 and 1965 (Hoffman *et al.*, 1989). Follow-up was for an average of 26 years. The incidence of breast cancer was determined from mailed questionnaires. The average dose to the breast was estimated to have been 0.13 Gy (0–1.59 Gy); some women had received over 600 spinal X-rays during the adolescent growth spurt and after. Eleven women developed breast cancer, whereas 6.0 would have been expected in the general population (SIR, 1.8; 90% CI, 1.0–3.0) [The Working Group noted that pregnancy risk factors could not be accounted for, raising the possibility that confounding could have contributed partially to the small number of observed cases. Women with severe scoliosis were less likely to marry than women in the general population, and they also had difficulty in becoming pregnant. As nulliparity is associated with an increased risk for breast cancer, it may confound the reported association.]

(ii)   Exposure in utero

The risks for cancer in childhood after exposure *in utero* have been studied (UNSCEAR, 1994; Doll & Wakeford, 1997). Prenatal X-rays were first associated with childhood leukaemia and cancer in the 1950s (Stewart *et al.*, 1958), and most of the subsequent studies showed a consistent 40% increase in the risk for childhood cancer (excluding leukaemia) associated with intrauterine exposure to low doses. These studies have been reviewed extensively (Committee on the Biological Effects of Ionizing Radiation, 1972, 1980; UNSCEAR, 1972, 1986, 1994). The evidence for an association comes from case–control studies of the use of X-rays for pelvimetry, while none of the cohort studies has demonstrated an excess risk (Court Brown *et al.*, 1960a; Boice & Miller, 1999). As a study of atomic bomb survivors who were exposed *in utero* showed no cases of childhood leukaemia, the causal nature of the association seen in the medical case–control studies has been questioned (Jablon & Kato, 1970).

The largest study of childhood cancer after prenatal exposure to X-rays is the Oxford Survey of Childhood Cancers, which is a national case–control study in the United Kingdom (Bithell & Stewart, 1975; Knox *et al.*, 1987; Muirhead & Kneale, 1989; Doll & Wakeford, 1997). The study was started in 1955 and, up to 1981, the mothers of 15 276 children with cancer and the same number of matched controls had been interviewed. The relative risks associated with exposure just before birth were about 1.4 for leukaemia and for all other childhood cancers, including Wilms tumour, neuroblastoma, brain cancer and non-Hodgkin lymphoma. It has been noted (Miller, 1969; UNSCEAR, 1994; Boice & Miller, 1999) that the similarity in the relative risks is unusual, given the difference in the incidence rates of these diverse tumours, their different origins and etiologies and the variation in risks for cancer after exposure to radiation in childhood and in adulthood (Thompson *et al.*, 1994; UNSCEAR, 1994; Pierce *et al.*, 1996). It is also peculiar that embryonic tumours could be induced by exposure only a few moments before birth, and that the incidences of tumours such as lymphomas would be increased, since they have not been convincingly associated with exposure to radiation. The 1.4-fold increase in the incidence of each form of childhood cancer in the British studies may hint at an underlying bias in the case–control studies that has eluded detection (Miller, 1969; Boice & Miller, 1999).

Initial criticisms of the Oxford Survey of Childhood Cancer included the potential for recall bias, in that the mothers of children with cancer might remember their experiences during pregnancy better than mothers of control children. These concerns were minimized when a large study in the USA was published in 1962 (MacMahon, 1962), which was based on medical records of X-ray examinations and not on the mother's recall of events some years in the past. An extension of the study published in 1984, however, no longer showed an excess risk for solid tumours related to prenatal X-ray, although the risk for leukaemia remained (Monson & MacMahon, 1984).

Case–control studies of childhood cancer in twins have generally shown associations with prenatal exposure (Harvey *et al.*, 1985; MacMahon, 1985; Mole, 1990), but cohort studies of twins showed no excess of childhood cancer, and most reported deficits of childhood leukaemia (Inskip *et al.*, 1991; Boice & Miller, 1999).

In 1997, Doll and Wakeford estimated that the excess risk associated with prenatal exposure to radiation was 6% per gray. Other interpretations of the same data, however, resulted in different conclusions about the causal nature of the association and the level of risk (Mole, 1974; MacMahon, 1989; Mole, 1990; Boice & Inskip, 1996; Boice *et al.*, 1996). The association is not questioned, but its etiological significance is. The medical profession has acted on the assumption that the association is causal, and X-rays for pelvimetry have been largely replaced by ultrasound procedures.

2.4   Occupational exposure

The earliest observations of the effects of γ- and X-rays on health were associated with occupational exposure. Case reports of skin cancer among early workers with X-rays were published soon after Röntgen's discovery of X-rays in 1895, and increased numbers of deaths from leukaemia among radiologists were reported in the 1940s (Doll, 1995; Miller, 1995).

Occupational exposure to ionizing radiation is common in medicine, the production of nuclear power, the nuclear fuel cycle, and military and industrial activities.

Workers in these industries who are potentially exposed to radiation are monitored for exposure with personal dosimetry systems.

Epidemiological studies of occupational exposure to radiation have been conducted for surveillance and to complement risk estimates from studies of populations exposed to high doses. Studies of individual facilities are rarely large enough to provide substantial information, as the doses are low. Therefore, mainly combined analyses and the largest individual studies are presented here. The discussion is also limited primarily to studies in which most of the subjects were monitored for external exposure and in which internal comparisons were made by dose.

2.4.1   Medical use of radiation

Studies of medical personnel exposed to radiation rarely had information on individual doses, and surrogate measures, such as first year worked or duration of work, were sometimes used. Generally, comparisons were made with population rates or a control group, and risk could not be quantified. The studies of early radiologists provide substantial evidence that radiation at high doses can cause leukaemia and other cancers. Before the hazards of excessive exposure to radiation were recognized, severe skin damage and low leukocyte counts were reported. The doses are estimated to have been of the order of many grays.

The first reports of an increased incidence of leukaemia among US radiologists were based on death notices published in *The Journal of the American Medical Association* (Henshaw & Hawkins, 1944; March, 1944). The report of March covered the years 1929–43 and showed a significant, tenfold increase in the proportional mortality ratio for leukaemia among radiologists, on the basis of eight cases. These findings were confirmed in similar analyses in the same journal in 1935–44 (Ulrich, 1946) and 1945–57 (Peller & Pick, 1952). A more formal analysis was conducted by Lewis (1963), who reported increased risks for leukaemia (SMR, 3.0; 95% CI, 1.5–5.2; $n = 12$), multiple myeloma (SMR, 5.0; 95% CI, 1.6–11.6; $n = 5$) and aplastic anaemia (SMR, 17; 95% CI, 4.7–44.5; $n = 4$) in 1948–61. In the most recent study, a cohort of 6524 radiologists was followed-up during 1920–69 (Matanoski *et al.*, 1975a,b), and the risk for leukaemia was found to be statistically significantly increased among those who had joined a radiological society in 1920–29 (1117 persons; SMR, 3.0) or 1930–39 (549 persons; SMR, 4.1) [confidence intervals not reported] when compared with the general population. No such increase was observed for other physicians.

In a study of cancer mortality in 1977 among 1338 British radiologists who had joined a British radiological society in 1897–1954, statistically significantly increased risks for cancers of the skin (SMR, 7.8; $n = 6$), lung (SMR, 2.2; $n = 8$) and pancreas (SMR, 3.2; $n = 6$) and for leukaemia (SMR, 6.15; $n = 4$) were observed among radiologists who entered the study before 1921 [confidence intervals not reported]. No significant excess of these cancers was observed among radiologists who had joined the society after 1920 (Smith & Doll, 1981).

Similarly, an increased incidence of cancer was reported in a cohort study of 27 011 Chinese radiologists and X-ray technologists in 1950–85 when compared with 25 000 other physicians in the same hospitals (Wang *et al.*, 1990a). The overall relative risk for leukaemia was 2.4 ($p < 0.05$; $n = 34$), which was seen mainly among those first employed before 1970, aged < 25 at initial employment and who had been employed for 5–14 years. Increased risks for cancers of the skin, oesophagus and liver were also observed, but the risks for the last two were thought to be related to other factors, such as alcohol consumption.

[The Working Group noted that the findings in different countries are consistent, and the association of risk with the year of first employment suggests that the excess of leukaemia is likely to be related to occupational exposure to radiation.]

No excess cancer mortality was observed in a cohort of 143 517 radiological technologists in the USA who had been certified during 1926–80; however, the risk for breast cancer was significantly elevated relative to all other cancers in a test for homogeneity of the SMRs (ratio of SMRs, 1.3; $p < 0.0001$). Significant risks were correlated with employment before 1940 (SMR, 1.5; 95% CI, 1.2–1.9), when the doses of radiation are likely to have been highest, and among women who had been certified as radiological technicians for more than 30 years (SMR, 1.4; CI, 1.2–1.7), for whom the cumulative exposure is likely to have been greatest (Doody *et al.*, 1998). The risk for breast cancer in women was not associated with surrogate measures of exposure in a nested case–control analysis within this cohort (Boice *et al.*, 1995).

2.4.2   *Clean-up of the Chernobyl nuclear reactor accident*

Between 600 000 and 800 000 workers ('liquidators') are thought to have parti-cipated in cleaning-up after the accident in the restricted 30-km zone around the Chernobyl power plants and in contaminated areas of Belarus and the Ukraine between 1986 and 1989 (200 000 in 1986–87) (Cardis *et al.*, 1996). They came from all areas of the former USSR, the largest numbers from the Russian Federation and Ukraine. Many are registered in the national Chernobyl registries in each country. A small proportion (around 36 000) were professional radiation workers from other nuclear research centres and power plants, but the great majority were military reservists, construction workers and others.

In most of the papers published to date, the mortality rates and sometimes the morbidity due to cancer of the liquidators have been compared only with those of the general population (Buzunov *et al.*, 1996; Cardis *et al.*, 1996; Okeanov *et al.*, 1996; Ivanov *et al.*, 1997a; Rahu *et al.*, 1997). An increased incidence of leukaemia was reported among Belarussian, Russian and Ukrainian liquidators who worked in the 30-km zone, but no excess was found in a small Estonian study with complete follow-up (Rahu *et al.*, 1997). These results are difficult to interpret, however, because of the different intensities of follow-up of the liquidators and the general population (Cardis *et al.*, 1996).

Ivanov *et al.* (1997b, 1998) reported the results of a cohort study of 169 372 emergency workers, including 119 000 (71%) for whom individual doses of external exposure were available. The mean age of the workers during their period of duty in the 30-km zone was 33.4 years. Of the 46 575 persons with the highest exposure, who were exposed in 1986, 4.5% have been assigned doses in excess of 250 mGy. In a nested case–control study of leukaemia within the subcohort of emergency workers with officially documented doses, no significant difference was seen in dose between 34 cases occurring more than two years after first exposure and 136 controls matched on date of birth (± 3 years) and region of residence (Ivanov *et al.*, 1997a). [The Working Group noted the uncertain dosimetry.]

2.4.3   *Nuclear industry workers*

These studies are summarized in Table 21.

(*a*)   *United Kingdom*

A combined study of three cohorts of nuclear industry workers in the United Kingdom (Carpenter *et al.*, 1994), including the Atomic Energy Authority (Fraser *et al.*, 1993), the Sellafield plant (Douglas *et al.*, 1994) and the Atomic Weapons Establishment (Beral *et al.*, 1988), covered 75 006 employees who had started work between 1946 and 1988; 40 761 had ever been monitored for exposure to radiation, and the rest formed an unexposed control group. The mean cumulative dose equivalent was 56.5 mSv. The mean duration of follow-up was 24 years. A lag of two years for leukaemia and 10 years for other cancers was assumed for dose–response analysis. There were 1884 deaths from cancer, of which 60 were from leukaemia. When information on social class was used to adjust for potential confounding, a statistically significant association was found between cumulative dose and leukaemia (regardless of exclusion or inclusion of chronic lymphocytic leukaemia), skin cancer (including melanoma; 10-year lag) and ill-defined and secondary neoplasms (10-year lag). The excess relative risk for leukaemia (excluding chronic lymphocytic leukaemia) was 4.2 per Sv (95% CI, 0.4–13), and the estimate for other cancers was −0.02 (−0.5, 0.6) (10-year lag).

In one of the largest studies on the association between cancer and exposure to radiation, a cohort of 124 743 persons working in nuclear energy production, the nuclear fuel cycle or production of atomic weapons were identified from the National Registry for Radiation Workers in the United Kingdom (Muirhead *et al.*, 1999), including all of those mentioned above and persons from several other facilities. Follow-up was begun between 1976 and 1983 and continued up to the end of 1992. Information on social class was available and adjusted for. The mean lifetime radiation dose equivalent was 30.5 mSv. The highest mean dose was that of Sellafield workers (87 mSv), who constituted half of all the workers and had a cumulative dose > 100 mSv (Douglas *et al.*, 1994). The only exposure for which information was

Table 21. Cohort studies of nuclear industry workers

Facility or database (reference)	No. of subjects	Mean dose (mSv)	ERR for all cancers per Sv (except as noted) (lag period = 10 years)	ERR for leukaemia per Sv (except as noted)
Sellafield, United Kingdom (Douglas et al., 1994)	14 282	128[a]	0.1 (90% CI, −0.4, 0.8)[b]	14 (90% CI, 1.9, 70.5)[c,d]
Atomic Energy Authority, United Kingdom (Fraser et al., 1993)	39 718	40	0.8 (95% CI, −1.0, 3.1)[b]	−4.2 (95% CI, −5.7, 2.6)[d]
Atomic Weapons Establishment, United Kingdom (Beral et al., 1988)	22 552	8	7.6 (95% CI, 0.4, 15)[e]	NR
National Registry of Radiological Workers, United Kingdom (Muirhead et al., 1999)	124 743	30.5	0.09 (90% CI, −0.28, 0.52)	2.55 (90% CI, −0.03, 7.2)[c,d]
Hanford site, USA (Gilbert et al., 1993a)	44 154	23	−0.1 (90% CI, < 0, 0.8)[e]	−1.1 (90% CI, < 0, 1.9)[d,e]
Oak Ridge X-10 and Y-12 plants, USA (Frome et al., 1997)	28 347[f]	10	1.45 (95% CI, 0.15, 3.5)	< 0 (95% CI, < 0, 6.5)[d]
Oak Ridge nuclear power plant, USA (Wing et al., 1991)	8 318	17	3.3 (95% CI, 0.9, 5.7)[e]	6.9 (95% CI, −15, 28)[e,g]
Atomic Energy Canada (Gribbin et al., 1993)	8 977	15	0.36 (90% CI, −0.46, 2.45)[e]	19 (90% CI, 0.14, 113)[d,e]
International collaborative study (Cardis et al., 1995)	95 673	40	−0.07 (90% CI, −0.4, 0.3)[b]	2.2 (90% CI, 0.1, 5.7)[c,d]

Table 21 (contd)

Facility or database (reference)	No. of subjects	Mean dose (mSv)	ERR for all cancers per Sv (except as noted) (lag period = 10 years)	ERR for leukaemia per Sv (except as noted)
Combined analyses				
Combined analysis of three facilities, United Kingdom (Carpenter et al., 1994)	75 006	56.5	0.03 (95% CI, −0.5, 0.7)	4.2 (95% CI, 0.4, 13)[c,d]
Combined analysis, USA (Gilbert et al., 1993b)	44 943	[27]	−0.0 (90% CI, <0, 0.8)	−1.0 (90% CI, <0, 2.2)[a,f]

ERR, excess relative risk; NR, not reported; < 0, negative value
[a] Muirhead et al. (1999) give 90 mSv
[b] Excluding leukaemia
[c] Excluding chronic lymphocytic leukaemia
[d] Lag period, 2 years
[e] % per 10 mSv
[f] Number of workers included in the dose–response analyses
[g] Lag period, 10 years

available was external radiation. This was lagged by two years for the analysis of leukaemia and by 10 years for other cancers. A total of 3598 deaths from cancer was observed in analyses without lagging, and 2929 in lagged analyses; leukaemia other than chronic lymphocytic leukaemia accounted for 90 and 89 deaths, respectively. No significant association was found between the dose of radiation and all cancers (ERR per Sv, 0.09; 90% CI, -0.28, 0.52; $n = 2929$) or leukaemia (other than chronic lymphocytic leukaemia; ERR per Sv, 2.55; 90% CI, -0.03, 7.2; $n = 89$). The only type of malignancy for which there was a significant association with radiation was multiple myeloma (ERR per Sv, 4.1; 90% CI, 0.03–15; $n = 35$), although a dose-dependent excess of 'ill-defined and secondary neoplasms' was reported (ERR per Sv, 2.4; 90% CI, 0.48–5.5; $n = 201$).

(b)   USA

The most informative study in the USA of workers at nuclear sites is a large combined analysis of 44 943 monitored workers (Gilbert et al., 1993b) at the Hanford nuclear site (Gilbert et al., 1993a), the Oak Ridge National Laboratory (Wing et al., 1991) and the Rocky Flats nuclear weapons site (Wilkinson et al., 1987). The mean length of follow-up was 19 years and the average dose was 27 mSv. There were 1871 deaths from cancer. For all cancer sites combined, the excess relative risk estimate was -0.0 per Sv (with an upper 90% confidence limit of 0.8). There were 67 deaths from leukaemia other than the chronic lymphocytic type, and the excess relative risk estimate was negative (-1.0 per Sv; upper 90% confidence limit, 2.2). Statistically significant excesses associated with the radiation dose were observed for cancers of the oesophagus and larynx and for Hodgkin disease, but these were interpreted as likely to be due to chance, as negative correlations with dose were found for the same number of sites. There was a statistically significant association between dose and cancer risk for people aged ≥ 75. [The Working Group noted that the combined analysis was dominated by the data for workers at the Hanford site.]

A cohort study of mortality among 15 727 employees at the Los Alamos National Laboratory, a nuclear research and development facility, between 1947 and 1990, who had been hired in 1943–77 showed an association between the dose of radiation and cancers of the oesophagus and brain and Hodgkin disease, but not for leukaemia or all cancers combined (Wiggs et al., 1994). [The Working Group noted that no risk estimates per unit dose were given.]

A cohort study of mortality among 106 020 persons employed in 1943–85 at the four nuclear plants in Oak Ridge, Tennessee, showed a slight excess of deaths from lung cancer among white male employees (Frome et al., 1997). In a dose–response analysis restricted to 28 347 white men at two plants who had received a mean dose of 10 mSv, significant positive relationships were found with deaths from all causes (ERR per Sv, 0.31; 95% CI, 0.16–1.01), deaths from all cancers (ERR per Sv, 1.45; 95% CI, 0.15–3.5; $n = 4673$) and lung cancer (ERR per Sv, 1.7; 95% CI, 0.03–4.9; $n = 1848$) after adjustment for age, year of birth, socioeconomic status, facility and length of employment; however, no information on smoking was available. For leukaemia, the excess relative risk per sievert was negative (upper 95% confidence limit, 6.5; $n = 180$).

(c)   Russian Federation

A cohort study of people who had worked at the Mayak nuclear complex in the early years of its operation showed an increased mortality rate from all cancers and from leukaemia (44 cases; 38 men) (Koshurnikova et al., 1996). The mortality of 8855 workers who were first employed between 1948 and 1958 at the nuclear reactors, at the Mayak fuel reprocessing plants and at the plutonium manufacturing complex was followed-up for an average of 36 years. The mean cumulative dose of external radiation was 1 Gy. A control group was formed of 9695 persons who were employed during the same period but whose radiation doses did not exceed the maximum permissible level [unspecified]. The excess relative risk for leukaemia was estimated to be 1.3 per Gy [confidence interval not reported] for 26 men in the reprocessing plants, but no estimates were available for the other two groups. Tokarskaya et al. (1997) and Koshurnikova et al. (1998) evaluated the risk for lung cancer in relation to external γ-ray dose (1.8 Gy) and internal dose from plutonium of male workers at the radiochemical and plutonium plants, who had received an average equivalent dose to the lung from plutonium of 6.6 Sv. No evidence of an association with external dose was found (ERR = −0.16 per Gy [CI not reported]; $n = 47$), but this may have been due to inadequate adjustment for plutonium dose and lack of information on smoking. [The Working Group noted that the study was potentially very informative because the doses were much higher than those of other occupational cohorts, but there is uncertainty about the adequacy of the dose estimates, and follow-up may have been selective. Further, in the absence of information on potential confounding by exposure to plutonium, the extent to which external radiation contributed to the increased cancer risks is difficult to estimate.]

(d)   International collaborative study

A combined cohort study of mortality from cancer among 95 673 nuclear industry workers in Canada (Gribbin et al., 1993), the United Kingdom (Carpenter et al., 1994) and the USA (Gilbert et al., 1993b) has been published (IARC Study Group on Cancer Risk among Nuclear Industry Workers, 1994; Cardis et al., 1995). The persons had been employed for at least six months and had been monitored for external exposure. The activities of the nuclear facilities included power production, research, weapons production, reprocessing and waste management. The mean cumulative dose was 40 mSv. Data on socioeconomic status were available for all except the Canadian workers, and adjustment was made for this variable in the analysis. The combined analysis covered 2 124 526 person–years and 3976 deaths from cancer. The risk for leukaemia other than chronic lymphocytic leukaemia was statistically significantly associated with the cumulative external dose of radiation (one-sided p value, 0.046).

The excess relative risk estimate for leukaemia other than the chronic lymphocytic type was 2.2 per Sv (90% CI, 0.1–5.7; $n = 119$). There was no excess risk for cancer at any other site, and the excess relative risk estimate for all cancers except the leukaemias was −0.07 per Sv (90% CI, −0.4, 0.3; $n = 3830$). Of the 31 specific cancer types other than leukaemia, only multiple myeloma was statistically significantly associated with the exposure ($p = 0.04$; ERR per Sv, 4.2; 90% CI, 0.3–14; $n = 44$).

2.4.4   *Various occupations*

An association between dose of radiation and the rate of mortality from cancer was found in a study of 206 620 Canadian radiation workers (Ashmore *et al.*, 1998) identified from the National Dose Registry, established in 1951. All workers except uranium miners who were monitored for exposure to radiation between 1951 and 1983 were included in the study. Most of the participants were medical (35%) or industrial (38%) workers and the remainder were employed in dentistry (21%) or nuclear power production (6%). The workers had been monitored with a film or thermoluminescent dosimeter. Nearly half (45%) of the workers had received doses below the recording threshold (usually 0.2 mSv), and the mean external dose was 6.3 mSv. The mean length of follow-up was 14 years. A statistically significant association between dose of radiation and death from any cancer was detected among men (% ERR per 10 mSv, 3.0; 90% CI, 1.1–4.9) but not among women (% ERR per 10 mSv, 1.5; 90% CI, −3.3, 6.3). In addition, a dose–response relationship was found with lung cancer among men (% ERR per 10 mSv, 3.6; 90% CI, 0.4–6.9). No significant association was found with other cancers, including leukaemia and cancers of the thyroid and breast, but a dose–response relationship was found for all causes of death among both men and women and for deaths from circulatory disease and accidents among men. [The Working Group noted that a strong association was found with causes of death other than cancer, which suggests possible confounding, perhaps by factors such as smoking. The mortality rate from cancer was only 68% of that predicted from national rates, suggesting ascertainment bias.]

2.5   **Environmental exposure**

2.5.1   *Natural sources*

Most studies of natural radiation are based on comparisons of cancer incidence or mortality among populations living in areas with different background levels of radiation. A direct effect of background radiation is unlikely to be observed since it is likely to be small in comparison with that due to other causes. Furthermore, large populations must be studied in order to obtain sufficient statistical power, and it could be difficult to maintain the same standards of diagnosis and registration for large populations and areas. The studies that have been conducted to investigate the risk for cancer from naturally occurring radiation have generally found no association, but they are not particularly informative because of their low power and because most are ecological studies, which are difficult to interpret causally. The overwhelmingly negative results do suggest, however, that the carcinogenic risk represented by the low natural levels of radiation is unlikely to be substantial. The most important studies are summarized in Table 22.

Court Brown *et al.* (1960b) studied mortality from leukaemia in Scotland and related it to residence at the date of death and estimated dose to the bone marrow. The substantial variation in rates among the 10 areas in Scotland was suggested to be due to incomplete ascertainment of cases, economic status or background radiation.

In a study of 369 299 persons living in western Ireland, 2756 outdoor and 145 indoor measurements of γ-radiation were performed (Allwright *et al.*, 1983). The mortality rates from cancer were not related to residence in regression analyses, and no risk was found in relation to background exposure.

The incidences of leukaemia and non-Hodgkin lymphoma among children who were < 15 years of age at the time of diagnosis were studied during 1969–83 in 459 county districts in England, Wales and Scotland (Muirhead *et al.*, 1991) in relation to indoor radon and terrestrial γ-radiation. The incidences were not found to increase significantly with dose rate. When essentially the same database was used to analyse 6691 cases of childhood leukaemia diagnosed between 1969 and 1983 (16.5% acute nonlymphocytic leukaemia) with respect to background γ-radiation (Richardson *et al.*, 1995), no association was found, but a positive association between leukaemia incidence and socioeconomic status was revealed.

In contrast to the studies of Muirhead *et al.* (1991) and Richardson *et al.* (1995), Gilman and Knox (1998) found increased mortality rates from childhood leukaemia and solid tumours in relation to exposure to radon and terrestrial γ-radiation. The study was based on the Oxford Survey of Childhood Cancers and comprised 9363 deaths from solid tumours (48%) and from leukaemia and malignant lymphoma (52%) among children < 15 years of age during the period 1953–64. Although indoor γ-radiation was associated with an increased risk, once radon was introduced into the regression model terrestrial γ-radiation did not contribute significantly to the risk.

Mortality from lung cancer was studied in an area of central Italy with high background radiation from outdoor sources of γ-radiation (2.4 mSv year^{-1}) and high doses of ^{226}Ra and ^{232}Th from building materials (Forastiere *et al.*, 1985). When villages on volcanic and non-volcanic soil were compared, no significant difference in mortality from lung cancer was noted after adjustment for tobacco sales. In an Italian case–control study, 44 men with acute myeloid leukaemia were compared with 211 male controls (Forastiere *et al.*, 1998) in relation to measurements of radon and indoor γ-radiation performed in 1993–94. A nonsignificantly decreased odds ratio was found for higher background exposure both to radon and to γ-radiation.

In an ecological study, standardized cancer rates for all 24 Swedish counties were correlated to the average background radiation based on measurements of γ-radiation in 1500 dwellings chosen at random (Edling *et al.*, 1982). Significant correlations

Table 22. Epidemiological studies of cancer associated with natural background radiation

Country/region (reference)	Characteristics of study	Main results
Scotland (Court Brown et al., 1960b)	Mortality from leukaemia in 10 major areas of Scotland compared with natural background radiation in four areas	An effect of radiation could not be ruled out, but social and economic factors were considered to be at least as important.
Irelan (Allwright et al., 1983)	Ecological study of cancer mortality rates and natural background radiation measured outdoors ($n = 2756$) and indoors ($n = 145$); highest and lowest doses differed by a factor of approximately 5 (McAulay & Colgan, 1980), and ~370 000 individuals included	No significantly elevated risk related to natural background radiation
United Kingdom (Muirhead et al., 1991; Richardson et al., 1995)	Incidence of childhood leukaemia in 459 county districts compared with exposure to indoor radon and γ-radiation and outdoor γ-radiation	No increased risk for leukaemia attributed to ionizing radiation, but a positive association of leukaemia incidence with socioeconomic status
United Kingdom (Gilman & Knox, 1998)	Mortality from childhood solid cancers and leukaemia in 1953–64 (9363 deaths) compared with residence, social class, radon and terrestrial γ-radiation	Increased incidences in areas of high socioeconomic status and in areas of high population density. Radon, but not significantly γ-radiation, affected the risk for dying from a solid tumour but not leukaemia or malignant lymphoma.
France (Tirmarche et al., 1988)*	Cancer mortality in seven 'départements' with high background γ-radiation compared with national rates	Increased mortality linked to background radiation only for childhood leukaemia, which was statistically significant in only one 'département'
Italy (Forastiere et al., 1985)	Lung cancer mortality in 31 villages in volcanic and non-volcanic areas in central Italy correlated to outdoor γ-radiation and cigarette sales	No significant difference in lung cancer mortality between volcanic and non-volcanic villages after adjustment for tobacco sales
Italy (Forastiere et al., 1998)	Five controls matched to each of 44 men who had died of acute myeloid leukaemia compared with indoor radon and γ-radiation	Nonsignificant decrease in odds ratio with increasing background radiation

Table 22 (contd)

Country/Region (reference)	Characteristics of study	Main results
Sweden (Stjernfeldt *et al.*, 1987)*	One control chosen for each of 15 cases of childhood cancer, and exposure to indoor à-radiation and radon measured	No difference in cumulative exposure to γ-radiation or radon daughters; low statistical power
Sweden (Edling *et al.*, 1982)	Cancer incidence in 24 Swedish counties correlated to γ-radiation measured in 1500 homes	Correlation for lung and pancreatic cancer but borderline correlation for leukaemia. Degree of urbanization and smoking most likely influenced the results.
Sweden (Flodin *et al.*, 1990)*	172 controls randomly selected for 86 cases of acute myeloid leukaemia; background radiation approximated from construction materials in homes and work places	Significantly increased risk for leukaemia when 'high-dose' exposure was contrasted to 'low-dose'. Selection of controls, approximation of exposure, and lack of information on number of cases of chronic lymphocytic leukaemia preclude firm conclusions.
Yangjiang, China (Tao & Wei, 1986; Wei *et al.*, 1990; Chen & Wei, 1991; Wei & Wang, 1994)	Ecological study of cancer mortality rates in thorium–monazite areas and a control area	Nonsignificantly lower rates of leukaemia, breast and lung cancer in the high background area but increased prevalence of stable chromosomal aberrations
Japan Noguchi *et al.*, 1986)	Correlation between background radiation and cancer mortality during 1950–78	Increased mortality correlated to background levels in some sites and negative correlations in others. Findings considered to be unrelated to radiation.
India (Nambi & Soman, 1987)	Cancer incidence in 5 Indian cities correlated to background γ-radiation of 0.3–1 mSv	Decreasing incidence with increasing background dose
USA (Mason & Miller, 1974)	Correlation of cancer mortality and altitude in 53 counties at an altitude > 3000 ft [> 900 m]	No significant difference in comparison with US national rates

Table 22 (contd)

Country/Region (reference)	Characteristics of study	Main results
USA (Amsel et al., 1982)	Relationship between altitude, urbanization, industrialization and cancer in 82 US counties	Generally, deficits in cancer mortality rates at high altitude
Connecticut, USA (Walter et al., 1986)	Cancer incidence related to background radiation, population density and socioeconomic status in data for 1935–74	No relationship with background radiation, but a high cancer incidence in areas of high population density
USA (Weinberg et al., 1987)	Correlation between cancer mortality, altitude and background irradiation in US cities at an altitude > 900 ft [> 250 m]	No overall correlation between background radiation and cancer or leukaemia

* Not described in text

were seen for cancers of the lung and pancreas in both men and women, but only a borderline correlation to leukaemia in men was seen. An association was found between degree of urbanization and γ-radiation. [The Working Group noted that cigarette smoking is more common in urban areas and among men, but no adjustment was made for smoking.]

In Yangjiang province, China, thorium-containing monazites have been washed down by rain from the nearby heights and raised the level of background radiation to three times that in adjacent areas of similar altitude. Several studies have been performed to derive indoor and outdoor doses, and individual doses have been measured with personal dosimeters. More than 80 000 individuals who live in the high background areas were estimated to receive an annual dose to the red bone marrow of 2.1 mSv, whereas the dose of those in the control area was 0.77 mSv. Nonsignificantly lower rates of mortality from all cancers and from leukaemia, breast cancer and lung cancer were found in the high background areas (Tao & Wei, 1986; Wei et al., 1990; Chen & Wei, 1991; Wei & Wang, 1994). Although a significantly higher risk for cancer of the cervix uteri was found in the high background area, it was considered not to be due to the ionizing radiation. Nevertheless, a higher frequency of stable chromosomal aberrations (translocations and inversions) was found in the high-dose area (see section 4.4.1). [The Working Group noted that, in contrast to the previous studies, migration was not a potential problem and that both indoor and outdoor exposures were considered.]

The correlation between background radiation and cancer mortality was studied in 46 of 47 prefectures of Japan for the period 1950–78 (Noguchi et al., 1986). Correlations were found only in women, with positive correlations for stomach cancer and uterine cancer and negative correlations for cancers of the breast, lung, pancreas and oesophagus. [The Working Group noted that only γ-radiation was considered and altitude was not taken into consideration.]

High natural background levels of radiation are also present in Kerala, India. Although studies have shown very little evidence for an excess cancer risk, they have been of limited quality. Cancer incidence and background γ-radiation were investigated in five Indian cities with background levels of 0.3–1 mSv (Nambi & Soman, 1987). A significantly decreased overall cancer incidence was observed with increasing dose, but the authors underlined the limited extent of cancer registration in India.

The association between cosmic radiation and cancer was investigated in two studies in the USA (Mason & Miller, 1974; Amsel et al., 1982), which found no increased risk for leukaemia or solid tumours in relation to altitude.

The relationship between background radiation, population density and cancer was studied with data from the Connecticut Tumor Registry for the period 1935–74 (Walter et al., 1986), and data from an airborne survey of γ-radiation to approximate the annual doses in 169 towns. No increased risks were found in relation to level of γ-radiation. [The Working Group noted that the advantages of the study were use of incidence rather than mortality data, the fairly high level of background radiation and a reasonable variation in exposure between towns.]

In order to study the simultaneous effects on mortality rates of altitude and terrestrial background radiation, all cities in the USA situated at an altitude > 900 feet [> 250 m] were identified in the metropolitan mortality report for 1959–61 (Weinberg et al., 1987), and information on background radiation, including cosmic radiation, was added. Background radiation did not appear to affect the rates of leukaemia or of cancers of the breast, intestine or lung. When altitude was added, the association was negative.

2.5.2   Releases into the environment

(a)   The Chernobyl accident

As noted above, the accident at the fourth unit of the Chernobyl nuclear power plant led to substantial contamination of large areas. [The dramatic increase in the incidence of thyroid cancer in persons exposed to radioactive iodine as children (Cardis et al., 1996) will be discussed during a forthcoming IARC Monographs meeting on radionuclides.] In a follow-up in the Ukraine, the incidences of leukaemia and lymphoma in the three most heavily contaminated regions (oblasts) were found to have increased during the period 1980–93 (Prisyazhniuk et al., 1995); however, the incidences of leukaemia (including chronic lymphocytic leukaemia) and other cancers in countries of the former USSR had shown an increasing trend before the accident, in 1981, which was most pronounced in the elderly (Prisyazhniuk et al., 1991). The findings are based on few cases, and increased ascertainment and medical surveillance are likely to have influenced them. [The Working Group emphasized the importance of taking the underlying increasing trend into account in interpreting the results of studies focusing on the period after the Chernobyl accident.]

In a study of the population of Kaluga oblast, the part of the Russian Federation nearest Chernobyl, in 1981–95, no statistically significant increase in trends of cancer incidence or mortality was seen after the accident, although a statistically significant increase in the incidence of thyroid cancer was observed in women (Ivanov et al., 1997c).

The European Childhood Leukaemia–Lymphoma Incidence Study was designed to address concerns about a possible increase in the risk for cancer in Europe after the Chernobyl accident. The results of surveillance of childhood leukaemia in cancer registry populations from 1980 up to the end of 1991 were reported by Parkin et al. (1993, 1996). During the period 1980–91, 23 756 cases of leukaemia were diagnosed in children aged 0–14 (655 × 10^6 person–years). Although there was a slight increase in the incidence of childhood leukaemia in Europe during the period studied, the overall geographical pattern of change bears no relation to estimated exposure to radiation from the Chernobyl fall-out.

All 888 cases of acute leukaemia diagnosed in Sweden in 1980–92, after the Chernobyl accident, in children aged 0–15 years, were examined in a population-based study in which place of birth and residence at the time of diagnosis were included (Hjalmars et al., 1994). A dose–response analysis showed no association between the degree of contamination and the incidence of childhood leukaemia.

Auvinen et al. (1994) reported on the incidence of leukaemia in Finland among children aged 0–14 in 1976–92 in relation to fall-out from the Chernobyl accident, measured as external exposure in 455 municipalities throughout the country. The incidence of childhood leukaemia did not increase over the period studied, and the excess relative risk in 1989–92 was not significantly different from zero.

The incidence of leukaemia among infants in Greece after exposure in utero as a consequence of the Chernobyl accident was found to be higher in children born to mothers who lived in areas with relatively greater contamination (Petridou et al., 1996). On the basis of 12 cases diagnosed in infants under the age of one year, a statistically significant increase in the incidence of infant leukaemia was observed (rate ratio, 2.6; 95% CI, 1.4–5.1). No significant difference in the incidence of leukaemia among 43 children aged 12–47 months born to presumably exposed mothers was found. [The Working Group was unclear why the authors chose to limit their analysis to infants, as there is little etiological reason for doing so.]

In a study of childhood leukaemia in relation to exposure in utero due to the Chernobyl accident based on the population-based cancer registry in Germany (Michaelis et al., 1997; Steiner et al., 1998), cohorts were defined as exposed or unexposed on the basis of date of birth and using the same selection criteria as Petridou et al. (1996). Overall, a significantly elevated risk was seen (RR, 1.5; 95% CI, 1.0–2.15; $n = 35$) for the exposed when compared with the unexposed cohort. The incidence was, however, higher among infants born in April–December 1987 (RR, 1.7; 95% CI, 1.05–2.7) than among those born between July 1986 and March 1987 (RR, 1.3; 95% CI, 0.76–2.2), although the exposure of the latter group in utero would have been greater than that of the former group. The authors concluded that the observed increase was not related to exposure to radiation from the Chernobyl accident.

(b)   Populations living around nuclear installations

A number of studies have been conducted of populations living near nuclear installations (Doll et al., 1994; UNSCEAR, 1994), and some have shown unexpected associations between exposure to radiation and cancer in either potentially exposed persons or their offspring.

A cluster of childhood leukaemias was reported around the Sellafield nuclear installation in the United Kingdom in 1983 (Black, 1984). Childhood leukaemia was subsequently reported to be occurring in excess in other regions of the United Kingdom where there were nuclear installations, although the incidence of all cancers was not increased (Forman et al., 1987). These observations were not replicated in Canada (McLaughlin et al., 1993b), France (Hill & Laplanche, 1990; Hattchouel et al., 1995),

Germany (Michaelis *et al.*, 1992) or the USA (Jablon *et al.*, 1991), although associations were reported around a reprocessing plant in France (Viel *et al.*, 1995; Pobel & Viel, 1997). More refined analyses in the United Kingdom gave little evidence that the incidence of childhood leukaemia was related to proximity to nuclear facilities, except for the Sellafield installation (Bithell *et al.*, 1994). Another study conducted in England and Wales showed that the incidence of childhood leukaemia was increased around sites selected for nuclear facility construction but in which the facilities had not been completed (Cook-Mozaffari *et al.*, 1989). An infectious agent associated with large migrations of people into these areas has been proposed as a possible explanation for the clusters (Kinlen *et al.*, 1991; Kinlen, 1993a). These ecological analyses are severely limited by the absence of information on individual doses of radiation, but they were probably lower than the dose of natural background radiation (Darby & Doll, 1987). [The Working Group noted that unknown factors associated with migration and selection of residence and occupation could play a major role in cancer occurrence.] Other studies around nuclear facilities have failed to provide clear insight into the reasons, other than chance or selection, for the apparent clusters of childhood cancer (MacMahon, 1992; Draper *et al.*, 1993).

A case–control study of leukaemia and non-Hodgkin lymphoma among children around Sellafield raised the possibility that exposure of the fathers who worked at the facility might explain the cluster. Four cases of leukaemia were seen among children whose fathers received doses $\geq$ 10 mSv within six months of conception (Gardner *et al.*, 1990). These findings were not replicated in a similar but smaller study at the Dounreay nuclear facility in Scotland (Urquhart *et al.*, 1991) or in two further surveys in Scotland (Kinlen, 1993b; Kinlen *et al.*, 1993) and one in Canada (McLaughlin *et al.*, 1993c). Further, a study of 10 363 children who were born to fathers who worked at the Sellafield facility included an evaluation of the geographical distribution in the county of Cumbria of the paternal dose received before conception. The paternal doses were consistently higher for fathers of children born outside Seascale, a village close to Sellafield where the original cluster was found. Since the incidence of child-hood leukaemia was not increased in these areas of West Cumbria, despite the higher preconception exposures, the authors concluded that paternal exposure to radiation before conception is unlikely to be a causal factor in childhood leukaemia (Parker *et al.*, 1993). The hypothesis was also not substantiated in further studies (Doll *et al.*, 1994; Committee on Medical Aspects of Radiation in the Environment, 1996).

A further study of cancer among the children of nuclear industry employees in the United Kingdom was conducted with a questionnaire approach (Roman *et al.*, 1999). Employees at three nuclear establishments were contacted, and 111 cancers (28 leukaemias) were reported among 39 557 children of male employees and 8883 children of female employees. The incidences of all cancers and of leukaemia were similar to those in the general population; however, the rate of leukaemia in children whose fathers had accumulated a preconceptual dose $\geq$ 100 mSv was significantly higher (5.8; 95% CI, 1.3–25) than that in children born before their fathers' employment in the nuclear industry, but this result is based on only three exposed cases. [The Working Group noted that two of these three cases were included in the study of Gardner *et al.* (1990) which generated the hypothesis, and should have been excluded in order that the study be considered an independent test of the hypothesis that paternal irradiation results in childhood leukaemia. Further, the approach used probably resulted in substantial under-ascertainment of the number of cases of childhood cancer because no effort was made to obtain information on children of workers who had died; ex-employees who were not on the pensions database were not contacted; ex-employees of one of the three nuclear establishments and persons over the age of 75 were not contacted at all; an unstated number of questionnaires was returned undelivered; and 18% of the male workers who received the questionnaires failed to return them. Comparison with a record linkage study that included all children of nuclear industry workers in the United Kingdom (Draper *et al.*, 1997) indicates that as many as two of every three childhood cancers may have been missed. The study is therefore susceptible to biases related to incomplete ascertainment of children with cancer and to the reasons for responding or failing to respond to the questionnaire.]

The nuclear reactor accident at Three-Mile Island, Pennsylvania (USA), released little radioactivity into the environment and resulted in doses to the population that were much lower than those received from the natural background. Any increase in the incidence of cancer would thus be expected to be negligible and undetectable (Upton, 1981). An ecological survey found no link between estimated patterns of radiation release and increased cancer rates (Hatch *et al.*, 1990; Jablon *et al.*, 1991). Other studies of the Three-Mile Island incident have given inconsistent results (Fabrikant, 1981; Wing *et al.*, 1997) and provide little evidence for an effect of radiation.

2.6   Issues in quantitative risk assessment

The wealth of data and the availability of quantitative estimates of biologically relevant measures of dose or exposure have led to the development of intricate approaches for estimating the magnitude of risks due to exposure to γ- and X-rays. These approaches, which have drawn on information obtained from both epidemiological and experimental studies, have then been used to estimate the risks from various exposures. In this section, several measures of risk are defined, problems and uncertainties in estimating those risks are discussed, and recent efforts of major national and international groups to provide quantitative risk estimates are summarized. Several estimates of risks from particular sources of exposure are given as illustrations.

2.6.1   *Measures of risk*

In general, summary measures of risk are based on the assumption that variation in risk among individuals within a population can be ignored (at least for certain purposes) and that the concept of an average risk for a population is meaningful. An important measure of risk is the lifetime risk that an individual will die from a cancer that has been caused by exposure to a carcinogenic agent such as radiation. The lifetime risk is sometimes referred to as the risk of exposure-induced death and differs from the excess lifetime risk (National Council on Radiation Protection and Measurements, 1997), which does not include deaths from cancers that would have occurred without exposure but which occur at a younger age because of the exposure (Thomas *et al.*, 1992). Such risks are dependent on dose and thus must be expressed as a function of dose. In the most commonly used linear model, the risk is often expressed per unit of dose. Lifetime risk estimates may depend on sex, age at exposure and the pattern of exposure over time. Approaches have been developed that allow estimation of sex-specific lifetime risks resulting from various patterns of exposure with regard to age and time. For example, the risk from single exposures at various ages or from continuous exposure over a specified period can be estimated. Lifetime risks also depend on many individual characteristics, but too little is known about such dependence for it to be taken into account. Rigorous definitions and interpretations of measures such as attributable risk and the probability of causation have been discussed extensively (Greenland & Robins, 1988). Only a broad definition is given here.

Once a model for estimating the lifetime risks of individuals has been developed, it can be applied to all individuals in a population (such as an entire country) to estimate the total number of cancers that are expected to occur as a result of exposure to various specified doses. Since risks often depend on sex and age at exposure, such estimates require demographic data on the population for which the risk estimates are being made. Like individual risks, population risks can be expressed as a function of dose, or per unit of dose for a linear model.

If estimates of the doses or distribution of doses received by a population from a particular source of radiation are available, the models for estimating lifetime risks can be applied to estimating the number of cancer deaths associated with exposure from the source. This number is sometimes expressed as a fraction of the total number of cancer deaths that have occurred in the population and is known as the attributable risk. A closely related quantity is the probability of causation, which is identical to the 'assigned share', which is the probability that a cancer that has already occurred in an individual was caused by radiation (Lagakos & Mosteller, 1986). Radiation risks are commonly measured in terms of cancer mortality, but all of the above measures can also be used to estimate the risk for non-fatal cancer. None of these measures reflects the age at which death from cancer occurs. An additional measure that takes account of age is the loss of life expectancy, which was defined and discussed by Thomas *et al.* (1992). This is sometimes expressed as the number of years of life lost per radiation-induced cancer.

2.6.2   *Problems and uncertainties in quantifying risks due to radiation*

Models or sets of assumptions are needed to estimate any of the quantities described above, and their development and application are described below in general terms. For more rigorous treatment, the reader is referred to Bunger *et al*. (1981), Thomas *et al.* (1992) or any of the documents describing the specific risk models summarized below.

The most recent attempts at risk assessment are based on epidemiological data, so that age-specific cancer mortality or incidence rates are estimated as a function of baseline rates and parameters that characterize the relationship between risk and exposure to radiation. The risk from radiation is usually expressed as a function of dose, age at the time of exposure, time since exposure, sex and sometimes other factors. These functions are then used in combination with data on the characteristics of the population.

A commonly used model takes the form:

$$\lambda\ (a,\ s,\ D,\ e,\ t) = \lambda\ (a,\ s)\ [1 + f\ (a,\ s,\ D,\ e,\ t)]$$

where $\lambda\ (a,\ s,\ D,\ e,\ t)$ is the age-specific rate for age (a), sex (s), dose (D), age at exposure (e) and time since exposure (t); $\lambda\ (a,\ s)$ is the baseline risk at age (a) and sex (s) and $f\ (a,\ s,\ D,\ e,\ t)$ is the ERR associated with a, s, D, e and t. A key feature of this model is that risks are expressed relative to the baseline rather than in absolute terms. If life-table methods are used, the age-specific risks $\lambda\ (a,\ s)$ and $\lambda f\ (a,\ s,\ D,\ e,\ t)$ can be applied to demographic data for the population for which risk estimates are being made to obtain lifetime risk estimates or any of the other measures described above. In this application, the baseline risks $\lambda\ (a,\ s)$ are usually derived for the population of interest (Committee on the Biological Effects of Ionizing Radiation (BEIR IV), 1988).

Because the populations and exposures for which risk estimates are desired nearly always differ from those for which epidemiological data are available, assumptions are required, many of which involve considerable uncertainty. Some of the more important assumptions are discussed below, and the approaches used to address these problems in specific risk assessments are described in section 2.6.4.

Most situations for which risk estimates are desired involve exposure to low doses and dose rates. Because the estimates obtained directly from epidemiological data on populations exposed to low doses are imprecise, it is necessary to extrapolate from risks estimated for persons exposed to higher doses and dose rates than those of direct interest. Specifically, the data on the atomic bomb survivors have played a strong role in developing models for risk estimation, and estimates based on those data tend to be driven by doses > 1 Gy, which is much higher than the doses for which risk estimates are needed, < 0.1 Gy. Although many epidemiological findings are compatible with a linear dose–response function in which risk is proportional to dose, other forms, such as a linear–quadratic relationship, cannot be excluded. Because experimental data have suggested that the risk per unit of dose is lower when radiation is received at low rates than when it is received at high rates, linear estimates of risk at low doses and dose rates are often reduced by a factor known as the dose-and-dose-rate-effectiveness factor. Although a factor of 2 has been used in several risk assessments, the magnitude of the factor, or whether it is needed at all, is uncertain. Because of the large uncertainty in the risks associated with exposures to < 0.1 Gy, some committees such as the Committee on the Biological Effects of Ionizing Radiations (BEIR V; 1990) have refrained from publishing estimates below this level and have noted the possibility that there is no risk at very low doses. Further discussion of this issue is given in section 2.7.

Although the risk for cancer associated with exposure to radiation has been found to depend on sex, age at exposure and the time between exposure and diagnosis or death, the available data are not adequate to determine the exact form and magnitude of such dependence, and risk estimates are usually based on relatively simple assumptions. For example, many estimates of the risk for solid tumours are based on the assumption that, for a given age at exposure, the ratio of the risk associated with radiation to the baseline risk, the ERR, remains constant as subjects are followed over time; however, some data suggest that this ratio declines over time, and populations have not yet been followed for their entire lifespans. The risks of people exposed at young ages are particularly uncertain, since follow-up of these persons is the least complete. The data on many cancer types indicate that the relative risk is greatest for people exposed early in life, but the magnitude of the increase and whether it persists throughout life is highly uncertain.

Another difficulty is that the baseline cancer risks of the population being studied may differ from those of the population for which risk estimates are desired. This has been a major concern in using data on Japanese survivors of the atomic bombings to estimate risks for white populations, especially for certain specific cancers, as the baseline rates of cancers of the breast, lung and colon are much lower in Japan than, for example, in the United Kingdom or the USA; in contrast, the rate of stomach cancer is much higher in Japan. In order to address this problem, some risk estimates (Committee on the Biological Effects of Ionizing Radiations (BEIR III), 1980) were based on the assumption that absolute risks do not depend on baseline risks, while others were based on the assumption that radiation risks are proportional to baseline risks (Committee on the Biological Effects of Ionizing Radiations (BEIR V), 1990). The risk for breast cancer can be estimated from the results of studies of white women (Abrahamson et al., 1991), but adequate data on non-Japanese populations are not available for many other cancers. The problem is less severe for leukaemia and for all solid tumours combined, since the baseline rates for these categories do not vary as greatly among countries.

A closely related problem is that smoking and other life-style factors may modify risks. This is especially important in estimating risks for individuals, but also affects population risks if these factors differ in the population used to develop the risk models and in that for which risk estimates are desired. In fact, these differences are probably part of the reason for differences among baseline rates in different countries.

Ideally, risk models should take account of the modifying effect of other exposures and life-style factors, but in practice too little is known to allow this.

Increasing attention is being given to quantifying the uncertainties in risk estimates. The sources of uncertainty include lack of knowledge about the correct assumptions, as discussed above, and these uncertainties must often be assessed subjectively. Sampling variation is another important source of uncertainty, but it differs from most other sources in that it can be quantified by reasonably rigorous statistical approaches, although it may be necessary to use Monte Carlo computer simulations to address the complex dependence of lifetime risk on the parameters that are estimated (Committee on the Biological Effects of Ionizing Radiations (BEIR V), 1990). Still other sources of uncertainty are possible errors and biases in the epidemiological data used, including errors in the estimated doses. Methods are available for addressing these uncertainties, but they are often difficult to apply and require a thorough understanding of the magnitude and nature of the errors.

2.6.3 *Lifetime risk estimates by national and international committees*

The vast literature relevant to radiation risk assessment is reviewed periodically by national and international committees, and several such reviews have included summary estimates of lifetime risks. In this section, the more recent efforts of UNSCEAR (1988, 1994), the Committee on the Biological Effects of Ionizing Radiations (BEIR V; 1990) and the ICRP (1991a) are briefly summarized.

(*a*) *UNSCEAR*

In their 1988 report, UNSCEAR provided estimates of lifetime risk that served as the basis for recommendations of the ICRP (1991a). Estimates were given for death from leukaemia, from all cancers except leukaemia and from several other types of cancer. For all cancers, separate estimates were given for the total population, for a working population aged 25–64 years and for an adult population aged ≥ 25. The estimates were based on the data on mortality among survivors of the atomic bombings during 1950–85, as presented by Shimizu *et al.* (1990). The lifetime risk estimates were based on demographic data for the population of Japan in 1982. Alternative estimates based on patients with ankylosing spondylitis or cervical cancer who were exposed to radiation were also given.

UNSCEAR (1988) used two approaches for extrapolating risks beyond the period for which follow-up data were available: an additive model, in which it was assumed that the absolute risk is constant over time, and a multiplicative model, in which it was assumed that the ratio of the radiation-induced cancer risk to the baseline risk (ERR) is constant over time. Because baseline risks increase as persons age, the multiplicative model generally results in larger estimates than the additive model. The additive model is no longer thought to be appropriate for solid tumours. For leukaemia, it was assumed that risks persist for 40 years after exposure, while for solid tumours it was assumed that the risks persist through the remainder of life. The estimates for most cancers were assumed not to depend on sex or age at exposure, but for leukaemia and the category 'all cancers except leukaemia' estimates based on age in categories of 0–9, 10–19 and ≥ 20 years were presented. The estimates were based on a linear model, but UNSCEAR recommended that the effects of low doses (< 0.2 Gy) and low dose rates (< 0.05 mGy/min) be reduced by a factor of 2–10, although no specific recommendation was made.

UNSCEAR (1994) presented lifetime risk estimates for leukaemia and several categories of solid tumour. The approach was similar to that used in 1988, in that the estimates were based on data on the mortality of atomic bomb survivors during 1950–87 and applied to the Japanese population in 1985 to obtain lifetime risks; however, the analyses used to derive the estimates were more refined than those used in 1988. In the model for leukaemia, the excess absolute risk was expressed as a linear–quadratic function of dose and was allowed to depend on sex, age at exposure (separate parameters estimated for 0–19, 20–34 and ≥ 35 years) and time since exposure (treated as a continuous variable that allowed the risk to decrease with time). Estimates were also presented for tumours of the oesophagus, stomach, colon, liver, lung, bladder, breast, ovary, other sites and all solid tumours. The ERRs were allowed to depend on sex and age at exposure, and the latter was treated as a continuous variable and evaluated separately for each cancer evaluated. The lifetime estimates were based on the assumption of constant relative risk, in which the ratio of the risk for radiation-induced cancer to the baseline risks was assumed to be constant over time. For the category of all solid tumours, lifetime risk estimates were also presented from two alternative models, in which the ERR was assumed to be constant for the first 45 years of follow-up and to then decline linearly with age. In the first alternative model, the risks were assumed to decline linearly until they reached the risk for exposure at the age of 50. In the second alternative model, the risks were assumed to decline linearly to reach zero risk at age 90. These alternatives yielded lifetime risks that were 20 and 30%, respectively, below those predicted by the constant relative risk model.

The resulting estimates of lifetime risk were compared with those given in the 1988 report by age-specific coefficients and multiplicative risk projection. The estimates for leukaemia were nearly identical in 1988 and 1994, whereas the 1994 estimate for all solid tumours based on the constant relative risk model was only slightly higher than that of 1988. UNSCEAR did not recommend that the estimates be modified but did recommend that the risks for solid tumours be reduced by a factor of about 2 for exposure to low doses (< 0.2 Sv).

(b)   Committee on the Biological Effects of Ionizing Radiations (BEIR V; 1990)

Unlike the models of UNSCEAR, those of BEIR V were developed for application to the population of the USA, and thus demographic data for the 1980 population were used in calculating lifetime risks. The BEIR V report provides estimates of the excess mortality from leukaemia and all cancers except leukaemia that would be expected to result from a single exposure to 0.1 Sv, from continuous lifetime exposure to 1 mSv per year and from continuous exposure to 0.01 Sv per year from the age of 18 until the age of 65, with separate estimates for men and women. Estimates of the number of excess deaths (with confidence intervals), the total years of life lost and the average years of life lost per excess death are given. For each exposure scenario, separate estimates are presented for leukaemia and for cancers of the breast, respiratory tract, digestive tract and other cancers, for each sex and for nine categories of age at exposure.

The estimates of BEIR V were based on models in which the ERR was expressed as a function of sex, age at exposure and time since exposure. Separate models were developed for leukaemia and the four categories of solid tumours listed above. The models were based primarily on analyses of data on the mortality of atomic bomb survivors, although the models for breast and thyroid cancers drew on data from several other epidemiological studies. The lifetime risk estimates were based on a multiplicative model in which the relative risks are assumed to be the same for the US population and Japanese survivors of the atomic bombings.

The ERR for leukaemia was found to depend on age at exposure and time since exposure, and separate estimates were made for each of several categories defined by these variables. The ERR for female breast cancer depended on time since exposure (treated as a continuous variable) and age at exposure (< 15, about 20 and ≥ 40 years); the risks increased and then declined with time since exposure and decreased with increasing age at exposure. The ERR for respiratory cancer depended on sex and time since exposure (treated as a continuous variable and indicating a decline with time) but not on age at exposure. The ERR for digestive cancers depended on sex and age at exposure (treated as a continuous variable with a decline starting at age 25) but not on time since exposure. For other cancers, the ERRs depended only on age at exposure (treated as a continuous variable with a decline starting at age 10), with no dependence on sex or time since exposure.

In order to estimate the risks for leukaemia at low doses and dose rates, a linear–quadratic model was used, which reduced the effect by a factor of 2 below the estimates that would have been obtained from a linear model. For cancers other than leukaemia, a linear model was used, with a non-specific recommendation to reduce the estimates obtained through linear extrapolation by a factor of 2–10 for doses received at low rates.

(c)   ICRP

ICRP (1991a) reviewed the estimates provided by UNSCEAR (1988) and by the BEIR V Committee (1990) and recommended use of the estimates obtained from the UNSCEAR age-specific additive model for leukaemia and from the UNSCEAR age-specific multiplicative model for all cancers other than leukaemia. ICRP also recommended that the linear risk estimates obtained from data on high doses be reduced by a factor of 2 for exposures to < 0.2 Gy or < 0.1 Gy h⁻¹. ICRP provided separate estimates for a working population and for the total population, including children.

ICRP was especially concerned with developing tissue weighting factors (w_T) to allow for their relative sensitivity to cancer. Such weighting factors are useful for estimating the detrimental effects of radiation received at non-uniform doses by various organs of the body (see section 1.4, Overall introduction). To develop these weighting factors, lifetime risks for several types of cancer were calculated from age-specific risk coefficients for the survivors of the atomic bombings. As the factors were to be applicable to the world population, separate calculations were made with reference populations from China, Japan, Puerto Rico, the United Kingdom and the USA on the basis of three sets of assumptions for projecting risks over time and across countries. In estimating risks for cancers of the thyroid, bone surface, skin and liver, ICRP (1991a) considered sources of data other than that on atomic bomb survivors. Other factors that were used in developing the weighting factors were the lethality of each type of cancer and the reduction in lifespan that would result.

(d)   Summary

Table 23 summarizes the lifetime risk estimates per 10^4 person–Gy for a population of all ages and each sex. The reasons for the differences among these estimates were discussed by Abrahamson *et al.* (1991) and Thomas *et al.* (1992). Table 24 shows the contributions of specific cancers to total mortality from cancer as proposed by ICRP and as used in developing the weighting factors.

2.6.4   *Estimates of risk due to specific sources of radiation*

Estimates of the risks attributable to specific sources of radiation are often of interest. As discussed in section 2.6.1, this requires that the magnitude of the doses be estimated. For a linear model, the total exposure, often referred to as the collective dose, may be sufficient. For exposures that vary by age or sex (such as medical and occupational exposure), information is required on such variation, since the risks depend on these factors. For exposures that involve non-uniform doses to various organs of the body, doses to specific organs are required. A few illustrative examples are given briefly below; for details, readers should consult the references indicated. The Working Group made no judgement about the validity of the methods used or the results obtained.

(a)   Natural background

Darby (1991) estimated the number of cancers expected to occur annually in relation to exposure to natural background ionizing radiation in the USA. The source of data on exposure was a report of the National Council on Radiation Protection and Measurements (1987a), which provided estimates of the effective dose equivalents received annually by an average member of the US population from various com-

Table 23. Estimates of lifetime risk for fatal cancer (excess deaths per 10^4 persons exposed to 1 Sv for a population of all ages and each sex)

Type of cancer	UNSCEAR (1988)[a]		BEIR V[b] (1990)	ICRP (1991a)
	Multiplicative[c]	Additive[d]		
Linear estimates[e]				
Leukaemia	97 (100)	93 (100)	[95]	100
All cancers except leukaemia	610 (970)	360 (320)	[695][f]	900
Total	707 (1070)	453 (420)	790	1000
Estimates for low dose and dose rate				
Leukaemia			47.5	50
All cancers except leukaemia				450

[a] The 1994 UNSCEAR report provided a linear–quadratic lifetime risk estimate of 110 for leukaemia after exposure to 1 Sv and linear estimates ranging from 750 to 1090 for solid tumours, but recommended continued use of the age-specific multiplicative estimates from the 1988 report. Based on constant (age-averaged) risk coefficients; those in parentheses were based on age-specific risk coefficients.
[b] Committee on the Biological Effects of Ionizing Radiations. Unlike estimates from other reports, those of BEIR V do not include radiation-induced cancer deaths in persons who would have died of cancer later.
[c] Based on a multiplicative model in which it is assumed that relative risks remain constant over time
[d] Based on an additive model in which it is assumed that the absolute risks remain constant over time
[e] Do not include modification for dose and dose rate reduction factors
[f] Sum of the BEIR V estimates for female breast cancer, respiratory cancer, digestive system cancers and other cancers

ponents of natural background radiation. The values used were 0.27 mSv from cosmic radiation, 0.22 mSv from terrestrial γ-radiation, 0.01 mSv from cosmogenic radio-nuclides, 2.0 mSv from inhaled radionuclides (mainly radon and its daughters) and 0.39 mSv from other radionuclides in the body. The first three sources irradiate the body uniformly, whereas the non-uniform nature of the remaining sources was taken into account in calculating the resulting effective dose equivalents. There is no important variation in such exposures by age or sex. The risk due to radon was eva-luated separately from those due to other sources, and only the non-radon sources were considered, which provided a total dose of about 1.0 mSv per person per year.

Darby (1991) applied the BEIR V model to data on US mortality rates and popu-lations in 1987 and estimated that each year about 6700 cancer deaths would be expected to occur in men and 7100 in women as a result of postnatal exposure to natural background radiation other than radon. She also estimated the numbers of deaths from leukaemia (men, 900; women, 700), respiratory cancers (men, 1800; women, 1800), female breast cancer (700), digestive cancers (men, 1300; women, 1900) and other cancers (men, 2700; women, 2000). These were then expressed as

**Table 24. Contribution of cancers in specific
organs to mortality from all cancers in a
general population**

Organ	Fatal probability coefficient (per 10^4 person–Sv)
Bladder	30
Bone marrow	50
Bone surface	5
Breast	20
Colon	85
Liver	15
Lung	85
Oesophagus	30
Ovary	10
Skin	2
Stomach	110
Thyroid	8
Remainder	50
Total	500

From ICRP (1991a)

attributable risks on the basis of the observation that they comprised 2.8% of all cancer deaths in men and 3.6% in women. She further noted that the BEIR V model for cancers other than leukaemia is based on linear extrapolation from risk estimates obtained from data on persons exposed to high doses and dose rates, and may require modification for application to the low doses and dose rates from natural background sources. If the risk estimates are halved to account for this modification, the attributable risks would be about 1.6% for men and 2.0% for women.

(b)   Medical diagnosis

Kaul *et al.* (1997) estimated the annual collective effective dose from medical diagnostic radiation in Germany in 1990–92 in order to evaluate the risk associated with such exposure. They first used health insurance and hospital records to estimate the number of examinations with X-ray and diagnostic medical procedures that had been conducted in the former Federal Republic of Germany. The effective doses from each type of procedure were then estimated, by thermoluminescent dosimetry for the X-ray procedures and information provided in ICRP publications (1991a,b) for the nuclear medical procedures. The collective dose was estimated by multiplying the effective doses associated with each type of examination by the estimated annual frequency of the procedure, and then summing over all procedures. Using this approach, Kaul *et al.* (1997) estimated an annual collective effective dose of about

115 000 person–Sv from X-ray diagnosis and 5000 person–Sv from diagnostic nuclear medicine for the former Federal Republic of Germany, which had a population of 65 million in 1992.

The risk calculations were based on ICRP recommendations (1991a), although the authors noted that the ICRP risk estimate of 5.2% per Sv (lifetime probability of radiation-induced fatal cancer) for a population covering all ages is not fully appropriate because medical exposures are much more frequent at older than at younger ages. By taking into consideration both the age-specific risk calculations provided in an appendix to the ICRP report (1991a) and information on the age distribution of the recipients of the procedures in Germany, they concluded that the estimate of 5.2% per Sv could be reduced by a factor of 0.6–0.7 to estimate the risk from diagnostic medical examinations. Use of a 0.6 reduction led to an estimate of approximately 0.5% for the average additional lifetime risk of fatal cancer attributable to medical irradiation, which can be compared with a 'spontaneous' total fatal cancer risk of 25%. [The Working Group calculated that the attributable risk would then be 0.5/25, or 2%.]

(c)   Dental radiography

White (1992) estimated the worldwide risk from dental radiography by adjusting the risk estimates from several sources so that they were all expressed in terms of full-mouth examinations and by substituting the ICRP (1991a) risk coefficient for the original risk coefficients, which were usually based on earlier data than used by ICRP. This standardization resulted in an average estimate of 2.5 fatal cancers per million full-mouth examinations. The worldwide risk was estimated on the basis of a United Nations report that 340 million dental radiographic procedures had been performed in 1980, with four films per procedure. The estimate of 2.5 fatal cancers per million full-mouth examinations was then converted to an estimate of 0.5 fatal cancers per million procedures, which resulted in an estimate of about 170 annual cancer fatalities world-wide due to dental radiography. White (1992) noted that the universal adoption of alternative films (E-speed films) and procedures (rectangular collimation) could reduce this estimate by a factor of 5.

(d)   Mammography

Mammographic screening and treatment can reduce the risk for fatal breast cancer, but since the radiation involved can cause breast cancer, the procedure also involves risk. Comparisons of the risks and benefits are clearly of interest. Mettler *et al.* (1996) estimated the annual risks and benefits for women in the USA who had annual mammographies beginning at the age of 35, 40 or 50. They used ERR coefficients specific for age at exposure obtained from data on atomic bomb survivors (Tokunaga *et al.*, 1994) but adjusted for differences in the baseline risks for breast cancer in Japan and the USA. The coefficients were applied to data on breast cancer incidence in 1973–90 in selected areas of the USA that are covered by cancer registries. Assumptions were made about the dose per mammography, the reduction in the risk for dying from breast cancer resulting from screening, the percentage of breast cancers that are fatal and the latency for breast cancer. On the basis of these assumptions and calculations, it was concluded that the benefits substantially outweigh the risks, with a 5% reduction in the rate of mortality from breast cancer with annual screening at the ages of 35–39 and a 25% reduction with screening at ages ≥ 40.

2.7   Other issues in epidemiological studies

The previous section dealt with quantitative issues in risk assessment. Other important epidemiological issues are the statistical power of a study to detect convincingly a cancer excess after exposure to radiation and other factors that modify the effect of radiation, such as age at the time of exposure.

The single most important study of radiation carcinogenesis in human populations is that of the Japanese atomic bomb survivors (Pierce *et al.*, 1996), as it is a long-term prospective cohort study in which a defined group of survivors have been followed forward in time since 1945 to determine their causes of death; more recently, cancer incidence has been evaluated (Thompson *et al.*, 1994). A single exposure to 2 Sv is estimated to double the risk, i.e. cause a 100% excess in the relative risk (RR, 2) for death from any solid tumour. The ability of epidemiological studies to detect such a twofold increase in risk is quite good. A single exposure to 1 Sv is estimated to be associated with a relative risk of about 1.4–1.5, and epidemiological methods are often sufficient to conclude causal associations of this magnitude. The excess absolute risk is about 10 extra cancers per year among 10 000 persons exposed to 1 Sv, and the lifetime risk is about 10% per Sv; i.e. 10 in 100 persons acutely exposed to 1 Sv of whole-body radiation would be predicted to develop a radiation-induced cancer sometime during their lifetime. At an exposure of only 0.1 Sv, the predicted relative risk is only 1.05, i.e. a 5% excess, and epidemiologists have difficulty in detecting such low risks. Sampling variability and inability to control for confounding factors provide 'noise' that swamps the small signal to be detected. Thus, estimates of effects at low doses are obtained by extrapolation from data on people exposed to high doses (Boice, 1996).

It is further assumed that estimates obtained from acute or brief exposures should be reduced by a factor of about 2 when exposure is spread over time and not instantaneous, although the possible range in the reduction factor is 2–10. Leukaemia is usually separated from other cancers because its minimum latency is shorter (about two years after exposure) and its mechanism of development may be different. The minimum latency before solid tumours appear after irradiation is about 5–10 years.

Summary estimates of risks associated with radiation can be used as guidelines for setting protection standards and health policy, although even estimates based on high doses are subject to uncertainty (National Council on Radiation Protection and Measurements, 1997). The five broad areas of uncertainty are: epidemiological uncertainties, dosimetric uncertainties, transfer of risk between populations, projection to a lifetime model and extrapolation to low doses or low dose rates. Risk varies by age at exposure, sex, time after exposure, dose rate, type of radiation, total dose and the presence of other factors such as cigarette smoke. Some cancers, such as chronic lymphocytic leukaemia, have not been associated with exposure to radiation (Boice, 1996). The convention of combining all cancers to obtain a global estimate of risk is a source of error as some cancers have not been associated with radiation and the sites of other cancers differ appreciably in their sensitivity to induction. At very low doses, radiation damage may be repaired, which might influence risk. In the absence of reliable data on the effects of low doses, it is often assumed that extrapolation to low doses should be linear and without a threshold. This assumption remains controversial, some people contending that a threshold does exist, others contending that the risks are higher than those estimated from a linear relationship and still others contending that low exposures may be beneficial (Fry *et al.*, 1998; Upton, 1999).

2.7.1   Scale of measurement

The scale of measurement is important in evaluating variation in the ability of radiation to induce specific cancers (tissue sensitivity) and the modifying effects of co-factors such as age. A relative scale is influenced by the baseline cancer incidence in the population being studied, and populations with different baselines have different risk coefficients. For example, the rate of naturally occurring breast cancer in Japan is much lower than that in western countries, and the relative risk for radiation-induced breast cancer per sievert is higher in Japanese atomic bomb survivors than in western women exposed to radiation (UNSCEAR, 1994). Differences in radiation-related relative rates between populations can thus be due to differences in the background incidence rates. On an absolute scale, the excess number of cancers occurring per person per year per dose is compared. If the relative risk for radiogenic cancers remains constant with this exposure, then the absolute risk will change at each follow-up period.

2.7.2   Complicating factors

Although perhaps more is known about radiation than any other carcinogen, with the possible exception of tobacco, there remain complicating factors which limit generalization of the findings (Table 25). Risk varies with dose, but not always in a linear fashion. The risk may be lower when low doses are delivered at low rates, but most of the evidence of effects comes from studies of high doses delivered at high rates. Risk depends on the sex of the individual exposed and the age at exposure. Risk varies by time since exposure. Exposure to high-LET radiation such as α-particles and neutrons appears to be associated with higher risks than exposure to low-LET radiation (X-rays, γ-rays and electrons). The presence of certain genetic, environmental or lifestyle factors may influence risk to an extent that is not yet well defined (Boice, 1996).

Table 25. Factors that complicate generalizations about estimates of risk associated with exposure to radiation

Factor	Comment
Dose dependence	Cell killing at high doses, repair at low doses
Dose rate	Higher risk for brief exposure, repair at low dose rates
Sex	Somewhat higher risk for women
Age	Somewhat higher risk for people exposed at a young age
Latency	Risk varies by time after exposure.
Co-factors	Smoking enhances the risk associated with radon and may potentiate the effect of radiotherapy; chemotherapy may interact with radiotherapy.
Genetic susceptibility	High-dose radiotherapy of susceptible patients may enhance their risk for malignancies, such as bone cancer after retinoblastoma.
Outcome	Cancer incidence may differ appreciably from cancer mortality, e.g. for the thyroid.
Background rates	Radiation risk varies for different cancers and in relation to the background rate (on a relative or absolute scale).
Tumour type	Cancer sites differ in inducibility, and some cancers have not been convincingly linked to radiation.
Cellular factors	Radiation damage can be repaired, but some errors occur. The extent of cellular repair at low doses is not known. The relevance of genomic instability and of the 'bystander effect' is yet to be determined

(a)   Dose

The dose of radiation to an organ is the most important consideration for risk estimation, and dose–response relationships must be understood since it is necessary to extrapolate from high doses. If the relationship were linear, extrapolation to lower doses would be straightforward. Over a broad range of doses in experimental and human studies, however, the relationship is not always linear, either at the highest or the lowest doses. For example, women who have been treated with radiation for cervical cancer have an increased risk of developing leukaemia, but the dose–response relationship is complex (Day & Boice, 1984; Boice et al., 1987; Blettner & Boice, 1991): the risk increases with doses up to about 4 Gy and decreases or levels off at higher doses (Figure 8). This reduction in risk at high doses has been attributable to cell killing, since so much energy is deposited into small volumes of bone marrow that the cells are destroyed or rendered incapable of division. Studies of atomic bomb survivors also show an apparent decrease in the risks for leukaemia and solid tumours at 2.5 Sv (Figures 4 and 5), although that may reflect dosimetric errors (Pierce et al., 1996). Other studies that have shown a decrease or levelling off of risk at high doses include those of women irradiated for mastitis in whom the risk for breast cancer declines (Shore et al., 1986), women irradiated for endometrial cancer in whom the

Figure 8. Dose–response relationships for leukaemia among women who have been treated with radiation for cervical cancer

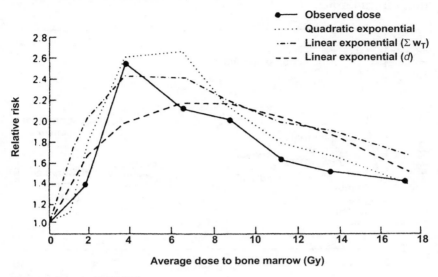

Adapted from Boice (1996)

risk for leukaemia reaches a plateau (Curtis *et al.*, 1994) and children given radio-therapy for cancer in whom the risk for thyroid cancer levels off and there is no increased risk for leukaemia (Tucker *et al.*, 1987b, 1991; Boice, 1996).

The risk coefficients and dose–response relationships for leukaemia vary appreciably among the populations studied. The data on atomic bomb survivors (Figure 4) show a linear–quadratic response to radiation in the low dose range (Preston *et al.*, 1994; Pierce *et al.*, 1996). Partial exposure of the body to high doses in medical procedures with various dose rates and various contributions of fractionation results in a variety of risk coefficients per gray (Figure 9). These differences among studies suggest a complex interplay between cell killing, fractionation, lengthened dose interval and neoplastic transformation in defining dose–response relationships.

For single whole-body exposures, the relationship between mortality from all cancers except leukaemia among the atomic bomb survivors is consistent with linearity up to about 3 Sv (Figure 10) (Pierce *et al.*, 1996). A significant excess is seen at 0.2–0.5 Sv, and is suggested down to 0.05 Sv; extrapolation to lower doses on the basis of a linear model appears reasonable. The authors caution, however, that reporting bias may have contributed to the shape of the dose–response curve at low doses in that Japanese physicians appeared to have been more likely to record cancer as the primary cause of death for people exposed to low doses than for those receiving high doses. The incidence data (Thompson *et al.*, 1994) are also consistent with linearity,

Figure 9. Relative risks for leukaemia by dose of radiation in survivors of the atomic bombings and patients receiving high doses in radiotherapy

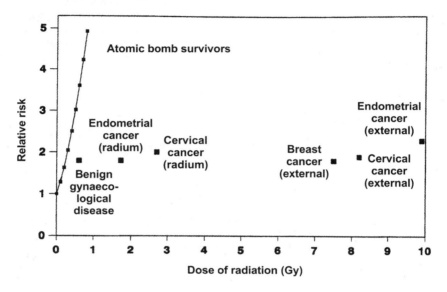

Adapted from Boice *et al.* (1996)

Figure 10. Dose–response relationship for all cancer except leukaemia among atomic bomb survivors

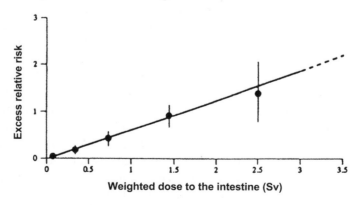

Adapted from Boice (1996)

although cancers of the breast and thyroid may disproportionally influence the aggregate data.

One complicating factor in estimating the risk associated with low doses is the extent to which neutrons (see separate monograph in this volume) may have influenced the shape of the dose–response curve. The bomb dropped on Hiroshima resulted in exposure to neutrons in addition to γ-rays. While the exact contribution of neutrons to the total dose is under investigation, the greater effectiveness of neutrons in causing cancer at low doses could be responsible for the seeming linearity of the dose–response curve. The larger the fraction of the total dose attributed to neutrons, the smaller will be the estimate of the risk attributable to photons. In the absence of exposure to neutrons, the dose–response relationships would be expected to be curvilinear, consistent with the majority of experimental data for exposure to γ-rays (Kellerer & Nekolla, 1997). Some analyses of the incidence of cancer among atomic bomb survivors indicate that a threshold or non-linear dose–response model is more suitable than a linear model for some cancers (Hoel & Li, 1998) and especially leukaemia (Little *et al.*, 1999) and skin cancer (Little *et al.*, 1997).

At very low doses, the relationship between cancer and exposure to radiation becomes blurred because the excess number of cancers at low doses predicted from studies of exposure to high doses is so much smaller than the spontaneous incidence, i.e. one in three persons is expected to develop cancer during his or her lifetime. Extrapolation of risks derived from studies of exposure to high doses to lower levels requires use of a model selected on the basis of the fundamental principles of radiation biology (UNSCEAR, 1993). The model used in radiation protection is the linear–quadratic function, which is a derivative of the linear non-threshold model with allowance for effects of low doses and low dose rates (Beninson, 1997; Sinclair, 1998; Upton, 1999).

Some scientists contend that linearity exaggerates the risk of low doses. They base their arguments on phenomena such as the ability of cellular mechanisms to repair damage to DNA induced by radiation, the absence of an excess risk for leukaemia among atomic bomb survivors exposed to low doses and among US military personnel who participated in nuclear tests, the absence of a risk for lung cancer in ecological studies of indoor exposure to radon, the absence of an excess risk for thyroid cancer among patients given ^{131}I, the absence of an excess of cancer in populations living in areas with high background radiation and others (Yalow, 1994; Cohen, 1995; Pollycove, 1995; Yalow, 1995; IAEA, 1997; Pollycove, 1998). They contend that epidemiological findings for people exposed to high doses at high rates should not be extrapolated to low doses, where the risk may be negligible or non-existent. These arguments are being considered by various scientific committees (Fry *et al.*, 1998; Upton, 1999).

(b)   *Dose rate*

Dose rate, i.e. the time over which a radiation dose is delivered, may influence risk in a variety of ways. In experimental animals, the risk per unit dose is usually greater at higher dose rates, for the same cumulative dose of low-LET radiation (Fry, 1992; UNSCEAR, 1993). It is thought that increasing the duration of exposure may increase the opportunity for cellular repair.

Perhaps the most thoroughly studied cancer with regard to the effects of fractionating low-LET radiation is that of the breast (Boice *et al*., 1979; Land *et al*., 1980; UNSCEAR, 1994). Large studies of patients with tuberculosis who were exposed to multiple chest fluoroscopies several times per month for three to five years in order to monitor lung collapse showed linear increases in the risk for breast cancer with increasing dose to the breast (Boice *et al*., 1991a; Howe & McLaughlin, 1996; Little & Boice, 1999). The age-specific absolute risk estimates were similar to those seen in studies of women irradiated for acute post-partum mastitis and among atomic bomb survivors. While fractionation did not seem to lower the risk for breast cancer measurably in the patients with tuberculosis, fractionation may well have influenced the risk for lung cancer. Despite an average cumulative dose of nearly 1 Gy, no excess lung cancers have been observed in these large series (Davis *et al*., 1989; Howe, 1995), and no excess risk for leukaemia has been reported after repeated chest fluoroscopies (Davis *et al*., 1989). Studies in experimental animals also indicate that the spectrum of tumour types may be different after protracted rather than brief exposure (see section 3; Fry, 1992; UNSCEAR, 1993; Upton, 1999).

Few studies have directly addressed the possible lowering of risk when exposure is protracted. No increase in the risk for thyroid cancer was seen in patients given diagnostic doses of ^{131}I, which has a half-life of only eight days, although the absence of risk may have been due to the older age of the patients when exposed or to the distribution of dose within the thyroid gland (Hall *et al*., 1996). Leukaemia did not occur in excess after ^{131}I treatment for hyperthyroidism (Holm *et al*., 1991; Ron *et al*., 1998b), although the dose to the bone marrow was small. Studies of working populations may provide useful guidance about the risks of low, protracted doses, although the number of excess cancers attributable to radiation is so far small and was of the order of 10 in a combined series of nearly 100 000 workers (Cardis *et al*., 1995).

ICRP (1991a) assumes a dose and dose rate effectiveness factor of 2 for radiation protection, i.e. the risk coefficients available for the atomic bomb survivors are reduced by half. The Committee on the Biological Effects of Ionizing Radiations (BEIR; 1990) and UNSCEAR (1988, 1993, 1994) indicate that a factor between 2 and 10 might be used, although a value closer to 3 has been suggested (UNSCEAR, 1993). Since the sites of cancer vary in their inducibility by radiation, they would also vary with respect to the protective effect of protraction. The factor for breast might be close to 1, whereas that for lung might be 10 (Howe, 1995; Boice, 1996; Howe &

McLaughlin, 1996). Perhaps the most important unanswered question in radiation epidemiology is the level of risk after prolonged as opposed to brief exposure.

(c) Age

Age at exposure can affect the response to radiation. In general, children appear to be at somewhat greater risk than adults. For example, women who were < 20 when they were exposed are at greater risk for breast cancer than women who were older, and little risk is associated with exposure after the menopause (Land *et al.*, 1980; Boice *et al.*, 1991b; UNSCEAR, 1994). The data on atomic bomb survivors show the dependence on age at exposure of the subsequent risk for breast cancer, children being at highest risk and women over the age of 40 at small or minimal risk (see Figure 6). The risk for radiogenic thyroid cancer appears to be concentrated almost entirely among children under the age of 15 (Ron *et al.*, 1995). Studies of atomic bomb survivors reveal little risk for radiation-induced thyroid cancer among those exposed after the age of 20 (Thompson *et al.*, 1994), and large studies of adult patients given diagnostic doses of ^{131}I show no increased risk for thyroid cancer (Hall *et al.*, 1996). Increased risks for thyroid cancer reported in other studies of adults were either not statistically significant (Boice *et al.*, 1988) or were seen after administration of extremely high doses (> 10 Sv) in the treatment of an underlying thyroid disorder (Ron *et al.*, 1998b). The risks for only a few cancers, such as of the lung, appear to be higher after exposure as an adult rather than as a child to the atomic bombs. Because no childhood population has been followed for life, however, it is not known whether the apparent differences in effects by age will continue to be seen.

(d) Sex

On a relative scale, women appear to be somewhat more sensitive to the carcinogenic effects of radiation than men for most cancer sites except perhaps leukaemia (Thompson *et al.*, 1994). Since the baseline risks for many cancers are lower for women than for men, however, the absolute risks tend to be more comparable by sex. The breast is one of the most important radiogenic sites in women: the risk coefficient is high, and there is no evidence that radiation causes breast cancer in males. Females, who are at higher risk for naturally occurring thyroid cancer than males, also seem to be at higher radiogenic risk for cancer at this site. Although increased rates of ovarian cancer have been seen, cancers of male genital organs have not been convincingly linked to exposure to ionizing radiation (UNSCEAR, 1988). In the data on cancer incidence among the atomic bomb survivors, women had approximately twice the relative risk for developing solid tumours when compared with men (Thompson *et al.*, 1994).

(e)   *Time*

The period of observation is also an important determinant of risk (UNSCEAR, 1994). As the expression of radiation-induced solid tumours takes many years, studies with a short follow-up period might find different risk coefficients than those with longer periods of observation. Leukaemia has a relatively short minimal latency, an increase in risk first appearing about two years after exposure (Figure 11). The pattern of risk over time is then somewhat wave-like, peaking after about 10 years and decreasing thereafter, but not to control levels (Preston *et al.*, 1994). Solid tumours appear to have a minimal latency of five to nine years, and the risk may remain high for much of a lifespan, although there might be a decrease in the relative risk for radiogenic solid tumours after long follow-up periods. Studies of patients with ankylosing spondylitis treated with radiotherapy showed a risk close to background after 25 years (Weiss *et al.*, 1994). Atomic bomb survivors who were exposed while young have a reduced relative risk with time (Pierce *et al.*, 1996), as do children treated with radiation for medical conditions (Little *et al.*, 1998b). Studies of cervical cancer patients treated with radiotherapy show no evidence for a decrease in risk after 30 years of observation (Figure 12), but the extremely high doses and the gynaeco-logical tumours involved do not allow any generalizations to be made (Boice *et al.*, 1988).

Figure 11. Relative risks for acute and nonlymphocytic leukaemia with time after irradiation

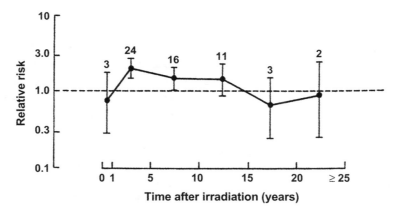

Adapted from Boice *et al.* (1996). The numbers of cases are shown above the upper confidence limits.

Figure 12. Observed:expected numbers of second primary cancers at or near the pelvis, by time since diagnosis of cervical cancer, for patients treated with and without radiation

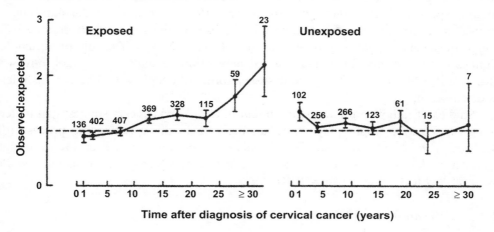

Adapted from Boice *et al.* (1996). The numbers of cases are shown above the upper confidence limits; 80% confidence intervals

(f)   Co-factors

(i)   Environmental

Co-factors are genetic, life-style or environmental conditions that influence a response to radiation. If co-factors differ appreciably between populations, it may be incorrect to extrapolate risk coefficients from one to the other. The risk estimates for the atomic bomb survivors were obtained after a brief exposure of a Japanese population with certain underlying disease rates who subsequently lived in a war-torn environment with severe malnutrition and poor sanitary conditions. Further, the striking excesses of mortality appear to be confined to a few cancer sites, such as the stomach, lung and breast, which account for about 70% of the total absolute risk (Pierce *et al.*, 1996). In addition, the convention of combining all cancers has little biological justification, given the different etiological and radiation risk coefficients for individual cancers.

Smoking is an important co-factor, and studies of patients with Hodgkin disease (van Leeuwen *et al.*, 1995) and small-cell lung cancer (Tucker *et al.*, 1997) suggest that continued use of tobacco after radiotherapy potentiates the risk for a second cancer in the lung. In a study of leukaemia among breast cancer patients, there appeared to be a multiplicative interaction between chemotherapy and radiotherapy (Curtis *et al.*, 1992).

(ii)   *Genetics*

An excess risk for skin cancers was seen in white but not black patients given radiotherapy for tinea capitis, suggesting that genetic factors act in concert with concomitant exposure to ultraviolet light (Shore *et al.*, 1984). Furthermore, the skin cancers in whites occurred on the face and around the edge of the scalp not covered by hair, suggesting that sunlight may potentiate the effects of X-rays. The role of ultraviolet light is not as evident for darker-skinned populations in Japan and Israel, however (Ron *et al.*, 1991, 1998a). The genetic susceptibility of people with inherited disorders is discussed in section 4.3.

Studies of radiotherapy in the treatment of childhood cancers suggest that underlying host factors might play an enhancing role in the carcinogenic process (de Vathaire *et al.*, 1992). Most studies of genetic susceptibility, however, involved high therapeutic doses to treat tumours, and it is unclear whether similar responses would occur at low levels of exposure (ICRP, 1999).

2.7.3   *Variations in risk by cancer site*

Variation in cancer risk coefficients is seen in the data on incidence among atomic bomb survivors (Thompson *et al.*, 1994; Preston *et al.*, 1994) and in compilations of organ-specific risks in various studies (UNSCEAR, 1994). The study of atomic bomb survivors has a distinct advantage, in that the risks can be averaged for the two sexes, all ages, for whole-body exposure on the same day and among subjects followed prospectively in the same manner. As 56% of the atomic bomb survivors were still alive in 1991 (Pierce *et al.*, 1996), however, the risk coefficients may change with further follow-up. In addition, the exposure was acute and not protracted, and studies in experimental animals suggest that the spectrum of tumour types is different after protracted and after brief exposure (Fry, 1992).

(*a*)   *Excess relative risk*

Table 26 shows a ranking of cancers by ERR, i.e. the relative risk minus 1.0, for exposure to 1 Gy. For example, if the relative risk for breast cancer after exposure to 1 Gy is 2.74, the ERR is 1.74. Only cancers linked to exposure to radiation are presented. Leukaemia is seen to be associated with by far the highest ERR per Gy, whereas the stomach, which was strongly affected by the atomic bombs, is associated with a very low ERR per Gy (Boice, 1996).

(*b*)   *Absolute excess risk*

The rankings change when an absolute scale is used (Table 27), reflecting the excess cancers per 10 000 persons per year per Gy. The estimate of absolute risk for breast cancer, for example, is 6.8×10^{-4} person–years Sv. Cancer of the female breast ranks first on an absolute scale, followed by cancers of the stomach and lung and then by leukaemia; cancers of the bladder and skin are at the lowest levels. These estimates are based on new data on cancer incidence among atomic bomb survivors, which have been collected since 1958, so that a minimal latency of about 12 years is incorporated into the estimates. The rankings might be different for populations with different baseline risks (Boice, 1996).

Table 26. Ranking of cancers by excess relative risk (ERR) at 1 Gy from data on atomic bomb survivors

Cancer site	ERR per Gy
Leukaemia	4.37
Breast	1.8
Thyroid	1.2
Lung	1.0
Ovary	1.0
Skin	1.0
Bladder	1.0
Colon	0.72
Liver	0.49
Stomach	0.32

Adapted from Boice (1996)

Table 27. Ranking of cancers in survivors of the atomic bombings by excess absolute risks

Cancer site	Excess cases per 10 000 persons per year per Gy
Breast	8.7
Stomach	4.8
Lung	4.4
Leukaemia	2.7
Colon	1.8
Thyroid	1.6
Liver	1.6
Bladder	1.2
Ovary	1.1
Skin	0.84

Adapted from Boice (1996)

(c)   *Attributable risk*

Sites can also be ranked by the percentage of tumours occurring in exposed survivors that could be related or attributable to exposure to the atomic bombings in 1945 (Table 28). These rankings are similar to those based on the ERR, since, as a first approximation, the attributable risk depends on the relative risk. More than half of the over 200 cases of leukaemia and 20–30% of the cancers of the breast, thyroid and skin could be attributable to exposure to radiation. The stomach has a very low attributable risk: only 6% of the over 1000 cases could be linked to exposure. For all solid tumours together, the attributable risk per cent is less than 10%, i.e. more than 90% of the cancers occurring in atomic bomb survivors were caused by factors other than atomic radiation (Boice, 1996). For all cancer deaths, the attributable risk is similar, about 8%, but for all deaths the attributable risk is about 1%. Overall, approximately 420 cancer deaths among the over 38 000 deaths among atomic bomb survivors can be attributed to the exposure to radiation received in 1945 (Pierce *et al.*, 1996).

Table 28. Ranking of cancers in survivors of the atomic bombings by attributable risk

Cancer site	Attributable risk (%)
Leukaemia	80
Breast	32
Thyroid	26
Skin	24
Lung	18
Ovary	18
Bladder	16
Colon	14
Liver	11
Stomach	8.5
Oesophagus	8.5

Adapted from Boice (1996)

(d)   *Relative tissue sensitivity*

Human tissues vary in their sensitivity to cancer induction by radiation (Committee on the Biological Effects of Ionizing Radiations (BEIR V), 1990; Thompson *et al.*, 1994; UNSCEAR, 1994; Weiss *et al.*, 1994; Boice, 1996; Boice *et al.*, 1996). Cancers that appear to be highly susceptible to radiation, with relatively high risk coefficients, include leukaemia and those of the premenopausal female breast and the childhood thyroid gland. The risks for these cancers are frequently increased in exposed populations.

Tissues that are apparently less susceptible or in which cancers are induced only at relatively high doses include the brain, bone, uterus, skin and rectum. Some cancers have not been linked convincingly to exposure to radiation; these include chronic lymphocytic leukaemia, Hodgkin disease, multiple myeloma, non-Hodgkin lymphoma (Boice, 1992) and cancers of the cervix, testis, prostate, pancreas and male breast.

3. Studies of Cancer in Experimental Animals

The ability of X-rays and γ-rays to induce neoplasms in experimental animals has been known for many years. The types and frequencies of radiation-induced tumours observed in experimental studies depend on the strain and species used, the total dose of radiation and whether the radiation is delivered as a single dose or over a longer time as either fractionated or low doses. Because the carcinogenic effects of X-rays and γ-rays are well recognized, most reports have emphasized the quantitative aspects of radiation carcinogenesis in experimental animals. This section is not meant to be comprehensive; the studies summarized are those that provide both qualitative and quantitative information and address critical issues in radiation carcinogenesis.

3.1 Carcinogenicity in adult animals

3.1.1 *Mice*

In a large series of studies, Upton *et al.* (1970) examined the induction of neoplasms in male and female RF/Un mice after irradiation with 250-kVp X-rays or ^{60}Co γ-rays over a range of doses and dose rates. Whole-body irradiation was initiated when the animals were 10 weeks of age, and the animals were allowed to live out their lifespan or were killed when moribund. All animals were fully necropsied, but only selected lesions were examined histopathologically, as needed to confirm diagnoses. A total of 4100 female and 2901 male mice were used, with 554 female and 623 male controls. The doses ranged from 0.25 to 4.5 Gy for acute X-irradiation and from ~1 Gy to 98.75 Gy for chronic ^{60}Co γ-irradiation. An increased frequency of all neoplasms was observed even at the lowest acute dose. The specific tumour types found included myeloid leukaemia and thymic lymphoma in both males and females, and an increased incidence of ovarian tumours was observed in females. As shown in Table 29, male mice exposed to X-rays were more sensitive to the induction of myeloid leukaemia than to thymic lymphoma, whereas females exposed to γ-rays were more sensitive to the induction of thymic lymphoma. Under conditions of a continuous low dose rate of ^{60}Co γ-irradiation for 23 h daily, the incidences of all neoplasms, myeloid leukaemia, thymic lymphoma and ovarian cancer were reduced when compared with acute X-irradiation. [The Working Group noted that the comparison of dose rate effects of X-rays and ^{60}Co γ-rays is complicated by the fact

Table 29. Incidences of leukaemia and lymphoma in male mice exposed to γ- and X-radiation

Exposure	Mean accumulated dose (Gy)	Average dose rate (mGy/min)	Myeloid leukaemia			Thymic lymphoma		
			Incidence		Mean age at death	Incidence		Mean age at death
			%	SE	(days)	%	SE	(days)
Control	0	–	4	1	463	4	1	502
X-rays	0.25	800	11	2	481	4	1	436
	0.5	800	12	2	481	6	2	334
	0.75	800	12	2	468	5	2	365
	1.0	800	22	3	407	5	2	363
	1.5	800	32	2	428	6	1	357
	3.0	800	42	3	370	15	2	309
	4.5	800	27	3	346	16	2	317
γ-rays	1.48	0.038	4	2	560	3	2	542
	1.53	0.106	6	2	582	4	2	408
	1.55	0.560	6	3	622	10	3	575
	3.29	0.038	10	3	597	3	2	598
	3.03	0.101	14	3	536	9	3	417
	3.08	0.159	12	4	473	10	4	433
	3.05	0.221	15	3	597	6	2	326
	3.15	0.570	10	3	487	5	3	472
	6.03	0.037	6	2	490	10	3	454
	6.21	0.098	10	4	533	12	4	401
	6.24	0.565	9	3	382	12	4	423
	58.1	0.115	5	4	679	26	7	382

From Upton *et al.* (1970); SE, standard error

that X-rays are slightly more effective than ^{60}Co γ-rays at low doses (relative biological effectiveness = 2). The frequency of myeloid leukaemia was reduced after exposure to a low dose rate, by a factor substantially greater than 2; it is therefore clear that the decreased effect is due to the lowering of the dose rate.]

Sensitivity to induction to myeloid leukaemia varies as a function not only of the sex of the animal but also of a number of other host factors, including genetic background, hormonal status, age, proliferative state of the bone marrow and the conditions under which the animals are maintained (Upton, 1968; Walburg & Cosgrove, 1969; Ullrich & Storer, 1979a).

One of the most comprehensive series of studies on the induction of cancer by γ-rays was reported by Ullrich and Storer (1979a,b,c). The induction of neoplastic disease was studied in male and female RFM/Un mice and in female BALB/c mice exposed to a range of doses of ^{137}Cs γ-rays at acute (0.4 Gy min^{-1}) and low dose rates (0.08 Gy per 20-h day). A total of 17 610 female and 1602 male RFM mice and 5659 female BALB/c mice were used; groups of 4762 female and 430 male RFM mice and 865 female BALB/c mice served as controls. The doses ranged from 0.1 to 3 Gy for the RFM mice and 0.5 to 2 Gy for BALB/c mice. As shown in Table 30, male and female RFM/Un mice showed dose-dependent increases in the frequencies of myeloid leukaemia and thymic lymphoma; females were more sensitive to the induction of thymic lymphoma. Significantly increased frequencies of thymic lymphomas were observed at doses as low as 0.25 Gy in both male and female RFM mice. Dose-dependent increased frequencies of ovarian, pituitary and Harderian gland tumours were observed in female RFM mice (Table 31), with an almost threefold increase in the frequency of ovarian cancer at 0.25 Gy. Higher doses were required to increase the frequencies of tumours at other sites. In male RFM mice, only the frequency of Harderian gland tumours was clearly increased in a dose-dependent manner, and males and females were equally sensitive to the induction of these tumours. Lowering the dose rate reduced the carcinogenic effectiveness of the radiation (Ullrich, 1983; Ullrich et al., 1987). In the same study, female BALB/c mice were not sensitive to the induction of leukaemia or lymphoma over the dose range used (0.5–2.0 Gy), but dose-dependent increased frequencies of ovarian tumours and significant increases in the frequencies of lung and mammary adenocarcinomas were observed even at the lowest dose. Again, lowering the dose rate markedly reduced the carcinogenic effect.

Table 30. Incidences of thymic lymphoma and myeloid leukaemia in γ-irradiated RFM/Un mice

Dose (Gy)	Incidence (% ± SE)							
	Thymic lymphoma				Myeloid leukaemia			
	Male		Female		Male		Female	
	Obs	Adj	Obs	Adj	Obs	Adj	Obs	Adj
0	6.6	6.6 ± 1.3	13.4	13.4 ± 0.6	1.3	1.3 ± 0.59	0.77	0.77 ± 0.14
0.1	6.5	6.5 ± 1.7	14.2	14.2 ± 0.63	0.86	0.8 ± 0.56	0.80	0.72 ± 0.15
0.25	9.6	9.6 ± 3.4	20.8	20.8 ± 1.3	1.2	1.2 ± 0.92	0.85	0.84 ± 0.30
0.5	12.9	9.1 ± 2.8	27.6	27.6 ± 1.2	3.6	4.5 ± 1.5	1.1	1.1 ± 0.32
1.0	9.2	15.9 ± 2.2	30.3	30.3 ± 1.3	9.2	9.1 ± 2.2	1.4	1.6 ± 0.41
1.5	20.2	20.3 ± 3.6	38.3	38.3 ± 1.2	9.5	10.2 ± 2.7	2.5	3.6 ± 0.76
2.0	NT	NT	44.4	44.4 ± 3.1	NT	NT	3.0	3.5 ± 0.78
3.0	25.8	25.9 ± 2.6	52.4	52.4 ± 1.3	17.7	19.5 ± 2.4	3.0	5.2 ± 0.56

From Ullrich & Storer (1979a). Obs, observed incidence; Adj, age-adjusted incidence; NT, not tested; SE, standard error

Table 31. Incidences of solid tumours in γ-irradiated female RFM/Un mice

Dose (Gy)	No. of animals	Incidence (% ± SE)						
		Ovarian tumours		Pituitary tumours		Harderian gland tumours	
		Obs	Adj	Obs	Adj	Obs	Adj
0	4014	2.4	2.4 ± 0.55	6.6	6.6 ± 0.87	1.2	1.2 ± 0.38
0.1	2827	2.2	2.0 ± 0.61	6.0	5.8 ± 1.0	1.5	1.3 ± 0.45
0.25	965	7.0	6.4 ± 1.7	6.2	5.5 ± 1.5	1.2	1.6 ± 0.88
0.5	1143	33.3	35.5 ± 2.8	8.0	9.1 ± 1.8	1.8	2.3 ± 1.0
1.0	1100	31.7	35.1 ± 1.9	8.2	9.5 ± 1.9	6.0	6.6 ± 1.6
0.15	1043	32.2	42.4 ± 3.0	6.5	9.4 ± 2.1	3.5	5.3 ± 1.7
0.2	333	28.8	43.9 ± 6.8	6.7	10.2 ± 4.1	8.5	15.4 ± 2.4
0.3	4133	27.2	47.8 ± 1.9	7.7	20.9 ± 1.8	7.5	16.2 ± 1.6

From Ullrich & Storer (1979b); Obs, observed incidence; Adj, age-adjusted incidence; SE, standard error

Subsequent studies by Ullrich and co-workers (Ullrich, 1983; Ullrich *et al.*, 1987) provided extensive data on the dose–response and time–dose relationships of ^{137}Cs γ-rays in the induction of both lung and mammary adenocarcinomas in female BALB/c mice at doses as low as 0.1 Gy. For mammary adenocarcinoma, a linear–quadratic dose–response relationship ($I = 7.7 + 0.035 D + 0.015 D^2$; where I = tumour incidence and D = dose) was observed over the 0–0.5-Gy dose range, while the response tended to flatten over the 0.5–2-Gy dose range. [The Working Group noted that the flattening is probably related to the effects of radiation on the ovary, since this organ is essentially ablated at doses ≥ 0.5 Gy.] Chronic exposure at a low dose rate (0.08 Gy day^{-1}) reduced the risk, while the effects of fractionated doses depended on the fraction size. In mice exposed chronically to ^{137}Cs γ-rays delivered at a dose rate of 0.01 Gy day^{-1} up to a total dose of 2 Gy, a linear dose–response relationship ($I = 7.7 + 0.035 D$) was seen for mammary tumours. [The Working Group noted that the linear term of this response was consistent with the linear–quadratic model for acute exposure.] When multiple small acute daily fractions of 0.01 Gy were given, the results were similar to those with the low dose rate, whereas the cancer incidence after the same total doses were delivered as 0.05-Gy daily fractions was similar to that after single acute doses. For lung adenocarcinomas, single exposure to ^{137}Cs γ-rays over a 0–2-Gy dose range showed a linear–quadratic dose–response relationship ($I = 11.8 + 0.041 D + 0.00043 D^2$). Delivery of γ-rays at a dose rate of 0.08 Gy day^{-1} resulted in a diminution of the D^2 portion of the dose–response curve, such that it was linear over the entire dose range ($I = 12.5 + 0.043 D$). When the doses were fractionated, the response was dependent on the dose per fraction. When the dose per fraction was < 0.5 Gy, the response was similar to that with low dose rates; when the dose per fraction was > 0.5 Gy, the tumour incidences were similar to those after acute exposure.

Grahn *et al.* (1992) reported the results of a large series of experiments with more than 8000 male and female B6CF$_1$ (C57BL/6JAn1 × BALB/CJAn1) hybrid mice, which were irradiated with ^{60}Co γ-rays at 0.225–7.88 Gy at high dose rates, at 0.225–24.6 Gy at low dose rates or in fractionation regimens. Increased frequencies of lymphoreticular tumours, tumours of the lung and Harderian gland and all epithelial tumours were observed in male mice, which appeared to increase as a linear function of dose. In addition, increased frequencies of ovarian tumours were observed in female mice [frequencies at each dose not reported]. Protraction or fractionation of the dose reduced the carcinogenic effects of the radiation.

Maisin *et al.* (1983) exposed 1267 male BALB/c mice to single doses of ^{137}Cs γ-rays at doses of 0.25–6 Gy. The incidences of thymic lymphoma were increased at 4 and 6 Gy. Maisin *et al.* (1988) examined the effects of acute and 8 × 3 h or 10 × 4 h fractionated doses of ^{137}Cs γ-rays over the same dose range in male C57BL/6 mice. While the greatest effect was to cause early death [considered by the Working Group to be due mainly to death from cancers], increased frequencies of leukaemia and all malignancies were found after acute doses of 4 and 6 Gy. Fractionation resulted in an earlier and more frequent appearance of tumours at 1–2 Gy, but the results were not statistically significant.

The induction of myeloid leukaemia in 951 male CBA/H mice exposed to 250-kVp X-rays at 0.25–6 Gy was compared with that in 800 controls. The frequency of myeloid leukaemia increased with increasing doses up to 3 Gy and then decreased at higher doses (Mole *et al.*, 1983).

Di Majo *et al.* (1996) examined the influence of sex on tumour induction by irradiation with 250-kVp X-rays (half-value layer, 1.5 mm Cu). After irradiation of 289 male and 259 female three-month-old CBA/Cne mice with doses of 1–7 Gy, increased incidences of myeloid leukaemia and malignant lymphomas were observed in males, and the incidence of Harderian gland tumours was increased in a dose-dependent manner and to a similar degree in males and females.

In 153 female RFM mice given a single localized thoracic X-irradiation at doses of 1–9 Gy, the incidence of pulmonary tumours at nine months increased as a linear–quadratic function of dose, but significant increases in the frequency of lung tumours over that in 88 controls and in the numbers of lung tumours per mouse were observed only at 6.5 and 9 Gy. While no data were available on low dose rates, experiments in which the doses were fractionated into two equal portions and given at intervals of 24 h or 30 days were conducted in 311 female RFM mice. A reduction in the carcinogenic effect was observed in animals given the high doses (6.5 and 9 Gy) at a 24-h interval, but no significant difference was observed with an interval of 30 days (Ullrich *et al.*, 1979; Ullrich, 1980).

Lung tumours developed in male and female SAS/4 mice after local exposure to thoracic X-rays at doses of 0.25–7.5 Gy (Coggle, 1988). A total of 557 male and 551 female mice were irradiated, and the animals were killed 12 months after irradiation and their lungs examined for tumours. As shown in Table 32, a dose-dependent increase in the frequency of lung tumours was found in both males and females with increasing frequencies over the range of 0.25–5 Gy.

Table 32. Incidences of primary lung tumours in SAS/4 mice given 200-kVp X-irradiation at 0.6 Gy/min

Sex	Dose (Gy)	No. of mice exposed	No. of mice with tumours	Incidence ± SE
Males	0	291	48	16.5 ± 2.2
	0.25	61	12	19.7 ± 5.1
	0.5	62	11	17.7 ± 4.8
	1.0	67	13	19.4 ± 4.8
	2.0	56	15	26.8 ± 5.9
	2.5	69	23	33.3 ± 5.7
	3.0	32	12	37.5 ± 8.6
	4.0	45	17	37.7 ± 7.2
	5.0	45	22	48.9 ± 7.5
	6.0	48	18	37.5 ± 7.0
	7.5	72	16	22.2 ± 4.9
Females	0	210	19	9.0 ± 2.0
	0.5	62	7	11.3 ± 4.0
	1.0	61	6	9.8 ± 3.8
	1.5	64	8	12.5 ± 4.1
	2.0	63	10	15.9 ± 4.1
	3.0	60	16	26.7 ± 5.7
	4.0	61	23	37.7 ± 6.2
	5.0	59	21	35.6 ± 6.2
	6.0	60	15	25.0 ± 5.6
	7.5	61	9	14.8 ± 4.5

From Coggle (1988); SE, standard error

3.1.2   *Genetically engineered mice*

Genetically engineered mice are used in radiation carcinogenesis mainly to study the genes that may affect susceptibility and as a means of elucidating mechanisms. Mice lacking the *p53* gene are useful because of the role of *p53* in damage recognition and response mechanisms. In addition, *p53* is known to be mutated in Li–Fraumeni syndrome, a genetic syndrome that affects sensitivity to radiation.

Thirty-three *p53* heterozygous (+/–) and 28 *p53* wild-type (+/+) mice were exposed by whole-body irradiation to 4 Gy of ^{60}Co γ-rays at 7–12 weeks of age and observed until they were moribund, when they were killed and autopsied. Eighteen null (–/–) and 14 heterozygous mice served as controls. None of the irradiated wild-type mice developed tumours within 80 weeks, but radiation significantly reduced the latency for tumour development (mainly lymphomas and sarcomas) in *p53* heterozygous mice. Approximately 90% of the heterozygous mice developed tumours with a mean latency of 40 weeks, before any of the unirradiated heterozygous mice developed tumours (mean latency, > 70 weeks). In the same study, a dose of 1 Gy of γ-rays given to two-day-old *p53* null (–/–) mice also decreased the latency for tumour development (Kemp *et al.*, 1994).

Radiation-induced thymic lymphoma has also been studied in Eμ-*pim*-1 mice. The *pim*-1 gene was discovered as a preferential proviral integration site in murine leukaemia virus-induced T-cell lymphomas (Cuypers *et al.*, 1984) and can act as an oncogene in mice (Van Lohuizen *et al.*, 1989). The transgenic mice have a low incidence of spontaneous T-cell lymphomas before the age of seven months but are highly susceptible to genotoxic carcinogens. In this study, groups of 12 female and 14 male heterozygous Eμ-*pim*-1 transgenic mice and 15 female and 11 male non-transgenic littermates, four to seven weeks of age, were irradiated with four fractions of 1.5 Gy of X-rays. The fractions were given one week apart for four weeks. Groups of 15 female and 11 male Eμ-*pim*-1 transgenic mice and 15 female and 16 male non-transgenic mice were irradiated with four fractions of 1 Gy of X-rays. Groups of 32 female and 31 male Eμ-*pim*-1 and 25 female and 38 male littermates were irradiated with four fractions of 0.5 Gy. Thirteen female and 12 male transgenic and 13 female and 11 male non-trans-genic mice served as controls. The animals were monitored for lymphoma development for 250 days after the last exposure. All 26 Eμ-*pim*-1 mice exposed to four fractions of 1.5 Gy of X-rays developed lymphomas within 250 days. At the lower doses per fraction, 20/22 effective mice developed lymphomas after exposure to four fractions of 1.0 Gy and 17/61 after exposure to four fractions of 0.5 Gy. In the non-transgenic litter-mates, 12/31, 6/31 and 0/62 irradiated mice developed lymphomas (Van der Houven van Oordt *et al.*, 1998).

3.1.3   *Rats*

A total of 398 female adult Sprague-Dawley rats were divided into seven groups and exposed to γ-rays at different ages: to single doses of 5 Gy at 40 days of age or 160 days of age or to four fractionated doses of 1.25 Gy; to eight fractions of 0.62 Gy; to 16 fractions of 0.3 Gy or to 32 fractions of 0.15 Gy at 40 days of age. One group was sham-irradiated. All of the fractionated doses of ^{60}Co γ-rays were delivered twice weekly at a dose rate of 0.40 Gy/min. The incidence of mammary tumours (adenocarcinomas, adenofibromas and fibroadenomas) was determined histologically up to the age of 1000 days. An increased frequency of mammary fibroadenomas and, to a lesser extent, adenocarcinomas, was observed, with 64 in controls and 92, 90, 96, 89, 85 and 87% with the different regimes, respectively. No significant difference between single and fractionated exposures was reported (Shellabarger *et al.*, 1966).

A total of 191 female adult Sprague-Dawley rats, 61–63 days of age, were given single whole-body doses of 0.28, 0.56 or 0.85 Gy of 250-kVp X-rays at a dose rate of 0.30 Gy min^{-1}. A group of 167 controls was available. The animals were observed over their lifespan (1033–1053 days) for the induction of mammary tumours, and the neo-plasms were identified histopathologically as adenocarcinomas or fibroadenomas. The incidences of mammary tumours were 67% in controls and 72, 77 and 79% in the irradiated groups, showing a dose-dependent increase in all mammary tumours and in particular in fibroadenomas. The principal effect of the irradiation was to cause an earlier time of onset of fibroadenomas, which was dose-dependent (Shellabarger *et al.*, 1980).

Groups of 40 control and low-dose and 20 mid- and high-dose female WAG/Rij, BN/Bi and Sprague-Dawley rats, eight weeks of age, were exposed by whole-body irradiation to a single dose of 300-kVp X-rays (Sprague-Dawley rats, 0.1, 0.3, 1 or 2 Gy; WAG/Rij and BN/bi rats, 0.5, 1 and 4 Gy [dose rate not given]). In another experiment, the numbers of animals in these groups were increased to 40 and 60, respectively. The animals were observed for life, and the mammary tumour incidences were determined by gross and histopathological observations. A dose-dependent increase in the incidence of all mammary tumours was observed: Sprague-Dawley rats, 30 (control), 70, 72, 75 and 86%; WAG/Rij rats, 27 (control), 26, 35 and 76%; and BN/Bi rats, 8 (control), 15, 86 and 88% (Broerse *et al.*, 1986, 1987).

Groups of 40 female WAG/Rij inbred rats were exposed to a single dose of 1 or 2 Gy of ^{137}Cs γ-radiation at 8, 12, 16, 22, 36 or 64 weeks of age at a dose rate of 0.75 Gy min^{-1} to study the effect of age at exposure. A group of 120 controls was available. The animals were observed for life, and tumours of the mammary gland were classified histologically as fibroadenoma or carcinoma. No statistically signi-ficant difference in the incidence of mammary tumours was found by age on the basis of crude incidences, but examination of normalized excess risk demonstrated a reduced risk after exposure at 64 weeks of age (Barstra *et al.*, 1998).

Lee *et al.* (1982) studied the induction of thyroid tumours in young, female Long-Evans rats after localized external irradiation of the thyroid glands with X-rays (250 kVp; half-value layer, 0.55 mm Cu) at estimated doses of 0.94, 4.1 or 10.6 Gy. The incidences of both follicular thyroid adenomas and carcinomas were increased with dose: 9/281 (control), 11/275, 35/282 and 74/267.

In 115 Sprague-Dawley rats, eight weeks of age, that received nerve isografts on the right posterior tibial nerve, exposure of the thigh region to 0 (control), 46, 66, 86 or 106 Gy ^{60}Co-γ radiation as 2-Gy fractions at a dose rate of 73 cGy/min, resulted in osteosarcomas and/or fibrous histiocytomas in 0/7 (controls), 0/20, 2/27, 2/20 and 8/41 rats in the respective groups (Tinkey *et al.*, 1998).

3.1.4   *Rabbits*

A group of 21 male and female Dutch rabbits were irradiated with 4.4–14.1 Gy of 2.5-MeV γ-rays at a dose rate of 17.6 Gy h^{-1}; a control group of 17 unirradiated rabbits was available. The animals were allowed to die naturally, and selected tissues were examined histologically. Tumours were found in 24% of controls, 75% at 4.4 Gy, 88% at 8.8–10.6 Gy and 56% at 11.5–14.1 Gy. The tumours included four osteosarcomas of the jaw, five fibrosarcomas of the dermis and six basal-cell tumours of the skin (Hulse, 1980).

3.1.5   *Dogs*

Groups of 120 male and female beagle dogs, aged 2 or 70 days, were exposed by whole-body irradiation to 0.88 or 0.83 Gy of ^{60}Co γ-rays, and a further group of 240 dogs received 0.81 Gy at 365 days of age; 360 controls were available. The animals were allowed to die naturally or were killed because of terminal illness. In 1343 dogs allowed to live out their life span, heritable lymphocytic thyroiditis with hypo-thyroidism was a major contributor to mortality. Of 86 dogs irradiated at 70 days of age, 25/86 had thyroid follicular adenomas and 10/86 had carcinomas, which repre-sented a significant increase ($p < 0.01$) over the 40/231 controls with adenomas and 16/231 with carcinomas. No significant increase in the incidence of thyroid tumours was found in dogs irradiated at 2 or 365 days of age. The irradiated dogs showed a consistent trend for a lower incidence of hypothyroidism when compared with controls. Hypothyroidal dogs had a significantly increased risk for thyroid neoplasia, including a greater risk for carcinomas, but no evidence was found in this group of a greater sensitivity to radiation-induced tumours (Benjamin *et al.*, 1991, 1997).

3.1.6   *Rhesus monkeys*

Twenty rhesus monkeys (*Macaca mulatta*), three years of age, were exposed by whole-body irradiation to doses of 4–8.6 Gy of X-rays (300 kVp; half-value layer, 3 mm Cu) at a dose rate of 0.3 Gy min^{-1}. A few hours after irradiation, most of the animals received intravenous grafts of 2–4 × 10^8 autologous bone-marrow cells. Between 7.5 and 15.5 years later, eight animals developed malignant tumours, comprising five adenocarcinomas of the kidney, two follicular carcinomas of the thyroid, two osteocarci-nomas and one glomus tumour of the subcutaneous tissues. No malignant tumours occurred in 21 controls within 18 years (Broerse *et al.*, 1981).

3.2   Prenatal exposure

3.2.1   *Mice*

C57BL/6 female mice, 10–14 weeks of age, were mated with WHT/Ht males of the same age overnight and removed next morning for timed pregnancies. Subsequently, 19 pregnant females were irradiated with approximately 2 Gy of X-rays (180 kVp, 20 mA with a filter of 0.7 mm Cu) at a dose rate of ~0.86 Gy min^{-1} on days 12 or 16–18 *post coitum*. A total of 573 male and female offspring were delivered and observed for life, and all suspected lesions or tumours were examined histopathologically. The control group consisted of 141 unirradiated C57BL/6 × WHT/Ht offspring of 19 mice. Significant increases were found in the incidences of tumours of the lung (both sexes), the pituitary gland (females) and the ovary of the offspring that had been irradiated on days 16–18 *post coitum* [statistical methods not given], whereas X-irradiation at day 12 *post coitum* did not increase the incidence of tumours in the offspring (Sasaki *et al.*, 1978a). In a study of 167 B6WF$_1$ (C57BL/6 × WHT/Ht) female mice irradiated 17 days *post coitum* with approximately 1.5 or 3 Gy of X-rays (200 kVp, 20 mA with a filter of 0.5 mm Al + 0.5 mm Cu) at a dose rate of 0.5–0.6 Gy min^{-1}, the offspring were allowed to die naturally. Significant increases were observed in the incidences of hepatocellular tumours in both male and female offspring in a dose-dependent manner (Table 33) [statistical method not given] (Sasaki *et al.*, 1978b).

A total of 410 C57BL/6 female × DBA/2 male fetuses were exposed to 0.2, 0.5, 1.0 or 2.0 Gy of ^{60}Co γ-rays on day 18 of gestation and were killed and autopsied when moribund or at two years of age. Tissues showing macroscopic alterations were submitted to histopathological examination. A group of 1009 historical controls was available. Tumours were found mainly in the lung, uterus and lymphoid tissues, and the total tumour incidence was significantly increased at 0.5, 1.0 and 2.0 Gy (Pearson's χ^2 test) (Lumniczky *et al.*, 1998).

In order to mimic human exposure to various carcinogenic and promoting agents in the diet and the environment, carcinogenic and/or promoting agents were given in some experiments postnatally after prenatal exposure to radiation. A total of 79 pregnant ICR mice, 9–11 weeks of age, were irradiated with 0.36 Gy of X-rays (180 kVp, 20 mA with a filter of 0.5 mm Cu) at the dose rate of 0.72 Gy min^{-1} on days 0, 2, 4, 6, 8, 10, 12, 14 or 16 of gestation. Then, 496 live offspring were treated with 5 μmol (g bw)$^{-1}$ of urethane, while 237 received distilled water, at 21 days of age. The mice were killed five months after the postnatal treatment, and tumour nodules in the lung were counted. As controls, 78 and 181 offspring of 26 unirradiated mice were similarly treated with urethane and water, respectively. No increase in the incidence of tumours was observed after prenatal X-irradiation alone, but both the incidence and the number of lung tumours per mouse were significantly increased when prenatal irradiation was coupled with postnatal urethane treatment on days 0–14 (except day 6) of gestation (χ^2 and Student's *t* test) (Nomura, 1984).

Table 33. Incidences of tumours in B6WF$_1$ (C57BL/6 × WHT/Ht) mice after prenatal exposure to X-radiation

Treated stage (dpc)	Sex	Dose (Gy)	No. of mice	Incidence (%)					Reference
				Total incidence	Lung tumour	Liver tumour	Ovarian tumour	Pituitary tumour	
12	Male	2	44	11**	5*	0	–	0	Sasaki et al. (1978a)
	Female		53	15**	4	0	0	0	
16–18	Male	2	126	73**	56**	17	–	1	
	Female		140	77	39**	10	14*	9*	
Control	Male	0	55	46	24	7	–	0	
	Female		77	65	17	7	1	1	
17	Male	3	22	–	–	46**	–	–	Sasaki et al. (1978b)
	Female		53	–	–	13*	–	–	
17	Male	1.5	39	–	–	28**	–	–	
	Female		53	–	–	8	–	–	
Control	Male		84	–	–	7	–	–	
	Female		129	–	–	1	–	–	

dpc, days *post coitum*. Significantly different from controls at *$p < 0.05$ and **$p < 0.01$

In a further study from the same laboratory, 289 fetuses of coat colour-mutant strains of PT and HT mice were exposed to 0, 0.3 or 1.03 Gy of X-rays at a dose rate of 0.54 Gy min^{-1} on day 10.5 of gestation. Offspring were examined for somatic mutations at six weeks of age, and then 139 offspring were treated with 12-O-tetradecanoylphorbol 13-acetate (TPA) and 150 with the acetone solvent. The mice were killed at 12 months of age, and the induced tumours were diagnosed histopathologically. Although a significant, linear dose-dependent increase in the incidence of somatic mutations was detected, no increase in tumour frequency was observed after prenatal irradiation alone. The incidences of skin tumours and hepatomas were increased in male offspring after prenatal irradiation and postnatal treatment with TPA (Table 34). When 59 PTHTF$_1$ fetuses were exposed to 1.03 Gy of X-rays at the low dose rate of 4.3 mGy min^{-1}, the mutant spot sizes and tumour incidences were about one-fifth of those produced by the dose rate of 0.54 Gy min^{-1} (Nomura et al., 1990).

Table 34. Induction of tumours in PTHTF$_1$ mice after irradiation in utero and postnatal treatment with TPA

Dose (Gy)	TPA	Tumour-bearing mice		Skin tumour[a]		Hepatoma in males		
		Incidence	%	Incidence	%	Incidence	%	Tumours per liver
1.03	+	14/47	29.8**	5/47	10.6*	8/23	34.8*	0.57
	–	3/49	6.1	0/49	0.0	1/25	4.0	0.04
0.3	+	6/38	15.8	1/38	2.6	4/20	20.0	0.20
	–	2/51	3.9	0/51	0.0	1/26	3.8	0.04
0	+	4/54	7.4	0/54	0.0	1/29	3.4	0.03
	–	3/50	6.0	0/50	0.0	1/22	4.5	0.05

From Nomura et al. (1990). TPA, 12-O-tetradecanoylphorbol 13-acetate
[a] Four squamous-cell carcinomas and two pigmented basal-cell carcinomas
*$p < 0.05$, **$p < 0.01$ when compared with untreated controls

In a separate study, 2241 male and female NMRI mouse fetuses were irradiated in utero with 0.2, 0.4, 0.8 or 1.6 Gy of X-rays (180 kVp, 10 mA with a filter of 0.3 mm Cu) at a dose rate of 0.6 Gy min^{-1} on day 15 of gestation. After birth, one subgroup at each dose received 45 mg (kg bw)$^{-1}$ N-ethyl-N-nitrosourea (ENU) at 21 days of age while another did not. All surviving animals were killed at 22 months. No significant increase in the incidence of tumours was observed in the offspring exposed to 0.2 or 0.8 Gy of X-radiation alone [0.4 and 1.6 Gy not tested], but significantly increased incidences of tumours of the liver, intestine, uterus and ovary were observed after prenatal exposure to 0.2, 0.4 or 0.8 Gy of X-rays in combination with postnatal treatment with ENU ($p < 0.05$–0.001; χ^2 test) when compared with ENU alone. In mice at 1.6 Gy in combination with ENU, the tumour incidences were often reduced (Schmahl, 1988).

3.2.2 Dogs

Groups of 60 male and 60 female beagles received mean doses of 0.16 or 0.83 Gy of ^{60}Co γ-radiation on day 8 (preimplantation), 28 (embryonic) or 55 (late fetal) *post coitum*. The offspring were allowed to die naturally, when they were examined histopathologically. As controls, 360 dogs were sham-irradiated. The tumours found predominantly in the offspring of irradiated and unirradiated bitches up to 16 years of age were malignant lymphoma, haemangiosarcoma and mammary carcinoma. Analysis of trends with increasing dose indicated that the incidences of both fatal malignancies and all neoplasms were significantly increased in the offspring of bitches irradiated on day 55 *post coitum*, while no significant increase was observed after exposure *in utero* at day 28 *post coitum*; however, the incidence of fatal haemangiosarcomas was significantly increased in the offspring of bitches exposed on day 8 *post coitum* (Peto's test) (Benjamin *et al.*, 1991).

3.3 Parental exposure

Male and female ICR mice were treated with X-rays (180 kVp, 20 mA with a filter of 0.5 mm Al + 0.5 mm Cu) at 0.36, 1.08, 2.16, 3.6 or 5.04 Gy at a dose rate of 0.72 Gy min^{-1} and mated with untreated mice at various intervals of days to examine the sensitivity of germ cells at different stages. About half of the pregnant mice were killed just before delivery (day 18 of gestation), and the others were allowed to deliver live offspring. Significant increases in the frequencies of dominant lethal mutations and congenital malformations were observed in a dose-dependent manner after exposure of the spermatozoa and spermatid stages to X-rays. Groups of 1529 and 1155 live offspring of male and female exposed parental mice were killed at eight months of age, and suspected tumours were diagnosed histopathologically. The control group consisted of 548 offspring of unirradiated mice. Significant increases in the incidences of total tumours were reported after paternal (153/1529, 10.0%) and maternal exposure (101/1155, 8.7%), when compared with controls (29/548, 5.3%; $p < 0.01$–0.005; χ^2 test). About 87% of the induced tumours were in the lung. At both germ-cell stages, the tumour incidence in the offspring increased in a nearly linear, dose-dependent mode after paternal exposure, and the increase was statistically significant at the high doses (χ^2 and t test). The sensitivity at the spermatogonial stage was about half that at the spermatid stage. No increase in the incidence of tumours was observed in offspring after maternal exposure to up to 1.08 Gy, but the incidence increased significantly at higher doses. When male and female parental mice were treated with doses of 0.36 Gy of X-rays at 2-h intervals, fractionation significantly reduced the carcinogenic effects of irradiation in offspring exposed at the spermatogonial and mature oocyte stages; however, no such reduction was observed when postmeiotic stages were treated. In another study, F_1 offspring of X-irradiated male mice were mated and their progeny were examined. Significantly higher incidences of tumours were observed in the F_2 generation of F_1 progeny that had tumours. The author suggested that germ-line alterations that caused tumours were transmitted to the next generation (Nomura, 1982).

In order to confirm these results, male mice of the N5 and LT strains were similarly treated with 5.04 Gy of X-rays at the spermatogonial or postmeiotic stage, respectively, and 229 irradiated and 244 unirradiated N5 offspring and 75 irradiated and 411 unirradiated LT offspring were killed at 12 months of age. A significant increase in the incidence of lymphocytic leukaemias was observed: N5 strain, 3.9% versus 0.4% in controls and LT strain, 5.3% versus 1.0% in controls ($p < 0.05$; χ^2 test) (Nomura, 1986, 1989).

Cattanach et al. (1995) used the experimental protocol of Nomura (1982) but a different strain of mice. Male BALB/cJ mice were treated with 2.5 or 5.0 Gy of X-rays (250 kVp, 14 mA, filter of 0.25 cm Cu) at a dose rate of 0.76 Gy min^{-1} and were mated with females of the same strain for one week and then new ones for a further week. All of the progeny obtained were therefore derived from irradiated spermatozoa and late spermatids. The study was carried out as a series of 21 replicate experiments over a one-year period in order to accommodate the maximum capacity of the histological laboratory (approximately 45 animals per week). The offspring of about 600 male mice at each dose were retained for examination for lung tumours at eight months of age, and offspring of 70 animals at each dose were retained for examination at 12 months. The total incidences of lung tumours were not significantly different in offspring from irradiated and unirradiated male parents. Nevertheless, the incidence of lung tumours changed significantly in all treated groups during the one-year study: adenocarcinomas were found only in the later experiments, while the incidence of benign adenomas declined over the first 8–10 replicates and then rose to yet higher rates than observed in the early series. The authors ascribed this effect to a seasonal change in the incidence of tumours in these mice.

The same group carried out a study in a different strain of mice, C3H/HeH. In a series of replicate studies over two years, male mice were exposed to 0, 2.5 or 5.0 Gy of X-rays and mated with untreated females in the same protocol as in the previous study. In 1381 offspring killed at 12 months of age, no significant increase in the incidence of lung tumours was observed. Again, a seasonal variation in tumour incidence was observed (Cattanach et al., 1998).

Groups of 27–28 male N5 mice were irradiated under conditions similar to those used by Nomura (1982, 1986) with 0 (control) or 5 Gy of X-rays (160 kVp, 18 mA, with a filter of 0.5 mm Cu + 10 mm Al) [dose rate not given] and mated 3, 7, 10 or 17 days after irradiation; 312 irradiated and 305 unirradiated offspring were observed until they were killed at one year of age. All tumours were examined histopathologically. The probability of dying from leukaemia (Kaplan-Meyer product-limit procedure) and overall survival (Cox–Mantel log-rank one-tailed test) were statistically significantly different ($p < 0.05$) in the offspring of X-ray-treated males and unirradiated controls. The incidences of leukaemia at one year of age were 11/165 (6.7%) in those exposed to X-rays and 10/305 (3.3%) in controls ($p = 0.07$, Fisher's exact test) (Daher *et al.*, 1998).

A lifetime experiment in CBA/J NCrj mice was carried out to examine whether paternal exposure to X-rays increases the risk for tumours. Male mice were exposed to 1 or 2 Gy of X-rays (100 kVp, 8 mA, with a filter of 1.7 mm Al + 0.2 mm Cu) at a dose rate of about 0.65 Gy min^{-1} and mated with unirradiated females one, three or nine weeks later. The 282 and 206 offspring of mice at 1 and 2 Gy were allowed to die naturally. A group of 631 unirradiated control offspring was available. The female offspring of males that had been exposed to 2 Gy of X-radiation one week before mating (spermatozoal stage) showed a trend towards a higher incidence of tumours of the haematopoietic system when compared with unirradiated offspring, and male offspring of these males had a somewhat higher incidence of broncho-alveolar adenocarcinomas. No increase in tumour incidence was observed in the offspring of males irradiated three or nine weeks before conception (Mohr *et al.*, 1999).

Further studies were carried out in which the offspring of irradiated parents were treated with chemical carcinogens or promoting agents. Significant increases in the frequencies of lung tumour nodules per mouse were observed in the offspring of X-irradiated ICR mice given urethane by subcutaneous injection postnatally (Nomura, 1983), and similar results were obtained with outbred Swiss mice given urethane intraperitoneally (Vorobtsova & Kitaev, 1988). The incidence of skin tumours was significantly increased in the offspring of parentally X-irradiated outbred SHR mice treated postnatally with TPA by dermal application (Vorobtsova *et al.*, 1993). Similar enhancing effects were not, however, observed when CBA/J male mice were irradiated and their offspring were treated postnatally with urethane by subcutaneous injection (Mohr *et al.*, 1999).

4. Other Data Relevant to an Evaluation of Carcinogenicity and its Mechanisms

4.1 Radiation syndromes: Early effects of whole-body irradiation

A hierarchy of health effects that appear sequentially after high doses of whole-body irradiation consists of the haematopoietic, gastrointestinal and central nervous syndromes, which are collectively referred to as the 'acute radiation syndromes' and have been extensively reviewed (Bond *et al.*, 1965; Young, 1987; UNSCEAR, 1988). The dose range over which these syndromes occur is shown in Table 35. The cutaneous radiation syndrome and the chronic radiation syndrome are now considered sufficiently distinct to be included in the list of radiation syndromes. The more severe

Table 35. Effects and outcomes after exposure to ionizing radiation

Dose range (Gy)	Prodromal effects	Tissue effects	Survival
0.5–1.0	Mild	Small decrease in blood cell count	$LD_{0/60}$ (normal subject)
2.0–3.5	Moderate	Moderate-to-severe damage (bone marrow)	$LD_{5/60}$–$LD_{50/60}$
3.5–5.5	Severe	Severe damage (bone marrow)	$LD_{90/60}$–$LD_{99/60}$[a] (death, 3.5–6 weeks)
5.5–7.5	Severe	Ablation (bone marrow)	Death, 2–3 weeks[a]
10–20	Severe	Severe damage (gastrointestinal)	Death, 5–12 days
100	Severe	Cerebrovascular damage	Death, within 2 days

Adapted from Young (1987)

[a] Treatment may increase survival by raising the dose that is lethal by 50% but to a lesser extent in the case of the gastrointestinal syndrome.

effects are preceded by a prodromal phase, which is mediated by a poorly understood effect on the autonomic system. Apart from the signs and the symptoms of the prodromal phase and the central nervous syndrome, the early effects of radiation are due to cell killing in tissues with rapid cell turnover such as the bone marrow and the gut. Cell killing is also the major determinant in tissues such as lung and skin that incur early deterministic effects, but later. The relative radiosensitivity of the clonogenic cells in various solid tissues is shown in Table 36.

Table 36. Radiosensitivity of clonogenic cells in solid tissues, as indicated by the D_0

Tissue	D_0 (Gy)	Reference
Jejunum	1.30	Withers & Elkind (1970)
Testis	1.36	Withers et al. (1974)
Kidney	1.53	Withers et al. (1986)
Skin	1.35	Withers (1967)
Colony-forming units (haematopoietic)	0.95	McCulloch & Till (1962)
Breast	1.22	Gould & Clifton (1979)
Thyroid	2.0	Mulcahy et al. (1980)

D_0, reciprocal of the final slope of the curve of survival as a function of dose, representing cell killing due to multiple events

Death from bone-marrow damage occurs at lower doses than death from damage to the gut and longer after exposure. This reflects differences in the cell kinetics and design of the two cell renewal systems and to some extent the inherent radiosensitivity of the stem cells. In the haematopoietic system, the lifespan of the functional cells varies with cell type: the megakaryocyte–platelet and leukocyte populations are at highest risk because of their short lifespan.

Two main types of cell death are induced by radiation: (1) death associated with mitosis because of DNA damage, in many cases causing chromosomal alterations that make the first or subsequent post-irradiation cell division lethal, and (2) death through apoptosis in interphase, in some cases before the irradiated cells reach mitosis and in other cases after they have undergone mitosis. The probability that a cell will die through apoptosis depends largely on the type of cell. For example, in some types of lymphocytes, damage to the cell membrane can trigger a cascade of enzymatic events that ultimately result in scission of the DNA strands. In contrast, apoptosis is not frequently induced in fibroblasts. While apoptosis may occur in non-cycling cells, most such cells remain functional even though they carry DNA damage that is lethal when the cell attempts division.

Individual cell loss may be random, but it is the overall effect of killing a critical number of cells that causes the deterministic effect, which may be expressed either early or late. In lung and especially skin, some effects, such as erythema, occur relatively soon after exposure, but others, such as fibrosis, are observed many months later.

4.2   Late deterministic effects of ionizing radiation

The late effects of radiation are not fully explained, and the relative importance of depletion of parenchymal cells, which directly affects the functional and proliferative capacity of tissues, and of damage to the microvasculature, which indirectly affects the parenchymal cells, is a matter of discussion. The initial model of late effects was based on radiation-induced changes in the microvasculature of organs. Endothelial cells can be lost as a result of interphase death or death associated with mitosis as the slowly cycling cells come into division. The loss of vascular integrity in turn leads to fibrosis and loss of parenchymal cells (Rubin & Casarett, 1968; Casarett, 1980). An alternative model (Withers, 1989) stresses the importance of the loss of functional subunits, the architectural arrangement of organs and their stem cells. For example, the nephron in the kidney consists of epithelial cells; if a sufficient number are killed, the functional unit is lost because it cannot be repopulated from neighbouring nephrons. The function of the kidney is critically compromised as the loss of functional subunits increases. Similarly, in the spinal cord, the functional subunit essential for myelination and therefore for the function of the neurons is the minimum number of glial cells required for maintaining the integrity of the myelin. It is clear that not only radiosensitivity but also the volume of tissue irradiated is important. Withers (1989) contended that the severity of a radiation-induced late effect in an organ is determined by the radiosensitivity of the stem cells and the arrangement into functional subunits. In those organs for which it has been determined, the radio-sensitivity of the stem cells is fairly similar, with the exception of the more radio-sensitive haematopoietic system. The most useful characteristic of the dose–response relationship is the $\alpha{:}\beta$ ratio (see section 5.1, Overall introduction), which is generally lower for late effects than for early effects and reflects the proportion of the damage repaired. The current approach to radiotherapy has gained from the idea that the quantal responses of tissues could be considered in terms of tissue-rescuing units (Hendry & Thames, 1986). It seems likely that damage to both the parenchymal cells and the microvasculature plays a role in the late deterministic effects, one being more important in some organs and less in others.

Most of the information about late effects comes from studies of patients undergoing radiotherapy. The success of radiotherapy comes at the risk of potential late effects, and dose fractionation is used to exploit the differential of repair and reco-very between normal and cancerous tissues (see Thames & Hendry, 1987).

Atomic bomb survivors constitute the largest population that has been exposed to whole-body irradiation; they have been monitored for almost five decades (Shimuzu *et al.*, 1999). During the period 1950–90, some 27 000 deaths occurred from causes other than cancer. The emphasis of the follow-up has been on diseases of the respi-ratory, cardiovascular and digestive systems, the rates of which increased 5–15% among people who received a dose of 1 Sv at these organs. This is a smaller increase than that for cancer. The most frequent causes of these deaths were stroke and heart disease, which accounted for about 54% of the total. It is not possible to distinguish statistically between a linear dose–response curve, a curvilinear response or the presence of a threshold. Late effects in the eye have also been studied, and the inci-dence of cataracts is discussed below.

The other relatively large population that has received whole-body irradiation is composed of patients who were exposed preparatory to bone-marrow transplantation. Late deterministic effects have been found in a number of tissues, including the lens of the eye, but no information is available on dose–response relationships, and the findings are confounded by prior chemotherapy in many patients. Future reviews of more homogeneous populations may provide more useful data.

The effects of radiation on organs for which some evidence of effects exists are described below.

4.2.1 *Skin*

The first reports of radiation-induced deterministic effects—erythema and radio-dermatitis—in the X-ray technicians and physicians involved in the early days of what would become radiology appeared within months of Röntgen's discovery of X-rays. The ease with which the effects of radiation on the skin could be detected made it the obvious indicator of exposure for the purposes of radiation protection.

In 1925, the concept of the 'tolerance dose' was introduced for use in setting limits on exposure to radiation, and was expressed as 1% of the threshold dose for inducing erythema per month for whole-body exposure to X-rays (Taylor, 1981). The ease with which effects could be detected in the skin proved to be of no advantage when it was realized that cancer could be induced by doses of penetrating radiation below those that induce deterministic effects in the skin. The classification of early and late deterministic effects in the skin is shown in Table 37.

Table 37. Radiation-induced deterministic effects in skin and time of appearance after exposure

Effect	Time of appearance after exposure
Early transient erythema	Hours
Main erythematous reaction	About 2 weeks
Dry desquamation	3–6 weeks
Moist desquamation	4 weeks
Late erythema	8–20 weeks
Secondary ulceration	10 weeks
Dermal necrosis	10 weeks
Dermal atrophy	26 weeks
Telangiectasia	52 weeks

From ICRP (1991c)

The tolerance of the skin depends on the area of the exposed field, the total dose, the fraction size and the interval between fractions. Unless the fields are large, erythema occurs only after exposure to 5–6 Gy or to about 12 Gy if the dose is fractionated; transient loss of hair may also occur. Moist desquamation may occur after a single dose of 18 Gy or after 40–50 Gy in about 25 fractions over about five weeks. The skin has a remarkably large capacity to recover from the damage induced by large total doses (tens of grays) if the dose is spread over a number of fractions, which allows time for repair of sublethal damage and for repopulation.

The early or acute effects of radiation on the skin include erythema, which occurs in varous phases. Erythema may be seen within hours of exposure of large fields to doses in the range used in radiotherapy, about 2 Gy, reflecting increased permeability of the capillaries and the early onset of inflammation. This phase is transient, and the erythema disappears within 24–48 h. The more significant phase, known as the main erythematous reaction, usually appears during the third week of a fractionated regimen. This phase is due to the inflammatory reaction that follows the death of cells in the basal layer of the epithelium. A few days after irradiation, cell proliferation may have stopped. Although the number of basal cells decreases, the integrity of the skin is maintained; however, dry desquamation may occur. With higher doses—about 30–40 Gy in multiple fractions—moist desquamation occurs. Desquamation is caused by inactivation of a critical number of clonogenic cells in the basal layer and follows within four to six weeks of exposure. Severe desquamation can lead to ulceration of the dermis. If the damage to the dermal vasculature is extensive, dermal necrosis may ensue within 10 or more weeks.

The responses to fractionated dose regimens are complex. In experimental studies of fractionated and prolonged irradiation of mouse skin, greater skin sensitivity was observed when 3-Gy fractions were given at an interval of 48 h than at either 6- or 24-h intervals. This effect was interpreted as the consequence of the increased radiosensitivity seen during the proliferative response induced by the radiation (Ruifrok *et al.*, 1994).

A different form of acute ulceration is found after exposure of extremely small areas of skin (and other epithelial surfaces) to very high doses, as occurs when 'hot' particles, such as the very small fragments of steel activated by neutron irradiation in a reactor, stick to the skin or in the nose, where they can remain unnoticed long enough to deliver an appreciable dose of β-particles and γ-rays. Within about two weeks of exposure, a pale, circular area surrounded by a halo of erythema is seen, which is quite distinct from other skin lesions induced by radiation. Ulceration follows when the overlying epidermis separates to reveal a small area of necrotic dermis. The evidence suggests that endothelial cells and fibroblasts in the superficial dermis are killed in interphase. The dosimetry for this type of radiation damage was established in experiments on pig skin *in vivo*. The median effective doses for the induction of moist desquamation by exposure to circular sources of ^{90}Sr (a high-energy β emitter) of various diameters were 27.5 Gy for a 22.5-mm source up to 75 Gy for a 5-mm source; the 2-mm and 1-mm sources induced acute necrosis within three weeks, at median effective doses of 125 and 275 Gy, respectively (Hopewell *et al.*, 1986).

Acute epithelial necrosis is induced by very-low-energy β-particles which cause interphase death in the suprabasal layer of the epidermis about 10 days after exposure. Radiation-induced lesions were studied in 56 workers, in particular firemen, at the Chernobyl facility who had incurred doses estimated to have been > 30 Gy at a depth of 150 mg cm^{-2} and over 200 Gy at about 70 mg cm^{-2}. The workers were exposed to high-activity fission products with a β-particle to γ-ray ratio of 10 to 30. Skin desquamation and subsequent infection in victims who received damage over 50% of their body surface area contributed to their deaths. All of these persons also had damage to their haematopoietic systems (UNSCEAR, 1988; Barabanova & Osanov, 1990).

Burns are induced by fall-out after detonation of nuclear weapons. For example, the doses to the skin received by Japanese fishermen exposed to the fall-out from one test were estimated to be 1.7–6.0 Gy. Erythema and necrosis were found in a few of the exposed men, and late effects were noted subsequently.

A late phase of erythema that gives the skin a dusky appearance is sometimes seen 8–20 weeks after exposure. It is seldom seen in patients receiving fractionated radiotherapy but was observed in victims of the Chernobyl accident who had received high doses 1.5 mm below the surface of the skin, where the deep dermal plexus of blood vessels is found. Loss of endothelial cells appears to be a major causal factor.

The other late effects of concern are dermal atrophy, telangiectasia and necrotic ulcer. The severity and the incidence of these lesions increase as the dose exceeds 30–40 Gy when given in fractions of 2 Gy. Dermal atrophy appears to develop in two phases, beginning 14–20 weeks after exposure and after about one year. The first phase is thought to be due to loss of endothelial cells, as in dermal necrosis (Hamlet & Hopewell, 1988), and to loss of fibroblasts (Withers *et al.*, 1980), a significant loss of endothelial cells sometimes preceding that of fibroblasts. The second phase involves degeneration of the smooth muscle of arterioles.

Telangiectasia may occur in patients treated with fractionated doses about one year or more after therapy. The incidence and the severity increase with time in a dose-dependent manner.

4.2.2 Lung

Radiation pneumonitis and fibrosis are the main deterministic effects in the lung. Three types of pulmonary cell are involved in the responses to radiation: type-1 and type-2 alveolar cells and endothelial cells; the last two undergo renewal and are targets for radiation-induced damage (see review by Travis, 1987). Radiation pneumonitis occurs in experimental animals and in humans about 80–180 days after exposure and, depending on the dose, may be fatal. The human lung is slightly more sensitive than that of mice, with estimated LD_{50} values of 9–10 Gy of external irradiation for humans and 12–15 Gy for mice. Radiation pneumonitis is characterized by interstitial oedema, infiltration of inflammatory cells and desquamation of alveolar epithelial cells. At high doses, an exudate is found in alveolar air spaces. An alveolar infiltrate can be detected radiologically, and opacification is detected by computerized tomography in a high percentage of patients within about 16 weeks of receiving fractionated doses. Dyspnoea is a symptom of pneumonitis in both humans and mice.

The effects of total dose, the number of fractions and the total period of treatment on the incidence of radiation-induced pneumonitis in patients undergoing radiotherapy are shown in Table 38.

Fibrosis, the main long-term effect of radiation on the lung, may occur in patients in whom pneumonitis has not been detected. The loss of volume and of diffusing capacity depend, as in other tissues, on the size of the radiation field. The histological changes include an increased amount of collagen which replaces the alveolar septa, a decrease in the number of functioning capillaries, atypical alveolar epithelial cells and loss of alveoli due to fibrotic changes which may lead to atelectasis. Lung fibrosis

Table 38. Incidence of radiation pneumonitis in patients undergoing radiotherapy, according to dose regimen

Total dose (Gy)	No. of fractions	Length of treatment (weeks)	Incidence of pneumonitis (%)
6–7	1		0 (threshold)
10	1		84
26.5	20	4	5
20	10	2–4	5
30.5	20	4	5
30.0	10	2	100

Data from Mah *et al.* (1987); UNSCEAR (1988)

may appear about one year after irradiation, and the changes are usually irreversible (Travis, 1987).

4.2.3   Gonads

(*a*)   Ovary

The ovary is a radiosensitive organ, but its radiosensitivity to the induction of sterility is age-dependent (Table 39). Radiation-induced ovarian failure gives rise not only to reduced fertility or sterility but also to reduction or cessation of hormone production, which may lead to premature menopause in younger women (Meistrich *et al.*, 1997). Amenorrhoea has been reported in 10% of patients exposed during childhood to 0.5 Gy to the ovaries and in about 66% exposed to 3.0 Gy (UNSCEAR, 1993). A dose of 1.0–1.5 Gy appears to be the threshold for an effect on fertility. Ovarian failure occurs in 40% of 20-year-old women and in 90% of 35-year-old women receiving a dose of 4.5 Gy. The effect is reduced by dose fractionation and protraction of radiotherapy (Meistrich *et al.*, 1997).

(*b*)   Testis

The germinative cells of the seminiferous tubules are highly radiosensitive, whereas the Sertoli cells, which provide support and nutrition for the spermatogonia, and the Leydig cells, the source of testicular hormones, are considerably more resistant. Irradiation may reduce fertility or induce temporary or permanent sterility but has little effect on libido. The response of the testis has been studied in patients undergoing radiotherapy, radiation workers, volunteers in state penitentiaries, victims of nuclear accidents and atomic bomb survivors (see Meistrich & Van Beek, 1990). The sperm count remains within the normal range for about eight weeks after irra-

Table 39. Minimum fractionated doses to the ovary that induce sterility

Dose (Gy)	Ovarian failure (%)	
	15–40 years of age	> 40 years of age
0.6	None	None
1.5	No risk	Small risk
2.5–5.0	60	100
5.0–8.0	60–70	NR
> 8.0	100	100

From Ash (1980) and Damewood & Grochow (1986);
NR, not reported

diation, but falls to its lowest level over the next three to eight months; aspermia may occur temporarily after a dose of about 0.2 Gy. The reduction in spermatogenesis is dose-dependent (Figure 13). A dose of 1.0 Gy causes aspermia in 90% of men. Fractionation does not reduce the effect and may increase it. The onset of recovery is also dose-dependent, occurring within about six months after a dose of 0.2 Gy but not until two years after a dose of 5 Gy. An analysis by Meistrich and Van Beek (1990) of the data obtained by Rowley *et al.* (1974) in a study of volunteers showed that type Ap and type B spermatogonia and early spermatocytes were the most radiosensitive cells and that late spermatocytes, spermatids and type Ad spermatogonia, considered to be the reserve stem cells, were somewhat less sensitive. It is difficult to estimate a threshold dose for temporary sterility, which depends on the time after exposure that fertility is assessed. A dose as low as 0.1 Gy has detectable effects in the young, and 0.15 Gy may cause oligospermia and temporary infertility in adults (UNSCEAR, 1993).

Two parameters have been used to assess the effect of radiation on the testis: loss of testicular weight and regeneration of the spermatogenic epithelium. The curve for loss of testicular weight as a function of dose has two components, and the logarithm of the loss of the radiosensitive component is linearly related to dose, with a D_0 of 0.9–1.0 Gy in mice, where D_0 represents cell killing due to multiple events (Kohn & Kallman, 1954; Alpen & Powers-Risius, 1981). The percentage of tubules that showed foci of repopulation by spermatogonial cells at 35–42 days after irradiation was used as a measure of stem-cell survival. At doses > 8 Gy, an exponential survival curve with a D_0 of 1.8 Gy was obtained (Withers *et al.*, 1974). It is not clear why the values for D_0 vary by a factor of two. A detailed assessment of the sensitivity of cells in the development stages of spermatogenesis in mice showed that the range of sensitivities is broad, but in general the sensitivity decreases from the intermediate spermatogonial stage to the mature sperm (see Table 40; Oakberg & Clark, 1964).

Figure 13. Percentages of men developing azoospermia after various single doses of radiation

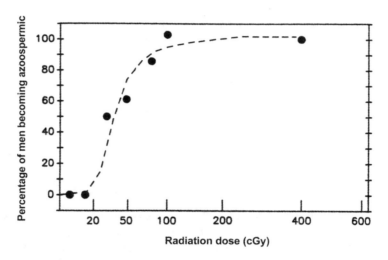

From Meistrich & Van Beek (1990). Doses are plotted after square-root transformation.

Table 40. Sensitivity of mouse spermatogenic cells to radiation

Cell type	LD_{50} (Gy)
Spermatogonia (types A_s, A_1–A_4)	2.0
Intermediate spermatogonia	0.2
Type B spermatogonia	1.0
Meiotic stages	2.0–9.0
Secondary spermatocytes	10.0
Spermatids	15.0
Spermatozoa	500.0

From Oakberg & Clark (1964); LD_{50}, median lethal dose

Although Leydig cells are generally considered to be relatively radioresistant, transient increases in serum follicular hormone concentrations were reported after exposure to doses as low as 0.2 Gy, while at 2.0 Gy the serum concentration of luteinizing hormone was increased. Both parameters are indicators of Leydig-cell dysfunction (Kinsella, 1989).

The outstanding features of the effects of radiation on the testis are the exquisite sensitivity of some testicular cells, the lack of sparing with fractionation and the long recovery time.

4.2.4   Kidney

Opinions about the relative radiosensitivity of the kidney vary (UNSCEAR, 1982). The importance of radiation-induced nephropathy and questions about whether the kidney should be shielded during whole-body irradiation before bone-marrow transplantation have renewed interest in the subject. The cells at risk in the three major components of the kidney, the renal tubules, the glomeruli and the complex, abundant vasculature, are mainly post-mitotic cells. This influences the response of the kidney to radiation and the sequelae. The late effects—nephritis, nephrosclerosis, tissue necrosis and fibrosis with subsequent hypertension and loss of renal function—are the main concerns (UNSCEAR, 1993).

Tests of renal function provide no evidence of renal damage during the first six months after radiotherapy with fractionated regimens of total doses < 23 Gy, but nephritis with signs and symptoms of renal damage may occur 6–12 months after treatment. Albuminuria and increased urea nitrogen in blood are common features. Renal failure and hypertension are later, more serious sequelae. The tolerance dose is about 23 Gy given in fractions over about five weeks to both kidneys. Doses of 20–24 Gy given over about four weeks may result in a 10–60% reduction in renal plasma flow and glomerular filtration rate.

The tolerance dose is lower in children than in adults, and radiation-induced nephropathy has been observed after bone-marrow transplantation in children. Anaemia, increased urinary creatinine concentrations and other signs of renal insufficiency have been observed after exposure to 12–14 Gy given in six to eight fractions. The precise contribution of radiation is difficult to assess because many such patients have had prior chemotherapy. It is also difficult to determine how much of the reduced tolerance, i.e. the delay before renal failure, is due to age or to chemotherapy. Experimental evidence in rats indicates that age is important and that tolerance increases with age at irradiation, within limits (Moulder & Fish, 1997).

The early histological changes seen in the kidneys after irradiation include hyperaemia, increased capillary permeability and interstitial oedema. The fine vasculature shows evidence of damaged endothelial cells and repopulation, which tends to occlude the lumen of the vessels. The glomerular arterioles are affected and blocked. The vascular occlusion and narrowing cause ischaemia in the cortex, and secondary degeneration of the tubular epithelium may follow. Damage to the tubules is the primary lesion, and dose–survival relationships have been determined in mice for the cells responsible for regeneration of the tubular epithelium. When regenerating tubules were scored in mice 60 weeks after irradiation, the D_0 was 1.53 Gy, which is comparable with that recorded for clonogenic cells in other tissues. The doses used in the assay (11–16 Gy) may, however, have damaged the vasculature (Withers *et al.*, 1986).

4.2.5   *Gastrointestinal tract*

The effects of radiation on the gastrointestinal tract have been the subject of extensive reviews (see e.g. Bond *et al.*, 1965; Becciolini, 1987; Potten & Hendry, 1995), from which the following descriptions are derived. Because the structure and the kinetics of cell turnover differ in the various regions of the gastrointestinal tract, the response to radiation also varies from one site to another.

(a)   *Oral cavity*

Effects on the oral mucosa provide a somewhat more sensitive indicator of radiation-induced damage than effects on the skin, and mucositis is widely used to assess the radiosensitivity of the oral cavity. The early changes are similar to those in the skin but occur sooner after exposure. In the second week of fractionated radio-therapy, dryness of the mouth and even dysphagia may occur. An interesting early effect is an alteration in sensitivity to taste, which appears to affect the taste of salt and bitter differentially from that of sour and sweet.

The late changes in the oral cavity are fibrosis in the submucosa, telangiectasia and fibrosis involving the mucous glands. Chronic ulcers of the mucosa can follow fibrosis in the vasculature. The environment of the oral cavity can be changed by exposure to radiation because the saliva from irradiated salivary glands is more acidic than normal, and dental caries may develop.

(b)   *Oesophagus*

Fractionated doses of 20–30 Gy can cause transient oesophagitis. Stricture may occur four to eight months after radiotherapy with doses of 30–65 Gy, depending on the fractionation regimen.

(c)   *Stomach*

Fractionated doses up to approximately 20 Gy have been used in the treatment of peptic ulcer. Irradiation suppressed gastric acidity for six months to many years and was well tolerated, but the risk for cancer increased subsequently. With conventional fractionated radiotherapy, the stomach can tolerate a dose of about 40 Gy, but the likelihood of ulceration and perforation increases rapidly above this dose. The delayed effects include dyspepsia, impaired gastric motility and chronic atrophic gastritis, due to fibrosis.

(d)   *Small intestine*

The small intestine is radiosensitive because the functional cells undergo rapid renewal and have a short lifespan. Studies in experimental animals indicate that damage to the intestinal epithelium occurs at doses > 1 Gy and that the degenerative changes are increasingly severe at doses of 5–10 Gy. Recovery depends on the survival of a sufficient number of clonogenic cells in the crypts before the villi and their vasculature lose their integrity. The acute radiation syndrome that occurs in humans after a single, high, whole-body irradiation is discussed in section 4.1. With fractionated radiotherapy, the probability of nausea, vomiting and diarrhoea is dependent on the dose per fraction and the frequency and number of fractions. Patients irradiated in the epigastric and abdominal regions experience nausea and vomiting, and when a dose of 25–30 Gy has been accumulated in radiation fields including the mid- and lower abdomen, loss of appetite, fatigue and diarrhoea are not uncommon. The malabsorption syndrome, involving reduced uptake of nutrients, may start during treatment and increase after therapy is completed. Patients vary in their sensitivity. Complications affecting the bowel after large-field abdominal radiotherapy have been reported to occur in 1% of patients receiving 35 Gy and in about 3% receiving higher doses. The late effects consist of excess collagen deposition in the submucosa and the typical radiation-induced changes in small vessels, such as intimal fibrosis (Becciolini, 1987).

(e)   Large intestine

Because the cell turnover rate is lower in the large intestine than in the small intestine, the former is less radiosensitive. Acute transient changes in the mucosal epithelium of both the colon and the rectum may occur with doses > 30–40 Gy. The rectum is relatively radioresistant, but rectal bleeding may occur 6–12 months after irradiation with fractionated doses totalling 60 Gy. The late changes include fibrosis, shortening of the colon and strictures. As in other tissues, late changes in the vasculature, such as endarteritis and fibrosis, are characteristic (Becciolini, 1987).

The survival curves for clonogenic cells of the jejunum and colon after irrradiation have been determined by the method introduced by Withers and Elkind (1970), which is based on the number of regenerating clones of crypt cells per cross-section of tissue three to four days after exposure to graded doses. The D_0 of the single-dose survival curve is about 1.3 Gy of 250-kVp X-rays. When the single-dose and the multiple-dose survival curves are separated, the 'shoulder' (see Figure 16, Overall introduction), assumed to indicate the amount of repair, is characterized by a D_q value between 4 and 4.5 Gy. Dose–survival curves for clonogenic cells in solid tissues can be determined experimentally only over a range of high doses, for example about 12–16 Gy in the jejunum. The survival curves for low doses must be obtained by reconstruction from data on fractionated doses.

4.2.6   Haematopoietic system

Death due to the acute radiation syndrome in the bone marrow is discussed in section 4.1. Depending on the dose, the prodromal stage is followed by the gastrointestinal syndrome; if the victim survives, the haematopoietic syndrome follows in the second week, and death may occur within two to three weeks after exposure to doses of 5.4–7.5 Gy and within four to six weeks after exposure to lower doses in the lethal range. The probability of death from bone-marrow damage depends on the treatment that is provided, more so than in any of the other syndromes. The prudent use of cytokines and growth factors has markedly improved the prospect of survival, although a fatal outcome becomes highly probable at doses ≥ 5.5 Gy. Survival of 10% of the haematopoietic progenitor cells is usually sufficient to prevent death.

The radiation-induced loss of the functional elements of the blood and the subsequent response depend on the cell type and the cell kinetics. The short lifespan of the neutrophils and platelets is reflected in the decreases in their number before that of the long-lived red cells. The radiosensitive subpopulations of lymphocytes are also affected shortly after exposure. Within 8–10 days, the decreases in granulocytes and platelets become critical, and, at doses in excess of 5 Gy, pancytopenia may follow (Figure 14). Haemorrhage and infection may exacerbate the condition (Wald, 1971).

The bone marrow can withstand higher total doses of radiation when the dose rate is lower, the dose is fractionated or the size of the radiation field is reduced. For example, patients irradiated with single doses < 10 Gy on either the upper or the lower half of the body can recover within about eight weeks. The effect is more severe after irradiation of the upper half of the body, where about 60% of the active bone marrow is found.

McCulloch and Till (1960) developed a technique for determining survival curves of colony-forming units that contain progenitor cells capable of producing erythrocytes, myelocytic elements and platelets. Erythrocytes predominated in the colonies that grew in the spleens of irradiated mice transplanted with bone marrow. When the bone-marrow cells were irradiated *in vivo*, the D_0 was 0.95 Gy, with a small shoulder on the survival curve (extrapolation number (*n*), 1.5; see Figure 16, Overall introduction). Both the D_0 and *n* were higher when the cells were exposed *in vitro*. The survival curves of colony-forming units in humans and mice are similar.

Information about the late effects of radiation on the bone marrow comes mainly from studies of patients undergoing radiotherapy and, to a lesser extent, from reports of accidental exposure. The decrease in progenitor cells may persist, and the duration of depletion is dose-dependent; the counts of circulating blood cells, especially lymphocytes, may be depressed for months. In general, accidental exposure to high but sublethal doses is followed by recovery of the bone marrow, as was also observed in the survivors of the atomic bombings. In the case of localized exposures to high total doses, aplasia is followed by replacement of the bone marrow with fat cells and fibrosis.

Figure 14. Counts (percentage of normal) of platelets, lymphocytes and neutrophils as a function of time after exposure to and dose of radiation during accidents

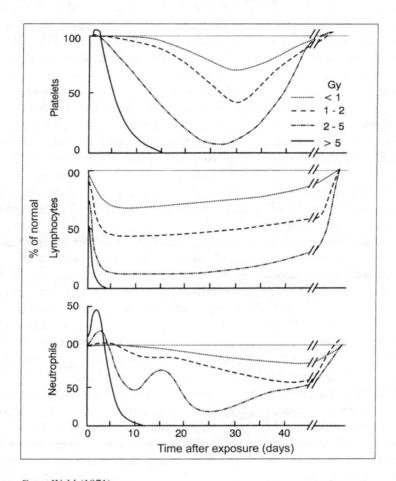

From Wald (1971)

4.2.7   *Central nervous system*

The developing brain is most sensitive to radiation during gestation. As early as 1929, recognition of the fact that proliferating cells are more radiosensitive than differentiated cells led Goldstein and Murphy (1929) to study children born to women exposed to pelvic irradiation during pregnancy. They found some effects on the central nervous system. Miller and Mulvihill (1956) reported that children exposed *in utero* to atomic bomb radiation had small head sizes, an indication of damage to the central nervous system.

Observation of severe mental retardation and reduced intelligence quotients in children exposed to radiation *in utero* indicated that the most sensitive periods are 8–15 and 16–25 weeks after fertilization (Otake & Schull, 1984, 1998). The number of neurons increases rapidly during weeks 8–15 of gestation, and proliferation of the neurons of the cerebral cortex is virtually complete by 16 weeks; by 26 weeks, the neurons are differentiated. Accordingly, no cases of severe mental retardation have been found among individuals exposed to radiation before 8 weeks or after 26 weeks of gestation. Some cell proliferation continues in the brain, particularly in the cerebellum, during the first two years of life, and the proliferating neurons are radiosensitive. Glial cells, which proliferate actively during the early years of life, retain the ability to divide. Loss of glial cells can lead to demyelinization. In the developing brain, neurons not only proliferate but also migrate to specific sites. This migration occurs mainly between weeks 7 and 10 and 13–15 of gestation and is virtually complete at 16 weeks. Exposure to radiation during weeks 8–16 of gestation is thus likely to interfere with this process. In a study with explants of the cerebral cortex from rat embryos at day 16 of gestation, a dose as low as 0.1 Gy affected neuronal migration (Fushiki *et al.*, 1993).

Most of the information on the effects of radiation on the brain postnatally comes from studies of patients—in particular, children treated for acute leukaemia. The degree of radiosensitivity depends on the effect and the age at exposure. In the adult brain, radiation-induced damage to the microvasculature is the major concern (for a review, see Gutin *et al.*, 1991). The acute central nervous syndrome (see section 4.1) occurs with doses of 20–100 Gy, and the survival time is about two days or less, but damage to the membranes and the vasculature rather than neuronal cell killing is involved. In contrast, neurons can be induced to fire (as detected by electroencephalography) by doses as low as 0.01 Gy.

Four types of late effect of radiation in the central nervous system have been described: leukoencephalopathy, mineralizing microangiopathy, cortical atrophy and cerebral necrosis. Leukoencephalopathy is not strictly an effect of radiation as it is the result of an interaction between radiation and methotrexate. It gives rise to demyelinization, multifocal necrosis and gliosis, but the grey matter and the basal ganglia are spared. The histological changes are reflected by reduced mental ability, ataxia, dementia and even death. Radiation doses of ≥ 20 Gy plus methotrexate will cause these lesions, but fractionated radiotherapy with 18–24 Gy alone does not. Mineralizing microangiopathy affects the cerebral grey matter and less frequently the cerebellum. It is assumed to be due to damage to the microvasculature, which leads to calcification, obstruction of the vessels and necrosis. Headaches, seizures, ataxia and defective muscle control have been noted. The condition is seen in children treated with a total dose of at least 20 Gy. Cortical atrophy, caused by focal necrosis with a loss of neurons from all layers, occurs in about 50% of patients receiving more than 30 Gy of fractionated radiotherapy to the entire brain. Cerebral necrosis, which involves an amorphous fibrin exudate, often in the junctional tissues between the white and grey matter, may appear 1–10 years after treatment. The incidence of cerebral necrosis increases rapidly at fractionated doses > 45 Gy (UNSCEAR, 1993).

The tolerance doses for brain damage are thus not known, but it is clear that the higher the dose per fraction the greater the probability of severe damage. In adults, a dose of 50 Gy to the brain in 2-Gy fractions over six weeks is considered to be critical, whereas the critical dose in children of three to five years of age is about 20% lower and that for younger children is even lower.

4.2.8   *Thyroid*

Hypothyroidism is the commonest late deterministic effect of radiation on the thyroid gland. It may be due to direct damage or, secondarily, to damage to the hypothalamic–pituitary axis (see UNSCEAR, 1993). Doses that are sufficient to affect function are more likely to be received during internal exposure from radionuclides such as ^{123}I, ^{125}I and ^{131}I for therapeutic treatment or as a result of a radiation accident.

Although there is conflicting evidence about the effect of age at the time of exposure, it is likely that the very young are more radiosensitive, as is the case for the induction of thyroid cancer (Ron, 1996). The activity of thyroid-stimulating hormone is frequently increased in children who have been irradiated for Hodgkin disease or brain tumours if the dose to the thyroid reaches about 24 Gy (Oberfield *et al.*, 1986), but no increase was found after exposure to 15 Gy (Glatstein *et al.*, 1971). Hypothyroidism was found in 20% of long-term survivors among children with acute leukaemia who received cranial or craniospinal irradiation with fractionated doses of a total of 18–25 Gy, the dose to the thyroid being about 3–8% of the total dose. No evidence of hypothyroidism has been found in children exposed to < 1 Gy (UNSCEAR, 1993). A study by DeGroot *et al.* (1983) indicated that chronic lymphocytic thyroiditis is relatively common in patients who received external irradiation in childhood. Hypothyroidism with increased serum levels of thyroid-stimulating hormone was found in 15% of patients who received < 30 Gy and in 68% of those who received higher doses (Kaplan *et al.*, 1983).

4.2.9   *Eye*

The ocular lens and the skin are the two tissues for which specific dose limits have been set for the prevention of deterministic effects of radiation. The occupational dose limits are 150 mSv year^{-1} and 500 mSv year^{-1}, respectively. The effects of radiation on these tissues were recognized soon after the discovery of X-rays. Much of the early literature on radiogenic cataracts was reviewed by Bendel *et al.* (1978), and the responses of the human eye were detailed by Merriam *et al.* (1972).

The lens is the most important radiosensitive structure in the eye, but it is not the only tissue affected. Keratitis and oedema of the cornea can occur after exposure to single doses of about 10 Gy, and damage to the lachrymal gland, the retina and the conjunctiva can be induced by higher doses (Merriam *et al.*, 1972).

The development and progression of the effects of radiation on the ocular lens can be studied by non-invasive techniques. While the mechanism of cataract induction by radiation is not known, the evidence indicates that cataracts are caused by damage of cells in the germinative zone, resulting in abnormal differentiation of the developing lens fibres. The latent period from the time of exposure to the appearance of opacities is consistent with the time required for the differentiation and migration of abnormal fibres. The long-held hypothesis that cell killing is central to the formation of lens opacities is being questioned, and damage to the genome of the epithelial cells has been proposed as an underlying principle (Worgul *et al.*, 1991). If this is so, cataract induction is probably a stochastic process with a threshold for a clinically significant lesion, and therefore differs from other deterministic effects. Like other deterministic effects, its incidence and severity increase with the dose of radiation.

The early stage of radiation-induced cataract is marked by changes in the posterior capsular area; subsequently, the anterior part of the lens is involved, and the posterior lesion expands. Opacities of the lens may develop and then cease to progress, and anecdotal accounts suggest that regression can occur. The latent period between exposure and detection of a cataract is dose-dependent but ranges from six months to several decades, with an average of two to three years (UNSCEAR, 1993).

Patients receiving radiotherapy are the main source of data for estimating the threshold dose for cataract induction and the increase in incidence with dose (Merriam *et al.*, 1972). The threshold single dose was estimated to be about 2 Gy, and the threshold for a dose fractionated over 3–13 weeks was estimated to be about 5.5 Gy. Further evidence of an effect of fractionation comes from studies of patients irradiated before bone-marrow transplantation: the incidence of cataract after a single dose of 10 Gy was 80%, while only 19% of patients who had received fractions of 2–4 Gy over six or seven days (total dose, 12–15 Gy) developed cataracts (Deeg *et al.*, 1984). At low doses above the threshold, the opacities are minimal and become static. The threshold dose for a progressive cataract is probably between 2.0 and 5.0 Gy.

In the survivors of the atomic bombings, the threshold dose for minimal opacities was reported to be 0.6–1.5 Gy, although the results are confounded by exposure of the survivors in Hiroshima not only to γ-rays but also to neutrons (see separate monograph; Otake & Schull, 1990). The data on radiation-induced cataracts in children treated for cancer are also confounded because in many cases the treatment consisted of a combination of radiotherapy and chemotherapy. Nevertheless, children appear to be more susceptible than adults. The data for the atomic bomb survivors also indicate age-dependency, the risk for cataract being two to three times higher in children under the age of 15 at the time of exposure than in older persons (UNSCEAR, 1993).

4.3 Radiation-sensitive disorders

Individuals who might be at enhanced risk for cancer caused by ionizing radiation include patients suffering from disorders that are associated with increased sensitivity to radiation at the cellular level. A paradigm of such disorders is xeroderma pigmentosum, in which enhanced sensitivity to the toxic effects of ultraviolet radiation (UV) parallels an enhanced risk for skin cancer after exposure to UV. The molecular mechanism underlying this phenomenon is reduced or absent repair of UV-induced DNA lesions, resulting in an increased frequency of mutations in the genome of cells from exposed parts of the body. These mutations can ultimately lead to cancer (see e.g. IARC, 1992). On the basis of this example, an enhanced risk for cancer induced by ionizing radiation might be expected in patients with a reduced capacity for repair of DNA damage and a smaller risk in those with conditions that result in disturbances in progression of the cell cycle. A further group of individuals who might be expected to show enhanced susceptibility to radiogenic cancer are those who have mutations of dominant tumour suppressor genes which are responsible for preventing the expansion of potentially malignant (initiated) cells. If radiation were to increase the number of these initiated cells, there would be an increased probability of their progression to frank tumours (for discussion, see National Radiological Protection Board, 1996).

4.3.1 *Ataxia telangiectasia*

The human genetic disorder ataxia telangiectasia is characterized by immunodeficiency, neurodegeneration, radiosensitivity and increased risks for developing a number of leukaemias and lymphomas and solid tumours (Boder, 1985; Sedgwick & Boder, 1991).

(*a*) *ATM gene and gene product*

The *ATM* gene ('mutated in ataxia telangiectasia') was identified by Savitsky *et al.* (1995). Full-length *ATM* cDNA was eventually cloned in two laboratories and shown to be capable of correcting aspects of the radiosensitivity of cells from patients with the disease as well as the defective cell-cycle checkpoints (Zhang *et al.*, 1997; Ziv *et al.*, 1997). Analysis of the *ATM* gene in patients with ataxia telangiectasia throughout the world showed over 300 mutations (see ataxia telangiectasia mutation database—http://www.vmmc.org/vmrc/atm.htm; P. Concannon and R. Gatti).

The ATM gene product is a highly phosphorylated nucleoprotein of about 370 kDa, which has a phosphatidylinositol 3-kinase (PI3) domain close to the C-terminus, through which it is related to a family of proteins involved in DNA damage recognition and/or cell cycle control (Hartley *et al.*, 1995; Anderson & Carter, 1996; Bentley *et al.*, 1996; Cimprich *et al.*, 1996). These proteins phosphorylate one or more substrates in response to DNA damage to activate signal transduction pathways and/or recruit proteins to sites of DNA repair. In the case of ATM, substrates such as TP53, c-Abl, RPA, mdm2 and PHAS-1 have been identified (Banin *et al.*, 1998; Canman *et al.*, 1998; Khanna *et al.*, 1998; Tibbetts *et al.*, 1999).

Immunoblotting studies showed that the ATM protein is located predominantly in the nucleus in proliferating cells (Chen & Lee, 1996; Keegan *et al.*, 1996; Lakin *et al.*, 1996; Brown *et al.*, 1997; Jung *et al.*, 1997; Watters *et al.*, 1997), although cell fractionation followed by immunoblotting revealed that 5–20% of ATM is in a microsomal fraction (Lakin *et al.*, 1996; Brown *et al.*, 1997; Watters *et al.*, 1997). Immunofluorescence studies confirmed that ATM is predominantly nuclear in fibroblasts, with relatively uniform distribution throughout the nucleus, except for nucleoli (Watters *et al.*, 1997). A distinct pattern of punctate labelling was seen in the cytoplasm, and immunoelectron microscopy showed that the protein is localized in 60–250-nm vesicles (Watters *et al.*, 1997) and co-localizes with β-adaptin to endosomes (Lim *et al.*, 1998).

(*b*)   *ATM and cell-cycle checkpoint control*

Cells from patients with ataxia telangiectasia are defective in activating both G_1/S and G_2/M phase checkpoints after irradiation, and DNA synthesis is inhibited to a lesser extent than in controls (Houldsworth & Lavin, 1980; Painter & Young, 1980; Scott & Zampetti-Bosseler, 1982; Nagasawa & Little, 1983; Beamish & Lavin, 1994).

Kastan *et al.* (1992) demonstrated that the response of the TP53 tumour suppressor protein in activating the G_1/S checkpoint after irradiation was defective in cells from patients with ataxia telangiectasia, and the induction of a number of *p53* effector genes was subsequently found to be reduced and/or delayed after irradiation (Canman *et al.*, 1994; Dulic *et al.*, 1994; Artuso *et al.*, 1995; Khanna *et al.*, 1995). Thus, *ATM* is initially activated in response to DNA damage by an unknown mechanism, which in turn activates *P53* (Shieh *et al.*, 1997; Siliciano *et al.*, 1997).

Cells from patients with ataxia telangiectasia are also characterized by radio-resistant DNA synthesis (Houldsworth & Lavin, 1980; Painter & Young, 1980) and a defective G_2/M checkpoint after irradiation (Nagasawa & Little, 1983; Ford *et al.*, 1984; Rudolph *et al.*, 1989). The reduced inhibition of DNA synthesis appears to be due to the failure of these cells to recognize and respond to the damage. Hyperphosphorylation of replication protein A is induced after irradiation in normal cells but is significantly delayed in cell lines from patients with ataxia telangiectasia (Liu & Weaver, 1993). When cells from patients with ataxia telangiectasia are irradiated in G_2 phase, they progress into mitosis with less delay than normal cells (Zampetti-Bosseler & Scott, 1981), but when they are irradiated in G_1 or S phase they progress through these phases unhindered and block irreversibly in the subsequent G_2/M phase (Beamish & Lavin, 1994).

(c)   Sensitivity to ionizing radiation

Clinical radiosensitivity in patients with ataxia telangiectasia was revealed when adverse reactions were observed during treatment with X-rays and other agents (Gotoff *et al.*, 1967; Morgan *et al.*, 1968; Feigin *et al.*, 1970). Increased sensitivity to radiation and radiomimetic agents was also demonstrated *in vitro* as reduced cell survival (Taylor *et al.*, 1975; Shiloh *et al.*, 1982a; Morris *et al.*, 1983; Shiloh *et al.*, 1983) and an increased frequency of chromosomal aberrations in cells from such patients after exposure to ionizing radiation (Higurashi & Cohen, 1973; Cohen *et al.*, 1975; Rary *et al.*, 1975). Defects in DNA repair in response to radiation damage were not found in early studies (Vincent *et al.*, 1975; Taylor *et al.*, 1976; Fornace & Little, 1980; Lavin & Davidson, 1981; Shiloh *et al.*, 1983), but a defect in potentially lethal damage repair was observed (Weichselbaum *et al.*, 1978; Cox *et al.*, 1981; Arlett & Priestley, 1983). Evidence was subsequently provided for a defect in DNA strand-break repair in cells from patients with ataxia telangiectasia. Cornforth and Bedford (1985) reported the existence of residual breaks in these cells, as demonstrated by premature chromatin condensation 24 h after irradiation. Foray *et al.* (1997) demonstrated that approximately 10% of double-strand breaks in such cells remained unrepaired for up to 72 h after irradiation. The exact nature of the lesion recognized by the ATM protein has not been identified, but it is likely to be some form of strand interruption (Taylor *et al.*, 1975; Chen *et al.*, 1978; Shiloh *et al.*, 1982b).

Since cells from patients with ataxia telangiectasia are defective in all cell-cycle checkpoints after irradiation and since they eventually accumulate and die in G_2/M, it was suggested that these cell-cycle anomalies could account for the radiosensitivity of these cells (Beamish & Lavin, 1994). The sensitivity is more likely to be due to a defect in the recognition and repair of specific lesions in DNA, with consequent effects on the cell cycle. Since radiosensitivity is observed in non-dividing cells from patients with ataxia telangiectasia, a repair defect is probably involved, rather than defective cell-cycle control (Jeggo *et al.*, 1998). Lack of correlation between *P53* status, G_1/S phase arrest and radiosensitivity in a variety of human cells and the fact that cells from $p53^{-/-}$ mice are more resistant to radiation (Lotem & Sachs, 1993; Lowe *et al.*, 1993; Clarke *et al.*, 1994) would appear to eliminate defective cell-cycle checkpoints as an explanation for sensitivy to radiation.

(d)   Cancers in patients with ataxia telangiectasia

A major hallmark of patients with ataxia telangiectasia is a predisposition to develop a range of lymphoid malignancies (Boder & Sedgwick, 1963). Around 10% of all such patients develop cancer, most of which are of the lymphoid type (Morrell *et al.*, 1986, 1990). The association between a defective thymus, immunodeficiency and the high frequency of lymphoid malignancies initially suggested that these tumours arose as a consequence of the immunodeficiency (Peterson *et al.*, 1964; Lévêque *et al.*, 1966; Miller & Chatten, 1967), but the observations that the spectrum of malignancies was not confined to those resulting from immunodeficiency and that chromosomal instability accompanied leukaemia in this syndrome provided an alternative explanation. Chromosomal rearrangements with specific breakpoints involving primarily chromosomes 7 and 14 are observed in up to 10% of T-lymphocytes from all patients with ataxia telangiectasia (Taylor *et al.*, 1996). The breakpoints are largely located in the vicinity of immunoglobulin heavy chain and *TCR* (T-cell receptor) genes, preferentially involving four regions, 7p13, 7q33-35, 14q11-12 and 14q32 (Hecht & Hecht, 1985). Clones capable of proliferation can be generated from translocations involving *TCR* genes and non-immune genes or inversions of chromosome 14, and these clones have been shown to develop into leukaemias (Taylor & Butterworth, 1986; Baer *et al.*, 1987; Davey *et al.*, 1988; Taylor *et al.*, 1992).

The lymphoid malignancies in patients with ataxia telangiectasia are of both B-cell and T-cell origin and include non-Hodgkin lymphoma, Hodgkin disease and several forms of leukaemia (Spector *et al.*, 1982; Hecht & Hecht, 1990). In a series of 119 patients with ataxia telangiectasia with neoplasms, 41% had non-Hodgkin lymphoma, 23% had leukaemia of any kind (usually acute lymphoblastic) and 10% had Hodgkin disease (Hecht & Hecht, 1990). In a smaller study in the United Kingdom of 17 children with ataxia telangiectasia, seven had leukaemias and 10 had lymphomas. The leukaemias were five T-cell acute lymphocytic leukaemias, a prolymphocytic leukaemia and a T-cell chronic lymphocytic leukaemia (Taylor *et al.*, 1996). In contrast, young adult patients with ataxia telangiectasia developed abnormal lymphocyte clones that converted with a high frequency into T-cell prolymphocytic leukaemia (Matutes *et al.*, 1991). Since the clonal expansions that give rise to lymphoid tumours in patients with ataxia telangiectasia are characterized by specific chromosomal breakpoints and rearrangements, it was considered likely that alterations in genes and/or their expression would contribute to the malignant phenotype. The breakpoints in chromosome 14 in patients with and without ataxia telangiectasia with T-prolymphocytic leukaemia occur in the vicinity of the *TCL-1* (T-cell leukaemia) locus (Baer *et al.*, 1987; Davey *et al.*, 1988; Mengle-Gaw *et al.*, 1988; Russo *et al.*, 1989; Virgilio *et al.*, 1993). *TCL-1* is expressed at high levels in leukaemia cells characterized by rearrangements of chromosome 14, suggesting that it is deregulated as a consequence of these changes (Virgilio *et al.*, 1994). Transcriptional activation of the *Tcl-1* proto-oncogene in transgenic mice caused the appearance of proleukaemic T-cell expansion expressing *Tcl-1*, and leukaemia developed after a long latency (Virgilio *et al.*, 1998). These results suggest that *TCL-1* plays an important role in the initiation of T-cell prolymphocytic leukaemia.

Overall, therefore, patients who are homozygous for *ATM* are cancer-prone, and their cells are hypersensitive to the induction of chromosomal damage and death by radiation, but they are not hypersensitive to other end-points such as inhibition of DNA synthesis and induction of *HPRT* mutations. There is no evidence that they are prone to radiogenic cancer.

(e)   ATM mutations in cancers in patients without ataxia telangiectasia

Clearly, the spectrum of leukaemias and lymphomas observed in patients with ataxia telangiectasia also occurs in the general population, albeit at low frequency. Since a higher incidence of these neoplasms is associated with loss of functional *ATM*, it was thought possible that sporadic cases of leukaemia, such as the rare T-cell pro-lymphocytic leukaemia, might show mutations in the *ATM* gene. Vorechovsky *et al.* (1997) used exon-scanning single-strand conformation polymorphism and described *ATM* mutations in 17/37 patients with T-cell prolymphocytic leukaemia. The pattern of mutations was complex, but most were missense mutations clustered in a region corresponding to the PI3-kinase domain of *ATM*. The mutations were predicted to interfere with either ATP binding or the catalytic activity of the ATM molecule. The pattern of mutations differed from those in patients with ataxia telangiectasia, the majority of which are predicted to give rise to truncated and unstable proteins (Gatti, 1998), and they did not tend to accumulate in specific regions of the molecule. Stilgenbauer *et al.* (1997) demonstrated loss of the q21–23 region of chromosome 11 (11q21–23) in 13/24 patients with T-cell prolymphocytic leukaemia. In six cases in which deletion of one *ATM* allele was shown, the second allele was also mutated and predicted to cause either absence, premature truncation or alteration of the ATM gene product. DNA fibre hybridization revealed structural lesions in both alleles of four T-cell prolymphocytic leukaemia samples (Yuille *et al.*, 1998). In a study of paired leukaemic and non-leukaemic cells, loss of heterozygosity at 11q22–23, including the *ATM* gene region, was detected in 10 of 15 cases. In cells from five T-cell prolympho-cytic leukaemias with loss of heterozygosity, immunoblotting revealed that the ATM protein was either absent or decreased in amount. These changes in ATM protein were reflected in nonsense, aberrant splicing and missense mutations in the second allele (Stoppa-Lyonnet *et al.*, 1998). These studies suggest that *ATM* is a tumour suppressor gene which, when inactivated, leads to the development of T-cell prolymphocytic leukaemia.

A second leukaemia seen frequently in patients with ataxia telangiectasia is B-cell chronic lymphocytic leukaemia (Taylor *et al.*, 1996). Loss of heterozygosity in the *ATM* gene was found in five of 36 cases (Starostik *et al.*, 1998), and reduced ATM protein (> 50%) was seen in 34% (38/111) of cases of this cancer. Patients with this deficiency had shorter survival times and more aggressive disease. Stankovic *et al.* (1999) detected mutations in the *ATM* gene in six of 32 patients and reduced or absent protein expression in eight of 20 tumours. There was no evidence of loss of hetero-zygosity in the region of the *ATM* gene, suggesting that the effect on ATM protein was due to a mutation within the gene. Germ-line mutations were detected in two of the six patients, indicating their *ATM* carrier status, whereas the frequency of *ATM* hetero-zygosity in the general population is 0.5–1% (Swift *et al.*, 1991; Easton, 1994). DNA sequence analysis revealed a mutated *ATM* gene in four of six patients with B-cell chronic lymphocytic leukaemia and an increased frequency of germ-line mutations (Bullrich *et al.*, 1999).

Loss of heterozygosity (loss of the wild-type allele leading to allelic imbalance) in the region of 11q23 has been reported in tumours of the cervix (Hampton *et al.*, 1994; Bethwaite *et al.*, 1995; Skomedal *et al.*, 1999), ovary (Gabra *et al.*, 1996), breast (Kerangueven *et al.*, 1997; Laake *et al.*, 1997; Rio *et al.*, 1998; Waha *et al.*, 1998), colon/rectum (Gustafson *et al.*, 1994; Uhrhammer *et al.*, 1998) and skin (melanoma) (Herbst *et al.*, 1995). While loss of heterozygosity in the 11q22–23 region is observed in T-cell acute lymphocytic leukaemia and ovarian cancer, no mutations in *ATM* have been reported in such cases (Takeuchi *et al.*, 1998; Koike *et al.*, 1999). These results suggest that epigenetic regulation of the *ATM* gene may play an important role in tumour development in some tissues. *ATM* is thus often mutated in some tumours that occur frequently in patients with ataxia telangiectasia but not in all.

(f) Radiosensitivity, ATM mutations and cancer risk in people heterozygous for ATM

Since ataxia telangiectasia is an autosomal recessive disorder, the *ATM* phenotype would not be expected to appear in gene carriers. Nevertheless, some penetrance does appear in carriers, namely intermediate sensitivity of their cells to ionizing radiation and increased risks for developing cancer and in particular breast cancer. Radiosensitivity of people heterozygous for *ATM* was first described by Chen *et al.* (1978), who used agar gel cloning and trypan blue exclusion to show that the radiosensitivity of six *ATM* heterozygous lymphoblastoid cell lines was intermediate between that of normal people and *ATM* homozygotes. Paterson and Smith (1979) subsequently described enhanced radiosensitivity, as determined by colony forming ability, and intermediate sensitivity to γ-radiation-induced DNA repair replication in fibroblasts from *ATM* heterozygotes. Such persons were subsequently reported to have greater radiosensitivity when taken as a group (Cole *et al.*, 1988). Dahlberg and Little (1995) demonstrated that the mean surviving fraction of irradiated control fibroblasts was significantly greater than that of *ATM* heterozygotes. Intermediate sensitivity in *ATM* heterozygotes has been shown in a number of other assays, including induction of chromosomal aberrations (Waghray *et al.*, 1990), production of micronuclei (Rosin & Ochs, 1986), flow cytometric analysis (Rudolph *et al.*, 1989; Lavin *et al.*, 1992) and by a cumulative labelling index (Nagasawa *et al.*, 1987). Heterozygotes as a group have been distinguished from controls by the radiosensitivity and accumulation of cells in the G_2 phase of the cell cycle (Shiloh *et al.*, 1986; Sanford & Parshad, 1990). A variety of measures of radiosensitivity distinguish *ATM* heterozygotes from controls, but there is considerable variation among heterozygotes and significant differences were found only when comparison was made between groups. None of the assays was specific for the detection of *ATM* heterozygotes.

Swift *et al.* (1991) concluded that diagnostic or occupational exposure to ionizing radiation probably increases the risk for breast cancer in women heterozygous for *ATM*. High doses of ionizing radiation, particularly before puberty, are known to increase the risk for breast cancer, but it is not yet known whether mammography leads to an increased risk for *ATM* carriers. A well-conducted mammographic examination involves an absorbed dose of about 0.3 cGy per breast, which, if applied annually over 35 years (between 40 and 75 years of age), would give rise to a lifetime radiation dose of 10.5 cGy—approximately the same as background radiation (Norman & Withers, 1992). An exposure of this order at the age of 40 would be estimated to increase the number of deaths from breast cancer by approximately 1/2000 women, which is insignificant when compared with the normal lifetime risk of 1/9 for breast cancer. If the increased sensitivity of *ATM* heterozygotes to radiogenic cancer were to parallel the hypersensitivity of their cells to radiation killing and the induction of chromosomal aberrations, i.e. an increase of 1.5–2-fold, a total dose of 10.5 cGy would not be expected to increase the lifetime risk for breast cancer in this group significantly. While the epidemiological studies point to a three- to fourfold increase in the risk for breast cancer, it is uncertain whether this is associated with mutation of the *ATM* gene.

(g)   *Cancer risk in* Atm$^{-/-}$ *mice*

Several murine models for ataxia telangiectasia have been developed by disrupting the mouse homologue, *Atm*, by gene targeting (Barlow *et al.*, 1996; Elson *et al.*, 1996; Xu *et al.*, 1996; Herzog *et al.*, 1998). Targeting led to loss of Atm protein, since truncated forms are highly unstable. In another model, deletion of nine nucleotides gave rise to a relatively stable, near full-length protein. Mice with a disturbed *Atm* gene showed disease characteristics similar in many respects to those of its human counterpart: growth retardation, mild neurological dysfunction, male and female infertility, immunodeficiency, sensitivity to cell killing by radiation and a predisposition to develop thymic lymphomas (Barlow *et al.*, 1996; Elson *et al.*, 1996; Xu *et al.*, 1996). In none of these studies in *Atm*$^{-/-}$ mice were the neurodegenerative changes seen in patients with ataxia telangiectasia reproduced, nor the ataxia and other abnormalities resulting from cerebellar changes. Kuljis *et al.* (1997) used electron microscopy to demonstrate the degeneration of several types of neuron in the cerebellar cortex of two-month-old *Atm*$^{-/-}$ mice. This process was accompanied by glial activation, deterioration of neutrophil structure and both presynaptic and postsynaptic degeneration, similar to observations made in patients with ataxia telangiectasia. Most *Atm*$^{-/-}$ mice also develop thymic lymphomas by three months of age (Barlow *et al.*, 1996; Elson *et al.*, 1996). These lymphomas grow rapidly, metastasize and lead to organ failure and death.

4.3.2   *Nijmegen breakage syndrome*

A number of syndromes have been described that overlap with ataxia telangiectasia in some of their clinical, cellular or molecular features (Byrne *et al.*, 1984; Lange *et al.*, 1993). Nijmegen breakage syndrome is an autosomal recessive condition characterized by immunodeficiency, chromosomal instability, sensitivity to cell killing by radiation and predisposition to cancer (Weemaes *et al.*, 1981; Shiloh, 1997). Documented cases of malignancy have been reported in 42 patients, including 12 lymphomas, one glioma, one rhabdomyosarcoma and one medulloblastoma (Van der Burgt *et al.*, 1996), and a significantly increased incidence of malignant neoplasms has been observed among persons heterozygous for the *NBS* (Nijmegen breakage syndrome) gene (Seemanová, 1990). The clinical presentation of this syndrome includes microcephaly, distinctive facial appearance, growth retardation and normal serum α fetoprotein, with none of the neuro-cutaneous manifestations seen in patients with ataxia telangiectasia (Chrzanowska *et al.*, 1995; Shiloh, 1997). The overwhelming majority of the 42 patients in the registry in Nijmegen in 1996 were detected in eastern Europe, particularly in Poland and the Czech Republic (Van der Burgt *et al.*, 1996).

Mapping of the *NBS* gene to chromosome 8q21 confirmed that the disease is genetically distinct from ataxia telangiectasia (Stumm *et al.*, 1995; Komatsu *et al.*, 1996; Matsuura *et al.*, 1997; Saar *et al.*, 1997; Cerosaletti *et al.*, 1998). The *NBS1* gene was cloned, and positional cloning showed a truncating mutation in patients with the syndrome (Matsuura *et al.*, 1998; Varon *et al.*, 1998). The gene product was designated 'nibrin' or p95 (Carney *et al.*, 1998).

Prior to its identification, nibrin/p95 was identified as part of a complex with four other components: hMre11 (Petrini *et al.*, 1995), hRad50 (Dolganov *et al.*, 1996) and two unidentified proteins of higher relative molecular mass. hMre11 and hRad50 are highly conserved between yeast and humans; in yeast, the phenotype of mutants includes hyper-recombination, sensitivity to DNA-damaging agents and DNA repair deficiency (Ajimura *et al.*, 1993; Game, 1993). This phenotype closely resembles that seen in Nijmegen breakage syndrome, suggesting that these patients have a defect in double-strand break repair. The hypothesis that hMre11 and hRad50 are involved in double-strand break repair is supported by the co-localization of these proteins in nuclear foci in response to breaks in DNA (Petrini *et al.*, 1995; Dolganov *et al.*, 1996). While Mre11, Rad50 and p95 co-immunoprecipitate as part of the same complex, Mre11 and Rad50 maintain a complex in the absence of p95 in cell extracts from patients with Nijmegen breakage syndrome, although radiation-induced foci are not evident.

These findings suggest that p95 is required for localization of the complex to damaged DNA. The hMre11–hRad50–p95 complex has magnesium-dependent single-strand DNA endonuclease and $5' \rightarrow 3'$ exonuclease activities, which could be important in recombination, repair and genetic instability (Lieber, 1997). Since the homologue of hMre11 in *Saccharomyces cerevisiae* has nuclease activity, it is likely that the corresponding human protein is responsible for these cleavages (Cao *et al.*, 1990).

Radiosensitivity is a uniform feature of Nijmegen breakage syndrome. The results of cytogenetic analyses by Conley *et al.* (1986), Taalman *et al.* (1989), Barbi *et al.* (1991) and Stoppa-Lyonnet *et al.* (1992), reviewed by Weemaes *et al.* (1994), showed that the percentage of chromosome 7 and 14 rearrangements was significantly higher in patients with this syndrome than in patients with ataxia telangiectasia. The hyper-sensitivity of cells from patients with Nijmegen breakage syndrome to X-rays and bleomycin was demonstrated by Taalman *et al.* (1983) and Jaspers *et al.* (1988). The D_0 values of the survival curves were of the same order as those reported for cells from patients with ataxia telangiectasia, and reduced inhibition of DNA synthesis after irradiation was noted. The basis for the radiosensitivy appeared to be distinct from that in cells from patients with ataxia telangiectasia, as fusion of these cells with cells from patients with Nijmegen breakage syndrome fully abolished the X-ray hypersensitivy of the former to cell killing (Jaspers *et al.*, 1988).

A defect in the S phase checkpoint in cells from patients with Nijmegen breakage syndrome was first described by Taalman *et al.* (1983), who showed that suppression of DNA synthesis by ionizing radiation was less effective in these cells than in control cells.

Abnormalities in the activation of the *p53*-inducible response to ionizing radiation have been documented in Nijmegen breakage syndrome cells, with a reduced response in fibroblast and lymphoblastoid lines after exposure to 5 Gy (Jongmans *et al.*, 1997). Studies of G_1–S cell-cycle progression in Nijmegen breakage syndrome cells after exposure to ionizing radiation produced conflicting results (Antoccia *et al.*, 1997; Jongmans *et al.*, 1997; Sullivan *et al.*, 1997; Tupler *et al.*, 1997; Yamazaki *et al.*, 1998), which may be due in part to differences in the cell types being studied. Increased accumulation in G_2 phase after exposure to ionizing radiation has also been reported (Seyschab *et al.*, 1992; Antoccia *et al.*, 1997; Jongmans *et al.*, 1997).

4.3.3 *Human severe combined immunodeficiency syndromes*

Bosma *et al.* (1983) first described a mouse mutant which had no detectable B or T lymphocytes. This severe combined immunodeficient (SCID) mouse was defective in recombination of the immunoglobulin heavy chain and *Tcr* genes and hyper-sensitive to ionizing radiation (Kim *et al.*, 1988; Biedermann *et al.*, 1991; Budach *et al.*, 1992), due to defective repair of double-strand breaks in DNA (Biedermann *et al.*, 1991), in which DNA protein kinase is involved (Blunt *et al.*, 1995; Araki *et al.*, 1997). To date, no human mutant in the catalytic subunit of DNA protein kinase has been described, but cell lines deficient in this protein and sensitive to radiation have been isolated from human tumours, including gliomas (Allalunis-Turner *et al.*, 1995). An extremely low level of ATM protein in these cells could also contribute to their radiosensitivity (Chan *et al.*, 1998), as dominant negative and anti-sense *ATM* constructs led to sensitization of normal control cells as a consequence of decreasing endogenous levels of ATM (Morgan *et al.*, 1997; Zhang *et al.*, 1998).

Human SCID includes a spectrum of X-linked and autosomal recessive disorders characterized by abnormalities in cellular and humoral immunity (Rosen *et al.*, 1984; Puck, 1994). These syndromes include X-linked SCID, adenosine deaminase deficiency, Swiss-type agammaglobulinaemia and atypical syndromes, Omenn syndrome, purine nucleoside phosphorylase deficiency and immunodeficiency with short limb dwarfism. SCID is usually classified into two general groups according to the presence (B^+ SCID) or absence (B^- SCID) of B cells (Fischer, 1992). Some 70% of patients represent the former group. The incidence of classical SCID is between one in 5×10^4 and one in 7.5×10^4 births; the disease is detected by the occurrence of severe bacterial, viral and fungal infections and is fatal unless treated by bone-marrow transplantation. Some rare cases of SCID have been reported in which pre-B and mature B cells are absent (Ichihara *et al.*, 1988).

Little information has been reported on human SCID. Cavazzana-Calvo *et al.* (1993) described increased sensitivity to radiation of granulocyte macrophage colony-forming units in three patients without mature T or B cells and a twofold sensitization of the cells to X-rays. The D_0 value of the survival curve for fibroblasts from one of these patients was the same as that observed for granulocyte macrophages, indicating that the basis for the radiosensitivity overlapped with the immune defect. In the same study, increased sensitivity to radiation was also observed for granulocyte macrophages in a patient with Omenn syndrome, which includes a restricted T-cell repertoire and no B cells, but cell survival was normal in a patient with X-linked SCID who lacked only T cells. In a follow-up study, Nicolas *et al.* (1998) demonstrated increased sensitivity to ionizing radiation in fibroblasts and bone-marrow precursor cells in T^- B^- SCID patients. Sproston *et al.* (1997) described variable radiosensitivity of fibroblasts in a variety of SCID disorders. SCID strains were significantly more sensitive to radiation at both low- and high-dose rates. The cells most sensitive to radiation were from patients with T^- B^- SCID (D_0, 0.60 Gy), at a dose comparable to that reported by Cavazzano-Calvo *et al.* (1993). Lymphoblastoid cells from two patients with X-linked agammaglobulinaemia showed radiosensitivity equivalent to that of cells from patients with ataxia telangiectasia (Huo *et al.* 1994). Overall, SCID patients with no detectable B cells (30% of patients) are the most severely affected and have abnormalities in immunoglobulin gene rearrangements (Schwarz *et al.*, 1991; Abe *et al.*, 1994). These irregular rearrangements were subsequently shown to be due to mutations in the V(D)J recombinases RAG1, RAG2 or both in approximately 50% of B^- SCID patients (McBlane *et al.*, 1995; Akamatsu & Oettinger, 1998).

4.3.4   *Adverse responses to radiotherapy*

Severe chemosensitivity and acute radiation reactions were observed in a patient being treated for acute lymphoblastic leukaemia (Plowman *et al.*, 1990). Fibroblasts from this individual were found to be indistinguishable from cells from patients with ataxia telangiectasia when exposed to ionizing radiation and were defective in repair of double-strand breaks in DNA (Plowman *et al.*, 1990; Badie *et al.*, 1995, 1997). The enhanced radiosensitivity was suggested to be due to a mutation in DNA ligase IV (Riballo *et al.*, 1999), as a patient was identified in whom DNA ligase was mutated in a conserved motif encompassing the active site. The defective protein was severely compromised in its ability to form a stable enzyme–adenylate complex. This individual, who appeared to be immunologically normal, had pronounced radiosensitivity, indicating that apparently normal individuals exist in the population who are radiosensitive due to a DNA-repair deficiency and may therefore be predisposed to leukaemia.

Individuals vary considerably in their ability to respond to radiation, as evidenced by the range of severity of the reactions of normal tissues of cancer patients exposed to radiotherapy; approximately 5% of patients show severe reactions (Norman *et al.*, 1988; Ribeiro *et al.*, 1993). Data on the survival of fibroblasts in culture have not predicted tissue sensitivity (West & Hendry, 1992; Budach *et al.*, 1998); only the adverse effects of radiotherapy in patients with ataxia telangiectasia (Gotoff *et al.*, 1967) were reflected in the hypersensitivity of the cells in culture to ionizing radiation (Taylor *et al.*, 1975; Chen *et al.*, 1978).

Chromosomal radiosensitivity has been observed in a number of syndromes characterized by a predisposition to cancer. Scott *et al.* (1998) drew attention to the importance of this characteristic as a biomarker for cancer, although sensitivity in these syndromes to various agents, including ionizing radiation, may not be the mechanism for cancer development. Using an assay to detect radiation-induced chromosomal damage in lymphocytes in G_2 phase, Scott *et al.* (1996) found that approximately 40% of an unselected series of breast cancer patients had elevated chromosomal radiosensitivity. Parshad *et al.* (1996) suggested that deficient DNA repair is a predisposing factor in breast cancer. When G_2/M cell-cycle arrest was determined 18–24 h after irradiation, lymphoblastoid cell lines from 22 of 108 breast cancer patients were shown to be radiation-sensitive (Lavin *et al.*, 1994), and in a rapid assay for micronucleus formation in lymphocytes exposed to γ-rays with delayed mitogenic stimulation, 12 of 39 breast cancer patients and 2 of 42 controls were found to be hypersensitive to radiation (Scott *et al.*, 1998). Thus, a substantial proportion of breast cancer patients showed cells that were sensitive to radiation *in vitro*. Severe clinical radiosensitivity, however, is observed in a considerably smaller proportion, approximately 5%, of breast cancer patients. Some of these patients may harbour a mutation in the *ATM* gene, particularly since there is substantial evidence that the sensitivity of at least some *ATM* heterozygotes to radiation is intermediate (Chen *et al.*, 1978; Shiloh *et al.*, 1986; Rudolph *et al.*, 1989; Waghray *et al.*, 1990; Lavin *et al.*, 1992). No mutations were found in the *ATM* gene in 16 breast cancer patients with severe acute reactions to radiotherapy (Appleby *et al.*, 1997) or in 15 patients who had developed severe late reactions to a standard radiotherapy schedule (Ramsay *et al.*, 1998), although the method used in the latter study would have missed up to 30% of non-truncating mutations, including missense mutations (Gatti, 1998). About 10% of *ATM* mutations are missense mutations. In this respect, it is of considerable interest that several rare allelic substitutions in *ATM* were observed in patients with various cancers but not ataxia telangiectasia (Vorechovsky *et al.*, 1997). It is unclear whether these changes affect the function of the ATM protein in such a way as to influence either radiation sensitivity or cancer susceptibility.

4.3.5   *Tumour suppressor gene disorders*

(*a*)   *Humans*

The term 'tumour suppressor gene' has been used to describe genes involved in growth control, differentiation and apoptosis, which undergo loss of function in the development of cancer (Stanbridge, 1990). Mutation in these genes would be expected to lead to a predisposition to cancer and a propensity to develop tumours in response to radiotherapy, but not necessarily to increased sensitivity of cells in culture.

(i)   *Retinoblastoma*

Retinoblastoma is the most common intraocular malignancy in children and has served as the prototypic example of genetic predisposition to cancer (see Knudson, 1984; Newsham *et al.*, 1998). Loss of one germ-line copy of *RB1* from all somatic cells predisposes to cancer in a dominant fashion because of the high probability of the loss of the remaining wild-type gene from a critical cell. It is estimated that 60% of cases are non-hereditary and unilateral, 15% are hereditary and unilateral, and 25% are hereditary and bilateral.

A significant proportion of children with the heritable bilateral form of retino-blastoma develop second cancers, most frequently bone and soft-tissue sarcoma. In an analysis of the treatment of 151 patients who developed a second neoplasm more than 12 months after the first, the second malignancy was considered to be associated with radiation in 61% of cases (Kingston *et al.*, 1987). A dose–response relationship for the induction of bone and soft-tissue sarcomas in patients with the heritable form of the disease who were treated by radiotherapy has been documented. The relative risks for soft-tissue sarcomas showed a step-wise increase for all dose categories and were statistically significant at 10–29.9 Gy and 30–59.9 Gy. An increased risk for all sarcomas combined was evident at doses > 5 Gy, rising to 10.7-fold at doses $\geq$ 60 Gy ($p < 0.05$) (Wong *et al.*, 1997). In a retrospective cohort study of mortality from second tumours among 1603 long-term survivors of retinoblastoma, follow-up was complete for 91% of the patients for a median of 17 years after diagnosis of the retinoblastoma. Of the 305 deaths, 167 were from retinoblastoma and 96 were from second primary tumours (relative risk, 30), with statistically significant excess mortality from second primary cancers of bone, connective tissue and malignant melanoma and benign and malignant neoplasms of the brain and meninges. Radiotherapy for retinoblastoma further increased the risk of dying from a second neoplasm (Eng *et al.*, 1993).

(ii)   *Li–Fraumeni syndrome*

Li–Fraumeni syndrome is a rare disorder with a high penetrance in respect of a range of tumour types. It is often associated with a germ-line mutation in the *p53* tumour suppressor gene (Malkin *et al.*, 1990; Malkin, 1998). Patients with Li–Fraumeni syndrome or with a similar familial pattern of cancer are at increased risk for second cancers after irradiation, many of the neoplasms occurring in the irradiated field. Patients with familial patterns of cancer similar to those of the syndrome are found to form a significant fraction of those who develop bone sarcoma or acute leukaemia after radiotherapy for rhabdomyosarcoma (Heyn *et al.*, 1993).

(iii)   *Naevoid basal-cell carcinoma syndrome*

The carcinogenic effects of ionizing radiation in patients with naevoid basal-cell carcinoma syndrome were recognized more than 50 years ago when a five-year-old boy was reported to have developed more than 1000 pigmented basal-cell lesions in the irradiated field after radiotherapy for thyroid enlargement. DNA synthesis is abnormally rapid in X-irradiated cells from such patients, and it has been suggested that this might be related to the susceptibility to cancer after exposure to X-rays (Fujii *et al.*, 1997). Taylor *et al.* (1975) and Stacey *et al.* (1989) reported no difference in survival between normal cells and those from patients with naevoid basal-cell carcinoma syndrome after exposure to γ-rays. Children with this syndrome who were treated for medulloblastoma developed multiple basal-cell carcinomas on irradiated skin (Atahan *et al.*, 1998; and see section 2.7).

(iv)   *BRCA1 and BRCA2*

Mutations in a small number of highly penetrant autosomal dominant genes are responsible for approximately 5% of breast and ovarian cancers (Szabo & King, 1995; Stratton & Wooster, 1996; Easton, 1997). Mutations in two of these genes, *BRCA1* and *BRCA2*, lead to early-onset breast cancer (Futreal *et al.*, 1994; Miki *et al.*, 1994). In families with multiple cases of both breast and ovarian cancer, *BRCA1* mutations are primarily responsible for the disposition, while they make a smaller contribution in families with breast cancer only (Easton *et al.*, 1993; Peto *et al.*, 1996). The prevalence of *BRCA1* mutations has been estimated to be 1/800 in western populations and that of *BRCA2* to be less (Peto *et al.*, 1996), although the prevalence can be as high as 1/100 in some inbred populations (Friend, 1996). The BRCA1 protein co-localizes in S-phase nuclei of human fibroblasts with Rad51 and interacts with this protein through a region encoded by exon 11 of *BCRA1* (Scully *et al.*, 1997). It shares this property with BRCA2 (Sharan *et al.*, 1997), which suggests that both proteins are involved in DNA repair and maintenance of genome integrity. In support of such a role, Gowen *et al.* (1998) demonstrated that *Brca1⁻/⁻* embryonic stem cells are defective in transcription-coupled repair of oxidative DNA damage and are hypersensitive to ionizing radiation and hydrogen peroxide. Whether the sensitivity to ionizing radiation arises as a consequence of a defect in transcription-coupled repair or is due to defective strand-break repair through the Rad51 pathway or to a combination of the two remains unclear. Further evidence for a role of the BRCA1 protein in DNA damage repair was reported by Husain *et al.* (1998), who showed that *BRCA1* is overexpressed in a cisplatin-resistant breast cancer cell line (MCF-7) and that inhibition of *BRCA1* with antisense vectors increased the sensitivity, decreased the efficiency of DNA repair and enhanced the rate of apoptosis. Ramus *et al.* (1999) showed that *p53* mutations are significantly more frequent in ovarian tumours with mutations in either *BRCA1* or *BRCA2* than in controls. These results support a model of BRCA-induced tumorigenesis in which loss of cell-cycle checkpoint control coupled with inefficient DNA repair is necessary for tumour development.

(v)   *Second tumours arising in response to radiotherapy*

Second malignant neoplasms occur at a higher frequency than expected after prior treatment with radiotherapy, particularly of childhood cancer (Tucker *et al.*, 1984; Hawkins *et al.*, 1987; de Vathaire *et al.*, 1989, 1999b). The studies of children with naevoid basal-cell carcinoma syndrome after being treated for medulloblastoma, discussed above, and other studies show that genetic background can influence the process of carcinogenesis in response to radiation. A case–control study has been reported in which 25 children from a cohort of 649 developed a second malignant neoplasm in response to radiotherapy during the period 1953–85. Children with one or more family relatives who had cancer had an odds ratio of 4.7 (95% CI, 1.3–17.1; $p = 0.02$) for a second malignant neoplasm when compared with children who had no family history of early-onset cancer. Thus, it is important to monitor children treated with radiotherapy, especially when there is a family history of early-onset cancer (Kony *et al.*, 1997).

(*b*)   *Experimental models*

Several animal models have been used to mimic cancer-predisposing conditions in humans in which radiation is implicated as a tumorigenic agent. These include inbred strains susceptible to the development of tumours (Storer *et al.*, 1988) and animals with mutations in known tumour suppressor genes (Friedberg *et al.*, 1998). In general, strains with a high spontaneous frequency of solid tumours also show an increased frequency of radiation-induced tumours (Storer *et al.*, 1988; Kemp *et al.*, 1994).

(i)   pr53 *gene*

Mutation of the *p53* gene is among the most frequent genetic alterations in human tumours (Hainaut *et al.*, 1998). The TP53 protein is important in maintenance of a normal cellular phenotype owing to its involvement in cell-cycle control, as a promoter of DNA repair and programmed cell death (Ko & Prives, 1996). *pr53* knock-out mice provide a dramatic demonstration of the role of *pr53* in experimental carcinogenesis: mice homozygous for a null *pr53* allele develop tumours at very high rates early in life, and the latent period for spontaneous tumours in *pr53* heterozygotes lies between that of the nulls and the wild types. The latent period for tumours in such mice can be significantly reduced by exposure to ionizing radiation (Kemp *et al.*, 1994), and the mice develop lymphoid tumours. The principal effect of *pr53* deficiency in the haematopoietic system of mice appears to be a constitutive abnormality that gives rise to an approximately 20-fold increase in the frequency of stable aberrations in *pr53* null mice and a 13-fold increase in *pr53* heterozygotes. The induction of stable aberrations was not increased by γ-rays, but *pr53* deficiency resulted in excess radiation-induced hyperploidy (> 10-fold the wild-type frequency) (Bouffler *et al.*, 1995).

(ii)   *Murine adenomatous polyposis coli gene*

Min (multiple intestinal neoplasia) is a mutant allele of the murine *Apc* (adenomatous polyposis coli) locus that contains an *N*-ethyl-*N*-nitrosourea-induced nonsense mutation at codon 850 (Su *et al.*, 1992; Moser *et al.*, 1995). Heterozygosity for this mutation in the Min mouse is analogous to the genetic condition of familial adenomatous polyposis in humans (Joslyn *et al.*, 1991; Nishisho *et al.*, 1991), in that it predisposes to intestinal neoplasia. γ-Irradiation has been shown to increase the number of intestinal adenomas per mouse (Luongo & Dove, 1996; Ellender *et al.*, 1997). While these tumours were not observed in irradiated or untreated wild-type animals, the adenomas in the irradiated Min mice depended on the *Min* mutation, and the exposure caused chromosomal deletions involving loss of the *Apc* gene (Luongo & Dove, 1996).

(iii)   *Eker rat*

The Eker rat strain is characterized by heterozygosity for a germ-line mutation in the *Tsc* 2 tumour suppressor gene, which predisposes this animal to spontaneous renal-cell carcinoma (Eker & Mossige, 1961). The corresponding mutation in humans is associated with tuberous sclerosis syndrome and leads to an increased incidence of renal cancers and of blastomas of the skin, heart and nervous system (Al-Saleem *et al.*, 1998). Exposure of Eker rats to 9 Gy of radiation caused an 11–12-fold increase in the incidence of renal tumours. When comparison was made with wild-type rats, the relative risk for developing renal-cell carcinomas after irradiation was 100-fold greater in the mutant animals (Hino *et al.*, 1993). This study has some deficiencies, however, because the wild-type animals were monitored for only 11 months, a short period for estimating life-time risk.

(iv)   *Brca2*

Although disruption of the *Brca2* gene in mice led to embryonic lethality, it was possible to establish that *Brca2* expression is transient and largely embryo-specific, with transcripts particularly prevalent in tissues with a high mitotic index. Evidence that the Brca2 protein might be involved in repair of damage to DNA stems from its ability to bind to the MmRad51 protein, a key component in the repair of double-strand breaks in DNA. Furthermore, homozygous mutants in these genes show developmental arrest at a similar stage, and their expression patterns are similar (Sharan *et al.*, 1997). In keeping with the radiosensitivity of MmRad51$^{-/-}$ embryos (Lim & Hasty, 1996), exposure of blastocysts from *Brca2*$^{-/-}$ embryos to 4 Gy of γ-rays led to complete ablation of the inner cell mass. It was not possible to distinguish between *Brca2*$^{+/-}$ and wild-type embryos. Because of the involvement of *Brca2* in DNA repair and the sensitivity to irradiation of *Brca2*$^{-/-}$ embryos, it will be of interest to determine whether heterozygous animals are susceptible to tumours.

4.4   Genetic and related effects

4.4.1   *Humans*

Evaluation of the hereditary effects associated with exposure of human populations to ionizing radiation has been a major concern of UNSCEAR. Many approaches have been used to formulate optimal predictions of the extent to which a given dose of ionizing radiation will increase the naturally occurring rate of mutation of germ cells in humans and how such an increase would affect the health of future generations.

(*a*)   *Background radiation*

The cytogenetic effects of chronic exposure to ionizing radiation have been studied among populations in areas with high background levels of natural radiation (see section 2.5.1). A group of 100 women aged 50–65 years living in Yangjiang County, China, with an annual whole-body dose of 0.18–0.28 cGy were compared with a control group of 100 women living in an area where the annual whole-body dose was 0.06–0.09 cGy. Peripheral blood lymphocytes were collected from all of the women and analysed for the presence of chromosomal aberrations. Overall and for each category of stable and unstable chromosomal aberrations, women in the area with high background radiation had more detectable abnormalities. The increase was statistically significant for unstable aberrations (dicentrics and rings; $p < 0.04$) and for the combination of stable and unstable aberrations ($p < 0.02$) (Wang *et al.*, 1990b).

Similar results were obtained in another study in the same region among people in a wider age group (15–65 years). The frequencies of dicentrics and rings were significantly higher in lymphocytes of inhabitants of the area with high background radiation than those from the area with low background exposure ($p < 0.05$). A higher frequency of stable aberrations was also reported among students aged 15–16 years ($p < 0.01$), and higher frequencies of stable and unstable aberrations were again found among women aged 50–65 years ($p < 0.05$ for both categories) (Chen & Wei, 1991).

(*b*) *Survivors of the atomic bombings*

The data on the survivors of the atomic bombings of Hiroshima and Nagasaki indicate that acute irradiation at moderate doses has a negligible adverse effect on the health of subsequent generations. Any minor effect that may be produced is so small that it is lost in the background noise of naturally occurring mutational effects: an increase above this background has not been demonstrated even by the refined epidemiological methods that have been used over the last five decades (Neel *et al.*, 1988; Neel, 1991; UNSCEAR, 1993). Information on the following types of adverse effect has been accumulated: untoward pregnancy outcome (congenital malforma-tions, stillbirths and neonatal deaths); deaths among children before reproductive age (exclusive of those resulting from a malignant tumour); cancer before the age of 20; increased frequencies of certain types of chromosomal abnormalities (balanced struc-tural rearrangements, abnormalities in sex chromosomes); increased frequencies of mutations affecting certain characteristics of proteins; altered sex ratios and impaired physical development of children.

Although some changes in these effects were noted in comparison with a control group, no statistically significant effect of parental irradiation has been found. The average combined dose of acute ionizing radiation to the gonads received by the parents was approximately 0.4 Sv (Neel *et al.*, 1988, 1990), which is similar to the dose that has been estimated to double the frequency of genetic effects in mice. This suggests that humans may be less sensitive to the genetic effects of radiation than mice. When it was assumed that some of the mutations did indeed result from the exposure to radiation from the atomic bombings, a doubling dose of 1.7–2.2 Sv was calculated (Neel *et al.*, 1990; Sankaranarayanan, 1996), whereas the doubling dose for severe genetic effects after long-term exposure was estimated to be approximately 4 Sv. The notion that ionizing radiation must have some genetic effect was strengthened by the observation of an increase in the frequency of chromosomal damage in the lym-phocytes of atomic bomb survivors (Awa, 1997).

(*c*) *Chernobyl accident*

(i) *Effects in somatic cells*

The accident in 1986 at the Chernobyl nuclear power station in the Ukraine resulted in acute irradiation from external and internal exposure to ^{131}I, with a half-life of eight days, and then to more stable isotopes, mainly ^{137}Cs. Between 1986 and 1992, peripheral blood samples were obtained from 102 workers who were on the site during the Chernobyl emergency or arrived there shortly thereafter to assist in the clean-up of radioactive contaminants and to isolate the damaged reactor. Blood was also taken from 13 unexposed individuals. The samples were analysed by flow cytometry with the allele-loss somatic mutation assay for glycophorin A (see Langlois *et al.*, 1986). The frequency of N/O variant red cells increased in proportion to the estimated exposure to radiation of each individual. The dose–response function derived for this population closely resembled that determined previously for atomic bomb survivors whose blood samples were obtained and analysed 40 years after exposure (Langlois *et al.*, 1993), which suggests comparable mutation induction per unit dose in these two populations and long-term persistence of the mutational damage. Measurements on multiple blood samples from each of 10 donors taken over seven years showed no significant change in N/O variant cell frequency, confirming the persistence of radiation-induced somatic mutations in long-lived bone-marrow stem cells (Jensen *et al.*, 1995).

A group of children exposed to the ionizing radiation released during the Chernobyl accident had an appreciable number of chromosomal breaks and rearrangements several years later, reflecting the persistence of the radiation-induced damage. The results suggested that the children were still being exposed to radioactive contamination from foods and other sources (Padovani *et al.*, 1993). In a follow-up study, 31 exposed children were compared with a control group of 11 children. All underwent measurements with whole-body counters and conventional cytogenetic analysis. The frequency of chromosomal aberrations in the exposed children was significantly greater than that in the control group, confirming the earlier report that a persistently abnormal cytogenetic pattern was still present many years after the accident (Padovani *et al.*, 1997).

A group of 125 workers involved in the initial clean-up operation (called 'liquidators', exposed mainly in 1986) and 42 people recovering from acute radiation sickness of second- and third-degree severity were examined in 1992–93 for cytogenetic effects. Increased frequencies of unstable and stable markers of exposure to radiation were found in all groups, showing a positive correlation with the initial exposure even as long as six to seven years after the accident. In a study of the mutagenic effects of long-term exposure to low levels of radiation, cytogenetic monitoring was also conducted among children, tractor drivers and foresters living in areas of the Ukraine contaminated by radionuclides released after the Chernobyl accident. All groups showed significantly increased frequencies of aberrant metaphases, chromosomal aberrations (both unstable and stable) and chromatid aberrations, and the number of aberrations in the children's cells correlated to the duration of exposure (Pilinskaya, 1996; see also section 2).

(ii)   *Heritable effects*

After the Chernobyl accident, germ-line mutations at human minisatellite loci were studied among children born in heavily polluted areas of the Mogilev district of Belarus (Dubrova *et al.*, 1996, 1997, 1998a,b). Many tandem-repeat minisatellite loci have a high spontaneous germ-line mutation rate, which allows detection of induced mutations in relatively small populations. Blood samples were collected from 79 families (father, mother, child) of children born between February and September 1994 whose parents had both lived in the Mogilev district since the time of the Chernobyl accident. The control sample consisted of 105 unirradiated white families in the United Kingdom, the children being matched by sex to the exposed group of offspring. The mutation frequency was found to be twice as high in the exposed families as in the control group. When the exposed families were divided into those that lived in an area with less than the median level of ^{137}Cs surface contamination and those that lived in more contaminated areas, the mutation rate in people in more contaminated areas was 1.5 times higher than that in those in the less contaminated areas. Since the blood samples for the control group were collected in the United Kingdom, it is conceivable that the increased mutation rate in the group in Mogilev might reflect intrinsic differences in minisatellite instability between these two white populations. It is also possible that the group in Mogilev was exposed to relatively high levels of other environmental contaminants, such as heavy metals, in addition to radioactive contamination.

(d)   Accident at Goiânia (Brazil)

A ^{137}Cs radiotherapy source (51×10^{12} Bq) was abandoned at a private hospital and picked up by a scrap dealer in Goiânia, Brazil, who destroyed the source capsule, thus releasing the radioactive material. The highest individual dose from internally deposited ^{137}Cs was accumulated at an initial rate of 0.25 Gy h^{-1}. The most highly exposed group received doses of 4–7 Sv, one receiving up to 10 Sv. The collective external dose amounted to 56 person–Sv and the internal dose to 4 person–Sv. Four people died within six weeks; of 112 000 people monitored, 249 showed detectable contamination, and 129 of them were found to have internal contamination and were referred for medical care. In order to estimate the absorbed radiation dose, the initial frequencies of chromosomal aberrations (dicentrics and rings) were determined in 110 exposed persons (Natarajan et al., 1991a,b; Ramalho & Nascimento, 1991; Ramalho et al., 1991; Straume et al., 1991), and some were followed cytogenetically in a search for parameters that could be used for retrospective radiation dosimetry. The frequencies of translocations detected years after the accident by fluorescence in situ hybridization were two to three times lower than the initial frequencies of dicentrics, the differences being larger at higher doses (> 1 Gy) (Ramalho et al., 1995; Natarajan et al., 1998; Ramalho et al., 1998). HPRT mutant frequencies were also monitored in T lymphocytes of this population, but no convincing increase in the mutation rate was detected (da-Cruz et al., 1996; Saddi et al., 1996; da-Cruz & Glickman, 1997; Skandalis et al., 1997).

4.4.2   Experimental systems

(a)   Mutations in vivo

Mice have been the main source of information on the genetic effects of ionizing radiation in mammals. Estimates of the spontaneous mutation rates for various genetic end-points are listed in Table 41, and those of induced mutation rates per centigray for the same end-points are given in Table 42, for both high and low dose rates of low-

LET radiation. The results for visible recessive mutations (specific locus test) indicate a conversion factor of 3 for acute to chronic irradiation (Russell & Kelly, 1982). This is the factor that has often been used to account for the difference between acute and protracted doses in humans, although a factor of 5–10 could equally well be proposed in view of the data shown in Table 42. The main results given in the tables are summarized in the text below.

Table 41. Estimated spontaneous mutation rates (mouse, unless otherwise indicated)

Genetic end-point and sex	Spontaneous rate
Dominant lethal mutations	
Both sexes	2×10^{-2}–10×10^{-2} per gamete
Recessive lethal mutations	
Both sexes	3×10^{-3} per gamete
Dominant visible mutations	
Male	
Skeletal	3×10^{-4} per gamete
Cataract	2×10^{-5} per gamete
Other	8×10^{-6} per gamete
Female	8×10^{-6} per gamete
Recessive visible mutations (seven-locus tester stock)	
Male	8×10^{-6} per locus
Female	2×10^{-6}–6×10^{-6} per locus
Reciprocal translocations (observed in meiotic cells)	
Male	
Mouse	2×10^{-4}–5×10^{-4} per cell
Rhesus monkey	8×10^{-4} per cell
Heritable translocations	
Male	1×10^{-4}–10×10^{-4} per gamete
Female	2×10^{-4} per gamete
Congenital malformations (observed *in utero* in late gestation)	
Both sexes	1×10^{-3}–5×10^{-3} per gamete
Aneuploidy (hyperhaploids)	
Female	
Preovulatory oocyte	2×10^{-3}–15×10^{-3} per cell
Less mature oocyte	3×10^{-3}–8×10^{-3} per cell

From Committee on the Biological Effects of Ionizing Radiations (BEIR V; 1990)

Table 42. Estimated induced mutation rates per cGy (mouse, unless otherwise indicated)

Genetic end-point, cell stage and sex	Low-LET radiation (dose rate)	
	High	Low
Dominant lethal mutations		
Postgonial, male	10×10^{-4} per gamete	5×10^{-4} per gamete
Gonial, male	10×10^{-5} per gamete	2×10^{-5} per gamete
Recessive lethal mutations		
Postgonial, male	1×10^{-4} per gamete	
Gonial, male	1×10^{-4} per gamete	
Dominant visible mutations		
Gonial, male	2×10^{-5} per gamete	
Skeletal	5×10^{-7} per gamete	
Cataract	$5–10 \times 10^{-7}$ per gamete	
Other	$5–10 \times 10^{-7}$ per gamete	1×10^{-7} per gamete
Postgonial, female	$5–10 \times 10^{-7}$ per gamete	
Recessive visible mutations (specific locus test)		
Postgonial, male	65×10^{-8} per locus	
Postgonial, female	40×10^{-8} per locus	$1–3 \times 10^{-8}$ per locus
Gonial, male	22×10^{-8} per locus	7×10^{-8} per locus
Reciprocal translocations		
Gonial, male		
Mouse	$1–2 \times 10^{-4}$ per cell	$1–2 \times 10^{-5}$ per cell
Rhesus monkey	2×10^{-4} per cell	
Marmoset	7×10^{-4} per cell	
Human	3×10^{-4} per cell	
Postgonial, female		
Mouse	$2–6 \times 10^{-4}$ per cell	
Heritable translocations		
Gonial, male	4×10^{-5} per gamete	
Postgonial, female	2×10^{-5} per gamete	
Congenital malformations		
Postgonial, female	2×10^{-4} per gamete	
Postgonial, male	4×10^{-5} per gamete	
Gonial, male	$2–6 \times 10^{-5}$ per gamete	
Aneuploidy (trisomy)		
Postgonial, female		
Preovulatory oocyte	6×10^{-4} per cell	
Less mature oocyte	6×10^{-5} per cell	

From Committee on the Biological Effects of Ionizing Radiations (BEIR V; 1990)

(i)   *Visible dominant mutations*

The mutations detected in the F_1 progeny of the irradiated generation comprise skeletal abnormalities, abnormalities of the lens (cataracts) and other dominant mutations.

The mutation rates for skeletal abnormalities in mice after single doses of X-rays were estimated to be 1×10^{-5} per gamete per cGy for spermatogonia and 3×10^{-5} per gamete per cGy for the post-spermatogonial cell stages (corrected for unirradiated controls) (Ehling, 1965, 1966). Another study showed a mutation rate in mouse spermatogonial cells of 2.3×10^{-5} per gamete per cGy induced by ^{137}Cs γ-rays (Selby & Selby, 1977) when the radiation was given in doses of 1–5 Gy separated by an interval of 24 h. This procedure is often used to increase the mutation yield while avoiding excessive cell killing (Russell, 1962).

In X- and γ-irradiated spermatogonia, the mutation rate for abnormalities of the lens was $3–13 \times 10^{-7}$ per gamete per cGy (Ehling, 1985; Graw *et al.*, 1986). No difference was observed between single and split-dose exposure. The mutation rate in post-spermatogonial stages appeared to be two- to fivefold higher than that in spermatogonia.

Other dominant mutations include those that result in changes in growth rate, coat colour, limb and tail structure, eye and ear size, hair texture and histocompatibility. No significant increase in mutation frequency at histocompatibility loci was detected in irradiated sperm or spermatogonia (Kohn & Melvold, 1976; Dunn & Kohn, 1981). This result could indicate reduced mutability of these loci or a greater susceptibility for lethal mutations than expected on the basis of known mutation rates for visible recessive mutations in mice.

The spontaneous rate of visible dominant mutations other than skeletal abnormalities and cataracts is approximately 8×10^{-6} per gamete per generation (see Table 41). Protracted treatment with ^{60}Co γ-rays yielded a spermatogonial mutation rate of 1.3×10^{-7} per gamete per cGy (Batchelor *et al.*, 1966). In X-irradiated female mice, the induced rates were between 5×10^{-7} and 10×10^{-7} per gamete per cGy for single doses of 2, 4 and 6 Gy (Lyon *et al.*, 1979). Studies with a different marker stock suggested a mutation rate as high as 3×10^{-6} per gamete per cGy, after two doses of 5 Gy of X-rays at a 24-h interval (Searle & Beechey, 1985, 1986).

(ii)   *Dominant lethal mutations*

Dominant lethal mutations are scored, essentially by their absence, in the F_1 progeny of an irradiated generation. Thus, a deficiency in the number of offspring is measured from conception to the time of weaning, i.e. as pre-implant or post-implant losses and reductions in litter size. Dominant lethal mutations are attributed to the induction of chromosomal aberrations that interfere with cell and tissue differentiation during fetal growth. These aberrations are generally eliminated during mitotic cell division and do not persist in stem-cell populations.

Post-gonial stage: In many studies, male mice were exposed to low-LET radiation at a high dose rate and mated during the first four to five weeks after exposure in order to obtain offspring derived from germ cells exposed at the postgonial stage. In general, mutation rates of about 10×10^{-4} per gamete per cGy were reported (Ehling, 1971; Schröder, 1971; Grahn et al., 1979, 1984; Kirk & Lyon, 1984), while the control value was $0.025–0.1 \times 10^{-4}$ per gamete per cGy. At low dose rates of radiation, mutation rates of 5×10^{-4} per gamete per cGy were observed (Grahn et al. 1979).

Few data are available on the induction of dominant lethal mutations in irradiated female mice. In one study, the average mutation rate 1–28 days after irradiation was similar to that seen in the male mice, 10×10^{-4} per gamete per cGy (Kirk & Lyon, 1982). In guinea-pigs, rabbits and hamsters, the rate of dominant lethal mutations in males appeared to be lower than that in male mice, but those in females were similar (Lyon, 1970; Cox & Lyon, 1975).

Stem-cell stage: Dominant lethal mutations generally do not persist in stem-cell populations because of chromosomal imbalance; however, balanced chromosomal translocations can be transmitted during the proliferative phase of gametogenesis, and such gametes behave like dominant lethal mutations. The average rate of mutations induced in spermatogonia by low-LET ionizing radiation at a high dose rate was reported to be 9×10^{-5} per gamete per cGy (Lüning & Searle, 1971). The dose-rate effect for γ-rays is significant, as the mutation rate fell to 3×10^{-5} per gamete per cGy with weekly exposures from 1.4×10^{-4} per gamete per cGy with continuous low-intensity exposure (Grahn et al., 1979).

(iii)   *Recessive autosomal and sex-linked lethal mutations*

Reviews of the rates of recessive autosomal lethal mutations in mice showed an average of 1×10^{-4} per gamete per cGy (Searle, 1974; Lüning & Eiche, 1976), but no information was available on the effects of dose rate.

The rate of sex-linked lethal mutations was first determined after the detection of a large inversion of the X chromosome. Two doses of 5 Gy of X-rays at a 24-h interval to the spermatogonia of mice gave a mutation rate of 3.7×10^{-6} per X chromosome per cGy (Lyon et al., 1982).

(iv)   *Visible recessive mutations*

Visible recessive mutations have been studied in the specific locus test (Russell, 1951) with seven stocks of mice bearing six coat-colour mutants and one structural (ears) mutant. Irradiated wild-type male or female mice are crossed with stock bearing these mutations, and new mutations at any of the marker loci are observed in the F_1 progeny. The spontaneous mutation rate in the tester stock is $8–8.5 \times 10^{-6}$ per locus, based on pooled data from the three principal laboratories where this test is conducted, for > 800 000 control F_1 mice. Most of the radiation-induced mutations examined at the molecular level appeared to be deletions (Bultman et al., 1991; Russell & Rinchik, 1993; Rinchik et al., 1994; Johnson et al., 1995; Shin et al., 1997).

The mutation rates induced in spermatogonia when male mice were exposed to low-LET radiation at a high dose rate was $21.9 \pm 1.9 \times 10^{-8}$ per locus per cGy with single doses of 3–7 Gy and $7.3 \pm 0.8 \times 10^{-8}$ per locus per cGy with 0.35–9 Gy of low dose-rate radiation (Russell & Kelly, 1982). In post-spermatogonial stages, the mutation rate reached $65–70 \times 10^{-8}$ per locus per cGy in progeny conceived four weeks after exposure of the male parent to 3 Gy of low dose-rate X-rays (Sega et al., 1978). The mutation rate was increased by fractionation of 1 Gy into two equal doses at a 24-h interval, but not by a larger number of fractions or a shorter interval (Russell, 1962).

The spontaneous rate of recessive visible mutations in female mice was estimated to be 1.4 or 5.6×10^{-6} per locus, depending on whether two or eight spontaneous events had been observed, as six events that occurred in one cluster could have been treated as one event (Russell, 1977). Exposure of mature oocytes to single doses of 0.5–6 Gy of X-rays at 0.5 Gy min^{-1} gave a mutation rate of 39×10^{-8} per locus per cGy in progeny conceived during the first week of exposure, whereas at lower dose rates values of $1–3 \times 10^{-8}$ per locus per cGy were observed. From these results it is clear that the dose-rate factor—the ratio of the mutation rates at high and low dose rates—for females is at least 10, whereas it is 3 for males (Lyon et al., 1979; Russell 1977; see Table 42).

(v)   *Somatic mutations*

Mouse spot assay: X-Radiation induced somatic coat colour mutations in C57BL × NB mice in a pioneering study by Russell and Major (1957). In a somewhat more recent system, somatic mutations were induced when embryos heterozygous for five recessive coat-colour genes from the cross C57BL/6 J Han × T-stock were X-irradiated with 1 Gy (Fahrig, 1975). The controls consisted of irradiated embryos resulting from wild-type C57BL × C57BL matings, which are homozygous for the genes under study, and untreated offspring of both matings. The colours of the spots on the adult fur were due either to expression of the recessive genes or were white because of cell killing. Irradiated offspring of the C57BL matings had only white spots, which were always midventral. No spots were seen in untreated offspring of either mating. After correction for the white midventral spots observed in C57BL matings, the frequency of expression of a recessive colour gene after C57BL/6 J Han × T-stock matings was about 11% for embryos irradiated 11 days after conception and about 1% for embryos irradiated 9 days after conception.

Loss of heterozygosity: Genetic alterations that result in loss of heterozygosity play an important role in the development of cancer. The underlying mechanisms are mitotic recombination, mitotic non-disjunction, gene conversion and deletion (Smith & Grosovsky, 1993). Such events occur not only in genetically unstable cancer cells but also in normal human and mouse somatic cells (Hakoda et al., 1991a,b). The mechanisms of loss of heterozygosity have been studied in mice rendered hetero-zygous for the autosomal *Aprt* gene by gene targeting (Van Sloun et al., 1998), which allows the study of mutations in both the *Aprt* and X-chromosomal *Hprt* loci *in vivo*. *Aprt*$^{+/-}$ mice received up to 3 Gy whole-body irradiation with X-rays, and seven weeks later the *Hprt* and *Aprt* mutant frequencies were determined in the same splenic T-lymphocyte cell population. A dose-dependent increase was observed in *Hprt* mutant frequency, but that for *Aprt* was no different from that of controls, even though clear induction of mutations at the *Aprt* locus was observed after treatment with chemical carcinogens. Molecular analysis indicated that 70% of these mutations were caused by loss of heterozygosity. The hemizygous *Hprt* locus appeared to be a better target for the recovery of X-ray-induced mutants than the heterozygous *Aprt* locus. This result is unexpected, as X-rays induce predominantly multilocus deletions (Hutchinson, 1995), and deletion of an essential flanking gene from a hemizygous locus would be more detrimental for the cell. The results also suggest that loss of heterozygosity might not occur after ionizing irradiation, at least at the *Aprt* locus in mice (Wijnhoven *et al.*, 1998).

(vi) *Minisatellite mutations*

Tandem repeat minisatellite loci in mice frequently have a high rate of germ-line mutations, and exposure to radiation increases the germ-line rate at a doubling dose comparable to that for other genetic end-points. The rate of induction cannot be explained by the occurrence of initial radiation damage within the minisatellite sequence, and suggests an unexpected mechanism involving radiation-induced damage elsewhere in the genome (Dubrova *et al.*, 1998a,b; Sadamoto *et al.*, 1994). Such minisatellite mutations have no known phenotypic effect or any direct relation to carcinogenesis. Their importance is that they illustrate the amplification of radiation-induced damage which results in the occurrence of mutation in a remote DNA sequence (Morgan *et al.*, 1996; Little *et al.*, 1997; see also section (c), below).

(vii) *Transgenic animals*

The development of transgenic mutagenesis systems has made it possible to study the mutagenic effects of ionizing radiation at both the molecular and the chromosomal level in the same animal. The responses of Big Blue® *LacI* transgenic mice to ionizing radiation were measured as induction of *LacI* mutations in the spleen. C57BL/6 Big Blue® transgenic mice were exposed to ^{137}Cs γ-rays at doses of 0.1–14 Gy and then allowed expression times of 2–14 days. Mutant plaques were analysed by restriction enzyme digestion. Of 34 mutations analysed, four were large-scale rearrangements, three of which were deletions within the *LacI* gene, while the fourth was a deletion that extended from within the α *LacZ* gene into downstream sequences. The other mutants did not involve major deletions (Winegar *et al.*, 1994).

The Big Blue® *LacI* transgenic mouse reporter system was also used to investigate mutation induction in the testis, spleen and liver after whole-body irradiation of the mice with ^{60}Co γ-rays. The spontaneous mutation frequencies were $6–17 \times 10^{-6}$. No statistically significant induction of mutation was observed in testis or spleen 35 days after exposure, although the mutation frequencies tended to be increased by approximately 1.5-fold. In the liver, however, the mutation frequencies were elevated approximately 4.5-fold after exposure to 1 Gy of ^{60}Co γ-rays. When the data for all organs were pooled, the mutation frequency was doubled, but no other significant increase was observed (Hoyes *et al.*, 1998).

[The Working Group noted that neither of these systems would detect the large, multilocus deletions that constitute the predominant radiation-induced mutations in mammalian cells.]

(b)   *Studies* in vivo/in vitro

The dynamics of the process of carcinogenesis and of the contribution of the initial carcinogenic insult to initiation and progression are difficult to study in intact animals and virtually impossible to study in humans. The main obstacles to understanding the fundamental processes involved in radiation-induced cancer in animal models until recently included the long latency and the complexity of the neoplastic process. In an effort to overcome these problems, animal models have been developed for the identification, isolation and characterization of radiation-altered or radiation-initiated cells from irradiated tissues shortly after exposure (Ethier & Ullrich, 1982; Clifton *et al.*, 1986; Adams *et al.*, 1987; Gould *et al.*, 1987). These 'in-vivo/in-vitro' systems have been used to show that initiation of cells by ionizing radiation is a frequent event, of the order of 10^{-2}, which is much greater than would be expected if initiation were the result of a simple mutation. Subsequent analysis of initiated cells and detailed study of their progression led to the hypothesis that a critical early event in radiation-induced carcinogenesis is the induction of widespread genomic instability, which is apparent from increased cytogenetic damage and increased mutation rates in the progeny of irradiated cells many cell doublings after exposure (Ullrich & Ponnaiya, 1998). Support for this hypothesis comes from a number of observations.

In one model involving transplantation of mammary tissue or mammary cells into syngeneic hosts (DeOme *et al.*, 1978; Medina, 1979), a differential effect of ionizing radiation was demonstrated on the growth of transplanted normal and hyperplastic mammary tissue (Faulkin *et al.*, 1983).

In an assay to determine the effects of exposure to γ-radiation at 0.5 or 1 Gy and of the time that the cells remained *in situ* after the treatment, mammary epithelial cells were isolated from BALB/cAnNBd mice at various times between 24 h and 52 weeks after irradiation *in vivo* and assayed for the growth of epithelial foci *in vitro*. The cell populations that emerged had increased growth potential *in vitro* and enhanced tumorigenic potential with increasing time *in situ* (Adams *et al.*, 1987).

In order to determine the radiation-induced transformation frequencies in sensitive BALB/C mice, in resistant C57BL mice and in resistant hybrid B6CF1 mice, independently of the host environment, ductal dysplasia was determined 10 or 16 weeks after injection of mammary epithelial cells from γ-irradiated (1 Gy from a ^{137}Cs source) donor mice into gland-free fat pads of recipient mice. The variations in radiation sensitivity of these mouse strains were shown to result from inherent differences in the sensitivity of the mammary epithelium to radiation-induced cell transformation (Ullrich *et al.*, 1996).

Cells of the EF42 cell line, derived from the mammary tissue of a female BALB/C mouse four weeks after γ-irradiation (1 Gy from a ^{137}Cs source), become neoplastic with time *in vitro* and *in vivo*. Before acquisition of the neoplastic phenotype, however, multiple mutations occur in *p53*. This finding suggests that the mutations are not caused directly by the radiation treatment but arise several cell generations later as a consequence of radiation-induced genomic instability (Selvanayagam *et al.*, 1995).

(*c*)   *Cellular systems*

(i)   *Genomic instability*

A characteristic of cancer cells is the presence of multiple mutations and chromosomal alterations. Although a single dose of ionizing radiation may induce a tumour, there is virtually no possibility that the changes needed to result in a malignant cell can be caused directly by a single exposure to the radiation. Nowell (1976) suggested that the chromosomal aberrations in cancer cells are associated with genomic instability. Loeb (1998) proposed that the acquisition of a mutator phenotype is central to cancer induction, in particular the genomic changes in tumour progression.

Radiation has been shown to induce genomic instability, a characteristic of which is the delay between exposure and the appearance of the effect, despite a number of mitotic divisions. Early observations of delayed heritable effects included small colony size of irradiated cells *in vitro* and a persistent reduction in the size of the cells that continued to grow *in vitro* (Sinclair, 1964).

The first report of delayed development of chromosomal aberrations was that of Weissenborn and Streffer (1988, 1989), who found that new aberrations were expressed in the second and third mitoses after exposure of one-cell mouse embryos to X-rays or neutrons. Pampfer and Streffer (1989) showed that irradiation of an embryo at the zygote stage induced genomic instability that later became apparent as chromatid and chromosome fragments in fibroblasts of fetal skin. In addition, delayed reduction in plating efficiency (Seymour *et al.*, 1986; Chang & Little, 1992) and delayed chromosomal alterations (Kadhim *et al.*, 1992, 1994, 1995; Marder & Morgan, 1993; Sabatier *et al.*, 1994) have been reported. Kadhim *et al.* (1992) found that α-particles were markedly more effective than X-rays in inducing delayed chromosomal aberrations in murine and human haematopoietic cells. In these experiments, 40–60% of the cells had chromosomal aberrations although only 10% of the surviving cells had been traversed by α-particles, indicating some indirect or 'bystander' effect. Marder and Morgan (1993) concluded that radiation-induced genomic instability probably results from deletion of a gene or genes responsible for genomic integrity.

Ponnaiya *et al.* (1997) showed that chromatid-type gaps and breaks appear in human epithelial MCF-10A cells as a delayed effect of irradiation. The aberrations were not found until about 20–35 cell population doublings after exposure to γ-rays.

The large number of cell doublings required to reveal genomic instability after exposure to X- or γ-rays may explain the reports of an absence of delayed chromosomal
changes after exposure to low-LET radiation. There appears to be a LET-dependent
difference in the time course of expression of radiation-induced genomic instability.

In mice, an association has been found between the probability of radiation-
induced chromatid-type aberrations and susceptibility for induction of mammary
cancer. Ullrich and Ponnaiya (1998) showed that BALB/c mice were more sensitive
than C57BL/6 mice to induction of mammary cancer by radiation and also to the
induction of delayed chromatid-type aberrations.

A possible role of genomic imprinting in the development of genomic instability
and radiation-induced mutations was discussed by Schofield (1998). Genomic
imprinting usually depends on post-replication modification of DNA, such as
methylation, which regulates which of the two alleles of a gene is expressed or
suppressed, depending on the gamete from which it was inherited. Thus, a cell
becomes hemizygous for the expression of certain key genes. For example, in radiosensitive mice that are predisposed to gastroschisis, its induction is closely linked to a
region on chromosome 7 in which a number of genes for imprinting are located.
Genomic instability is thus apparently associated with the development of the malfor-
mation: it occurs only in the predisposed mouse strain and is transmitted to the next
generation. Genomic instability therefore contributes to radiation-induced carcinogenesis and to other effects such as malformations.

The evidence for the induction by radiation of chromosomal instability is
compelling, but the susceptibility of cell lines is clearly influenced by their genetic
background. Neither the target, which appears to be large, nor the mechanism(s) of
induction has been identified unequivocally. The probability of induction depends on
the LET of the radiation; dose-dependence has been reported (Limoli *et al.*, 1999).
Delayed appearance of *hprt* mutations has also been demonstrated after exposure to
low-LET radiation *in vitro* in several systems (Little *et al.*, 1990; Harper *et al.*, 1997;
Loucas & Cornforth, 1998).

The possibility that radiation-induced genomic instability contributes to radiation-
induced carcinogenesis has important mechanistic implications. The characteristic
delay between the event that initiates genomic instability and its expression is consistent with the long latent period between exposure to radiation and the appearance of a
tumour. Better understanding of this phenomenon will be required before the implications of genomic instability for extrapolation of epidemiological findings to low-
level exposures are fully understood.

(ii)   *Cell transformation*

Ionizing radiation was one of the first agents to be used in cell transformation
systems (Borek & Sachs, 1966), and there is now an extensive literature (reviewed by
Hall & Hei, 1985; Kakunaga & Yamasaki, 1985; Hall & Hei, 1990; Suzuki, 1997). The
initial studies were carried out with primary Syrian hamster embryo cells, a fibroblast

cell system that has the advantage that the effects of radiation on initial immortalization (or transformation) and the other changes required for neoplastic transformation can be studied. Because of technical problems with these primary cells, the C3H/10T½ cell line developed by Reznikoff *et al.* (1973a,b) has been used more extensively. Very high transformation frequencies were obtained in C3H/10T½ and C3H/3T3 cells when the frequencies were expressed per initial number of cells plated (Terzaghi & Little, 1976), indicating that even dishes with very few cells would eventually yield a neoplastically transformed clone. The actual neoplastic transformation process appears to be delayed and a change occurs in a large proportion of cells even after very low doses, so that there is a finite probability that one of their descendants will have a transformed phenotype (Kennedy *et al.*, 1980). This may be an expression of induced genetic instability, and its mechanism is still obscure.

Human primary cells have proven very difficult to transform neoplastically. Human keratinocytes (Rhim *et al.*, 1990, 1993) and bronchial cells (Hei *et al.*, 1994) immortalized by SV40 and papilloma virus, respectively, have been used to study neoplastic transformation. These systems have the advantage that the cells are human and epithelial, but they are immortalized and therefore do not allow study of the initial change in the carcinogenic process.

In a human hybrid cell system, HeLa × skin fibroblasts, the appearance of transformed foci is associated with apoptosis which begins about eight days after irradiation. The authors suggested that the instability process has two relevant outcomes: induction of apoptotic death and neoplastic transformation of a small subset of survivors. These survivors were shown to have lost fibroblast chromosomes 11 and 14, and the authors suggested that tumour suppressor gene loci might be located on these chromosomes. The yield of transformants was found to be modulated by serum batch and this was correlated with the extent of delayed death, possibly reflecting altered expression of the induced genetic instability (Mendonca *et al.*, 1995, 1998a,b).

The results obtained with the human hybrid system can be as difficult to understand as those from earlier systems. For example, cells exposed to a dose of 1 cGy (which is too low to induce either cell killing or neoplastic transformation) and held for 24 h at 37 °C before plating, showed fewer transformants on subsequent incubation than unirradiated cells (Redpath & Antoniono, 1998). This confirmed an earlier result with a specific clone of C3H/10T½ cells (Azzam *et al.*, 1996).

Little work has been done to elucidate the type of initial radiation damage that leads ultimately to cell transformation. Obe *et al.* (1992) argued that double-strand DNA breaks are the critical lesion, citing the results of Zajac-Kaye and Ts'o (1984), who showed that application of DNase I in liposomes to Syrian hamster embryo cells led to foci of transformed cells that gave rise to tumours when injected into newborn hamsters, and the work of Bryant and Riches (1989) who treated C3H/10T½ cells with the restriction enzyme *Pvu*II in the presence of inactivated Sendai virus and observed that the cells became morphologically altered.

While cell transformation systems may be useful for revealing the potential of radiation to induce changes that may be associated with carcinogenesis, it is not clear how some of the observations obtained *in vitro* should be extrapolated to the situation *in vivo*.

(iii)   *Chromosomal damage*

Three classes of chromosomal aberration are known to occur in somatic and germ cells: numerical aberrations, chromosomal breaks and structural rearrangements (Savage, 1976, 1979). Numerical and structural aberrations are associated with congenital abnormalities and neoplasia in humans. Numerical aberrations in germ cells occur as a result of nondisjunction during female gametogenesis. In normal somatic cells, the frequency of changes in chromosome number is low and difficult to estimate, but in cancer cells such changes are rather common (Holliday, 1989). A single-strand break induced before DNA replication gives rise to a chromosomal break at the following mitosis. When breakage occurs after the S phase or during G_2, it will be observed as a chromatid break, but many such breaks rejoin rapidly and go unnoticed. Single-strand breaks, both chromosomal and chromatid, are readily induced by ionizing radiation, and their number increases linearly with dose. Unrepaired breaks generally result in cell death in normal (as opposed to transformed) cells.

Structural chromosomal rearrangements are the result of inappropriate joining of radiation-induced breaks at one or more sites. They comprise simple unstable forms such as rings and dicentrics, simple stable forms including inversions, interstitial deletions and translocations, and also more complex combinations. The conventional assumption has been that two sites of radiation damage are necessary to produce simple exchange aberrations, either linearly with dose by a single track or proportional to the square of the dose by pairs of tracks (ICRP, 1991a; see also section 3.4, Overall introduction). Alternatively, some evidence suggests that simple chromosomal exchanges result from single tracks, due to recombination with undamaged DNA, and that multiple-track damage can lead to more complex chromosomal aberrations (Goodhead *et al.*, 1993; Chadwick & Leenhouts, 1998; Griffin *et al.*, 1998). The ability of X- and γ-radiation to induce all types of chromosomal damage has been documented extensively (see UNSCEAR, 1988; Committee on the Biological Effects of Ionizing Radiations (BEIR V), 1990; UNSCEAR, 1993). Dose–response curves for dicentrics, the most useful aberration for dosimetric purposes, were reported by Lloyd and Purrott (1981).

Although ionizing radiation induces more DNA single-strand breaks than double-strand breaks, several observations indicate that double-strand breaks of variable complexity are the major lesions responsible for the induction of chromosomal aberrations. Direct evidence that simple double-strand breaks can lead to chromosomal aberrations comes from experiments in which restriction endonucleases were introduced into cells. Although restriction enzymes produce only simple double-strand breaks (with blunt or cohesive ends), the induction of chromosomal aberrations was efficient and the observed aberration patterns were similar to those induced by ionizing radiation (Bryant, 1984; Natarajan & Obe, 1984). The structural chromosomal aberrations seen at metaphase are of two types: chromosome-type aberrations and chromatid-type aberrations. Ionizing radiation induces chromosome-type aberrations in cells exposed in G_0 or G_1 phase of the cell cycle and chromatid-type aberrations in cells exposed in the S or G_2 phase (Savage, 1976).

Since human T lymphocytes have a long lifetime—a small proportion survive for decades—and the rate of replacement is rather slow, the frequency of structural chromosomal aberrations can serve as an indicator of the dose received by the exposed individual. In early work, the frequency of dicentric chromosomes at the first metaphase after stimulation of human T cells was determined. With the introduction of fluorescent *in situ* hybridization and chromosome-specific probes, it became possible to quantify the frequency of chromosomal translocations accurately (Natarajan *et al.*, 1996), and these approaches were used to estimate past exposure during radiation accidents (see section 4.4.1; Natarajan *et al.*, 1991a,b; UNSCEAR, 1993; Natarajan *et al.*, 1998). The development of additional chromosome arm-specific probes as well as specific probes for telomeres allowed detailed analysis of the spectrum of ionizing radiation-induced chromosomal aberrations in humans cells *in vivo* as well as *in vitro* (Natarajan *et al.*, 1996; Boei *et al.*, 1997, 1998a,b).

(iv)   *Mutagenicity*

Ionizing radiation has held a special place in mutation research ever since Muller (1927) demonstrated that X-rays induce hereditary effects in the fruit fly, *Drosophila melanogaster*. His was the first report on the induction of germ-cell mutations by a toxic, exogenous agent. Since that time, many studies have shown that ionizing radiation is mutagenic in essentially all experimental systems in which it has been examined (see extensive reviews of UNSCEAR, 1988; Committee on the Biological Effects of Ionizing Radiations (BEIR V), 1990; UNSCEAR, 1993).

In most mammalian systems, the predominant mutations induced by ionizing radiation are deletions, which range in size from extensive regions visible by microscopy to single nucleotides. Southern blotting, a technique used frequently for detecting deletions, is sensitive for deletions of more than about 100 nucleotides (Southern, 1975).

Base-pair substitution mutations have been shown to be induced by ionizing radiation in bacteria (Bridges *et al.*, 1967), mediated by the same SOS system that is involved in mutation induction by ultraviolet light and most other DNA damaging agents (Bridges *et al.*, 1968). The mutation rates at various loci ranged from 1.5×10^{-11} to 1.5×10^{-10} per cell per cGy. While such rates are readily measured in bacteria, mammalian cells are much more sensitive to the lethal effect of radiation; thus, a mutation rate of the order of 10^{-10} per cell per cGy would cause increases in the mutation frequency that are too small to be measured at doses at which cell survival is sufficiently good.

The first demonstration of the mutagenic action of ionizing radiation in mammalian cells was *Hprt* deficiency in Chinese hamster cells (Bridges *et al.*, 1970). The observation has since been confirmed and extended (for a review, see Thacker, 1992). Various mammalian somatic cell systems have been used to compare the spectrum of radiation-induced mutations with that of spontaneous mutations. The genetic loci most commonly used for mutation analysis in human cells are those encoding *HPRT* (Albertini *et al.*, 1982), adenine-phosphoribosyltransferase (*APRT*; Grosovsky *et al.*, 1986), a histocompatibility gene (*HLA-A*; Janatipour *et al.*, 1988), thymidine kinase (*TK*; Yandell *et al.*, 1990) and dihydrofolate reductase (*DHFR*; Urlaub & Chasin, 1980). Another method for detecting mutations in humans is an assay of loss of the allele for glycophorin A, a surface protein of erythrocytes (Langlois *et al.*, 1986). Ionizing radiation does not significantly increase the frequency of ouabain-resistant mutants, which are believed to be due to base-pair substitutions (Thacker *et al.*, 1978).

Depending on the test system used, 80–97% of the spontaneous *HPRT* and *APRT* mutations are base-pair changes. The percentages are only 50–60% at the *HLA-A* locus and 5–20% at the *TK* locus because mitotic recombination contributes substantially to the spontaneous mutation spectra at these loci. With a few exceptions, most radiation-induced mutations in cultured cells are deletions and other gross changes that are visible in Southern-blot patterns: at the *Hprt* or *HPRT* locus, mutations of this type constitute 70–90% of those in Chinese hamster ovary cells, 50–85% of those in TK6 human lymphoid cells and 50–75% of those in human T lymphocytes, and deletions constitute 60–80% of *TK* mutations in the TK6 cell line, 80% at the *HLA-A* locus in T lymphocytes and 100% at the *Dhfr* locus in Chinese hamster ovary cells. Of the radation-induced changes in *Aprt* in Chinese hamster ovary cells, only 16–20% consisted of deletions or other changes. Mutations that do not show aberrant Southern blot patterns may, of course, still be small deletions (Sankaranarayanan, 1991).

The results of a study in which *Hprt* and *Aprt* mutations were analysed after exposure of two Chinese hamster ovary cell lines (*Aprt*$^{+/-}$ and Aprt$^{+/0}$, respectively) to ionizing radiation strongly suggested that radiation-induced mutational events often consist of deletions of more than 40 kilobases (the length of the *Hprt* gene) and that the difference in the frequency at the two loci in the two types of cell lines was due to the presence of essential sequences close the respective target genes, a deletion of which would be lethal to the cell (Bradley *et al.*, 1988).

Spontaneous and induced *Aprt* deficiencies were studied in the mouse P19H22 embryonal carcinoma cell line, which contains two distinct chromosome 8 homo-logues, one derived from *Mus domesticus* and the other from *M. musculus*. The cell line also contains a deletion for the *M. musculus Aprt* allele, which is located on chromo-some 8. The large majority (> 95%) of the spontaneous and γ-radiation-induced mutants showed *Aprt* gene loss, indicating that relatively large deletions had occurred and that homozygosity for these regions is not a lethal event. Loss of heterozygosity for adjacent markers was found to be a common event in cells with *Aprt* gene loss (Turker *et al.*, 1995).

In Chinese hamster ovary K1 cells and 10T5 cells, a K1 derivative containing the bacterial gene xanthine-guanine phosphoribosyl transferase *(Gpt)*, mutants were analysed at the *Gpt*, *Hprt* and *Tk* loci. After X-irradiation, the mutation rates at the *Tk* and *Gpt* loci were 8–10 times higher than that at the *Hprt* locus. The greater sensitivity of the *Tk* locus compared to that of the *Hprt* locus to mutation induction by ionizing radiation is likely to be due, at least in part, to the recovery of an additional class of mutants, possibly ones containing larger mutational events giving rise to small colonies. Approximately half of the X-ray-induced *Tk* mutants were small-colony mutants (Schwartz *et al.*, 1991).

Reduction of the radiation dose rate generally diminishes the severity of the biological effect per unit dose. The influence of dose rate on the mutagenicity of ionizing radiation has been investigated extensively in cultured cells. In his review, Thacker (1992) concluded that the results of studies in cells and animals indicated that a reduction in dose rate could reduce mutagenic effectiveness by a factor of 2–4, with some notable exceptions. Changing the dose rate of low-LET radiation had no effect in certain cell types, such as human TK6 cells and certain repair-deficient rodent cell lines or for certain types of mutation. Thacker (1992) concluded that, insofar as it was possible, there was no deviation from linearity in the dose–response relationship measured at low doses and low dose rates, but the errors were inevitably large in such measurements.

(v)   *DNA damage*

Ionizing radiation may act directly on the cellular molecules or indirectly through water molecules. The high energy (typically megavolts) of an incident particle or electromagnetic wave ultimately results in a large number of small energy deposits (typically 60–100 eV), each of which provides energy for one or a small number of ionizations. As a result, electrons, charged and neutral radicals and non-radical species are generated. In aqueous media these are e_{aq}^-, $^\bullet H$, $^\bullet OH$, H_{aq}^+ and H_2O_2, and they react with nearby molecules in a very short time, leading to breakage of chemical bonds or oxidation of the affected molecules. The hydroxyl radical in particular is highly reactive and is also the most active mutagen generated by ionizing radiation.

The major effects of ionizing radiation on DNA are the induction of base damage, breaks of either single strands or both strands and more complex combinations. Double-strand breaks and damage of varying complexity are considered to be biologically more important because repair of this type of damage is much more difficult, and erroneous rejoining of broken ends may occur (see e.g. Sikpi *et al.*, 1992; Jenner *et al.*, 1993; Goodhead, 1994; Prise, 1994; Löbrich *et al.*, 1995, 1998). These so-called 'misrepairs' may result in mutations, chromosomal aberrations or cell death. The types, frequencies and extent of repair of these lesions depend on the dose, the dose rate and the LET of the radiation. Most cells can survive a dose of about 1.5 Gy low-

LET radiation, despite the fact that hundreds of DNA strand breaks are induced in each cell. This means that repair processes play an important role in the cellular response to radiation (see e.g. Cole *et al.*, 1988).

The active oxygen species produced when ionizing radiation interacts with water are comparable to those that are generated continuously by the metabolic processes of aerobic organisms. Double-stranded DNA breaks may be produced, but rarely, by the active oxygen species associated with metabolism. Instead, oxidative damage is induced in individual nucleotides. In some cases, this leads to the removal of a base, which results in an apurinic or apyrimidinic site. These sites, if not removed by the relevant endonuclease repair system, can be mutagenic because an incorrect nucleotide will be incorporated into the opposite strand (Schaaper *et al.*, 1982).

Free radical-induced DNA damage associated with exposure to ionizing radiation may give rise to a number of oxidized purines, of which $7H$-8-oxoguanine and $7H$-8-oxoadenine predominate. In a detailed quantum-mechanical study to assess the tautomeric preferences of the bases in aqueous solution, the 6,8-diketo form of guanine and the 6-amino-8-keto form of adenine were the major species. The estimated free energies of hydration indicate that mutagenically significant amounts of minor tautomeric forms exist in the aqueous phase and may be responsible for induction of both transversion and transition mutations (Venkateswarlu & Leszczynski, 1998).

Minor oxidative lesions induced in DNA by exposure to ionizing radiation are 5-hydroperoxymethyl-2'-deoxyuridine and its decomposition products 5-hydroxymethyl-2'-deoxyuridine and 5-formyl-2'-deoxyuridine. The first compound was a more potent mutagen than the other two in *Salmonella typhimurium*, the TA100 strain being the most sensitive (Patel *et al.*, 1992).

Because of the ubiquitous presence of nucleotide damage resulting from endogenously generated active oxygen species, living organisms have evolved a comprehensive array of DNA repair systems to deal with such damage (see Friedberg *et al.*, 1995). At low doses of radiation, the yield of active oxygen species would be small in comparison with those occurring spontaneously, and most of the resulting nucleotide damage (base damage and single-strand breaks) would be expected to be removed by repair processes. This is consistent with the accumulated evidence that multiple damaged sites, including double-strand breaks, are responsible for the effects of ionizing radiation on DNA (Goodhead, 1988; see also section 3.4, Overall introduction). Such damage presents a severe and often insurmountable challenge to the cellular repair systems. Because of the non-homogeneity of the energy deposition and the ensuing clustered damage, the effects of radiation are quite different from those induced by endogenously generated active oxygen species.

5. Summary of Data Reported and Evaluation

5.1 Exposure data

The greatest exposure of the general population to X-rays and γ-rays comes from natural terrestrial radiation. The next most significant source is the use of X-rays and radiopharmaceuticals in various diagnostic and therapeutic procedures. Exposures from the atmospheric testing of nuclear weapons have diminished, and only small contributions to the collective human dose are made by the generation of electrical energy by nuclear reactors, by accidental releases from nuclear facilities and radioactive devices and by occupational exposure during medical uses, commercial nuclear fuel cycles, nuclear industrial sources, military activities and the clean-up of nuclear or radiation accidents. The latter contributions are important, however, as they can result in significant exposure of groups of individuals.

The most important exposures to X- and γ-rays from the point of view of the determination of cancer risk in humans are from the past use of atomic weapons and from the medical uses of radiation.

With regard to the overall exposure of the population, the variation in individual doses over time, place and conditions of exposure makes it difficult to summarize mean individual doses accurately, although some indications are possible. Most exposures are measured in units of absorbed dose (Gy) in individual organs, but they are compared in units of effective dose (Sv) in order to account for effects in all the organs, which differ in radiosensitivity (and for differences in radiation quality when appropriate). The average annual effective dose from X- and γ-rays from natural sources is about 0.5 mSv, with elevated values up to about 5 mSv. Medical procedures in developed countries result in an annual effective dose of about 1–2 mSv, of which about two-thirds comes from diagnostic radiography. Possible exposures in medicine vary widely, however, ranging from several hundred millisieverts from frequent diagnostic procedures to several sieverts from therapeutic procedures. The annual effective doses to monitored workers are commonly in the range of 1–10 mSv.

5.2 Human carcinogenicity data

The carcinogenic effects of ionizing radiation in human populations have been studied extensively. Evidence for causal associations comes primarily from epidemiological studies of survivors of the atomic bombings in Japan and patients exposed to radiation for medical reasons. Epidemiological studies of populations exposed to lower doses of radiation were considered but were determined not to be informative for this evaluation.

In epidemiology, associations between exposure and disease are most often accepted as causal when there is consistency across many studies conducted by different investigators using different methods; when the association is strong; and when there is evidence of a dose–response gradient, with risk increasing as the level of exposure increases. These three important causal criteria are satisfied for exposure to radiation and the induction of cancer.

Perhaps most important is that the association between radiation and cancer has been found consistently in many different populations exposed at different times and in different countries throughout the world. Among survivors of the atomic bombings in Hiroshima and Nagasaki, who were exposed primarily to γ-rays, excess numbers of cases of leukaemia and other cancers have been observed up to 45 years after exposure. Excess numbers of cases of leukaemia and other cancers have also been observed among patients treated with X-rays or γ-rays for malignant or benign diseases. Important evidence comes from studies of women in 15 countries who were irradiated for cervical cancer and persons who were irradiated for ankylosing spondylitis in the United Kingdom. Excess risks for cancer were also found among children irradiated for an enlarged thymus gland in the USA, for ringworm of the scalp in Israel and for skin haemangioma in Sweden. Increased numbers of breast cancers have been observed in patients in Canada and the USA who received frequent chest fluoroscopic X-rays for tuberculosis. There are well over 100 studies of patient populations in which excess numbers of cancers have been linked to radiotherapy. Pioneering medical radiologists practising shortly after the discovery of X-rays in 1895 had increased rates of leukaemia and other cancers in studies conducted in the United Kingdom, the USA and, later, in China.

Strong associations between exposure to radiation and several types of cancer have been reported. Exposure to radiation at sufficiently high doses has increased the risk of developing leukaemia by over fivefold. Even higher relative risks have been reported for thyroid cancer following irradiation during childhood. Greater than twofold increases in the risk for breast cancer have been seen after irradiation before the menopause.

Since in many studies the dose of radiation received by individuals was estimated with considerable accuracy, dose–response relationships could be evaluated. An increase in the risk for leukaemia with increasing dose was seen among atomic bomb survivors over a broad range of doses and among patients given radiotherapy for cervical cancer. Dose–response relationships for thyroid cancer have been demonstrated following irradiation in childhood for various conditions and among atomic bomb survivors. Dose–response relationships for breast cancer have been demonstrated among atomic bomb survivors, women treated for acute post-partum mastitis and benign breast conditions and patients who received many chest fluoroscopies. A dose–response relationship was also demonstrated for the combined category of all cancers among the survivors of the atomic bombings.

The level of cancer risk after exposure to X-rays or γ-rays is modified by a number of factors, in addition to radiation dose, including the age at which exposure occurs, the length of time over which the radiation is received and the sex of the exposed person. The level of cancer risk also varies with time since exposure. The sensitivity of tissues to the carcinogenic effects of ionizing radiation differs widely. Cancers that appear to be readily inducible by X- and γ-rays include leukaemia, breast cancer in women exposed before the menopause, cancer of the thyroid gland among people exposed during childhood and some gastrointestinal tumours, including those of the stomach and colon. Some tissues in which cancer is induced only rarely or at relatively high doses include bone, soft tissue, uterus, skin and rectum. A number of cancers, such as chronic lymphocytic leukaemia, have not been linked to exposure to X- or γ-rays.

While there is some variation in the level of risk for specific cancers seen in epidemiological studies of populations exposed to X- and γ-rays, the consistency of the association, the strength of the association and the dose–response relationships all provide strong evidence that X-rays and γ-rays cause cancer in humans.

5.3   Animal carcinogenicity data

X-Rays and γ-rays have been tested for carcinogenicity at various doses and under various conditions in mice, rats, rabbits, dogs and rhesus monkeys. They have also been tested by exposure of mice and dogs *in utero* and by parental exposure of mice.

In adult animals, the incidences of leukaemia and of a variety of neoplasms including mammary, lung and thyroid tumours were increased in a dose-dependent manner with both types of radiation. When sufficient data were available over a range of doses and dose rates, the dose–response relationship was generally consistent with a linear–quadratic model, while lowering the dose rate resulted in a diminution of the quadratic portion of the curve. The effects of fractionation of the dose were highly dependent on fractionation size. Most importantly, low dose fractions were equivalent to low dose rates with respect to carcinogenic effectiveness.

Prenatal exposure of mice to X-rays in two studies and to ^{60}Co γ-rays in one study and of dogs to ^{60}Co γ-rays at late fetal stages resulted in significant increases in the incidences of lung and liver tumours in mice and malignant lymphoma, haemangiosarcoma and mammary carcinoma in dogs. Exposure at early fetal stages, however, did not increase the incidence of tumours in the offspring of either species. Parental effects in mice appear to depend on the strain tested. Parental exposure of mice of four strains to X-rays resulted in increased incidences of lung tumours and leukaemia in the offspring; however, studies with two other strains of mice showed no increase in the incidence of neoplasms.

5.4   Other relevant data

Exposure to radiation may result in effects on tissues and organs that are known as deterministic effects, which are distinct from cancer and genetic effects, known as stochastic effects. Deterministic effects increase in both incidence and severity with increasing dose and are not recognized below a threshold dose. The dose-dependent increase in severity and the fact that the damage must reach a critical or threshold level to be detected distinguish deterministic effects from stochastic effects, for which, by convention for radiation protection purposes, there is no threshold and which do not increase in severity with increasing dose.

Deterministic effects, in general, result from cell killing. In the case of rapidly proliferating tissues, such as the gastrointestinal and haematopoietic systems, the effects may be early, occurring within a matter of days to a few weeks after high doses at high dose rates. Doses that kill critical numbers of clonogenic or stem cells may result in loss of the integrity of tissues and death. The loss of cells may be severe but not lethal, and in both cases the damage to these and other proliferating cell systems is reflected in clinical syndromes that result from impairment of organ function. Depending on the rates of cell renewal, radiation-induced damage is expressed at different times. In humans, death from damage to the gut may occur within about 10 days, whereas death from damage to the pulmonary system may occur only after six months. The information about deterministic effects comes from studies of humans exposed accidentally, to the atomic bombs or to radiotherapy. Much of the under-standing of the underlying mechanisms and kinetics comes from studies in experi-mental animals. The need to understand deterministic effects led to studies of cell kinetics and the development of methods of studying cell survival and repair and the recovery of stem cells *in vivo* in the major tissues. Tissues affected early after expo-sure to radiation may also show late effects months or years after irradiation. Other tissues, such as those of the central nervous system and kidney, do not show effects until quite late after irradiation. Clinically, the former class of tissues is called 'early responding' and the latter, 'late responding'.

The damage that appears late may result from lesions incurred at the time of exposure but which are not expressed for many months. If the cells are renewed slowly and die only when attempting mitosis, the timing of the critical damage reflects the cell renewal rate. The function of some cell populations is affected indirectly by damage to blood vessels and by the fibrosis that replaces damaged tissue.

The success of radiotherapy depends on the differential between the killing of cancer cells and of cells of normal tissues. Recovery of normal tissues depends on repair of sublethal damage and repopulation. Fractionation of the dose increases the probability of recovery of the normal tissue more than recovery of the cancer cells. The total dose, the dose per fraction and the interval between fractions influence the effect of fractionation. The probability of late effects is determined mainly by the dose per fraction. Lowering the dose rate also reduces the effect. The degree and time of expression of injury vary among tissues and organs, depending on the radiosensitivity of the stem cells, which varies by a factor of about 2, and cell renewal rates, which vary many-fold. Cell survival is influenced by many genes, especially those concerned with repair of sublethal damage and also by *p53*, a tumour suppressor gene. Data on cell survival are frequently fitted by the so-called linear–quadratic model.

In the two large populations that received total-body irradiation—the atomic bomb survivors and patients receiving bone-marrow transplantation—the rates of non-cancer adverse effects in a number of organs, including the lens, increased at about 1 Sv.

Radiation-induced deterministic effects were first reported in the skin, and effects such as erythema are still used as an indicator of individual patients' reponse to radiation.

When the radiation field is restricted, as in the case of radiotherapy, and the doses are fractionated, many tissues can maintain their integrity and function even when receiving total doses up to 20–30 Gy; however, the gonads, the lens of the eye and the developing brain are highly radiosensitive.

Cellular hypersensitivity to radiation is shown in several (primarily two) rare, heritable cancer-prone disorders of DNA processing, but evidence that such individuals are prone to radiogenic cancer is lacking. Some normal members of the general population, including persons heterozygous for the *ATM* gene, can be made more sensitive to cell killing and induction of chromosomal damage by exposure to radiation. There is no evidence that they are at increased risk for radiogenic cancer. Individuals heterozygous for tumour suppressor gene mutations would be expected to be hypersensitive to both radiogenic and spontaneous cancer, and this hypothesis is borne out by the results of several studies in humans and experimental animals.

The induction of chromosomal aberrations, particularly dicentrics, in human lymphocytes has been well established *in vitro* and has been used as a biological dosimeter in a variety of situations of exposure in which induction of aberrations has occurred. The persons exposed include inhabitants of areas with a high background level of natural radiation, survivors of the atomic bombings, workers involved in cleaning-up after the accident at the Chernobyl nuclear reactor in Chernobyl, Ukraine, and people accidentally exposed to a discarded source of ^{137}Cs in Goiânia, Brazil. An increase in the number of minisatellite mutations has been reported in the children of parents living in a region heavily polluted by the Chernobyl accident. The lack of availability of appropriate local controls and possible confounding by heavy metal pollution indicate that this result should be treated with some caution.

Most of the data available on effects in mammals come from experiments with mice. The effects of ionizing radiation can be divided into two categories: those in germ cells, which become visible in the offspring of exposed mice, and those in somatic cells, determined directly in the exposed animals. X- and γ-radiation induce dominant lethal mutations, recessive autosomal mutations and sex-linked recessive lethal mutations. The germ cells have been most extensively studied, and a clear picture is available of the sensitivity of the germ cells of male mice during the various stages of development. The rate of germ-cell minisatellite mutations in mice was increased after exposure to ionizing radiation, with a doubling dose comparable to that for other genetic end-points. Recessive coat-colour mutations were seen in mice when embryos were treated with X-rays *in utero* two and nine days after conception.

Mutations were also induced by ionizing radiation in somatic cells of exposed mice, both in endogenous genes (*Hprt* and *Aprt*) of T lympocytes isolated from the spleen and in transgenic mice carrying a marker gene in which mutation rates can be determined in all cells of the body, provided enough DNA can be isolated from the organ or cell type of interest. Ionizing radiation was reported not to induce loss of heterozygosity at the *Aprt* locus in mice.

A number of in-vivo/in-vitro systems have been developed in which mammary, thyroid and tracheal cells are isolated and examined after exposure of the whole animal or are exposed *in vitro* and introduced into the whole animal. Studies with these systems have shown that: (i) X- and γ-radiation initiate many more cells than tumours develop; (ii) strain differences in susceptibility for radiation-induced mammary cancers are related to the sensitivity of the cells more than to host factors; and (iii) the late changes in chromosomes and multiple mutations in the *p53* tumour suppressor gene associated with the development of neoplasms suggest that genomic instability is an early event induced by radiation.

Chromosomal aberrations, gene mutations and reduced plating efficiency have been shown to occur in various systems many cell generations after exposure to radiation, indicating the induction of persistent genomic instability.

Ionizing radiation induces neoplastic transformation *in vitro* in mammalian cells, including human cells. While this indicates a potential for carcinogenicity, it is not clear to what extent these observations made *in vitro* can be extrapolated to the situation *in vivo*.

Ionizing radiation induces gene mutations in a wide variety of cellular systems. The predominant mutations are deletions resulting in gene inactivation. Chromosomal aberrations are induced in all eukaryotic systems that have been examined.

Although ionizing radiation can give rise to many different types of nucleotide damage in DNA through the active oxygen species that it generates, double-stranded DNA breaks and more complex lesions are believed to be largely responsible for its biological effects.

5.5   Evaluation

There is *sufficient evidence* in humans for the carcinogenicity of X-radiation and γ-radiation.

There is *sufficient evidence* in experimental animals for the carcinogenicity of X-radiation and γ-radiation.

Overall evaluation

X-radiation and γ-radiation are *carcinogenic to humans (Group 1)*.

6. References

Abe, T., Tsuge, I., Kamachi, Y., Torii, S., Utsumi, K., Akahori, Y., Ichihara, Y., Kurosawa, Y. & Matsuoka, H. (1994) Evidence for defects in V(D)J rearrangements in patients with severe combined immunodeficiency. *J. Immunol.*, **152**, 5504–5513

Abrahamson, A., Bender, M.A., Boecker, B.B., Gilbert, E.S. & Scott, B.R. (1991) *Health Effects Models for Nuclear Power Plant Accident Consequence Analysis. Modifications of Models Resulting from Recent Reports on Health Effects of Ionizing Radiation* (NUREG/CR-4214, Rev. 1, Part II, Addendum 1, LMF-132), Washington DC, United States Nuclear Regulatory Commission

Adams, L.M., Ethier, S.P. & Ullrich, R.L. (1987) Enhanced *in vitro* proliferation and *in vivo* tumorigenic potential of mammary epithelium from BALB/c mice exposed *in vivo* to γ-radiation and/or 7,12-dimethylbenz[*a*]anthracene. *Cancer Res.*, **47**, 4425–4431

Ahsan, H. & Neugut, A.I. (1998) Radiation therapy for breast cancer and increased risk for esophageal carcinoma. *Ann. intern. Med.*, **128**, 114–117

Ajimura, M., Leem, S.H. & Ogawa, H. (1993) Identification of new genes required for meiotic recombination in *Saccharomyces cerevisiae*. *Genetics*, **133**, 51–66

Akamatsu, Y. & Oettinger, M.A. (1998) Distinct roles of RAG1 and RAG2 in binding the V(D)J recombination signal sequences. *Mol. cell Biol.*, **18**, 4670–4678

Albertini, R.J., Castle, K.L. & Borcherding, W.R. (1982) T-cell cloning to detect the mutant 6-thioguanine-resistant lymphocytes present in human peripheral blood. *Proc. natl Acad. Sci. USA*, **79**, 6617–6621

Alderson, M.R. & Jackson, S.M. (1971) Long term follow-up of patients with menorrhagia treated by irradiation. *Br. J. Radiol.*, **441**, 295–298

Allalunis-Turner, M.J., Zia, P.K.Y., Barron, G.M., Mirzayans, R. & Day, R.S, III (1995) Radiation-induced DNA damage and repair in cells of a radiosensitive human malignant glioma cell line. *Radiat. Res.*, **144**, 288–293

Allwright, S.P.A., Colgan, P.A., McAulay, I.R. & Mullins, E. (1983) Natural background radiation and cancer mortality in the Republic of Ireland. *Int. J. Epidemiol.*, **12**, 414–418

Alpen, E.L. & Powers-Risius, P. (1981) The relative biological effect of high-*Z*, high-LET charged particles for spermatogonial killing. *Radiat. Res.*, **88**, 132–143

Al-Saleem, T., Wessner, L.L., Scheithauer, B,W., Patterson, K., Roach, E.S., Dreyer, S.J., Fujikawa, K., Bjornsson, J., Berstein, J. & Henske, E.P. (1998) Malignant tumors of the kidney, brain, and soft tissues in children and young adults with the tuberous sclerosis complex. *Cancer*, **83**, 2208–2216

Amsel, J., Waterbor, J.W., Oler, J., Rosenwaike, I. & Marshall, K. (1982) Relationship of site-specific cancer mortality rates to altitude. *Carcinogenesis*, **3**, 461–465

Anderson, C.W. & Carter, T.H. (1996) The DNA-activated protein-kinase DNA-PK. *Curr. Top. Microbiol. Immunol.*, **217**, 91–111

Andersson, M., Storm, H.H. & Mouridsen, H.T. (1991) Incidence of new primary cancers after adjuvant tamoxifen therapy and radiotherapy for early breast cancer. *J. natl Cancer Inst.*, **83**, 1013–1017

Anspaugh, L.R., Ricker, Y.E., Black, S.C., Grossman, R.F., Wheeler, D.L., Church, B.W. & Quinn, V.E. (1990) Historical estimates of external gamma exposure and collective external gamma exposure from testing at the Nevada test site. II. Test series after Hardtack II, 1958, and summary. *Health Phys.*, **59**, 525–532

Antoccia, A., Ricordy, R., Maraschio, P., Prudente, S. & Tanzarella, C. (1997) Chromosomal sensitivity to clastogenic agents and cell cycle perturbations in Nijmegen breakage syndrome lymphoblastoid cell lines. *Int. J. Radiat. Biol.*, **71**, 41–49

Appleby, J.M., Barber, J.B.P., Levine, E., Varley, J.M., Taylor, A.M.R., Stankovic, T., Heighway, J., Warren, C. & Scott, D. (1997) Absence of mutations in the *ATM* gene in breast cancer patients with severe responses to radiotherapy. *Br. J. Cancer*, **76**, 1546–1549

Arai, T., Nakano, T., Fukuhisa, K., Kasamatsu, T., Tsunematsu, R., Masubuchi, K., Yamauchi, K., Hamada, T., Fukuda, T. & Noguchi, H. (1991) Second cancer after radiation therapy for cancer of the uterine cervix. *Cancer*, **67**, 398–405

Araki, R., Fujimori, A., Hamatani, K., Mita, K., Saito, T., Mori, M., Fukumura, R., Morimyo, M., Muto, M., Itoh, M., Tatsumi, K. & Abe, M. (1997) Nonsense mutation at Tyr-4046 in the DNA-dependent protein kinase catalytic subunit of severe combined immune deficiency mice. *Proc. natl Acad. Sci. USA*, **94**, 2438–2443

Arlett, C.F. & Priestley, A. (1983). Defective recovery from potentially lethal damage in some human fibroblast cell strains. *Int. J. Radiat. Biol.*, **43**, 157–167

Artuso, M., Esteve, A., Brésil, H., Vuillaume, M. & Hall, J. (1995) The role of the ataxia telangiectasia gene in the p53, WAF1/CIPl(p21)- and GADD45-mediated response to DNA damage produced by ionizing radiation. *Oncogene*, **8**, 1427–1435

Ash, P. (1980) The influence of radiation on fertility in man. *Br. J. Radiol.*, **53**, 271–278

Ashmore, J.P., Krewski, D., Zielinski, J.M., Jiang, H., Semenciw, R. & Band, P.R. (1998) First analysis of mortality and occupational radiation exposure based on the National Dose Registry of Canada. *Am. J. Epidemiol.*, **148**, 564–574

Atahan, I.L., Yildiz, F., Ozyar, E., Uzal, D. & Zorlu, F. (1998) Basal cell carcinomas developing in a case of medulloblastoma associated with Gorlin's syndrome. *Pediatr. Hematol. Oncol.*, **15**, 187–191

Auvinen, A., Hakama, M., Arvela, H., Hakulinen, T., Rahola, T., Suomela, M., Söderman, B. & Rytömaa T. (1994) Fallout from Chernobyl and incidence of childhood leukaemia in Finland, 1976–92. *Br. med. J.*, **309**, 151–154

Awa, A. (1997) Analysis of chromosome aberrations in atomic bomb survivors for dose assessment: Studies at the Radiation Effects Research Foundation from 1968 to 1993. *Stem Cells*, **15** (Suppl. 2), 163–173

Azzam, E.I., de Toledo, S.M., Raaphorst, G.P. & Mitchel, R.E. (1996) Low-dose ionizing radiation decreases the frequency of neoplastic transformation to a level below the spontaneous rate in C3H 10T1/2 cells. *Radiat. Res.*, **146**, 369–373

Badie, C. Iliakis, G., Foray, N., Alsbeih, G., Pantellias, G.E., Okayasu, R., Cheong, N., Russell, N.S., Begg, A.C., Arlett., C.F. & Malaise, E.P. (1995) Defective repair of DNA double-strand breaks and chromosome damage in fibroblasts from a radiosensitive leukemia patient. *Cancer Res.*, **55**, 1232–1234

Badie, C., Goodhardt, M., Waugh, A., Doyen, N., Foray, N., Calsou, P., Singleton, B., Gell, D., Salles, B., Jeggo, P., Arlett, C.F. & Malaise, E.-P. (1997) A DNA double-strand break defective fibroblast cell line (180BR) derived from a radiosensitive patient represents a new mutant phenotype. *Cancer Res.*, **57**, 4600–4607

Baer, R., Heppell, A., Taylor, A.M.R., Rabbitts, P.H., Bouiller, B. & Rabbitts, T.H. (1987) The breakpoint of an inversion of chromosome 14 in a T-cell leukemia: Sequences downstream of the immunoglobulin heavy chain locus are implicated in tumorigenesis. *Proc. natl Acad. Sci. USA*, **84**, 9069–9073

Banin, S., Moyal, L., Shieh, S.-Y., Taya, Y., Anderson, C.W., Chessa, L., Smorodinsky, N.I., Prives, C., Reiss, Y., Shiloh, Y. & Ziv, Y. (1998) Enhanced phosphorylation of p53 by ATM in response to DNA damage. *Science*, **281**, 1674–1677

Barabanova, A. & Osanov, D.P. (1990) The dependence of skin lesions on the depth-dose distribution of β-irradiation of people in the Chernobyl nuclear power plant accident. *Int. J. Radiat. Biol.*, **57**, 775–782

Baral, E., Larsson, L.-E. & Mattsson, B. (1977) Breast cancer following irradiation of the breast. *Cancer*, **40**, 2905–2910

Barbi, G., Scheres, J.M.J.C., Schindler, D., Taalman, R.D.F.M., Rodens, K., Mehnert, K., Müller, M. & Seyschab, H. (1991) Chromosome instability and X-ray hypersensitivity in a microcephalic and growth-retarded child. *Am. J. med. Genet.*, **40**, 44–50

Barlow, C., Hirotsune, S., Paylor, R., Liyanage, M., Eckhaus, M., Collins, F., Shiloh, Y., Crawley J.N., Reid, T., Tagle, D. & Wynshaw-Boris, A. (1996) *Atm*-deficient mice: A paradigm of ataxia-telangiectasia. *Cell*, **86**, 159–171

Barstra, R.W., Bentvelzen, P.A.., Zoetelief, J., Mulder, A.H., Broerse, J.J. & van Bekkum, D.W. (1998) Induction of mammary tumors in rats by single-dose gamma irradiation at different ages. *Radiat. Res.*, **150**, 442–450

Basco, V.E., Coldman, A.J., Elwood, J.M. & Young, M.E.J. (1985) Radiation dose and second breast cancer. *Br. J. Cancer*, **52**, 319–325

Batchelor, A.L., Phillips, R.J.S. & Searle, A.G. (1966) A comparison of the mutagenic effectiveness of chronic neutron- and gamma irradiation of mouse spermatogonia. *Mutat. Res.*, **3**, 218–229

Beamish, H. & Lavin, M.F. (1994) Radiosensitivity in ataxia-telangiectasia: Anomalies in radiation-induced cell cycle delay. *Int. J. Radiat. Biol.*, **65**, 175–184

Beaty, O., III, Hudson, M.M., Greenwald, C., Luo, X., Fang, L., Wilimas, J.A., Thompson, E.I., Kun, L.E. & Pratt, C.B. (1995) Subsequent malignancies in children and adolescents after treatment for Hodgkin's disease. *J. clin. Oncol.*, **13**, 603–609

Becciolini, A. (1987) Relative radiosensitivities of the small and large intestine. *Adv. Radiat. Biol.*, **12**, 83–128

Bendel, I., Schüttmann, W. & Arndt, D. (1978) Cataract of lens as late effect of ionizing radiation in occupationally exposed persons. In: *Late Effects of Biological Effects of Ionizing Radiation*, Vol. 1, Vienna, International Atomic Energy Agency, pp. 309–319

Beninson, D. (1997) Risk of radiation at low doses. *Health Phys.*, **71**, 122–125

Benjamin, S.A., Saunders, W.J., Angleton, G.M. & Lee, A.C. (1991) Radiation carcinogenesis in dogs irradiated during prenatal and postnatal development. *J. Radiat. Res.*, **Suppl. 2**, 86–103

Benjamin, S.A., Saunders, W.J., Lee, A.C., Angleton, G.M., Stephens, L.C. & Mallinckrodt, C.H. (1997) Non-neoplastic and neoplastic thyroid disease in beagles irradiated during prenatal and postnatal development. *Radiat. Res.*, **147**, 422–430

Bentley, N.J., Holtzman, D.A., Flaggs, G., Keegan, K.S., DeMaggio, A., Ford, J.C., Hoekstra, M. & Carr, A.M. (1996) The *Schizosaccharomyces pombe rad3* checkpoint gene. *EMBO J.*, **15**, 6641–6651

Beral, V., Fraser, P., Carpenter, L., Booth, M., Brown, A. & Rose, G. (1988) Mortality of employees of the Atomic Weapons Establishment, 1951–82. *Br. med. J.*, **297**, 757–770

Bethwaite, P.B., Koreth, J., Herrington, C.S. & McGee, J.O. (1995) Loss of heterozygosity occurs at the D11S29 locus on chromosome 11q23 in invasive cervical carcinoma. *Br. J. Cancer*, **71**, 814–818

Bhatia, S., Robison, L.L., Oberlin, O., Greenberg, M., Bunin, G., Fossati-Bellani, F. & Meadows, A.T. (1996) Breast cancer and other second neoplasms after childhood Hodgkin's disease. *New Engl. J. Med.*, **334**, 745–751

Biedermann, K.A., Sun, J., Giacca, A.J., Tosto, L.M. & Brown, J.M. (1991) *Scid* mutation in mice confers hypersensitivity to ionizing radiation and a deficiency in DNA double-strand break repair. *Proc. natl Acad. Sci. USA*, **88**, 1394–1397

Bithell, J.F. & Stewart, A.M. (1975) Pre-natal irradiation and childhood malignancy: A review of British data from the Oxford Survey. *Br. J. Cancer*, **31**, 271–287

Bithell, J.F., Dutton, S.J., Draper, G.J. & Neary, N.M. (1994) Distribution of childhood leukaemias and non-Hodgkin's lymphomas near nuclear installations in England and Wales. *Br. med. J.*, **309**, 501–505

Black, D. (1984) *Investigation of the Possible Increased Incidence of Cancer in Western Cumbria,* London, Her Majesty's Stationery Office

Blayney, D.W., Longo, D.L., Young, R.C., Greene, M.H., Hubbard, S.M., Postal, M.G., Duffey, P.L. & DeVita, V.T., Jr (1987) Decreasing risk of leukemia with prolonged follow-up after chemotherapy and radiotherapy for Hodgkin's disease. *New Engl. J. Med.*, **316**, 710–714

Blettner, M. & Boice, J.D., Jr (1991) Radiation dose and leukaemia risk: General relative risk techniques for dose–response models in a matched case–control study. *Stat. Med.*, **10**, 1511–1526

Bliss, P., Kerr, G.R. & Gregor, A. (1994) Incidence of second brain tumours after pituitary irradiation in Edinburgh 1962–1990. *Clin. Oncol.*, **6**, 361–363

Blunt, T., Finnie, N.J., Taccioli, G.E., Smith, G.C.M., Demengeot, J., Gottlieb, T.M., Mizuta, R., Varghese, A.J., Alt, F.W., Jeggo, P.A. & Jackson, S.P. (1995) Defective DNA-dependent protein kinase activity is linked to V(D)J recombination and DNA repair defects associated with the murine *scid* mutation. *Cell*, **80**, 813–823

Boder, E. (1985) Ataxia-telangiectasia: An overview. In: Gatti, R.A. & Swift, M., eds, *Ataxia-telangiectasia: Genetics, Neuropathology, and Immunology of a Degenerative Disease of Childhood.* New York, Alan R. Liss, pp. 1–63

Boder, E. & Sedgwick, R.P. (1963) Ataxia-telangiectasia. A review of 101 cases. In: Walsh, G., ed., *Little Club Clinics in Developmental Medicine*, No. 8, London, Heinemann Medical Books, pp. 110–118

Boei, J.J.W.A., Vermeulen, S. & Natarajan, A.T. (1997) Differential involvement of chromosomes 1 and 4 in the formation of chromosomal aberrations in human lymphocytes after X-irradiation. *Int. J. Radiat. Biol.*, **72**, 139–145

Boei, J.J.W.A., Vermeulen, S., Fomina, J. & Natarajan, A.T. (1998a) Detection of incomplete exchanges and interstitial fragments in X-irradiated human lymphocytes using a telomeric PNA probe. *Int. J. Rad. Biol.*, **73**, 599–603

Boei, J.J.W.A., Vermeulen, S. & Natarajan, A.T. (1998b) Dose–response curves for X-ray induced interchanges and inter-arm intrachanges in human lymphocytes using arm-specific probes for chromosome 1. *Mutat. Res.,* **404**, 45–53

Boice, J.D., Jr (1992) Radiation and non-Hodgkin's lymphoma. *Cancer Res.*, **52**, 5489–5491

Boice, J.D., Jr (1996) Risk estimates for radiation exposure. In: Hendee, W.R. & Edwards, F.M., eds, *Health Effects of Exposure to Low-level Ionizing Radiation*, Philadelphia, Institute of Physics Publishing, pp. 237–268

Boice, J.D., Jr (1997) Radiation epidemiology: Past and present. In: Boice, J.D., Jr, ed., *Implications of New Data on Radiation Cancer Risk* (NCRP Proceedings No. 18), Bethesda, MD, National Council on Radiation Protection and Measurements, pp. 7–28

Boice, J.D., Jr & Inskip, P.D. (1996) Radiation-induced leukemia. In: Henderson, E.S., Lister, T.A. & Greaves, M.F., eds, *Leukemia*, 6th Ed., Philadelphia, W.B. Saunders, pp. 195–209

Boice, J.D., Jr & Miller, R.W. (1999) Childhood and adult cancer after intrauterine exposure to ionizing radiation. *Teratology*, **59**, 227–233

Boice, J.D., Jr, Land, C.E., Shore, R.E., Norman, J.E. & Tokunaga, M. (1979) Risk of breast cancer following low-dose radiation exposure. *Radiology,* **131**, 589–597

Boice, J.D., Jr, Storm, H.H., Curtis, R.E., Jensen, O.M., Kleinerman, R.A., Jensen, H.S., Flannery, J.T. & Fraumeni, J.F., Jr, eds (1985a) Multiple primary cancers in Connecticut and Denmark. *Natl Cancer Inst. Monogr.*, **68**

Boice, J.D., Jr, Day, N.E., Andersen, A., Brinton, L.A., Brown, R., Choi, N.W., Clarke, E.A., Coleman, M.P., Curtis, R.E., Flannery, J.T., Hakama, M., Hakulinen, T., Howe, G.R., Jensen, O.M., Kleinerman, R.A., Magnin, D., Magnus, K., Makela, K., Malker, B., Miller, A.B., Nelson, N., Patterson, C.C., Pettersson, F., Pompe-Kirn, V., Primic-Žakelk, M., Prior, P., Ravnihar, B., Skeet, R.G., Skjerven, J.E., Smith, P.G., Sok, M., Spengler, R.F., Storm, H.H., Stovall, M., Tomkins, G.W.O. & Wall, C. (1985b) Second cancers following radiation treatment for cervical cancer. An international collaboration among cancer registries. *J. natl Cancer Inst.*, **74**, 955–975

Boice, J.D., Jr, Blettner, M., Kleinerman, R.A., Stovall, M., Moloney, W.C., Engholm, G., Austin, D.F., Bosch, A., Cookfair, D.L., Krementz, E.T., Latourette, H.B., Peters, L.J., Schulz, M.D., Lundell, M., Pettersson, F., Storm, H.H., Bell, C.M.J., Coleman, M.P., Fraser, P., Palmer, M., Prior, P., Choi, N.W., Hislop, T.G., Koch, M., Robb, D., Robson, D., Spengler, R.F., von Fournier, D., Frischkorn, R., Lochmüller, H., Pompe-Kirn, V., Rimpela, A., Kjørstad, K., Pejovic, M.H., Sigurdsson, K., Pisani, P., Kucera, H. & Hutchison, G.B. (1987) Radiation dose and leukemia risk in patients treated for cancer of the cervix. *J. natl Cancer Inst.*, **79**, 1295–1311

Boice, J.D., Jr, Engholm, G., Kleinerman, R.A., Blettner, M., Stovall, M., Lisco, H., Moloney, W.C., Austin, D.F., Bosch, A., Cookfair, D.L., Krementz, E.T., Latourette, H.B., Merrill, J.A., Peters, L.J., Schulz, M.D., Storm, H.H., Björkholm, E., Pettersson, F., Bell, C.M.J., Coleman, M.P., Fraser, P., Neal, F.E., Prior, P., Choi, N.W., Hislop, T.G., Koch, M., Kreiger, N., Robb, D., Robson, D., Thomson, D.H., Lochmüller, H., von Fournier, D., Firschkorn, R., Kjørstad, K.E., Rimpela, A., Pejovic, M.-H., Pompe Kirn, V., Stankusova, H., Berrino, F., Sigurdsson, K., Hutchison, G.B. & MacMahon, B. (1988) Radiation dose and second cancer risk in patients treated for cancer of the cervix. *Radiat. Res.*, **116**, 3–55

Boice, J.D., Jr, Blettner, M., Kleinerman, R.A., Engholm, G., Stovall, M., Lisco, H., Austin, D.F., Bosch, A., Harlan, L., Krementz, E.T., Latourette, H.B., Merrill, J.M., Peters, L.J.,

Schulz, M.D., Wactawski, J., Storm, H.H., Björkholm, E., Pettersson, F., Bell, C.M.J., Coleman, M.P., Fraser, P., Neal, F.E., Prior, P., Choi, N.W., Hislop, T.G., Koch, M., Kreiger, N., Robb, D., Robson, D., Thomson, D.H., Lochmüller, H., von Fournier, D., Frischkorn, R., Kjørstad, K.E., Rimpelä, A., Pejovick, M.-H., Pompe Kirn, V., Stankusova, H., Pisani, P., Sigurdsson, K., Hutchison, G.B. & MacMahon, B. (1989) Radiation dose and breast cancer risk in patients treated for cancer of the cervix. *Int. J. Cancer*, **44**, 7–16

Boice, J.D., Jr, Morin, M.M., Glass, A.G., Friedman, G.D., Stovall, M., Hoover, R.N. & Fraumeni, J.F., Jr (1991a) Diagnostic X-ray procedures and risk of leukemia, lymphoma, and multiple myeloma. *J. Am. med. Assoc.*, **265**, 1290–1294

Boice, J.D., Jr, Preston, D., Davis, F.G. & Monson, R.R. (1991b) Frequent chest X-ray fluoro-scopy and breast cancer incidence among tuberculosis patients in Massachusetts. *Radiat. Res.*, **125**, 214–222

Boice, J.D., Jr, Harvey, E.B., Blettner, M., Stovall, M. & Flannery, J.T. (1992) Cancer in the contralateral breast after radiotherapy for breast cancer. *New Engl. J. Med.*, **326**, 781–785

Boice, J.D., Jr, Mandel, J.S. & Doody, M.M. (1995) Breast cancer among radiologic techno-logists. *J. Am. med. Assoc.*, **274**, 394–401

Boice, J.D., Jr, Land, C.E. & Preston, D.L. (1996) Ionizing radiation. In: Schottenfeld, D. & Fraumeni, J.F., Jr, eds, *Cancer Epidemiology and Prevention*, 2nd Ed., New York, Oxford University Press, pp. 319–354

Boivin, J.-F., Hutchison, G.B., Evans, F.B., Abou-Daoud, K.T. & Junod, B. (1986) Leukemia after radiotherapy for first primary cancers of various anatomic sites. *Am. J. Epidemiol.*, **123**, 993–1003

Boivin, J.-F., Hutchison, G.B., Zauber, A.G., Bernstein, L., Davis, F.G., Michel, R.P., Zanke, B., Tan, C.T.C., Fuller, L.M., Mauch, P. & Ultmann, J.E. (1995) Incidence of second cancers in patients treated for Hodgkin's disease. *J. natl Cancer Inst.*, **87**, 732–741

Bond, V.P., Fliedner, T.M. & Archambeau, J.O. (1965) *Mammalian Radiation Lethality: A Disturbance in Cellular Kinetics*, New York, Academic Press

Borek, C. & Sachs, L. (1966) In vitro cell transformation by X-irradiation. *Nature*, **210**, 276–278

Bosma, G.C., Custer, R.P. & Bosma, M.J. (1983) A severe combined immunodeficiency mutation in the mouse. *Nature*, **301**, 527–530

Bouffler, S.D., Kemp, C.J., Balmain, A. & Cox, R. (1995) Spontaneous and ionizing radiation-induced chromosomal abnormalities in *p53*-deficient mice. *Cancer Res.*, **55**, 3883–3889

Bougrov, N.G., Goksu, H.Y., Hasakell, E., Degteva, M.O., Meckbach, R. & Jacob, P. (1998) Issues in the reconstruction of environmental doses on the basis of thermoluminescence measurements in the Techa riverside. *Health Phys.*, **75**, 574–583

Brada, M., Ford, D., Ashley, S., Bliss, J.M., Crowley, S., Mason, M., Rajan, B. & Traish, D. (1992) Risk of second brain tumour after conservative surgery and radiotherapy for pituitary adenoma. *Br. med. J.*, **304**, 1343–1346

Bradley, W.E., Belouchi, A. & Messing, K. (1988) The aprt heterozygote/hemizygote system for screening mutagenic agents allows detection of large deletions. *Mutat. Res.*, **199**, 131–138

Bridges, B.A., Dennis, R.E. & Munson, R.J. (1967) Mutation in *Escherichia coli* B/r WP2 try⁻ by reversion or suppression of a chain-terminating codon. *Mutat. Res.*, **4**, 502–504

Bridges, B.A., Law, J. & Munson, R.J. (1968) Mutagenesis in *Escherichia coli*. II. Evidence for a common pathway for mutagenesis by ultraviolet light, ionizing radiation and thymine deprivation. *Mol. Gen. Genet.*, **103**, 266–273

Bridges, B.A., Huckle, J. & Ashwood-Smith, M.J. (1970) X-ray mutagenesis of cultured Chinese hamster cells. *Nature*, **226**, 184–185

Brill, A.B., Tomonaga, M. & Heyssel, R.M. (1962) Leukemia in man following exposure to ionizing radiation. A summary of the findings in Hiroshima and Nagasaki, and a comparison with other human experience. *Ann. intern. Med.*, **56**, 590–609

Broerse, J.J., Hollander, C.F. & Van Zwieten, M.J. (1981) Tumor induction in rhesus monkeys after total body irradiation with X-rays and fission neutrons. *Int. J. Radiat. Biol.*, **40**, 671–676

Broerse, J.J., Hennen, L.A. & Solleveld, H.A. (1986) Actuarial analysis of the hazard for mammary carcinogenesis in different rat strains after X- and neutron irradiation. *Leukemia Res.*, **10**, 749–754

Broerse, J.J., Hennen, L.A., Klapwijk, W.M. & Solleveld, H.A. (1987) Mammary carcinogenesis in different rat strains after irradiation and hormone administration. *Int. J. Radiat. Biol.*, **51**, 1091–1100

Brown, K.D., Ziv, Y., Sadanandan, S.N., Chessa, L., Collins, F.S., Shiloh, Y. & Tagle, D. (1997) The ataxia-telangiectasia gene product, a constitutively expressed nuclear protein that is not upregulated following genome damage. *Proc. natl Acad. Sci. USA*, **94**, 1840–1845

Bryant, P.E. (1984) Enzymatic restriction of mammalian cell DNA using Pvu II and Bam H1: Evidence for the double strand break origin of chromosomal aberrations. *Int. J. Radiat. Biol.*, **46**, 57–65

Bryant, P.E. & Riches, A.C. (1989) Oncogenic transformation of murine C3H 10T1/2 cells resulting from DNA double-strand breaks induced by a restriction endonuclease. *Br. J. Cancer*, **60**, 852–544

Budach, W., Hartford, A., Gioioso, D., Freeman, J., Taghian, A. & Suit, H.D. (1992) Tumors arising in SCID mice share enhanced radiation sensitivity of SCID normal tissues. *Cancer Res.*, **52**, 6292–6296.

Budach, W., Classen, J., Belka, C. & Bamberg, M. (1998) Clinical impact of predictive assays for acute and late radiation morbidity. *Strahlenther. Onkol.*, **174** (Suppl. 3), 20–24

Bullrich, F., Rasio, D., Kitada, S., Starostik, P., Kipps, T., Keating. M., Albitar, M., Rees, J.C. & Croce, C.M. (1999) *ATM* mutations in B-cell chronic lymphocytic leukemia. *Cancer Res.*, **59**, 24–27

Bultman, S.J., Russell, L.B., Gutierrez-Espeleta, G.A. & Woychik, R.P. (1991) Molecular characterization of a region of DNA associated with mutations at the *agouti* locus in the mouse. *Proc. natl. Acad. Sci. USA*, **88**, 8062–8066

Bundesamt für Strahlenschutz (1998) *Radioactivity in the Environment in the Federal Republic of Germany 1994–1995* (BfS-SCHR-16/98), Bremerhafen (in German)

Bundesministerium für Umwelt, Naturschutz und Reaktorsicherheit (BMU) (1999) *Environmental Policy, Environmental Radioactivity and Radiation Exposure in the Year 1996*, Bonn (in German)

Bunger, B.M., Cook, J.R. & Barrick, M.K. (1981) Life table methodology for evaluating radiation risk: An application based on occupational exposures. *Health Phys.*, **40**, 439–455 van der Burgt, I., Chrzanowska, K.H., Smeets, D. & Weemaes, C. (1996) Nijmegen breakage syndrome. *J. med. Genet.*, **33**, 153–156

Burkart, W. (1996) Radioepidemiology in the aftermath of the nuclear program of the former Soviet Union: Unique lessons to be learnt. *Radiat. Environ. Biophys.*, **35**, 65–73

Burkart, W. & Kellerer, A., eds (1994) A first assessment of radiation doses and health effects in workers and communities exposed since 1948 in the Southern Urals. *Sci. total Environ.*, **142**, 1–125

Buzunov, V., Omelyanetz, N., Strapko, N., Ledoschuk, B., Krasnikova, L. & Kartushin, G. (1996) Chernobyl NPP accident consequences cleaning up participants in Ukraine— Health status epidemiologic study—main results. In: Karaoglou, A., Desmet, G., Kelly, G.N. & Menzel, H.G., eds, *The Radiological Consequences of the Chernobyl Accident* (Proceedings of the First International Conference, Minsk, Belarus, 18–22 March 1996), Luxembourg, Office for Official Publications of the European Communities, pp. 871–878

Byrne, E., Hallpike, J.F., Manson, J.I., Sutherland, G.R. & Thong, Y.H. (1984) Ataxia-without-telangiectasia. Progressive multisystem degeneration with IgE deficiency and chromosomal instability. *J. neurol. Sci.*, **66**, 307–317

Caldwell, G.G., Kelley, D., Zack, M., Falk, H. & Heath, C.W., Jr (1983) Mortality and cancer frequency among military nuclear test (Smoky) participants, 1957 through 1979. *J. Am. med. Assoc.*, **250**, 620–624

Canman, C.E., Wolff, A.C., Chen, C.-Y., Fornace, A.J., Jr & Kastan, M.B. (1994) The p53 dependent G_1 cell cycle checkpoint pathway and ataxia-telangiectasia. *Cancer Res.*, **54**, 5054–5058

Canman, C.E., Lim, D-S., Cimprich, K.A., Taya, Y., Tamai, K., Sakaguchi, K., Appella, E., Kastan, M.B. & Siliciano, J.D. (1998) Activation of the ATM kinase by ionizing radiation and phosphorylation of p53. *Science*, **281**, 1677–1679

Cao, L., Alani, E. & Kleckner, N. (1990) A pathway for generation and processing of double-strand breaks during meiotic recombination in *S. cerevisiae. Cell*, **61**, 1089–1101

Cardis, E., Gilbert, E.S., Carpenter, L., Howe, G., Kato, I., Armstrong, B.K., Beral, V., Cowper, G., Douglas, A., Fix, J., Fry, S.A., Kaldor, J., Lavé, C., Salmon, L., Smith, P.G., Voelz, G.L. & Wiggs, L.D. (1995) Effects of low doses and low dose rates of external ionizing radiation: Cancer mortality among nuclear industry workers in three countries. *Radiat. Res.*, **142**, 117–132

Cardis, E., Anspaugh, L., Ivanov, V.K., Likhtarev, I.A., Mabuchi, K., Okeanov, A.E. & Prisyazhniuk, A.E. (1996) Estimated long term health effects of the Chernobyl accident, In: *One Decade after Chernobyl: Summing up the Consequences of the Accident*, Vienna, International Atomic Energy Agency, pp. 241–279

Carney, J.P., Maser, R.S., Olivares, H., Davis, M.E., Le Beau, M., Yates, J.R., III, Hays, L., Morgan, W.F. & Petrini, J.H.J. (1998) The hMre 11/hRad50 protein complex and Nijmegen breakage syndrome: Linkage of double-strand break repair to the cellular DNA damage response. *Cell*, **93**, 477–486

Carpenter, L., Higgins, C., Douglas, A., Fraser, P., Beral, V. & Smith, P. (1994) Combined analysis of mortality in three United Kingdom nuclear industry workforces, 1946–1988. *Radiat. Res.*, **138**, 224–238

Casarett, G.W. (1980) *Radiation Histopathology*, Boca Raton, FL, CRC Press

Cattanach, B.M., Patrick, G., Papworth, D., Goodhead, D.T., Hacker, T., Cobb, L. & Whitehill, E. (1995) Investigation of lung tumour induction in BALB/cJ mice following paternal X-irradiation. *Int. J. Radiat. Biol.*, **67**, 607–615

Cattanach, B.M., Papworth, D., Patrick, G., Goodhead, D.T., Hacker, T., Cobb, L. & Whitehill, E. (1998) Investigation of lung tumour induction of C3H/HeH mice, with and without tumour promotion with urethane, following paternal X-irradiation. *Mutat. Res.*, **403**, 1–12

Cavazzana-Calvo, M., Le Diest, F., De Saint Basile, G., Papadopoulo, D., De Villartay, J.P. & Fischer, A. (1993) Increased radiosensitivity of granulocyte macrophage colony-forming units and skin fibroblasts in human autosomal recessive severe combined immuno-deficiency. *J. clin. Invest.*, **91**, 1214–1218

Cerosaletti, K.M., Lange, E., Stringham, H.M., Weemaes, C.M.R., Smeets, D., Sölder, B., Belohradsky, B.H., Taylor, A.M.R., Karnes, P., Elliott, A., Komatsu, K., Gatti, R.A., Boehnke, M. & Concannon, P. (1998) Fine localization of the Nijmegen breakage syndrome gene to 8q21: Evidence for a common founder haplotype. *Am. J. hum. Genet* **63**, 125–134

Chadwick, K.H. & Leenhouts, H.P. (1998) Radiation induced chromosome aberrations: Some biophysical considerations. *Mutat. Res.*, **404**, 113–117

Chan, D.W., Gately, D.P., Urban, S., Galloway, A.M., Lees-Miller, S.P., Yen, T. & Allalunis-Turner, J. (1998) Lack of correlation between ATM protein expression and tumour cell radiosensitivity. *Int. J. Radiat. Biol.*, **74**, 217–224

Chang, W.P. & Little, J.B. (1992) Delayed reproductive death as a dominant phenotype in cell clones surviving X-irradiation. *Carcinogenesis*, **13**, 923–928

Chen, G. & Lee, E.Y.H.P. (1996) The product of the *ATM* gene is a 370 kDa nuclear phospho-protein. *J. biol. Chem.*, **271**, 33693–33697

Chen, D.-Q. & Wei, L.-X. (1991) Chromosome aberration, cancer mortality and hormetic phenomena among inhabitants in areas of high background radiation in China. *J. Radiat. Res.*, **32** (Suppl. 2), 46–53

Chen, P.C., Lavin, M.F., Kidson, C. & Moss, D. (1978) Identification of ataxia telangiectasia heterozygotes, a cancer prone population. *Nature*, **274**, 484–486

Chrzanowska, K.H., Kleijer, W.J., Krajewska-Walasek, M., Bialecka, M., Gutkowska, A., Goryluk-Kozakiewicz, B., Michalkiewicz, J., Stachowski, J., Gregorek, H., Lysón-Wojciechowska, G., Janowicz, W. & Józwiak, S. (1995) Eleven Polish patients with microcephaly, immunodeficiency, and chromosomal instability: The Nijmegen breakage syndrome. *Am. J. med. Genet.*, **57**, 462–471

Cimprich, K.A., Shin, T.B., Keith, C.T. & Schreiber, S.L. (1996) cDNA cloning and gene mapping of a candidate human cell cycle checkpoint protein. *Proc. natl Acad. Sci. USA*, **93**, 2850–2855

Clarke, E.A., Kreiger, N. & Spengler, R.F. (1984) Second primary cancer following treatment for cervical cancer. *Can. med. Assoc. J.*, **131**, 553–556

Clarke, A.R., Gledhill, S., Hooper, M.L., Bird, C.C. & Wyllie, A.H. (1994) p53 dependence of early apoptotic and proliferative responses within the mouse intestinal epithelium following gamma-irradiation. *Oncogene*, **9**, 1767–1773

Clifton, K.H., Tanner, M.A. & Gould, M.N. (1986) Assessment of radiogenic cancer initiation frequency per clonogenic rat mammary cell in vivo. *Cancer Res.*, **46**, 2390–2395

Coggle, J.E. (1988) Lung tumour induction in mice after X-rays and neutrons. *Int. J. Radiat. Biol.*, **53**, 585–598

Cohen, B.L. (1995) Test of the linear-no threshold theory of radiation carcinogenesis for inhaled radon decay products. *Health Phys.*, **68**, 157–174

Cohen, M.M., Shaham, M., Dagan, J., Shmueli, E. & Kohn, G. (1975) Cytogenetic investigations in families with ataxia-telangiectasia. *Cytogenet. cell. Genet.*, **15**, 338–356

Cole, J., Arlett, C.F., Green, M.H.L., Harcourt, S.A., Priestley, A., Henderson, L., Cole, H., James, S.E. & Richmond, F. (1988) Comparative human cellular radiosensitivity: II. The survival following gamma-irradiation of unstimulated (G_0) T-lymphocytes, T-lymphocyte lines, lymphoblastoid cell lines and fibroblasts from normal donors, from ataxia-telangiectasia patients and from ataxia-telangiectasia heterozygotes. *Int. J. Radiat. Biol.*, **54**, 929–943

Commission of the European Communities (1993) *Radiation Atlas. Natural Sources of Ionizing Radiation in Europe* (Report EUR 14470), Luxembourg

Committee on Medical Aspects of Radiation in the Environment (1996) *Fourth Report. The Incidence of Cancer and Leukaemia in Young People in the Vicinity of the Sellafield Site, West Cumbria: Further Studies and an Update of the Situation since the Publication of the Report of the Black Advisory Group in 1984*, London, Her Majesty's Stationery Office

Committee on the Biological Effects of Ionizing Radiations (BEIR I) (1972) *The Effects on Populations of Exposure to Low Levels of Ionizing Radiation*, Washington DC, National Academy Press

Committee on the Biological Effects of Ionizing Radiations (BEIR III) (1980) *The Effects on Populations of Exposure to Low Levels of Ionizing Radiation: 1980*, Washington DC, National Academy Press

Committee on the Biological Effects of Ionizing Radiations (BEIR IV) (1988) *Health Risks of Radon and other Internally Deposited Alpha-emitters*, Washington DC, National Academy Press

Committee on the Biological Effects of Ionizing Radiations (BEIR V) (1990) *Health Effects of Exposure to Low Levels of Ionizing Radiation*, Washington DC, National Academy Press

Committee on the Biological Effects of Ionizing Radiations (BEIR VII) (1998) *Health Effects of Exposure to Low Levels of Ionizing Radiations. Time for Reassessment?* Washington DC, National Academy Press

Conard, R.A., Paglia, D.E., Larsen, R.P., Sutow, W.W., Dobyns, B.M., Robbins, J., Krotosky, W.A., Field, J.B., Rall, J.E. & Wolff, J. (1980) *Review of Medical Findings in a Marshallese Population Twenty-six Years after Accidental Exposure to Radioactive Fallout* (Brookhaven National Laboratory Report BNL 51261), Springfield, VA, National Technical Information Service

Conley, M.E., Spinner, N.B., Emanuel, B.S., Nowell, P.C. & Nichols, W.W. (1986) A chromosome breakage syndrome with profound immunodeficiency. *Blood*, **67**, 1251–1256.

Cook-Mozaffari, P., Darby, S. & Doll, R. (1989) Cancer near potential sites of nuclear installations. *Lancet*, **ii**, 1145–1147

Cornforth, M.N. & Bedford, J.S. (1985) On the nature of a defect in cells from individuals with ataxia-telangiectasia. *Science*, **227**, 1589–1591

Court Brown, W.M. & Doll, R. (1957) *Leukaemia and Aplastic Anaemia in Patients Irradiated for Ankylosing Spondylitis*, London, Her Majesty's Stationery Office

Court Brown, W.M., Doll, R. & Hill, A.B. (1960a) Incidence of leukemia after exposure to diagnostic radiation *in utero*. *Br. med. J.*, **5212**, 1539–1545

Court Brown, W.M., Doll, R., Spiers, F.W., Duffy, B.J. & McHugh, M.J. (1960b) Geographical variation in leukaemia mortality in relation to background radiation and other factors. *Br. med. J.*, **5188**, 1753–1759

Cox, B.D. & Lyon, M.F. (1975) X-ray induced dominant lethal mutations in mature and immature oocytes of guinea pigs and golden hamsters. *Mutat. Res.*, **28**, 421–436

Cox, R., Masson, W.K., Weichselbaum, R.R., Nove, J. & Little, J.B. (1981) The repair of potentially lethal damage in X-irradiated cultures of normal and ataxia telangiectasia human fibroblasts. *Int. J. Radiat. Biol.*, **39**, 357–365

Crick, M.J. & Linsley, G.S. (1984) An assessment of the radiological impact of the Windscale reactor fire, October 1957. *Int. J. Radiat. Biol.*, **46**, 479–506

da-Cruz, A.D. & Glickman, B.W. (1997) Nature of mutation in the human *hprt* gene following in vivo exposure to ionizing radiation of cesium-137. *Environ. Mol. Mutag.*, **30**, 385–395

da-Cruz, A.D., Curry, J., Curado, M.P. & Glickman, B.W. (1996) Monitoring *hprt* mutant frequencies over time in T-lymphocytes of people accidentally exposed to high doses of ionizing radiation. *Environ. mol. Mutag.*, **27**, 165–175

Curtis, R.E. (1997) Second cancers following radiotherapy for cancer. In: Boice, J.D., Jr, ed., *Implications of New Data on Radiation Cancer Risk* (NCRP Proceedings No. 18), Bethesda, MD, National Council on Radiation Protection and Measurements, pp. 79–94

Curtis, R.E., Boice, J.D., Jr, Stovall, M., Flannery, J.T. & Moloney, W.C. (1989) Leukemia risk following radiotherapy for breast cancer. *J. clin. Oncol.*, **7**, 21–29

Curtis, R.E., Boice, J.D., Jr, Stovall, M., Bernstein, L., Greenberg, R.S., Flannery, J.T., Schwartz, A.G., Weyer, P., Moloney, W.C. & Hoover, R.N. (1992) Risk of leukemia after chemotherapy and radiation treatment for breast cancer. *New Engl. J. Med.*, **326**, 1745–1751

Curtis, R.E., Boice, J.D., Jr, Stovall, M., Bernstein, L., Holowaty, E., Karjalainen, S., Langmark, F., Nasca, P.C., Schwartz, A.G., Schymura, M.J., Storm, H.H., Toogood, P., Weyer, P. & Moloney, W.C. (1994) Relationship of leukemia risk to radiation dose following cancer of the uterine corpus. *J. natl Cancer Inst.*, **86**, 1315–1324

Curtis, R.E., Rowlings, P.A., Deeg, H.J., Shriner, D.A., Socié, G., Travis, L.B., Horowitz, M.M., Witherspoon, R.P., Hoover, R.N., Sobocinski, K.A., Fraumeni, J.F., Jr & Boice, J.D., Jr (1997) Solid cancers after bone marrow transplantation. *New Engl. J. Med.*, **336**, 897–904

Cuypers, H.T. Selten, G., Quint, W., Zijlstra, M., Maandag, E.R., Boelens, W., van Wezenbeek, P., Melief, C. & Berns, A. (1984) Murine leukemia virus-induced T-cell lymphomagenesis: Integration of proviruses in a distinct chromosomal region. *Cell*, **37**, 141–150

Cuzick, J. & De Stavola, B. (1988) Multiple myeloma—A case control study. *Br. J. Cancer*, **57**, 516–520

van Daal, W.A.J., Goslings, B.M., Hermans, J., Ruiter, D.J., Sepmeyer, C.F., Vink, M., Van Vloten, W.A. & Thomas, P. (1983) Radiation-induced head and neck tumours: Is the skin as sensitive as the thyroid gland? *Eur. J. Cancer clin. Oncol.*, **19**, 1081–1086

Daher, A., Varin, M., Lamontagne, Y. & Oth, D. (1998) Effect of pre-conceptional external or internal irradiation of N5 male mice and the risk of leukemia in their offspring. *Carcinogenesis*, **19**, 1553–1558

Dalhberg, W.K. & Little, J.B. (1995) Response of dermal fibroblast cultures from patients with unusually severe responses to radiotherapy and from ataxia telangiectasia heterozygotes to fractionated radiation. *Clin. Cancer Res.*, **1**, 785–790

Damber, L., Larsson, L.-G., Johansson, L. & Norin, T. (1995) A cohort study with regard to the risk of haematological malignancies in patients treated with X-rays for benign lesions in the locomotor system. I. Epidemiological analyses. *Acta oncol.*, **34**, 713–719

Damewood, M.D. & Grochow, L.B. (1986) Prospects for fertility after chemotherapy or radiation for neoplastic disease. *Fertil. Steril.*, **45**, 443–459

Darby, S.C. (1991) Contribution of natural ionizing radiation to cancer mortality in the United States. In: Brugge, J., Curran, T., Harlow, E. & McCormick, F., eds, *Origins of Human Cancer: A Comprehensive Review*, Cold Spring Harbor, NY, Cold Spring Harbor Laboratory Press, pp. 183–190

Darby, S.C. & Doll, R. (1987) Fallout, radiation doses near Dounreay, and childhood leukaemia. *Br. med. J.*, **294**, 603–607

Darby, S.C., Doll, R., Gill, S.K. & Smith, P.G. (1987) Long-term mortality after a single treatment course with X-rays in patients treated for ankylosing spondylitis. *Br. J. Cancer*, **55**, 179–190

Darby, S.C., Kendall, G.M., Fell, T.P., O'Hagan, J.A., Muirhead, C.R., Ennis, J.R., Ball, A.M., Dennis, J.A. & Doll, R. (1988) A summary of mortality and incidence of cancer in men from the United Kingdom who participated in the United Kingdom's atmospheric nuclear weapon tests and experimental programmes. *Br. med. J.*, **296**, 332–338

Darby, S.C., Kendall, G.M., Fell, T.P., Doll, R., Goodill, A.A., Conquest, A.J., Jackson, D.A. & Haylock, R.G. (1993) Further follow up of mortality and incidence of cancer in men from the United Kingdom who participated in the United Kingdom's atmospheric nuclear weapon tests and experimental programmes. *Br. med. J.*, **307**, 1530–1535

Darby, S.C., Reeves, G., Key, T., Doll, R. & Stovall, M. (1994) Mortality in a cohort of women given X-ray therapy for metropathia haemorrhagica. *Int. J. Cancer*, **56**, 793–801

Davey, M.P., Bertness, V., Nakahara, K., Johnson, J.P., McBride, O.W., Waldmann, T.A. & Kirsch, I.R. (1988) Juxtaposition of the T-cell receptor α-chain locus (14q11) and a region (14q32) of potential importance in leukaemogenesis by a 14:14 translocation in a patient with T-cell chronic lymphocytic leukaemia and ataxia-telangiectasia. *Proc. natl Acad. Sci. USA*, **85**, 9287–9291

Davis, F.G., Boice, J.D., Jr, Hrubec, Z. & Monson, R.R. (1989) Cancer mortality in a radiation-exposed cohort of Massachusetts tuberculosis patients. *Cancer Res.*, **49**, 6130–6136

Day, N.E. & Boice, J.C., Jr, eds (1984) *Second Cancers in Relation to Radiation Treatment for Cervical Cancer: Results of a Cancer Registry Collaboration* (IARC Scientific Publications No. 52), Lyon, IARC Press

Deeg, H.J., Storb, R. & Thomas, E.D. (1984) Bone marrow transplantation: a review of delayed complications. *Br. J. Haematol.*, **57**, 185–208

DeGroot, L.J., Reilly, M., Pinnamaneni, K. & Refetoff, S. (1983) Retrospective and prospective study of radiation-induced thyroid disease. *Am. J. Med.*, **74**, 852–862

Degteva, M.O., Kozheurov, V.P. & Vorobiova, M.I. (1994) General approach to dose reconstruction in the population exposed as a result of the release of radioactive wastes into the Techa River. *Sci. total Environ.*, **142**, 49–61

Degteva, M.O., Kozheurov, V.P., Burmistrov, D.S., Vorobyova, M.I., Valchuk, V.V., Bougrov, N.G. & Shishkina, H.A. (1996) An approache to dose reconstruction for the Urals population. *Health Phys.*, **71**, 71–76

DeOme, K.B., Miyamoto, M.J., Osborn, R.C., Guzman, R.C. & Lum, K. (1978) Detection of inapparent nodule-transformed cells in the mammary gland tissues of virgin female BALB/cfC3H mice. *Cancer Res.*, **38**, 2103–2111

Di Majo, V., Coppola, M., Rebessi, S., Saran, A., Pazzaglia, S., Pariset, L. & Covelli, V. (1996) The influence of sex on life shortening and tumor induction in CBA/Cne mice exposed to X rays or fission neutrons. *Radiat. Res.*, **146**, 81–87

Dolganov, G.M., Maser, R.S., Novikov, A., Tosto, L., Chong, S., Bressan, D.A. & Petrini, J.H.J. (1996) Human Rad50 is physically associated with human Mre11: Identification of a conserved multiprotein complex implicated in recombinational DNA repair. *Mol. cell. Biol.*, **16**, 4832–4841

Doll R. (1995) Hazards of ionising radiation: 100 years of observations on man. *Br. J. Cancer*, **72**, 1339–1349

Doll, R. & Wakeford, R. (1997) Risk of childhood cancer from fetal irradiation. *Br. J. Radiol.*, **70**, 130–139

Doll, R., Evans, H.J. & Darby, S.C. (1994) Paternal exposure not to blame. *Nature*, **367**, 678–680

Doody, M.M., Mandel, J.S., Lubin, J.H. & Boice, J.D., Jr (1998) Mortality among United States radiologic technologists, 1926–90. *Cancer Causes Control*, **9**, 67–75

Douglas, A.J., Omar, R.Z. & Smith, P.G. (1994) Cancer mortality and morbidity among workers at the Sellafield plant of British Nuclear Fuels. *Br. J. Cancer*, **70**, 1232–1243

Draper, G.J., Stiller, C.A., Cartwright, R.A., Craft, A.W. & Vincent, T.J. (1993) Cancer in Cumbria and in the vicinity of the Sellafield nuclear installation, 1963–1990. *Br. med. J.*, **306,** 89–94

Draper, G.J., Little, M.P., Sorahan, T., Kinlen, L.J., Bunch, K.J., Conquest, A.J., Kendall, G.M., Kneale, G.W., Lancashire, R.J., Muirhead, C.R., O'Connor, C.M. & Vincent, T.J. (1997) Cancer in the offspring of radiation workers: A record-linkage study. *Br. Med. J.*, **315**, 1181–1188

Dubrova, Y.E., Nesterov, V.N., Krouchinsky, N.G., Ostapenko, V.A., Neumann, R., Neil, D.L. & Jeffreys, A.J. (1996) Human minisatellite mutation rate after the Chernobyl accident. *Nature*, **380**, 683–686

Dubrova, Y.E., Nesterov, V.N., Krouchinsky, N.G., Ostapenko, V.A., Vergnaud, G., Giraudeau, F., Buard, J. & Jeffreys, A.J. (1997) Further evidence for elevated human minisatellite mutation rate in Belarus eight years after the Chernobyl accident. *Mutat. Res.*, **381**, 267–278

Dubrova,Y.E., Plumb, M., Brown, J. & Jeffreys, A.J. (1998a) Radiation-induced germline instability at minisatellite loci. *Int. J. Radiat. Biol.*, **74**, 689–96

Dubrova,Y.E., Plumb, M., Brown, J., Fennelly, J., Bois, P., Goodhead, D. & Jeffreys, A.J. (1998b) Stage specificity, dose response, and doubling dose for mouse minisatellite germline mutation induced by acute radiation. *Proc. natl. Acad. Sci. USA*, **95**, 251–255

Dulic, V., Kaufmann, W.K., Wilson, S.J., Tlsty, T.D., Lees, E., Harper, J.W., Elledge, S.J. & Reed, S.I. (1994) p53-dependent inhibition of cyclin-dependent kinase activities in human fibroblasts during radiation-induced G_1 arrest. *Cell*, **76**, 1013–1023

Dunn, G.R. & Kohn, H.I. (1981) Some comparisons between induced and spontaneous mutation rates in mouse sperm and spermatogonia. *Mutat. Res.*, **80**, 159–164

Easton, D.F. (1994) Cancer risks in A-T heterozygotes. *Int. J. Radiat. Biol.*, **6**, 177–182

Easton, D.F. (1997) Breast cancer genes—What are the real risks? *Nat. Gen.*, **16**, 210–211

Easton, D.F., Bishop, T., Ford, D. & Crockford, G.P. and the Breast Cancer Linkage Consortium (1993) Genetic linkage analysis in familial breast and ovarian cancer: Results from 214 families. *Am. J. Hum. Genet.*, **52**, 678–701

Edling, C., Comba, P., Axelson, O. & Flodin, U. (1982) Effects of low-dose radiation— A correlation study. *Scand. J. Work Environ. Health*, **8** (Suppl. 1), 59–64

Ehling, U.H. (1965) The frequency of X-ray-induced dominant mutations affecting the skeleton of mice. *Genetics*, **51**, 723–732

Ehling, U.H. (1966) Dominant mutations affecting the skeleton in offspring of X-irradiated male mice. *Genetics*, **54**, 1381–1389

Ehling, U.H. (1971) Comparison of radiation- and chemically-induced dominant lethal mutations in male mice. *Mutat. Res.*, **11**, 35–44

Ehling, U.H. (1985) The induction and manifestation of hereditary cataracts. In: Woodhead, A.V., Shellaberger, C.J., Bond, V. & Hollaender, A., eds, *Assessment of Risk from Low-level Exposure to Radiation and Chemicals*, New York, Plenum, pp. 345–367

Eker, R. & Mossige, J. (1961) A dominant gene for renal adenomas in the rat. *Nature*, **189**, 858–859

Ellender, M., Larder, S.M., Harrison, J.D., Cox, R. & Silver, A.R.J. (1997) Radiation-induced intestinal neoplasia in a genetically-predisposed mouse (Min). *Radioprotection*, **32**, 287–288

Elson, A., Wang, Y., Daugherty, C.J., Morton, C.C., Zhou, F., Campos-Torres, J. & Leder, P. (1996) Pleiotropic defects in ataxia-telangiectasia protein-deficient mice. *Proc. natl Acad. Sci. USA*, **83**, 13084–13089

Eng, C., Li, F.P., Abramson, D.H., Ellsworth, R.M., Wong, F.L., Goldman, M.B., Seddon, J., Tarbell, N. & Boice, J.D., Jr (1993) Mortality from second tumors among long-term survivors of retinoblastoma. *J. natl Cancer Inst.*, **85**, 1121–1128

Ethier, S.P. & Ullrich, R.L. (1982) Detection of ductal dysplasia in mammary outgrowths derived from carcinogen-treated virgin female BALB/c mice. *Cancer Res.*, **42**, 1753–1760

Fabrikant, J.I. (1981) Health effects of the nuclear accident at Three Mile Island. *Health Phys.*, **40**, 151–161

Fahrig, R. (1975) A mammalian spot test: Induction of genetic alterations in pigment cells of mouse embryos with x-rays and chemical mutagens. *Mol. Gen. Genet.*, **138**, 309–314

Faulkin, L.J., Mitchell, D.J., Cardiff, R.D., Rosenblatt, L.S. & Goldman, M. (1983) Effects of X irradiation on the growth of normal and hyperplastic mouse mammary gland transplants. *Radiat. Res.*, **94**, 390–403

Favus, M.J., Schneider, A.B., Stachura, M.E., Arnold, J.E., Ryo, U.Y., Pinsky, S.M., Colman, M., Arnold, M.J. & Frohman, L.A. (1976) Thyroid cancer occurring as a late consequence of head-and-neck irradiation. Evaluation of 1056 patients. *New Engl. J. Med.*, **294**, 1019–1025

Fegan, C., Robinson, H., Thompson, P., Whittaker, J.A. & White, D. (1995) Karyotypic evolution in CLL: Identification of a new sub-group of patients with deletions of 11q and advanced progressive disease. *Leukemia*, **9**, 2203–2208

Fehr, P.E. & Prem, M.D. (1973) Post irradiation sarcoma of the pelvic girdle following therapy for squamous cell carcinoma of the cervix. *Am. J. Obstet. Gynecol.*, **116**, 192–200

Feigin, R.D., Vietti, T.J., Wyatt, R.G., Kaufmann, D.G. & Smith, C.H., Jr (1970) Ataxia-telangiectasia with granulocytopenia. *J. Pediatr.*, **77**, 431–438

Fischer, A. (1992) Severe combined immunodeficiencies. *Immunodefic. Rev.*, **3**, 83–100

Fjälling, M., Tisell, L.-E., Carlsson, S., Hansson, G., Lundberg, L.-M. & Odén, A. (1986) Benign and malignant thyroid nodules after neck irradiation. *Cancer*, **58**, 1219–1224

Flodin, U., Fredriksson, M., Persson, B. & Axelson, O. (1990) Acute myeloid leukemia and background radiation in an expanded case–referent study. *Arch. environ. Health*, **45**, 364–366

Folley, J.H., Borges, W. & Yamasaki, T. (1952) Incidence of leukemia in survivors of the atom bomb in Hiroshima and Nagasaki, Japan. *Am. J. Med.*, **13**, 311–321

Forastiere, F., Valesini, S., Arca, M., Magliola, M.E., Michelozzi, P. & Tasco, C. (1985) Lung cancer and natural radiation in an Italian province. *Sci. total Environ.*, **45**, 519–526

Forastiere, F., Sperati, A., Cherubini, G., Miceli, M., Biggeri, A. & Axelson, O. (1998) Adult myeloid leukaemia, geology, and domestic exposure to radon and γ radiation: A case control study in central Italy. *Occup. environ. Med.*, **55**, 106-110

Foray, N., Priestley, A., Alsbeih, G., Badie, C., Capulas, E.P., Arlett, C.F. & Malaise, E.P. (1997) Hypersensitivity of ataxia-telangiectasia fibroblasts to ionizing radiation is associated with a repair deficiency of DNA double-strand breaks. *Int. J. Radiat. Biol.*, **72**, 271–283

Ford, M.D., Martin, L. & Lavin, M.F. (1984) The effects of ionizing radiation on cell cycle progression in ataxia telangiectasia. *Mutat. Res.*, **125**, 115–122

Forman, D., Cook-Mozaffari, P., Darby, S., Davey, G., Stratton, I., Doll, R. & Pike, M. (1987) Cancer near nuclear installations. *Nature,* **329,** 499–505

Fornace, A.J., Jr & Little, J.B. (1980) Normal repair of DNA single-strand breaks in patients with ataxia-telangiectasia. *Biochim. biophys. Acta*, **607**, 432–437.

Fraser, P., Carpenter, L., Maconochie, N., Higgins, C., Booth, M. & Beral, V. (1993) Cancer mortality and morbidity in employees of the United Kingdom Atomic Energy Authority. *Br. J. Cancer,* **67,** 615–624

Friedberg, E.C., Walker, G.C. & Siede, W. (1995) *DNA Repair and Mutagenesis*, Washington DC, American Society for Microbiology (ASM) Press

Friedberg, E.C., Meira, L.B. & Cheo, D.L. (1998) Database of mouse strains carrying targeted mutations in genes affecting cellular responses to DNA damage. Version 2. *Mutat. Res.*, **407**, 217–226

Friend, S.H. (1996) Breast cancer susceptibility testing: Realities in the post-genomic era. *Nature Genet.*, **13**, 16–17

Frome, E.L., Cragle, D.L., Watkins, J.P., Wing, S., Shy, C.M., Tankersley, W.G. & West, C.M. (1997) A mortality study of employees of the nuclear industry in Oak Ridge, Tennessee. *Radiat Res.*, **148**, 64–80 (erratum *Radiat. Res.*, 1997, **148**, 297–298)

Fry, R.J.M. (1992) The role of animal experiments in estimates of radiation risk. In: Nygaard, O.F., Sinclair, W.K. & Lett, J.T., eds, *Advances in Radiation Biology*, Vol. 16, *Effects of Low Dose Rate Radiation*, San Diego, Academic Press, pp. 181–197

Fry, R.J., Grosovsky, A., Hanawalt, P.C., Jostes, R.F., Little, J.B., Morgan, W.F., Oleinick, N.L. & Ullrich, R.L. (1998) The impact of biology on risk assessment—Workshop of the

National Research Council's Board on Radiation Effects Research. *Radiat. Res.*, **150**, 695–705

Fujii, K., Suzuki, N., Ishijima, S., Kita, K., Sonoda, T., Dezawa, M., Sugita, K. & Niimi, H. (1997) Abnormal DNA synthesis activity induced by X-rays in nevoid basal cell carcinoma syndrome cells. *Biochem. Biophys. Res. Commun.*, **240**, 269–272

Fürst, C.J., Lundell, M., Holm, L.-E. & Silfversward, C. (1988) Cancer incidence after radiotherapy for a skin hemangioma: A retrospective cohort study in Sweden. *J. natl Cancer Inst.*, **80**, 1387–1392

Fürst, C.J., Silfversward, C. & Holm, L.-E. (1989) Mortality in a cohort of radiation treated childhood skin hemangiomas. *Acta oncol.*, **28**, 789–794

Fürst, C.J., Lundell, M. & Holm, L.-E. (1990) Tumors after radiotherapy for skin hemangioma in childhood. A case–control study. *Acta oncol.*, **29**, 557–562

Fushiki, S., Matsushita, K. & Schull, W.J. (1993) Decelerated migration of neocortical neurones in explant culture after exposure to radiation. *NeuroReproduction*, **5**, 353–356

Futreal, A., Liu, Q., Shattuck-Eidens, D., Cochran, C., Harshman, K., Tavtigian, S., Bennett, L.M., Haugen-Strano, A., Swensen, J., Miki, Y., Eddington, K., McClure, M., Frye, C., Weaver-Feldhaus, J., Ding, W., Gholami, Z., Söderkvist, P., Terry, L., Jhanwar, S., Berchuck, A., Iglehart, J.D., Marks, J., Ballinger, D.G., Barrett, J.C., Skolnick, M.H., Kamb, A. & Wiseman, R. (1994) *BRCA1* mutations in primary breast and ovarian carcinomas. *Science*, **266**, 120–122

Gabra, H., Watson, J.E.V., Taylor, K.J., Mackay, J., Leonard, R.C.F., Steel, C.M., Porteous, D.J. & Smyth, J.F. (1996) Definition and refinement of a region of loss of heterozygosity at 11q23.3-q24.3 in epithelial ovarian cancer associated with poor prognosis. *Cancer Res.*, **56**, 950–954

Game, J.C. (1993) DNA double-strand breaks and the *RAD50-RAD57* genes in *Saccharomyces. Cancer Biol.*, **4**, 73–83

Gardner, M.J., Snee, M.P., Hall, A.J., Powell, C.A., Downes, S. & Terrell, J.D. (1990) Results of a case–control study of leukaemia and lymphoma among young people near Sellafield nuclear plant in west Cumbria. *Br. med. J.*, **300**, 423–429

Gatti, R.A. (1998) Ataxia-telangiectasia. In: Vogelstein, B. & Kinzler, K.W., eds, *The Genetic Basis of Human Cancer*, New York, McGraw-Hill, pp. 275–300

Gilbert, E.S., Omohundro, E., Buchanan, J.A. & Holter, N.A. (1993a) Mortality of workers at the Hanford site: 1945–1986. *Health Phys.*, **64**, 577–590

Gilbert, E.S., Cragle, D.L. & Wiggs, L.D. (1993b) Updated analyses of combined mortality data for workers at the Hanford Site, Oak Ridge National Laboratories, and Rocky Flats Nuclear Weapons Plant. *Radiat. Res.*, **136**, 408–421

Gilman, E.A. & Knox, E.G. (1998) Geographical distribution of birth places of children with cancer in the UK. *Br. J. Cancer*, **77**, 842–849

Glanzmann, C., Veraguth, A. & Lütolf, U.M. (1994) Incidence of second solid cancer in patients after treatment of Hodgkin's disease. *Strahlenther. Onkol.*, **170**, 140–146

Glatstein, E., McHardy-Young, S., Brast, N., Eltringham, J.R. & Kriss, J.P. (1971) Alterations in serum thyrotrophin (TSH) and thyroid function following radiotherapy in patients with malignant lymphoma. *J. clin. Endocrinol.*, **32**, 833–841

Goldstein, L. & Murphy, D.P. (1929) Etiology of the congenital nervous and immune deficiencies in newborns resulting from in utero exposure to radiation. Part 2. Defective children born after post-conception pelvic irradiation. *Am. J. Roentgenol.*, **22**, 322–331

Goodhead, D.T. (1988) Spatial and temporal distribution of energy. *Health Phys.*, **55**, 231–240

Goodhead, D.T. (1994) Initial events in the cellular effects of ionizing radiations: Clustered damage in DNA. *Int. J. Radiat. Biol.*, **65**, 7–17

Goodhead, D.T., Thacker, J. & Cox, R. (1993) Weiss Lecture. Effects of radiations of different qualities on cells: Molecular mechanisms of damage and repair. *Int. J. Radiat. Biol.*, **63**, 543–556

Gotoff, S.P., Amirmokri, E. & Liebner, E.J. (1967) Ataxia-telangiectasia. Neoplasia, untoward response to X-irradiation, and tuberous sclerosis. *Am. J. Dis. Child.*, **114**, 617–625

Gould, M.N. & Clifton, K.H. (1979) Evidence for a unique *in situ* component of the repair of radiation damage. *Radiat. Res.*, **77**, 149–155

Gould, M.N., Watanabe, H., Kamiya, K. & Clifton, K.H. (1987) Modification of expression of the malignant phenotype in radiation-initiated cells. *Int. J. Radiat. Biol. relat. Stud. Phys. chem. Med.*, **51**, 1081–1090

Gowen, L.C., Avrutskaya, A.V., Latour, A.M., Koller, B.H. & Leadon, S.A. (1998) BRCA1 required for transcription-coupled repair of oxidative DNA damage. *Science*, **281**, 1009–1012

Grahn, D., Frystak, B.H., Lee, C.H., Russell, J.J. & Lindenbaum, A. (1979) Dominant lethal mutations and chromosome aberrations induced in male mice by incorporated ^{239}Pu and by external fission neutron and gamma irradiation. In: *Biological Implications of Radionuclides Released by Nuclear Industries*, Vol. I, Vienna, International Atomic Energy Agency, pp. 163–184

Grahn, D., Carnes, B.A., Farrington, B.H. & Lee, C.H. (1984) Genetic injury in hybrid male mice exposed to low doses of ^{60}Co gamma-rays or fission neutrons. I. Response to single doses. *Mutat. Res.*, **129**, 215–229

Grahn, D., Lombard, L.S. & Carnes, B.A. (1992) The comparative tumorigenic effects of fission neutrons and cobalt-60 gamma rays in the B6CF$_1$ mouse. *Radiat. Res.*, **129**, 19–36

Graw, J., Favor, J., Neuhauser-Klaus, A. & Ehling, U.H. (1986) Dominant cataract and recessive specific locus mutation in offspring of X-irradiated male mice. *Mutat. Res.*, **159**, 47–54

Green, B.M.R., Hughes, J.S., Lomas, P.R. & Janssens, A. (1992) Natural radiation atlas of Europe. *Radiat. Protect. Dosim.*, **45**, 491–493

Greenland, S. & Robins, J.M. (1988) Conceptual problems in the definition and interpretation of attributable fractions. *Am. J. Epidemiol.*, **128**, 1185–1197

Gribbin, M.A., Weeks, J.L. & Howe, G.R. (1993) Cancer mortality (1956–1985) among male employees of Atomic Energy of Canada Limited with respect to occupational exposure to external low-linear-energy-transfer ionizing radiation. *Radiat. Res.*, **133**, 375–380

Griem, M.L., Kleinerman, R.A., Boice, J.D., Jr, Stovall, M., Shefner, D. & Lubin, J.H. (1994) Cancer following radiotherapy for peptic ulcer. *J. natl Cancer Inst.*, **86**, 842–849

Griffin, C.S., Hill, M.A., Papworth, D.G., Townsend, K.M., Savage, J.R. & Goodhead, D.T. (1998) Effectiveness of 0.28 keV carbon K ultrasoft X-rays at producing simple and complex chromosome exchanges in human fibroblasts in vitro detected using FISH. *Int. J. Radiat. Biol.*, **73**, 591–598

Grosovsky, A.J., Drobetsky, E.A., deJong, P.J. & Glickman, B.W. (1986) Southern analysis of genomic alterations in gamma-ray-induced aprt⁻ hamster cell mutants. *Genetics*, **113**, 405–415

Gusev, B.I., Abylkassimova, Z.N. & Apsalikov, K.N. (1997) The Semipalatinsk nuclear test site: A first assessment of the radiological situation and the test-related radiation doses in the surrounding territories. *Radiat. Environ. Biophys.*, **36**, 201–204

Gustafson, C.E., Young, J., Leggett, B., Searle, J. & Chenevix-Trench, G. (1994) Loss of heterozygosity on the long arm of chromosome 11 in colorectal tumours. *Br. J. Cancer*, **70**, 395–397

Gutin, P., Leibel, S. & Sheline G., eds (1991) *Radiation Injury to the Nervous System*, New York, Raven Press

Hainaut, P., Hernandez, T., Robinson, A., Rodriguez-Tome, P., Flores, T., Hollstein, M., Harris, C.C. & Montesano, R. (1998) IARC database of p53 gene mutations in human tumors and cell lines: Updated compilation, revised formats and new visualisation tools. *Nucl. Acids Res.*, **26**, 205–213

Hakoda, M., Kamatani, N., Ohtsuka, S. & Kashiwazaki, S. (1991a) Germline and somatic mutations leading to adenine phosphoribosyltransferase (APRT) deficiency. *Adv. Exp. Med. Biol.*, **309B**, 87–90

Hakoda, M., Yamanaka, H., Kamatani, N. & Kamatani, N. (1991b) Diagnosis of heterozygous states for adenine phosphoribosyltransferase deficiency based on detection of in vivo somatic mutants in blood T cells: Application to screening of heterozygotes. *Am. J. Hum. Genet.*, **48**, 552–562

Hall, E.J. & Hei, T.K. (1985) Oncogenic transformation with radiation and chemicals. *Int. J. Radiat. Biol. Relat. Stud. Phys. chem. Med.*, **48**, 1–18

Hall, E.J. & Hei, T.K. (1990) Modulating factors in the expression of radiation-induced oncogenic transformation. *Environ. Health Perspect.*, **88**, 149–155

Hall, P., Mattsson, A. & Boice, J., Jr (1996) Thyroid cancer after diagnostic administration of iodine-131. *Radiat. Res.*, **145**, 86–92

Hallquist, A., Hardell, L., Degerman, A., Wingren, G. & Boquist, L. (1994) Medical diagnostic and therapeutic ionizing radiation and the risk for thyroid cancer: A case–control study. *Eur. J. Cancer Prev.*, **3**, 259–267

Hamlet, R. & Hopewell, J.W. (1988) A quantitative assessment of changes in the dermal fibroblast population of pig skin after single doses of X-rays. *Int. J. Radiat. Biol.*, **54**, 675–682

Hampton, G.M., Penny, L.A., Baergen, R.N., Larson, A., Brewer, C., Liao, S., Busby-Earle, R.M.C., Williams, A.W.R., Steel, C.M., Bird, C.C., Stanbridge, E.J. & Evans, G.A. (1994) Loss of heterozygosity in cervical carcinoma: Subchromosomal localization of a putative tumor-suppressor gene to chromosome 11q22–q24. *Proc. natl Acad. Sci. USA*, **91**, 6953–6957

Hancock, S.L., Cox, R.S. & McDougall, I.R. (1991) Thyroid diseases after treatment of Hodgkin's disease. *New Engl. J. Med.*, **325**, 599–605

Hancock, S.L., Tucker, M.A. & Hoppe, R.T. (1993) Breast cancer after treatment of Hodgkin's disease. *J. natl Cancer Inst.*, **85**, 25–31

Hanford, J.M., Quimby, E.H. & Frantz, V.K. (1962) Cancer arising many years after radiation therapy. Incidence after irradiation of benign lesions in the neck. *J. Am. med. Assoc.*, **181**, 404–410

Harper, K., Lorimore, S.A. & Wright, E.G. (1997) Delayed appearance of radiation-induced mutations at the Hprt locus in murine hemopoietic cells. *Exp. Hematol.*, **25**, 263–269

Hartley, K.O., Gell, D., Smith, G.C.M., Zhang, H., Divecha, N., Connelly, M.A., Admon, A., Lees-Miller, S.P., Anderson, C.W. & Jackson, S.P. (1995) DNA-dependent protein kinase catalytic subunit: A relative of phosphatidylinositol 3-kinase and the ataxia telangiectasia gene product. *Cell*, **82**, 849–856

Harvey, E.B. & Brinton, L.A. (1985) Second cancer following cancer of the breast in Connecticut, 1935–82. *Natl Cancer Inst. Monogr.*, **68**, 99–112

Harvey, E.B., Boice, J.D., Jr, Honeyman, M. & Flannery, J.T. (1985) Prenatal X-ray exposure and childhood cancer in twins. *New Engl. J. Med.*, **312**, 541–545

Hatch, M.C., Beyea, J., Nieves, J.W. & Susser, M. (1990) Cancer near the Three Mile Island nuclear plant: Radiation emissions. *Am. J. Epidemiol.*, **132**, 397–412

Hattchouel, J.-M., Laplanche, A. & Hill, C. (1995) Leukaemia mortality around French nuclear sites. *Br. J. Cancer*, **71**, 651–653

Hawkins, M.M., Draper, G.J. & Kingston, J.E. (1987) Incidence of second primary tumours among childhood cancer survivors. *Br. J. Cancer*, **56**, 339–347

Hawkins, M.M., Kinnier Wilson, L.M., Stovall, M.A., Marsden, H.B., Potok, M.H., Kingston, J.E. & Chessells, J.M. (1992) Epipodophyllotoxins, alkylating agents, and radiation and risk of secondary leukaemia after childhood cancer. *Br. med. J.*, **304**, 951–958

Hawkins, M.M., Kinnier Wilson, L.M., Burton, H.S., Potok, M.H.N., Winter, D.L., Marsden, H.B. & Stovall, M.A. (1996) Radiotherapy, alkylating agents, and risk of bone cancer after childhood cancer. *J. natl Cancer Inst.*, **88**, 270–278

Hecht, F. & Hecht, B.K. (1985) Ataxia-telangiectasia breakpoints in chromosome rearrangements reflect genes important to T and B lymphocytes. In: Gatti, R.A. & Swift, M., eds, *Ataxia Telangiectasia: Genetics, Neuropathology, and Immunology of a Degenerative Disease of Childhood*, New York, Alan R. Liss, pp. 189–195

Hecht, F. & Hecht, B.K. (1990) Cancer in ataxia-telangiectasia patients. *Cancer Genet. Cytogenet.*, **46**, 9–19

Hei, T.K., Piao, C.Q., Willey, J.C., Thomas, S. & Hall, E.J. (1994) Malignant transformation of human bronchial epithelial cells by radon-simulated alpha-particles. *Carcinogenesis*, **15**, 431–437

Hempelmann, L., Pifer, J.W., Burke, G.J., Terry, R. & Ames, W.R. (1967) Neoplasms in persons treated with X-rays in infancy for thymic enlargement. A report on the third follow-up survey. *J. natl Cancer Inst.*, **38**, 317–341

Hendry, J.H. & Thames, H.D. (1986) The tissue-rescuing unit. *Br. J. Radiol.*, **59**, 628–630

Henry-Amar, M. (1983) Second cancers after radiotherapy and chemotherapy for early stages of Hodgkin's disease. *J. natl Cancer Inst.*, **71**, 911–916

Henshaw, P.S. & Hawkins, J.W. (1944) Incidence of leukemia in physicians. *J. natl Cancer Inst.*, **4**, 339–346

Herbst, R.A., Larson, A., Weiss, J., Cavenee, W.K., Hampton, G.M. & Arden, K.C. (1995) A defined region of loss of heterozygosity at 11q23 in cutaneous malignant melanoma. *Cancer Res.*, **55**, 2494–2496

Herzog, K.-H., Chong, M.J., Kapsetaki, M., Morgan, J.I. & McKinnon, P.J. (1998) Requirement for Atm in ionizing radiation-induced cell death in the developing central nervous system. *Science*, **280**, 1089–1091

Heyn, R., Haeberlen, V., Newton, W.A., Ragab, A.H., Raney, R.B., Tefft, M., Wharam, M., Ensign, L.G. & Maurer, H.M. (1993) Second malignant neoplasms in children treated for rhabdomyosarcoma (Intergroup Rhabdomyosarcoma Study Committee). *J. Clin. Oncol.*, **11**, 262–270

Higurashi, M. & Cohen, P.E. (1973) *In vitro* chromosomal radiosenstivity in 'chromosomal breakage syndromes'. *Cancer*, **32**, 380–383

Hildreth, N.G., Shore, R.E., Hempelmann, L.H. & Rosenstein, M. (1985) Risk of extrathyroid tumors following radiation treatment in infancy for thymic enlargement. *Radiat. Res.*, **102**, 378–391

Hildreth, N.G., Shore, R.E. & Dvoretsky, P.M. (1989) The risk of breast cancer after irradiation of the thymus in infancy. *New Engl. J. Med.*, **321**, 1281–1284

Hill, C. & Laplanche, A. (1990) Overall mortality and cancer mortality around French nuclear sites. *Nature*, **347**, 755–757

Hino, O., Klein-Szanto, A.J., Freed, J.J., Testa, J.R., Brown, D.Q., Vilensky, M., Yeung, R.S., Tartof, K.D. & Knudson, A.G. (1993) Spontaneous and radiation-induced renal tumors in the Eker rat model of dominantly inherited cancer. *Proc. natl Acad. Sci. USA*, **90**, 327–331

Hjalmars, U., Kulldorff, M. & Gustafsson, G. on behalf of the Swedish Child Leukaemia Group (1994) Risk of acute childhood leukaemia in Sweden after the Chernobyl reactor accident. *Br. med. J.*, **309**, 154–157

Hoel, D.G. & Li, P. (1998) Threshold models in radiation carcinogenesis. *Health Phys.*, **75**, 241–250

Hoffman, D.A., Lonstein, J.E., Morin, M.M., Visscher, W., Harris, S.H., III & Boice, J.D., Jr (1989) Breast cancer in women with scoliosis exposed to multiple diagnostic X rays. *J. natl Cancer Inst.*, **81**, 1307–1312

Holliday, R. (1989) Chromosome error propagation and cancer. *Trends Genet.*, **5**, 42–45

Holm, L.-E., Hall, P., Wiklund, K., Lundell, G., Berg, G., Bjelkengren, G., Cederquist, E., Ericsson, U.-B., Hallquist, A., Larsson, L.-G., Lidberg, M., Lindberg, S., Tennvall, J., Wicklund, H. & Boice, J.D., Jr (1991) Cancer risk after iodine-131 therapy for hyperthyroidism. *J. natl Cancer Inst.*, **83**, 1072–1077

Hopewell, J.W., Coggle, J.E., Wells, J., Hamlet, R., Williams, J.P. & Charles, M.W. (1986) The acute effects of different energy beta-emitters on pig and mouse skin. *Br. J. Radiol.*, **Suppl. 19**, 47–51

Horwich, A. & Bell, J. (1994) Mortality and cancer incidence following radiotherapy for seminoma of the testis. *Radiother. Oncol.*, **30**, 193–198

Houldsworth, J. & Lavin, M.F. (1980) Effect of ionizing radiation on DNA synthesis in ataxia telangiectasia cells. *Nucleic Acids Res.*, **8**, 3709–3720

van der Houven van Oordt, C.W., Schouten, T.G., van Krieken, J.H., van Dierendonck, J.H., van der Eb, A.J. & Breuer, M.L. (1998) X-ray-induced lymphomagenesis in Eμ-*pim*-1 transgenic mice: An investigation of the co-operating molecular events. *Carcinogenesis*, **19**, 847–853

Howe, G.R. (1995) Lung cancer mortality between 1950 and 1987 after exposure to fractionated moderate-dose-rate ionizing radiation in the Canadian fluoroscopy cohort study and a comparison with lung cancer mortality in the atomic bomb survivors study. *Radiat. Res.*, **142**, 295–304

Howe, G.R. & McLaughlin, J. (1996) Breast cancer mortality between 1950 and 1987 after exposure to fractionated moderate-dose-rate ionizing radiation in the Canadian fluoroscopy cohort study and a comparison with breast cancer mortality in the atomic bomb survivors study. *Radiat. Res.*, **145**, 694–707

Hoyes, K.P., Wadeson, P.J., Sharma, H.L., Hendry, J.H. & Morris, I.D. (1998) Mutation studies in lacI transgenic mice after exposure to radiation or cyclophosphamide. *Mutagenesis*, **13**, 607–612

Hrubec, Z., Boice, J.D., Jr, Monson, R.R. & Rosenstein, M. (1989) Breast cancer after multiple chest fluoroscopies: Second follow-up of Massachusetts women with tuberculosis. *Cancer Res.*, **49**, 229–234

Huda, W. & Sourkes, A.M. (1989) Radiation doses from chest X-rays in Manitoba (1979 and 1987). *Radiat. Prot. Dosim.*, **28**, 303–308

Hulse, E.V. (1980) Tumor incidence and longevity in neutron and gamma irradiated rabbits, with an assessment of RBE. *Int. J. Radiat. Biol.*, **37**, 633–652

Huo, Y.K., Wang, Z., Hong, J.-H., Chessa, L., McBride, W.H., Perlman, S.L. & Gatti, R.A. (1994) Radiosensitivity of ataxia-telangiectasia, X-linked agammaglobulinemia, and related syndromes using a modified colony survival assay. *Cancer Res.*, **54**, 2544–2547

Husain, A., He, G., Venkatraman, E.S. & Spriggs, D.R. (1998) *BRCA1* up-regulation is associated with repair-mediated resistance to *cis*-diamminedichloroplatinum(II). *Cancer Res.*, **58**, 1120–1123

Hutchinson, F. (1995) Analysis of deletions induced in the genome of mammalian cells by ionizing radiation. *J. Mol. Biol.*, **254**, 372–380

IAEA (International Atomic Energy Agency) (1988) *The Radiological Accident in Goiânia*, Vienna

IAEA (International Atomic Energy Agency) (1997) *Low Doses of Ionizing Radiation: Biological Effects and Regulatory Control* (IAEA-TECDOC-976), Vienna

IAEA (International Atomic Energy Agency) (1998) *Planning the Medical Response to Radiological Accidents* (Safety Report Series No. 4), Vienna

IARC (1987) *IARC Monographs on the Evaluation of Carcinogenic Risks to Humans*, Suppl. 7, *Overall Evaluations of Carcinogenicity: An Update of IARC Monographs Volumes 1 to 42*, Lyon, IARC Press

IARC (1992) *IARC Monographs on the Evaluation of Carcinogenic Risk to Humans*, Vol. 55, *Solar and Ultraviolet Radiation*, Lyon, IARC Press

IARC Study Group on Cancer Risk among Nuclear Industry Workers (1994) Direct estimates of cancer mortality due to low doses of ionising radiation: An international study. *Lancet*, **344**, 1039–1043

Ichihara, Y., Matsuoka, H., Tsuge, I., Okada, J., Torii, S., Yasui, H. & Kurosawa, Y. (1988) Abnormalities in DNA rearrangements of immunoglobulin gene loci in precursor B cells derived from a X-linked agammaglobulinemia patient and a severe combined immunodeficiency patient. *Immunogenetics*, **27**, 330–337

Ichimaru, M., Ishimaru, T. & Belsky, J.L. (1978) Incidence of leukemia in atomic bomb survivors belonging to a fixed cohort in Hiroshima and Nagasaki, 1950–71. Radiation dose, years after exposure, age at exposure, and type of leukemia. *J. Radiat. Res.*, **19**, 262–282

ICRP (International Commission on Radiological Protection) (1991a) *1990 Recommendations of the International Commission on Radiological Protection* (ICRP Publication 60; *Annals of the ICRP*, Vol. 21), Oxford, Pergamon Press

ICRP (International Commission on Radiological Protection) (1991b) *Addendum 1 to ICRP Publication 53. Radiation Dose to Patients from Radiopharmaceuticals*, Oxford, Pergamon Press

ICRP (International Commission on Radiological Protection) (1991c) *The Biological Basis for the Dose Limitation in the Skin* (ICRP Publication 59; *Annals of the ICRP*, Vol. 22, No. 2), Oxford, Pergamon Press

ICRP (International Commission on Radiological Protection) (1999) *Genetic Susceptibility to Cancer* (ICRP Publication 79), Amsterdam, Elsevier Science

Inskip, P.D., Monson, R.R., Wagoner, J.K., Stovall, M., Davis, F.G., Kleinerman, R.A. & Boice, J.D., Jr (1990a) Cancer mortality following radium treatment for uterine bleeding. *Radiat. Res.*, **123**, 331–344

Inskip, P.D., Monson, R.R., Wagoner, J.K., Stovall, M., Davis, F.G., Kleinerman, R.A. & Boice, J.D., Jr (1990b) Leukemia following radiotherapy for uterine bleeding. *Radiat. Res.*, **122**, 107–119

Inskip, P.D., Harvey, E.B., Boice, J.D., Jr, Stone, B.J., Matanoski, G., Flanneru, J.T. & Fraumeni, J.F., Jr (1991) Incidence of childhood cancer in twins. *Cancer Causes Control*, **2**, 315–324

Inskip, P.D., Kleinerman, R.A., Stovall, M., Cookfair, D.L., Hadjimichael, O., Moloney, W.C., Monson, R.R., Thompson, W.D., Wactawski-Wende, J., Wagoner, J.K. & Boice, J.D., Jr (1993) Leukemia, lymphoma, and multiple myeloma after pelvic radiotherapy for benign disease. *Radiat. Res.*, **135**, 108–124.

Inskip, P.D., Stovall, M. & Flannery, J.T. (1994) Lung cancer risk and radiation dose among women treated for breast cancer. *J. natl Cancer Inst.*, **86**, 983–988

Inskip, P.D., Ekbom, A., Galanti, M.R., Grimelius, L. & Boice, J.D., Jr (1995) Medical diagnostic X rays and thyroid cancer. *J. natl Cancer Inst.*, **87**, 1613–1621

Ivanov, V.K., Tsyb, A.F., Konogorov, A.P., Rastopchin, E.M. & Khait, S.E. (1997a) Case–control analysis of leukaemia among Chernobyl accident emergency workers residing in the Russian Federation, 1986–1993. *J. Radiat. Prot.*, **17**, 137–157

Ivanov, V.K., Tsyb, A.F., Gorsky, A.I., Maksyutov, M.A., Rastopchin, E.M., Konogorov, A.P., Korelo, A.M., Biryukov, A.P. & Matyash, V.A. (1997b) Leukaemia and thyroid cancer in emergency workers of the Chernobyl accident: Estimation of radiation risks (1986–1995). *Radiat. environ. Biophys.*, **36**, 9–16

Ivanov, V.K., Tsyb, A.F., Nilova, E.V., Efendiev, V.F., Gorsky, A.I., Pitkevich, V.A., Leshakov, S.Y. & Shiryaev, V.I. (1997c) Cancer risks in the Kaluga oblast of the Russian Federation 10 years after the Chernobyl accident. *Radiat. environ. Biophys.*, **36**, 161–167

Ivanov, V.K., Rastopchin, E.M., Gorsky, A.I. & Ryvkin, V.B. (1998) Cancer incidence among liquidators of the Chernobyl accident: Solid tumors, 1986–1995. *Health Phys.*, **74**, 309–315

Jablon, S. & Kato, H. (1970) Childhood cancer in relation to prenatal exposure in atomic-bomb radiation. *Lancet*, **ii**, 1000–1003

Jablon, S., Hrubec, Z. & Boice, J.D., Jr (1991) Cancer in populations living near nuclear facilities. A survey of mortality nationwide and incidence in two states. *J. Am. med. Assoc.*, **265**, 1403–1408

Jacobsen, G.K., Mellemgaard, A., Engelholm, S.A. & Møller, H. (1993) Increased incidence of sarcoma in patients treated for testicular seminoma. *Eur. J. Cancer*, **29A**, 664–668

Janatipour, M., Trainor, K.J., Kutlaca, R., Bennett, G., Hay, J., Turner, D.R. & Morley, A.A. (1988) Mutations in human lymphocytes studied by an HLA selection system. *Mutat. Res.*, **198**, 221–226

Janower, M.L. & Miettinen, O.S. (1971) Neoplasms after childhood irradiation of the thymus gland. *J. Am. med. Assoc.*, **215**, 753–756

Jaspers, N.G.J., Gatti. R.A., Baan, C., Linssen, P.C.M.L. & Bootsma, D. (1988) Genetic complementation analysis of ataxia telangiectasia and Nijmegen breakage syndrome: A survey of 50 patients. *Cytogenet. Cell Genet.*, **49**, 259–263

Jeggo, P.A., Carr, A.M. & Lehmann, A.R. (1998) Splitting the ATM: Distinct repair and checkpoint defects in ataxia-telangiectasia. *Trends Genet.*, **14**, 312–316

Jenner, T.J., de Lara, C.M., O'Neill, P. & Stevens, D.L. (1993) The induction and rejoining of DNA double strand breaks in V79-4 mammalian cells by γ- and α-irradiation. *Int. J. Radiat. Biol.*, **64**, 265–273

Jensen, R.D. & Miller, R.W. (1971) Retinoblastoma: Epidemiologic characteristics. *New Engl. J. Med.*, **285**, 307–311

Jensen, R.H., Langlois, R.G., Bigbee, W.L., Grant, S.G., Moore, D., 2nd, Pilinskaya, M., Vorobtsova, I. & Pleshanov, P. (1995) Elevated frequency of glycophorin A mutations in erythrocytes from Chernobyl accident victims. *Radiat. Res.*, **141**, 129–135

Johansson, L., Larsson, L.-G. & Damber, L. (1995) A cohort study with regard to the risk of haematological malignancies in patients treated with X-rays for benign lesions in the locomotor system. II. Estimation of absorbed dose in the red bone marrow. *Acta oncol.*, **34**, 721–726

Johnson, D.K., Stubbs, L.J., Culiat, C.T., Montgomery, C.S., Russell, L.B. & Rinchik, E.M. (1995) Molecular analysis of 36 mutations at the mouse pink-eyed dilution (p) locus. *Genetics*, **141**, 1563–1571

Johnson, J.C., Thaul, S., Page, W.F. & Crawford, H. (1997) Mortality of veteran participants in the CROSSROADS nuclear test. *Health Phys.*, **73**, 187–189

Jongmans, W., Vuillaume, M., Chrzanowska, K., Smeets, D., Sperling, K. & Hall, J. (1997) Nijmegen breakage syndrome cells fail to induce the p53-mediated DNA damage response following exposure to ionizing radiation. *Mol. cell. Biol.*, **17**, 5016–5022

Joslyn, G., Carlson, M., Thliveris, A., Albertsen, H., Gelbert, L., Samowitz, W., Groden, J., Stevens, J., Spirio, L., Robertson, M., Sargeant, L., Krapcho, K., Wolff, E., Burt, R., Hughes, J.P., Warrington, J., McPherson, J., Wasmuth, J., Le Paslier, D., Abderrahim, H., Cohen, D., Leppert, M. & White, R. (1991) Identification of deletion mutations and three new genes at the familial polyposis locus. *Cell*, **66**, 601–613

Jung, M., Kondratyev, A., Lee, S., Dimtchev, A. & Dritschilo, A. (1997) *ATM* gene product phosphorylates IκB-α. *Cancer Res.*, **57**, 24–27

Kadhim, M.A., Macdonald, D.A., Goodhead, D.T., Lorimore, S.A., Marsden, S.J. & Wright, E.G. (1992) Transmission of chromosomal instability after plutonium alpha-particle irradiation. *Nature*, **355**, 738–740

Kadhim, M.A., Lorimore, S.A., Hepburn, M.D., Goodhead, D.T., Buckle, V.J. & Wright, E.G. (1994) Alpha-particle-induced chromosomal instability in human bone marrow cells. *Lancet*, **344**, 987–988

Kadhim, M.A., Lorimore, S.A., Townsend, K.M., Goodhead, D.T., Buckle, V.J. & Wright, E.G. (1995) Radiation-induced genomic instability: Delayed cytogenetic aberrations and apoptosis in primary human bone marrow cells. *Int. J. Radiat. Biol.*, **67**, 287–293

Kakunaga, T. & Yamasaki, H., eds (1985) *Transformation Assay of Established Cell Lines: Mechanisms and Application* (IARC Scientific Publications No. 67), Lyon, IARC Press

Kaldor, J.M., Day, N.E., Band, P., Choi, N.W., Clarke, E.A., Coleman, M.P., Hakama, M., Koch, M., Langmark, F., Neal, F.E., Pettersson, F., Pompe-Kirn, V., Prior, P. & Storm, H.H. (1987) Second malignancies following testicular cancer, ovarian cancer and Hodgkin's disease: An international collaborative study among cancer registries. *Int. J. Cancer*, **39**, 571–585

Kaldor, J.M., Day, N.E., Clarke, E.A., Van Leeuwen, F.E., Henry-Amar, M., Fiorentino, M.V., Bell, J., Pedersen, D., Band, P., Assouline, D., Koch, M., Choi, W., Prior, P., Blair, V., Langmark, F., Pompe-Kirn, V., Neal, F., Peters, D., Pfeiffer, R., Karjalainen, S., Cuzick, J., Sutcliffe, S.B., Somers, R., Pellae-Cosset, B., Pappagallo, G.L., Fraser, P., Storm, H. & Stovall, M. (1990a) Leukemia following Hodgkin's disease. *New Engl. J. Med.*, **322**, 7–13

Kaldor, J.M., Day, N.E., Pettersson, F., Clarke, E.A., Pedersen, D., Mehnert, W., Bell, J., Høst, H., Prior, P., Karjalainen, S., Neal, F., Koch, M., Band, R., Choi, W., Pompe-Kirn, V., Arslan, A., Zanén, B., Belch, A.R., Storm, H., Kittelmann, B., Fraser, P. & Stovall, M. (1990b) Leukemia following chemotherapy for ovarian cancer. *New Engl. J. Med.*, **322**, 1–6

Kaldor, J.M., Day, N.E., Bell, J., Clarke, E.A., Langmark, F., Karjalainen, S., Band, P., Pedersen, D., Choi, W., Blair, V., Henry-Amar, M., Prior, P., Assouline, D., Pompe-Kirn, V., Cartwright, R.A., Koch, M., Arslan, A., Fraser, P., Sutcliffe, S.B., Høst, H., Hakama, M. & Stovall, M. (1992) Lung cancer following Hodgkin's disease: A case–control study. *Int. J. Cancer*, **52**, 677–681

Kaldor, J.M., Day, N.E., Kittelmann, B., Pettersson, F., Langmark, F., Pedersen, D., Prior, P., Neal, F., Karjalainen, S., Bell, J., Choi, W., Koch, M., Band, P., Pompe-Kirn, V., Garton, C., Staneczek, W., Zarén, B., Stovall, M. & Boffetta, P. (1995) Bladder tumours following chemotherapy and radiotherapy for ovarian cancer: A case–control study. *Int. J. Cancer*, **63**, 1-6

Kaplan, M.M., Garnick, M.B., Gelber, R., Li, F.P., Cassady, J.R., Sallan, S.E., Fine, W.E. & Sack, M.J. (1983) Risk factors for thyroid abnormalities after neck irradiation for childhood cancer. *Am. J. Med.*, **74**, 272–280

Karlsson, P., Holmberg, E., Johansson, K.-A., Kindblom, L.-G., Carstensen, J. & Wallgren, A. (1996) Soft tissue sarcoma after treatment for breast cancer. *Radiother. Oncol.*, **38**, 25–31

Karlsson, P., Holmberg, E., Lundberg, L.M., Nordborg, C. & Wallgren, A. (1997) Intracranial tumors after radium treatment for skin hemangioma during infancy—A cohort and case–control study. *Radiat. Res.*, **148**, 161–167

Karlsson, P., Holmberg, E., Lundell, M., Mattsson, A., Holm, L.-E. & Wallgren, A. (1998) Intracranial tumors after exposure to ionizing radiation during infancy. A pooled analysis of two Swedish cohorts of 28,008 infants with skin hemangioma. *Radiat. Res.*, **150**, 357–364

Kastan, M.B., Zhan, O., El-Deiry, W.S., Carrier, F., Jacks, T., Walsh, W.V., Plunkett, B.S., Vogelstein, B. & Fornace, A.J. (1992) A mammalian cell cycle checkpoint pathway utilizing *p53* and *GADD45* is defective in ataxia-telangiectasia. *Cell*, **71**, 587–597

Kaul, A., Bauer, B., Bernhardt, J., Nosske, D. & Veit, R. (1997) Effective doses to members of the public from diagnostic application of ionizing radiation in Germany. *Eur. Radiol.*, **7**, 1127–1132

Keegan, K.S., Holtzman, D.A., Plug, A.W., Christenson, E.R., Brainerd, E.E., Flaggs, G., Bentley, N.J., Taylor, E.M., Meyn, M.S., Moss, S.B., Carr, A.M., Ashley, T. & Hoekstra, M.F. (1996) The Atr and Atm protein kinases associate with different sites along meiotically pairing chromosomes. *Genes Dev.*, **10**, 2423–2437

Kellerer, A.M. & Nekolla, E. (1997) Neutron versus gamma-ray risk estimates. Inferences from the cancer incidence and mortality data in Hiroshima. *Radiat. Environ. Biophys.*, **36**,73–83

Kemp, C.J., Wheldon, T. & Balmain, A. (1994) *p53*-Deficient mice are extremely susceptible to radiation-induced tumorigenesis. *Nature Genet.*, **8**, 66–69

Kennedy, A.R., Fox, M., Murphy, G.R. & Little, J.B. (1980) Relationship between X-ray exposure and malignant transformation in C3H 10T1/2 cells. *Proc. natl Acad. Sci. USA*, **77**, 7262–7266

Kerangueven, F., Eisinger, F., Noguchi, T., Allione, F., Wargniez, V., Eng, C., Padberg, G., Theillet, C., Jacquemier, J., Longy, M., Sobol, H. & Birnbaum, D. (1997) Loss of heterozygosity in human breast carcinomas in the ataxia telangiectasia, Cowden disease and *BRCA1* gene regions. *Oncogene*, **14**, 339–347

Khanna, K.K., Beamish, H., Yan, J., Hobson, K., Williams, R., Dunn, I. & Lavin, M.F. (1995) Nature of G1/S cell cycle checkpoint defect in ataxia-telangiectasia. *Oncogene*, **11**, 609–618

Khanna, K.K., Keating, K.E., Kozlov, S., Scott, S., Gatei, M., Hobson, K., Taya, Y., Gabrielli, B., Chan, D., Lees-Miller, S.P. & Lavin, M.F. (1998) ATM associates with and phosphorylates p53: Mapping the region of interaction. *Nature Genet.*, **20**, 398–400

Khoo, V.S., Liew, K.H., Crennan, E.C., D'Costa, I.M. & Quong, G. (1998) Thyroid dysfunction after mantle irradiation of Hodgkin's disease patients. *Australas. Radiol.*, **42**, 52–57

Kim, M.-G., Schuler, W., Bosma, M.J. & Marcu, K.B. (1988) Abnormal recombination of *Igh* D and J gene segments in transformed pre-B cells of *scid* mice. *J. Immunol.*, **141**, 1341–1347

Kingston, J.E., Hawkins, M.M., Draper, G.J., Marsden, H.B. & Kinnier Wilson, L.M. (1987) Patterns of multiple primary tumours in patients treated for cancer during childhood. *Br. J. Cancer*, **56**, 331–338

Kinlen, L.J. (1993a) Childhood leukaemia and non-Hodgkin's lymphoma in young people living close to nuclear reprocessing sites. *Biomed. Pharmacother.*, **47**, 429–434

Kinlen, L.J. (1993b) Can paternal preconceptional radiation account for the increase of leukaemia and non-Hodgkin's lymphoma in Seascale? *Br. med. J.*, **306**, 1718–1721

Kinlen, L.J., Hudson, C.M. & Stiller, C.A. (1991) Contacts between adults as evidence for an infective origin of childhood leukaemia: An explanation for the excess near nuclear establishments in West Berkshire. *Br. J. Cancer*, **64**, 549–554

Kinlen, L.J., Clarke, K. & Balkwill, A. (1993) Paternal preconceptional radiation exposure in the nuclear industry and leukaemia and non-Hodgkin's lymphoma in young people in Scotland. *Br. med. J.*, **306**, 1153–1158

Kinsella, T. (1989) Effects of radiotherapy and chemotherapy on testicular function. In: Burger, E.J., Jr, Scialli, A.E., Tardiff, R.G. & Zenick, H., eds, *Sperm Measures and Reproductive Success*, *Prog. clin. biol. Res.*, **302**, New York, Alan Liss, pp. 157–171

Kirk, K.M. & Lyon, M.F. (1982) Induction of congenital anomalies in offspring of female mice exposed to varying doses of X-rays. *Mutat. Res.*, **106**, 73–83

Kirk, K.M. & Lyon, M.F. (1984) Induction of congenital malformations in the offspring of male mice treated with X-rays at pre-meiotic and post-meiotic stages. *Mutat. Res.*, **125**, 75–85

Knox, E.G., Stewart, A.M., Kneale, G.W. & Gilman, E.A. (1987) Prenatal irradiation and childhood cancer. *J. Soc. Radiol. Prot.*, **7**, 177–189

Knudson, A.G., Jr (1984) Genetic predisposition to cancer. *Cancer Detect. Prev.*, **7**, 1–8

Ko, L.J. & Prives, C. (1996) p53: Puzzle and paradigm. *Genes Dev.*, **10**, 1054–1072

Kohn, H.I. & Kallman, R.F. (1954) Testes weight loss as a quantitative measure of X-ray injury in the mouse, hamster and rat. *Br. J. Radiol.*, **27**, 586–591

Kohn, H.I. & Melvold, R.W. (1976) Divergent X-ray-induced mutation rates in the mouse for H and '7-locus' groups of loci. *Nature*, **259**, 209–210

Koike, M., Takeuchi, S., Park, S., Hatta, Y., Yokota, J., Tsuruoka, N. & Koeffler, H.P. (1999) Ovarian cancer: Loss of heterozygosity frequently occurs in the ATM gene, but structural alterations do not occur in this gene. *Oncology*, **56**, 160–163

Komatsu, K., Matsumura, S., Tauchi, H., Endo, S., Kodama, S., Smeets, D., Weemaes, C. & Oshimura, M. (1996) The gene for Nijmegen breakage syndrome (V2) is not located on chromosome 11. *Am. J. hum. Genet.*, **58**, 885–888

Kony, S.J., de Vathaire, F., Chompret, A., Shamsaldim, A., Grimaud, E., Raquin, M.-A., Oberlin, O., Brugières, L., Feunteun, J., Eschwège, F., Chavaudra, J., Lemerle, J. & Bonaïti-Pellié, C. (1997) Radiation and genetic factors in the risk of second malignant neoplasms after a first cancer in childhood. *Lancet*, **350**, 91–95

Koshurnikova, N.A., Bysogolov, G.D., Bolotnikova, M.G., Khohryakov, V.F., Kreslov, V.V., Okatenko, P.V., Romanov, S.A. & Shilnikova, N.S. (1996) Mortality among personnel who worked at the Mayak complex in the first years of its operation. *Health Phys.*, **71**, 90–93

Koshurnikova. N.A., Bolotnikova, M.G., Ilyin, L.A., Keirim-Markus, I.B., Menshikh, Z.S., Okatenko, P.V., Romanov, S.A., Tsvetkov, V.I. & Shilnikova, N.S. (1998) Lung cancer risk due to exposure to incorporated plutonium. *Radiat. Res.*, **149**, 366–371

Kossenko, M.M., Degteva, M.O., Vyushkova, O.V., Preston, D.L., Mabuchi, K. & Kozheurov, V.P. (1997) Issues in the comparison of risk estimates for the population in the Techa River region and atomic bomb survivors. *Radiat. Res.*, **148**, 54–63

Kozheurov, V.P. & Degteva, M. (1994) Dietary intake evaluation and dosimetric modelling for the Techa River residents based on in vivo measurements of strontium-90 in teeth and skeleton. *Sci. total Environ.*, **142**, 63–72

Kuljis, R.O., Xu, Y., Aguila, M.C. & Baltimore, D. (1997) Degeneration of neurons, synapses, and neuropil and glial activation in a murine *Atm* knockout model of ataxia-telangiectasia. *Proc. natl Acad. Sci. USA*, **94**, 12688–12693

Laake, K., Ødegård, Å., Andersen, T.I., Bukholm, I.K., Kåresen, R., Nesland, J.M., Ottestad, L., Shiloh, Y. & Børresen-Dale, A.-L. (1997) Loss of heterozygosity at 11q23.1 in breast carcinomas: Indication for involvement of a gene distal and close to ATM. *Genes Chromosomes Cancer*, **18**, 175–180

Lagakos, S.W. & Mosteller, F. (1986) Assigned shares in compensation for radiation-related cancers. *Risk Anal.*, **6**, 345–357

Lakin, N.D., Weber, P., Stankovic, T., Rottinghus, S.T., Taylor, A.M.R. & Jackson, S.P. (1996) Analysis of the ATM protein in wild-type and ataxia-telangiectasia cells. *Oncogene*, **13**, 2707–2716

Land, C.E., Boice, J.D., Jr, Shore, R.E., Norman, J.E. & Tokunaga, M. (1980) Breast cancer risk from low-dose exposures to ionizing radiation: Results of parallel analysis of three exposed populations of women. *J. natl Cancer Inst.*, **65**, 353–376

Land, C.E., Hayakawa, N., Machado, S.G., Yamada, Y., Pike, M.C., Akiba, S. & Tokunaga, M. (1994a) A case–control interview study of breast cancer among Japanese A-bomb survivors. I. Main effects. *Cancer Causes Control*, **5**, 157–165

Land, C.E., Hayakawa, N., Machado, S.G., Yamada, Y., Pike, M.C., Akiba, S. & Tokunaga, M. (1994b) A case–control interview study of breast cancer among Japanese A-bomb survivors. II. Interactions with radiation dose. *Cancer Causes Control*, **5**, 167–176

Land, C.E., Saku, T., Hayashi, Y., Takahara, O., Matsuura, H., Tokuoka, S., Tokunaga, M. & Mabuchi, K. (1996) Incidence of salivary gland tumors among atomic bomb survivors, 1950–1987. Evaluation of radiation-related risk. *Radiat. Res.*, **146**, 28–36

Lange, E., Gatti, R.A, Sobel, E., Concannon, P. & Lange, K. (1993) How many A-T genes? In: Gatti, R.A. & Painter, R.B., eds, *Ataxia-telangiectasia*, Heidelberg, Springer-Verlag, pp. 37–54

Langlois, R.G., Bigbee, W.L. & Jensen, R.H. (1986) Measurements of the frequency of human erythrocytes with gene expression loss phenotypes at the glycophorin A locus. *Hum. Genet.*, **74**, 353–362

Langlois, R.G., Akiyama, M., Kusunoki, Y., DuPont, B.R., Moore, D.H., 2nd, Bigbee, W.L., Grant, S.G. & Jensen, R.H. (1993) Analysis of somatic cell mutations at the glycophorin A locus in atomic bomb survivors: A comparative study of assay methods. *Radiat. Res.*, **136**, 111–117

Lavin, M.F. & Davidson, M. (1981) Repair of strand breaks in superhelical DNA of ataxia telangiectasia lymphoblastoid cells. *J. Cell Sci.*, **48**, 383–391

Lavin, M.F., Le Poidevin, P. & Bates, P. (1992) Enhanced levels of radiation-induced G2 phase delay in ataxia telangiectasia heterozygotes. *Cancer Genet. Cytogenet.*, **60**, 183–187

Lavin, M.F., Bennett, I., Ramsay, J., Gardiner, R.A., Seymour, G.J., Farrell, A. & Walsh, M. (1994) Identification of a potentially radiosensitive subgroup among patients with breast cancer. *J. natl Cancer Inst.*, **86**, 1627–1634

Lee, W., Chiacchierini, R.P., Shleien, B. & Telles, N.C. (1982) Thyroid tumors following ^{131}I or localized X-irradiation to the thyroid and pituitary glands in rats. *Radiat. Res.*, **92**, 307–319

van Leeuwen, F.E., Klokman, W.J., Stovall, M., Hagenbeek, A., van den Belt-Dusebout, A.W., Noyon, R., Boice, J.D., Jr, Burgers, J.M. & Somers, R. (1995) Roles of radiotherapy and smoking in lung cancer following Hodgkin's disease. *J. natl Cancer Inst.*, **87**, 1530–1537

Lévêque, B., Debauchez, C.I., Desbois, J.-C., Feingold, J., Barbet, J. & Marie, J. (1966) [Immunological and lymphocytic anomalies in the ataxia telangiectasia syndrome: Analysis of personal observations.] *Ann. Pediatr.*, **13**, 2710–2725 (in French)

Le Vu, B., de Vathaire, F., Shamsaldin, A., Hawkins, M.M., Grimaud, E., Hardiman, C., Diallo, I., Vassal, G., Bessa, E., Campbell, S., Panis, X., Daly-Schveitzer, N., Lagrange, J.-L., Zucker, J.-M., Eschwège, F., Chavaudra, J. & Lemerle, J. (1998) Radiation dose, chemotherapy and risk of osteosarcoma after solid tumours during childhood. *Int. J. Cancer*, **77**, 370–377

Levy, A.R., Goldberg, M.S., Hanley, J.A., Mayo, N.E. & Poitras, B. (1994) Projecting the lifetime risk of cancer from exposure to diagnostic ionizing radiation for adolescent idiopathic scoliosis. *Health Phys.*, **66**, 621–633

Lewis, E.B. (1963) Leukemia, multiple myeloma and aplastic anemia in American radiologists. *Science,* **142**, 1492–1494

Li, F.P., Cassady, J.R. & Barnett, R.N. (1974) Cancer mortality following irradiation in infancy for hemangioma. *Radiology*, **113**, 177–178

Lieber, M.R. (1997) The FEN-1 family of structure-specific nucleases in eukaryotic DNA replication, recombination and repair. *Bioessays*, **19**, 233–240

Lim, D.-S. & Hasty, P. (1996) A mutation in mouse *rad51* results in an early embryonic lethal that is suppressed by a mutation in *p53*. *Mol. Cell Biol.*, **16**, 7133–7143

Lim, D.-S., Kirsch, D.G., Canman, C.E., Ahn, J.H., Ziv, Y., Newman, L.S., Darnell, R.B., Shiloh, Y. & Kastan, M.B. (1998) ATM binds to β-adaptin in cytoplasmic vesicles. *Proc. natl Acad. Sci. USA*, **95**, 10146–10151

Limoli, C.L., Corcoran, J.J., Milligan, J.R., Ward, J.F. & Morgan, W.F. (1999) Critical target and dose and dose-rate responses for the induction of chromosomal instability by ionizing radiation. *Radiat. Res.*, **151**, 677–685

Lindberg, S., Karlsson, P., Arvidsson, B., Holmberg, E., Lunberg, L.M. & Wallgren, A. (1995) Cancer incidence after radiotherapy for skin haemangioma during infancy. *Acta oncol.*, **34**, 735–740

Linos, A., Gray, J.E., Orvis, A.L., Kyle, R.A., O'Fallon, M. & Kurland, L.T. (1980) Low dose radiation and leukemia. *New Engl. J. Med.*, **302**, 1101–1105

Little, M.P. & Boice, J.D., Jr (1999) Comparison of breast cancer incidence in the Massachusetts tuberculosis fluoroscopy cohort and in the Japanese atomic bomb survivors. *Radiat. Res.*, **151**, 218–224

Little, J.B., Gorgojo, L. & Vetrovs, H. (1990) Delayed appearance of lethal and specific gene mutations in irradiated mammalian cells. *Int. J. Radiat. Oncol. Biol. Phys.*, **19**, 1425–1429

Little, J.B., Nagasawa, H., Pfenning, T. & Vetrovs, H. (1997) Radiation-induced genomic instability: Delayed mutagenic and cytogenetic effects of X rays and alpha particles. *Radiat. Res.*, **148**, 299–307

Little, M.P., de Vathaire, F., Shamsaldin, A., Oberlin, O., Campbell, S., Grimaud, E., Chavaudra, J., Haylock, R.G.E. & Muirhead, C.R. (1998a) Risks of brain tumour following treatment for cancer in childhood: Modification by genetic factors, radiotherapy and chemotherapy. *Int. J. Cancer*, **78**, 269–275

Little, M.P., De Vathaire, F., Charles, M.W., Hawkins, M.M. & Muirhead, C.R. (1998b) Variations with time and age in the risks of solid cancer incidence after radiation exposure in childhood. *Stat. Med.*, **17**, 1341–1355

Little, M.P., Weiss, H.A., Boice, J.D., Jr, Darby, S.C., Day, N.E. & Muirhead, C.R. (1999) Risks of leukemia in Japanese atomic bomb survivors, in women treated for cervical cancer and in patients treated for ankylosing spondylitis. *Radiat. Res.*, **152**, 280–292

Liu, V.F. & Weaver, D.T. (1993) The ionizing radiation-induced replication protein A phosphorylation response differs between ataxia telangiectasia and normal human cells. *Mol. Cell Biol.*, **13**, 7222–7231

Lloyd, D.C. & Purrott, R.J. (1981) Chromosome aberration analysis in radiological protection dosimetry. *Rad. Protect. Dosim.*, **1**, 19–28

Löbrich, M., Rydberg, B. & Cooper, P.K. (1995) Repair of X-ray-induced DNA double-strand breaks in specific *Not* I restriction fragments in human fibroblasts: Joining correct and incorrect ends. *Proc. natl Acad. Sci. USA*, **92**, 12050–12054

Löbrich, M., Cooper, P.K. & Rydberg, B. (1998) Joining of correct and incorrect DNA ends at double-strand breaks produced by high-linear energy transfer radiation in human fibroblasts. *Radiat. Res.*, **150**, 619–626

Loeb, L.A. (1998) Cancer cells exhibit a mutator phenotype. *Adv. Cancer Res.*, **72**, 25–56

van Lohuizen, M., Verbeek, S., Krimpenfort, P., Domen, J., Saris, C., Radaszkiewicz, T. & Berns, A. (1989) Predisposition to lymphomagenesis in *pim*-1 transgenic mice: Cooperation with *c-myc* and *N-myc* in murine leukemia virus-induced tumours. *Cell*, **56**, 673–682

Lotem, J. & Sachs, L. (1993) Hematopoietic cells from mice deficient in wild-type p53 are more resistant to induction of apoptosis by some agents. *Blood*, **82**, 1092–1096

Loucas, B.D. & Cornforth, M.N. (1998) Postirradiation growth in HAT medium fails to eliminate the delayed appearance of 6-thioguanine-resistant clones in EJ30 human epithelial cells. *Radiat. Res.*, **149**, 171–178

Lowe, S.W., Schmitt, E.M., Smith, S.W., Osborne, B.A. & Jacks, T. (1993) p53 is required for radiation-induced apoptosis in mouse thymocytes. *Nature*, **362**, 847–849

Lumniczky, K., Antal, S., Unger, E., Wunderlich, L., Hidvegi, E.J. & Safrany, G. (1998) Carcinogenic alterations in murine liver, lung, and uterine tumors induced by in utero exposure to ionizing radiation. *Mol. Carcinog.*, **21**, 100–110

Lundell, M. & Holm, L.-E. (1995) Risk of solid tumors after irradiation in infancy. *Acta oncol.*, **34**, 727–734

Lundell, M. & Holm, L.-E. (1996) Mortality from leukemia after irradiation in infancy for skin hemangioma. *Radiat. Res.*, **145**, 595–601

Lundell, M., Hakulinen, T. & Holm, L.-E. (1994) Thyroid cancer after radiotherapy for skin hemangioma in infancy. *Radiat. Res.*, **140**, 334–339

Lundell, M., Mattsson, A., Hakulinen, T. & Holm, L.-E. (1996) Breast cancer after radiotherapy for skin hemangioma in infancy. *Radiat. Res.*, **145**, 225–230

Lundell, M., Mattson, A., Karlsson, P., Holmberg, E., Gustafsson, A. & Holm, L.-E. (1999) Breast cancer risk after radiotherapy in infancy. A pooled analysis of two Swedish cohorts of 17 202 infants. *Radiat. Res.*, **151**, 626-632

Lüning, K.G. & Eiche, A. (1976) X-ray-induced recessive lethal mutations in the mouse. *Mutat. Res.*, **34**, 163–174

Lüning, K.G. & Searle, A.G. (1971) Estimates of the genetic risks from ionizing radiation. *Mutat. Res.*, **12**, 291–304

Luongo, C. & Dove, W.F. (1996) Somatic genetic events linked to the *Apc* locus in intestinal adenomas of the Min mouse. *Genes Chromosomes Cancer*, **17**, 194–198

Lyon, M.F. (1970) X-ray induced dominant lethal mutation in male guinea-pigs, hamsters and rabbits. *Mutat. Res.*, **10**, 133–140

Lyon, M.F., Phillips, R.J.S. & Fisher, G. (1979) Dose–response curves for radiation-induced gene mutations in mouse oocytes and their interpretation. *Mutat. Res.*, **63**, 161–173

Lyon, M.F., Phillips, R.J.S. & Fisher, G. (1982) Use of an inversion to test for induced X-linked lethals in mice. *Mutat. Res.*, **92**, 217–228

Mabuchi, K., Soda, M., Ron, E., Tokunaga, M., Ochikubo, S., Sugimoto, S., Ikeda, T., Terasaki, M., Preston, D.L. & Thompson, D.E. (1994) Cancer incidence in atomic bomb survivors. Part I: Use of the tumor registries in Hiroshima and Nagasaki for incidence studies. *Radiat. Res.*, **137** (Suppl. 2), S1–S16

MacMahon, B. (1962) Prenatal X-ray exposure and childhood cancer. *J. natl Cancer Inst.*, **28**, 1173–1191

MacMahon, B. (1985) Prenatal X-ray exposure and twins. *New Engl. J. Med.*, **312**, 576–577

MacMahon, B. (1989) Some recent issues in low-exposure radiation epidemiology. *Environ. Health Perspect.*, **81**, 131–135

MacMahon, B. (1992) Leukemia clusters around nuclear facilities in Britain. *Cancer Causes Control*, **3**, 283–288

Mah, K., Van Dyk, J., Keane, T. & Poon, P.Y. (1987) Acute radiation-induced pulmonary damage: A clinical study on the response to fractionated radiation therapy. *Int. J. Radiat. Oncol. Biol. Phys.*, **13**, 179–188

Maier, U., Ehrenböck, P.M. & Hofbauer, J. (1997) Late urological complications and malignancies after curative radiotherapy for gynecological carcinomas: A retrospective analysis of 10,709 patients. *J. Urol.*, **158**, 814–817

Maisin, J.R., Wambersie, A., Gerber, G.B., Gueulette, J., Mattelin, G. & Lambiet-Collier, M. (1983) Life shortening and disease incidence in BALB/c mice following a single d(50)-Be neutron or gamma exposure. *Radiat. Res.*, **94**, 374–389

Maisin, J.R., Wambersie, A., Gerber, G.B., Mattelin, G., Lambiet-Collier, M., De Coster, B. & Gueulette, J. (1988) Life shortening and disease incidence in C57BL mice after single and fractionated gamma and high-energy neutron exposure. *Radiat. Res.*, **113**, 300–317

Malkin, D. (1998) The Li-Fraumeni syndrome. In: Vogelstein, B. & Kinzler, K.W., eds, *The Genetic Basis of Human Cancer*, New York, McGraw-Hill, pp. 393–407

Malkin, D., Li, F.P., Strong, L.C., Fraumeni, J.F., Jr, Nelson, C.E., Kim, D.H., Kassel, J., Gryka, M.A., Bischoff, F.Z., Tainsky, M.A. & Friend, S.H. (1990) Germ line p53 mutations in a familial syndrome of breast cancer, sarcomas, and other neoplasms. *Science*, **250**, 1233–1238

March, H.C. (1944) Leukemia in radiologists. *Radiology*, **43**, 275–278

Marder, B.A. & Morgan, W.F. (1993) Delayed chromosomal instability induced by DNA damage. *Mol.Cell Biol.*, **13**, 6667–6677

Marshall, E. (1984) Juarez: An unexpected radiation accident. *Science*, **223**, 1152–1154

Mason, T.J. & Miller, R.W. (1974) Cosmic radiation at high altitudes and US cancer mortality, 1950–1969. *Radiat. Res.*, **60**, 302–306

Matanoski, G.M., Seltser, R., Sartwell, P.E., Diamond, E.L. & Elliott, E.A. (1975a) The current mortality rates of radiologists and other physician specialists: Deaths from all causes and from cancer. *Am. J. Epidemiol.*, **101**, 188–198

Matanoski, G.M., Seltser, R., Sartwell, P.E., Diamond, E.L. & Elliott, E.A. (1975b) The current mortality rates of radiologists and other physician specialists: Specific causes of death. *Am. J. Epidemiol.*, **101**, 199–210

Matsuo, T., Tomonaga, M., Bennett, J.M., Kuriyama, K., Imanaka, F., Kuramoto, A., Kamada, N., Ichimaru, M., Finch, S.C., Pisciotta, A.V. & Ishimaru, T. (1988) Reclassification of leukemia among A-bomb survivors in Nagasaki using French–American–British (FAB) classification for acute leukemia. *Jpn. J. clin. Oncol.*, **18**, 91–96

Matsuura, S., Weemaes, C., Smeets, D., Takami, H., Kondo, N., Sakamoto, S., Yano, N., Nakamura, A., Tauchi, H., Endo, S., Oshimura, M. & Komatsu, K. (1997) Genetic mapping using microcell-mediated chromosome transfer suggests a locus for Nijmegen breakage syndrome at chromosome 8q21-24. *Am. J. hum. Genet.*, **60**, 1487–1494

Matsuura, K., Balmukhanov, T., Tauchi, H., Weemaes, C., Smeets, D., Chrzanowska, K., Endou, S., Matsuura, S. & Komatsu, K. (1998) Radiation induction of p53 in cells from Nijmegen breakage syndrome is defective but not similar to ataxia-telangiectasia. *Biochem. biophys. Res. Commun.*, **26**, 602–607

Mattsson, A., Rudén, B.-I., Hall, P., Wilking, N. & Rutqvist, L.E. (1993) Radiation-induced breast cancer: Long-term follow-up of radiation therapy for benign breast disease. *J. natl Cancer Inst.*, **85**, 1679–1685

Mattsson, A., Ruden, B.I., Palmgren, J. & Rutqvist, L.E. (1995) Dose- and time-response for breast cancer risk after radiation therapy for benign breast disease. *Br. J. Cancer*, **72**, 1054–1061

Mattsson, A., Hall, P., Rudén, B.-I. & Rutqvist, L.E. (1997) Incidence of primary malignancies other than breast cancer among women treated with radiation therapy for benign breast disease. *Radiat. Res.*, **148**, 152–160

Matutes, E., Brito-Babapulle, V., Swansbury, J., Ellis, J., Morilla, R., Dearden, C., Sempere, A. & Catovsky, D. (1991) Clinical and laboratory features of 78 cases of T-prolymphocytic leukaemia. *Blood*, **78**, 3269–3274

Maxon, H.R., Saenger, E.L., Thomas, S.R., Buncher, C.R., Kereiakes, J.G., Shafer, M.L. & McLaughlin, C.A. (1980) Clinically important radiation-associated thyroid disease. A controlled study. *J. Am. med. Assoc.*, **244**, 1802–1805

Maxon, H.R., Saenger, E.L., Buncher, C.R., Thomas, S.R., Kereiakes, J.C., Shafer, M.L. & McLaughlin, C.A. (1981) Radiation-associated carcinoma of the salivary glands: A controlled study. *Ann. Otol.*, **90**, 107–109

McBlane, J.F., van Gent, D.C., Ramsden, D.A., Romeo, C., Cuomo, C.A., Gellert, M. & Oettinger, M.A. (1995) Cleavage at a V(D)J recombination signal requires only RAG1 and RAG2 proteins and occurs in two steps. *Cell*, **83**, 387–395

McCulloch, E.A. & Till, J.E. (1960) The radiation sensitivity of normal mouse bone marrow cells, determined by quantitative marrow transplantation into irradiated mice. *Radiat. Res.*, **13**, 115–125

McCulloch, E.A. & Till, J.E. (1962) The sensitivity of cells from normal mouse bone marrow to γ-radiation *in vitro* and *in vivo*. *Radiat. Res.*, **16**, 822–832

McLaughlin, J.R., Kreiger, N., Sloan, M.P., Benson, L.N., Hilditch, S. & Clarke, E.A. (1993a) An historical cohort study of cardiac catheterization during childhood and the risk of cancer. *Int. J. Epidemiol.*, **22**, 584–591

McLaughlin, J.R., Clarke, E.A., Nishri, E.D. & Anderson, T.W. (1993b) Childhood leukemia in the vicinity of Canadian nuclear facilities. *Cancer Causes Control*, **4**, 51–58

McLaughlin, J.R., King, W.D., Anderson, T.W., Clarke, E.A. & Ashmore, J.P. (1993c) Paternal radiation exposure and leukemia in offspring: The Ontario case–control study. *Br. med. J.*, **307**, 959–965

Medina, D. (1979) Serial transplantation of chemical carcinogen-induced mouse mammary ductal dysplasias. *J. natl Cancer Inst.*, **62**, 397–405

Meistrich, M.L. & Van Beek, M.E.A.B. (1990) Radiation sensitivity of the human testis. *Adv. Radiat. Biol.*, **14**, 227–268

Meistrich, M.L., Vassilopoulou-Sellin, R. & Lipshultz, L.I. (1997) Gonadal dysfunction. In: De Vita, V.T., Jr, Hellman, S. & Rosenberg S.A., eds, *Principles and Practices of Oncology*, 5th Ed., Philadelphia, PA, J.B. Lippincott Raven, pp. 2758–2773

Mendonca, M.S., Fasching, C.L., Srivatsan, E.S., Stanbridge, E.J. & Redpath, J.L. (1995) Loss of a putative tumor suppressor locus after gamma-ray-induced neoplastic transformation of HeLa x skin fibroblast human cell hybrids. *Radiat. Res.*, **143**, 34–44

Mendonca, M.S., Temples, T.M., Farrington, D.L. & Bloch, C. (1998a) Evidence for a role of delayed death and genomic instability in radiation-induced neoplastic transformation of human hybrid cells. *Int. J. Radiat. Biol.*, **74**, 755–64

Mendonca, M.S., Howard, K., Fasching, C.L., Farrington, D.L., Desmond, L.A., Stanbridge, E.J. & Redpath, J.L. (1998b) Loss of suppressor loci on chromosomes 11 and 14 may be required for radiation-induced neoplastic transformation of HeLa x skin fibroblast human cell hybrids. *Radiat. Res.*, **149**, 246–55

Mengle-Gaw, L., Albertson, D.G., Sherrington, P.D. & Rabbitts, T.H. (1988) Analysis of a T-cell tumor-specific breakpoint cluster at human chromosome 14q32. *Proc. natl Acad. Sci. USA*, **85**, 9171–9175

Merriam, G.R., Jr, Szechter, A. & Focht, E.F. (1972) The effects of ionising radiation on the eye. *Front. Rad. Ther. Oncol.*, **6**, 346–385

Mettler, F.A., Jr, Hempelmann, L.H., Dutton, A.M., Pifer, J.W., Toyooka, E.T. & Ames, W.R. (1969) Breast cancer neoplasms in women treated with X-rays for acute postpartum mastitis. A pilot study. *J. natl Cancer Inst.*, **43**, 803–811

Mettler, F.A., Jr, Upton, A., Kelsey, C.A., Ashby, R.N., Rosenberg, R.D. & Linver, M.N. (1996) Benefits versus risks from mammography: A critical reassessment. *Cancer*, **77**, 903–909

Michaelis, J., Keller, B., Haaf, G. & Kaatsch, P. (1992) Incidence of childhood malignancies in the vicinity of West German nuclear power plants. *Cancer Causes Control*, **3**, 255–263

Michaelis, J., Kaletsch, U., Burkart, W. & Grosche, B. (1997) Infant leukaemia after the Chernobyl accident (Letter to the Editor). *Nature*, **387**, 246

Miki, Y., Swensen, J., Shattuck-Eidens, D., Futreal, P.A., Harshman, K., Tavtigian, S., Liu, Q., Cochran, C., Bennett, L.M., Ding, W., Bell, R., Rosenthal, J., Hussey, C., Tran, T., McClure, M., Frye, C., Hattier, T., Phelps, R., Haugen-Strano, A., Katcher, H., Yakumo, K., Gholami, Z., Shaffer, D., Stone, S., Bayer, S., Wray, C., Bogden, R., Dayananth, P., Ward, J., Tonin, P., Narod, S., Bristow, P.K., Norris, F.H., Helvering, L., Morrison, P., Rosteck, P., Lai, M., Barrett, J.C., Lewis, C., Neuhausen, S., Cannon-Albright, L., Goldgar, D., Wiseman, R., Kamb, A. & Skolnick, M.H. (1994) A strong candidate for the breast and ovarian cancer susceptibility gene *BRCA1. Science*, **266**, 66–71

Miller, R.W. (1969) Delayed radiation effects in atomic-bomb survivors. *Science*, **166**, 569–574

Miller, K.M. (1992) Measurements of external radiation in United States dwellings. *Radiat. Protect. Dosim.*, **45**, 535–539

Miller, R.W. (1995) Delayed effects of external radiation exposure: A brief history. *Radiat. Res.*, **144**, 160–169

Miller, M.E. & Chatten, J. (1967) Ovarian changes in ataxia telangiectasia. *Acta paediatr. scand.*, **56**, 559–561

Miller, R.W. & Mulvihill, J.J. (1956) Small head size after atomic irradiation. *Teratology*, **14**, 355–358

Miller, A.B., Howe, G.R., Sherman, G.J., Lindsay, J.P., Yaffe, M.J., Dinner, P.J., Risch, H.A. & Preston, D.L. (1989) Mortality from breast cancer after irradiation during fluoroscopic examinations in patients being treated for tuberculosis. *New Engl. J. Med.*, **321**, 1285–1289

Modan, B., Chetrit, A., Alfandary, E. & Katz, L. (1989) Increased risk of breast cancer after low-dose irradiation. *Lancet*, **i**, 629–631

Mohr, U., Dasenbrock, C., Tillmann, T., Kohler, M., Kamino, K., Hagemann, G., Morawietz, G., Campo, E., Cazorla, M., Fernandez, P., Hernandez, L., Cardesa, A. & Tomatis, L. (1999) Possible carcinogenic effects of X-rays in a transgenerational study with CBA mice. *Carcinogenesis*, **20**, 325–332

Mole, R.H. (1974) Antenatal irradiation and childhood cancer: Causation or coincidence? *Br. J. Cancer*, **30**, 199–208

Mole, R.H. (1990) Childhood cancer after prenatal exposure to diagnostic x-ray examinations in Britain. *Br. J. Cancer,* **62**, 152–168

Mole, R.H., Papworth, D.G. & Corp, M.J. (1983) The dose–response of X-ray induction of myeloid leukaemia in male CBA/H mice. *Br. J. Cancer*, **47**, 285–291

Møller, H., Mellemgaard, A., Jacobsen, G.K., Pedersen, D. & Storm, H.H. (1993) Incidence of second primary cancer following testicular cancer. *Eur. J. Cancer*, **29A**, 672–676

Monson, R.R. & MacMahon, B. (1984) Prenatal X-ray exposure and cancer in children. In: Boice, J.D., Jr & Fraumeni, J.F., Jr, eds, *Radiation Carcinogenesis: Epidemiology and Biological Significance*, New York, Raven Press, pp. 97–105

Morales, M.D., González, F.A., Villegas, A., del Potro, E., Díaz Mediavilla, J., Martínez, R., Alvarez, A. & Colomé, J.A. (1992) [Second neoplasms as a late complication of the treatment of Hodgkin's disease]. *Sangre*, **37**, 429–433 (in Spanish)

Morgan, J.L., Holcomb, T.M. & Morrissey, R.W. (1968) Radiation reaction in ataxia-telangiectasia. *Am. J. Dis. Child.*, **116**, 557–558

Morgan, W.F., Day, J.P., Kaplan, M.I., McGhee, E.M. & Limoli, C.L. (1996) Genomic instability induced by ionizing radiation. *Radiat. Res.*, **146**, 247–258

Morgan, S.E., Lovly, C., Pandita, T.K., Shiloh, Y. & Kastan, M. (1997) Fragments of ATM which have dominant-negative or complementing activity. *Mol. cell. Biol.*, **17**, 2020–2029

Morrell, D., Cromartie, E. & Swift, M. (1986) Mortality and cancer incidence in 263 patients with ataxia-telangiectasia. *J. natl Cancer Inst.*, **77**, 89–92

Morrell, D., Chase, C.L. & Swift, M. (1990) Cancers in 44 families with ataxia-telangiectasia. *Cancer Genet. Cytogenet.*, **50**, 119–123

Morris, C., Mohamed, R. & Lavin, M.F. (1983) DNA replication and repair in ataxia-telangiectasia cells exposed to bleomycin. *Mutat. Res.*, **112**, 67–74

Moser, A.R., Luongo, C., Gould, K.A., McNeley, M.K., Shoemaker, A.R. & Dove, W.F. (1995) *Apc^{Min}* : A mouse model for intestinal and mammary tumorigenesis. *Eur. J. Cancer*, **31A**, 1061–1064

Moulder, J.E. & Fish, B.L. (1997) Age dependence of radiation nephropathy in the rat. *Radiat. Res.*, **147**, 340–353

Muirhead, C.R. & Kneale, G.W. (1989) Prenatal irradiation and childhood cancer. *J. Radiol. Prot.*, **9**, 209–212

Muirhead, C.R., Butland, B.K., Green, B.M.R. & Draper, G.J. (1991) Childhood leukaemia and natural radiation (Letter to the Editor). *Lancet*, **337**, 503–504

Muirhead, C.R., Goodill, A.A., Haylock, R.G.E., Vokes, J., Little, M.P., Jackson, D.A., O'Hagan, J.A., Thomas, J.M., Kendall, G.M., Silk, T.J., Bingham, D. & Berridge, G.L.C. (1999) Occupational radiation exposure and mortality: Second analysis of the National Registry for Radiation Workers. *J. Radiol. Prot.*, **19**, 3–26

Mulcahy, R.T., Gould, M.N. & Clifton, K.H. (1980) The survival of thyroid cells: *in vivo* irradiation and *in situ* repair. *Radiat. Res.*, **84**, 523–528

Muller, H.J. (1927) Artificial transmutation of the gene. *Science*, **66**, 84–87

Nagasawa, H. & Little, J.B. (1983) Comparison of kinetics of X-ray-induced cell killing in normal, ataxia-telangiectasia and hereditary retinoblastoma fibroblasts. *Mutat. Res.*, **109**, 297–308

Nagasawa, H., Kraemer, K. H., Shiloh, Y. & Little J.B. (1987) Detection of ataxia telangiectasia heterozygous cell lines by postirradiation cumulative labelling index: Measurements with coded samples. *Cancer Res.*, **47**, 398–402

Nambi, K.S.V. & Soman, S.D. (1987) Environmental radiation and cancer in India. *Health Phys.*, **52**, 653–657

Nandakumar, A., Davis, S., Moolgavkar, S., Witherspoon, R.P. & Schwartz, S.M. (1991) Myeloid leukaemia following therapy for a first primary cancer. *Br. J. Cancer*, **63**, 782–788

Natarajan, A.T. & Obe, G. (1984) Molecular mechanisms involved in the production of chromosomal aberrations. III. Restriction endonucleases. *Chromosoma*, **90**, 120–127

Natarajan, A.T., Ramalho, A.T., Vyas, R.C., Bernini, L.F., Tates, A.D., Ploem, J.S., Nascimento, A.C. & Curado, M.P. (1991a) Goiania radiation accident: Results of initial dose estimation and follow up studies. *Prog. clin. Biol. Res.*, **372**, 145–553

Natarajan, A.T., Vyas, R.C., Wiegant, J. & Curado, M.P. (1991b) A cytogenetic follow-up study of the victims of a radiation accident in Goiania, Brazil. *Mutat. Res.*, **247**, 103–111

Natarajan, A.T., Boei, J.J.W.A., Vermeulen, S. & Balajee, A.S. (1996) Frequencies of X-ray induced pericentric inversions and centric rings in human blood lymphocytes detected by FISH using chromosome arm specific probes. *Mutat. Res.*, **372**, 1–7

Natarajan, A.T., Santos, S.J., Darroudi, F., Hadjidikova, V., Vermeulen, S., Chatterjee, S., Van den Berg, M., Grigorova, M., Sakamoto-Hojo, E.T., Granath, F., Ramalho, A.T. & Curado, M.P. (1998) [137]Cesium-induced chromosome aberrations analyzed by fluorescence in situ hybridization: Eight years follow up of the Goiânia radiation accident victims. *Mutat. Res.*, **400**, 299–312

National Council on Radiation Protection and Measurements (1987a) *Exposure of the Population in the United States and Canada from Natural Background Radiation* (NCRP Report No. 94), Bethesda, MD

National Council on Radiation Protection and Measurements (1987b) *Genetic Effects from Internally Deposited Radionuclides* (NCRP Report No. 89), Bethesda, MD

National Council on Radiation Protection and Measurements (1989) *Exposure of the US Population from Diagnostic Medical Radiation* (NCRP Report No. 100), Bethesda, MD

National Council on Radiation Protection and Measurements (1997) *Uncertainties in Fatal Cancer Risk Estimates Used in Radiation Protection* (NCRP Report No. 126), Bethesda, MD

National Radiological Protection Board (1991) *Committed Equivalent Organ Doses and Committed Effective Doses from Intakes of Radionuclides* (NRPB-R245), Chilton, Oxfordshire

National Radiological Protection Board (1996) *Risk from Deterministic Effects of Ionizing Radiation* (Documents of the NRPB Vol. 7, No. 3), Chilton, Oxfordshire

Neel, J.V. (1991) Update on the genetic effects of ionizing radiation. *J. Am. med. Assoc.*, **266**, 698–701

Neel, J.V., Satoh, C., Goriki, K., Asakawa, J., Fujita, M., Takahashi, N., Kageoka, T. & Hazama, R. (1988) Search for mutations altering protein charge and/or function in children of atomic bomb survivors: Final report. *Am. J. hum. Genet.*, **42**, 663–676

Neel, J.V., Schull, W.J., Awa, A.A., Satoh, C., Kato, H., Otake, M. & Yoshimoto, Y. (1990) The children of parents exposed to atomic bombs: Estimates of the genetic doubling dose of radiation for humans. *Am. J. hum. Genet.*, **46**, 1053–1072

Neglia, J.P., Meadows, A.T., Robison, L.L., Kim, T.H., Newton, W.A., Ruymann, F.B., Sather, H.N. & Hammond, G.D. (1991) Second neoplasms after acute lymphoblastic leukemia in childhood. *New Engl. J. Med.*, **325**, 1330–1336

Neugut, A.I., Murray, T., Santos, J., Amols, H., Hayes, M.K., Flannery, J.T. & Robinson, E. (1994) Increased risk of lung cancer after breast cancer radiation therapy in cigarette smokers. *Cancer*, **73**, 1615–1620

Neugut, A.I., Ahsan, H. & Antman, K.H. (1997a) Incidence of malignant pleural mesothelioma after thoracic radiotherapy. *Cancer*, **80**, 948–950

Neugut, A.I., Ahsan, H., Robinson, E. & Ennis, R.D. (1997b) Bladder carcinoma and other second malignancies after radiotherapy for prostate carcinoma. *Cancer*, **79**, 1600–1604

Newsham, I.F., Hadjistilianov, T. & Cavenee, W.K. (1998) Retinoblastoma. In: Vogelstein, B. & Kinzler, K.W., eds, *The Genetic Basis of Human Cancer*, New York, McGraw-Hill, pp. 363–391

Nicolas, N., Moshous, D., Cavazzan-Calvo, M., Papadopoulo, D., de Chasseval, R., Le Deist, F., Fischer, A. & de Villartay, J.-P. (1998) A human severe combined immunodeficiency (SCID) condition with increased sensitivity to ionizing radiations and impaired V(D)J rearrangements defines a new DNA recombination/repair deficiency. *J. exp. Med.*, **188**, 627–634

Nishisho, I., Nakamura, Y., Miyoshi, Y., Miki, Y., Ando, H., Horii, A., Koyama, K., Utsunomiya, J., Baba, S., Hedge, P., Markham, A., Krush, A.J., Petersen, G., Hamilton, S.R., Nilbert, M.C., Levy, D.B., Bryan, T.M., Preisinger, A.C., Smith, K.J., Su, L.-K., Kinzler, K.W. & Vogelstein, B. (1991) Mutations of chromosome 5q21 genes in FAP and colorectal cancer patients. *Science*, **253**, 665–669

Noguchi, K., Shimizu, M. & Anzai, I. (1986) Correlation between natural radiation exposure and cancer mortality in Japan (I). *J. Radiat. Res.*, **27**, 191–212

Nomura, T. (1982) Parental exposure to X rays and chemicals induces heritable tumours and anomalies in mice. *Nature*, **296**, 575–577

Nomura, T. (1983) X-ray-induced germ-line mutation leading to tumors. Its manifestation in mice given urethane post-natally. *Mutat. Res.*, **121**, 59–65

Nomura, T. (1984) Induction of persistent hypersensitivity to lung tumorigenesis by in utero X-radiation in mice. *Environ. Mutag.*, **6**, 33–40

Nomura, T. (1986) Further studies on X-ray and chemically induced germ-line alterations causing tumors and malformations in mice. In: Ramel, C., Lambert, B. & Magnusson, J., eds, *Genetic Toxicology of Environmental Chemicals, Part B: Genetic Effects and Applied Mutagenesis*, New York, Alan R. Liss, pp. 13–20

Nomura, T. (1989) Role of radiation-induced mutations in multigeneration carcinogenesis. In: Napalkov, N.P., Rice, J.M., Tomatis, L. & Yamasaki, H., eds, *Perinatal and Multigeneration Carcinogenesis* (IARC Scientific Publications No. 96), Lyon, IARC, pp. 375–387

Nomura, T., Nakajima, H., Hatanaka, T., Kinuta, M. & Hongyo, T. (1990) Embryonic mutation as a possible cause of in utero carcinogenesis in mice revealed by postnatal treatment with 12-*O*-tetradecanoylphorbol-13-acetate. *Cancer Res.*, **50**, 2135–2138

Norman, A. & Withers, H.R. (1992) Mammography screening for A-T heterozygotes. *Cell Biol.*, **77**, 137–140

Norman, A., Kagan, A.R. & Chan, S.L. (1988) The importance of genetics for the optimization of radiation therapy. A hypothesis. *Am. J. clin. Oncol.*, **11**, 84–88

Nowell, P.C. (1976) The clonal evolution of tumor cell populations. *Science*, **194**, 23–28

Oakberg, E.F. & Clark, E. (1964) Species comparisons of radiation response of the gonads. In: Carlson, W.D. & Gassner, F.X., eds, *Effects of Ionizing Radiation on the Reproductive System*, New York, Pergamon Press, pp. 11–24

Obe, G., Johannes, C. & Schulte-Frohlinde, D. (1992) DNA double-strand breaks induced by sparsely ionizing radiation and endonucleases as critical lesions for cell death, chromosomal aberrations, mutations and oncogenic transformation. *Mutagenesis*, **7**, 3–12

Oberfield, S.E., Allen, J.C., Pollack, J., New, M.I. & Levine, L.S. (1986) Long-term endocrine sequelae after treatment of medulloblastoma: Prospective study of growth and thyroid function. *J. Pediatr.*, **108**, 219–223

Okeanov, A.E., Cardis, E., Antipova, S.I., Polyakov, S.M., Sobolev, A.V. & Bazulko, N.V. (1996) Health status and follow-up of the liquidators in Belarus. In: Karaoglou, A., Desmet, G., Kelly, G.N. & Menzel, H.G., eds, *The Radiological Consequences of the Chernobyl Accident* (Proceedings of the First International Conference, Minsk, Belarus, 18–22 March 1996), Luxembourg, Office for Official Publications of the European Communities, pp. 851–859

Otake, M. & Schull, W.J. (1984) *In utero* exposure to A-bomb radiation and mental retardation: A reassessment. *Br. J. Radiol.*, **57**, 409–414

Otake, M. & Schull, W.J. (1990) Radiation-related posterior lenticular opacities in Hiroshima and Nagasaki atomic bomb survivors based on the DS86 dosimetry system. *Radiat. Res.*, **121**, 3–13

Otake, M., & Schull, W.J. (1998) Radiation-related brain damage and growth retardation among the prenatally exposed atomic bomb survivors. *Int. J. Radiat. Biol.*, **74**, 159–171

Padovani, L., Caporossi, D., Tedeschi, B., Vernole, P., Nicoletti, B. & Mauro, F. (1993) Cytogenetic study in lymphocytes from children exposed to ionizing radiation after the Chernobyl accident. *Mutat. Res.*, **319**, 55–60

Padovani, L., Stronati, L., Mauro, F., Testa, A., Appolloni, M., Anzidei, P., Caporossi, D., Tedeschi, B. & Vernole, P. (1997) Cytogenetic effects in lymphocytes from children exposed to radiation fall-out after the Chernobyl accident. *Mutat. Res.*, **395**, 249–254

Painter, R.B. & Young, B.R. (1980) Radiosensitivity in ataxia-telangiectasia: A new explanation. *Proc. natl Acad. Sci. USA*, **77**, 7315–7317

Pampfer, S. & Streffer, C. (1989) Increased chromosome aberration levels in cells from mouse fetuses after zygote X-irradiation. *Int. J. Radiat. Biol.*, **55**, 85–92

Parker, L., Craft, A.W., Smith, J., Dickinson, H., Wakeford, R., Binks, K., McElveney, D., Scott, L. & Slovak, A. (1993) Geographical distribution of preconceptual radiation doses to fathers employed at the Sellafield nuclear station. *Br. med. J.*, **307**, 966–971

Parkin, D.M., Cardis, E., Masuyer, E., Friedl, H.P., Hansluwka, H., Bobev, D., Ivanov, E., Sinnaeve, J., Augustin, J., Plesko, I., Storm, H.H., Rahu, M., Karjalainen, S., Bernard, J.L., Carli, P.M., L'Huillier, M.C., Lutz, J.M., Schaffer, P., Schraub, S., Michaelis, J., Möhner, M., Staneczek, W., Vargha, M., Crosignani, P., Magnani, C., Terracini, B., Kriauciunas, R., Coebergh, J.W., Langmark, F., Zatonski, W., Merabishvili, V., Pompe-Kirn, V., Barlow, L., Raymond, L., Black, R., Stiller, C.A. & Bennett, B.G. (1993) Childhood leukaemia following the Chernobyl accident: The European Childhood Leukaemia–Lymphoma Incidence Study (ECLIS). *Eur. J. Cancer*, **29A**, 87–95

Parkin, D.M., Clayton, D., Black, R.J., Masuyer, E., Friedl, H.P., Ivanov, E., Sinnaeve, J., Tzvetansky, C.G., Geryk, E., Storm, H.H., Rahu, M., Pukkala, E., Bernard, J.L., Carli, P.M., L'Huillier, M.C., Ménégoz, F., Schaffer, P., Schraub, S., Kaatsch, P., Michaelis, J., Apjok, E., Schuler, D., Crosignani, P., Magnani, C., Terracini, B., Stengrevics, A., Kriauciunas, R., Coebergh, J.W., Langmark, F., Zatonski, W., Tulbure, R., Boukhny, A., Merabishvili, V., Plesko, I., Kramárová, E., Pompe-Kirn, V., Barlow, L., Enderlin, F., Levi, F., Raymond, L., Schüler, G., Torhorst, J., Stiller, C.A., Sharp, L. & Benett, B.G. (1996) Childhood leukaemia in Europe after Chernobyl: 5 year follow-up. *Br. J. Cancer*, **73**, 1006–1012

Parshad, R., Price, F.M., Bohr, V.A., Cowans, K.H., Zujewski, J.A. & Sanford, K.K. (1996) Deficient DNA repair capacity, a predisposing factor in breast cancer. *Br. J. Cancer*, **74**, 1–5

Patel, U., Bhimani, R. & Frenkel, K (1992) Mechanism of mutagenicity by 5-hydroperoxymethyl-2'-deoxyuridine, an intermediate product of ionizing radiation, in bacteria. HPMdU bacterial mutagenicity and oxidation of DNA bases. *Mutat. Res.*, **283**, 145–156

Paterson, M.C. & Smith, P.J. (1979) Ataxia-telangiectasia: An inherited human disorder involving hypersensitivity to ionizing radiation and related DNA-damaging chemicals. *Ann. Rev. Genet.*, **13**, 291–318

Pearce, N., Winkelmann, R., Kennedy, J., Lewis, S., Purdie, G., Slater, T., Prior, I. & Fraser, J. (1997) Further follow-up of New Zealand participants in United Kingdom atmospheric nuclear weapons tests in the Pacific. *Cancer Causes Control*, **8**, 139–145

Peller, S. & Pick, P. (1952) Leukemia and other malignancies in physicians. *Am. J. med. Sci.*, **224**, 154–159

Peterson, R.D.A., Kelly, W.D. & Good, R.A. (1964) Ataxia-telangiectasia: Its association with a defective thymus, immunological-deficiency disease, and malignancy. *Lancet*, **i**, 1189–1193

Peto, J., Easton, D.F., Matthews, F.E., Ford, D. & Swerdlow, A.J. (1996) Cancer mortality in relatives of women with breast cancer: The OPCS Study. Office of Population Censuses and Surveys. *Int. J. Cancer*, **65**, 275–283

Petridou, E., Trichopoulos, D., Dessypris, N., Flytzani, V., Haidas, S., Kalmanti, M., Koliouskas, D., Kosmidis, H., Piperopoulou, R. & Tzortzatou, F. (1996) Infant leukaemia after *in utero* exposure to radiation from Chernobyl. *Nature*, **382**, 352–353

Petrini, J.H.J., Walsh, M.E., DiMare, C., Chen, X.-N., Korenberg, J.R. & Weaver, D.T. (1995) Isolation and characterization of the human *MRE11* homologue. *Genomics*, **29**, 80–86

Pettersson, F., Fotiou, S., Einhorn, N. & Silfverswärd, C. (1985) Cohort study of the long-term effect of irradiation for carcinoma of the uterine cervix. Second primary malignancies in the pelvic organs in women irradiated for cervical carcinoma at Radiumhemmet 1914–1965. *Acta radiol. oncol.*, **24**, 145–151

Pettersson, F., Ryberg, M. & Malker, B. (1990) Second primary cancer after treatment of invasive carcinoma of the uterine cervix, compared with those arising after treatment for in situ
carcinomas. An effect of irradiation? A cancer registry study. *Acta obstet. gynecol. scand.*,
69, 161–174

Pierce, D.A., Shimizu, Y., Preston, D.L., Vaeth, M. & Mabuchi, K. (1996) Studies of the mortality of atomic bomb survivors. Report 12, Part I. Cancer: 1950–1990. *Radiat. Res.*, **146**, 1–27

Pilinskaya, M.A. (1996) The results of selective cytogenetic monitoring of Chernobyl accident
victims in the Ukraine. *Health Phys.*, **71**, 29–33

Plowman, P.N., Bridges, B.A., Arlett, C.F., Hinney, A. & Kingston, J.E. (1990) An instance of
clinical radiation morbidity and cellular radiosensitivity, not associated with ataxia-telangiectasia. *Br. J. Radiol.*, **63**, 624–628

Pobel, D. & Viel, J.-F. (1997) Case–control study of leukaemia among young people near La
Hague nuclear reprocessing plant: The environmental hypothesis revisited. *Br. med. J.*,
314, 101–106

Pollycove, M. (1995) The issue of the decade: Hormesis. *Eur. J. Nucl. Med.*, **22**, 399–401

Pollycove, M. (1998) Nonlinearity of radiation health effects. *Environ. Health Perspectives*,
106 (Suppl. 1), 363–368

Ponnaiya, B., Cornforth, M.N. & Ullrich, R.L. (1997) Induction of chromosomal instability in
human mammary cells by neutrons and gamma rays. *Radiat. Res.*, **147**, 288–294

Potish, R.A., Dehner, L.P., Haselow, R.E., Kim, T.H., Levitt, S.H. & Nesbit, M. (1985) The
incidence of second neoplasms following megavoltage radiation for pediatric tumors.
Cancer, **56**, 1534–1537

Potten, C.S & Hendry, J. H., eds (1995) *Radiation and Gut*, Amsterdam, Elsevier

Pottern, L.M., Kaplan, M.M., Larsen, P.R., Silva, J.E., Koenig, R.J., Lubin, J.H., Stovall, M. &
Boice, J.D., Jr (1990) Thyroid nodularity after childhood irradiation for lymphoid hyperplasia: A comparison of questionnaire and clinical findings. *J. clin. Epidemiol.*, **43**,
449–460

Preston, D.L., Kusumi, S., Tomonaga, M., Izumi, S., Ron, E., Kuramoto, A., Kamada, N.,
Dohy, H., Matsuo, T., Nonaka, H., Thompson, D.E., Soda, M. & Mabuchi, K. (1994)
Cancer incidence in atomic bomb survivors. Part III: Leukemia, lymphoma and multiple
myeloma, 1950–1987. *Radiat. Res.*, **137**, S68–S97

Preston-Martin, S., Paganini-Hill, A., Henderson, B.E., Pike, M.C. & Wood, C. (1980) Case–
control study of intracranial meningiomas in women in Los Angeles County, California. *J.
natl Cancer Inst.*, **65**, 67–73

Preston-Martin, S., Thomas, D.C., Yu, M.C. & Henderson, B.E. (1989) Diagnostic radiography
as a risk factor for chronic myeloid and monocytic leukaemia (CML). *Br. J. Cancer*, **59**,
634–644

Pride, G.L. & Buchler, D.A. (1976) Carcinoma of vagina 10 or more years following pelvic
irradiation therapy. *Am. J. Obstet. Gynecol.*, **127**, 513–517

Prise, K.M. (1994) Use of radiation quality as a probe for DNA lesion complexity. *Int. J.
Radiat. Biol.*, **65**, 43–48

Prisyazhniuk, A.E., Pjatak, O.A., Buzanov, V.A., Reeves, G.K. & Beral, V. (1991) Cancer in the
Ukraine, post-Chernobyl (Letter to the Editor). *Lancet*, **338**, 1334–1335

Prisyazhniuk, A.E., Gristchenko, V., Zakordonets, V., Fouzik, N., Slipeniuk, Y. & Ryzhak, I. (1995) The time trends of cancer incidence in the most contaminated regions of the Ukraine before and after the Chernobyl accident. *Radiat. environ. Biophys.*, **34**, 3–6

Puck, J.M. (1994) Molecular basis for three X-linked immune disorders. *Hum. mol. Genet.*, **3**, 1457–1461

Rahu, M., Tekkel, M., Veidebaum, T., Pukkala, E., Hakulinen, T., Auvinen, A., Rytömaa, T., Inskip, P.D. & Boice, J.D., Jr (1997) The Estonian study of Chernobyl cleanup workers: II. Incidence of cancer and mortality. *Radiat. Res.*, **147**, 653–657

Ramalho, A.T. & Nascimento, A.C. (1991) The fate of chromosomal aberrations in ^{137}Cs-exposed individuals in the Goiânia radiation accident. *Health Phys.*, **60**, 67–70

Ramalho, A.T., Nascimento, A.C., Littlefield, L.G., Natarajan, A.T. & Sasaki, M.S. (1991) Frequency of chromosomal aberrations in a subject accidentally exposed to ^{137}Cs in the Goiânia (Brazil) radiation accident: Intercomparison among four laboratories. *Mutat. Res.*, **252**, 157–160

Ramalho, A.T., Curado, M.P. & Natarajan, A.T. (1995) Lifespan of human lymphocytes estimated during a six year cytogenetic follow-up of individuals accidentally exposed in the 1987 radiological accident in Brazil. *Mutat. Res.*, **331**, 47–54

Ramalho, A.T., Costa, M.L. & Oliveiria, M.S. (1998) Conventional radiation–biological dosimetry using frequencies of unstable chromosome aberrations. *Mutat. Res.*, **404**, 97–100

Ramsay, J., Birrell, G. & Lavin, M. (1998) Testing for mutations of the ataxia telangiectasia gene in radiosensitive breast cancer patients. *Radiother. Oncol.*, **47**, 125–128

Ramus, S.J., Bobrow, L.G., Pharoah, P.D., Finnigan, D.S., Fishman, A., Altaras, M., Harrington, P.A., Gayther, S.A., Ponder, B.A. & Friedman, L.S. (1999) Increased frequency of TP53 mutations in BRCA1 and BRCA2 ovarian tumours. *Genes Chromosomes Cancer*, **25**, 91–96

Rary, J.M., Bender, M.A. & Kelly, T.E. (1975) A 14/14 marker chromosome lymphocyte clone in ataxia-telangiectasia. *J. Hered.*, **66**, 33–35

Redpath, J.L. & Antoniono, R.J. (1998) Induction of an adaptive response against spontaneous neoplastic transformation in vitro by low-dose gamma radiation. *Radiat. Res.*, **149**, 517–20

Refetoff, S., Harrison, J., Karanfilski, B.T., Kaplan, E.L., De Groot, L.J. & Bekerman, C. (1975) Continuing occurrence of thyroid carcinoma after irradiation to the neck in infancy and childhood. *New Engl. J. Med.*, **292**, 171–175

Reznikoff, C.A., Brankow, D.W. & Heidelberger, C. (1973a) Establishment and characterization of a cloned line of C3H mouse embryo cells sensitive to postconfluence inhibition of division. *Cancer Res.*, **33**, 3231–3238

Reznikoff, C.A., Bertram, J.S., Brankow, D.W. & Heidelberger, C. (1973b) Quantitative and qualitative studies of chemical transformation of cloned C3H mouse embryo cells sensitive to postconfluence inhibition of cell division. *Cancer Res.*, **33**, 3239–3249

Rhim, J.S., Yoo, J.H., Park, J.H., Thraves, P., Salehi, Z. & Dritschilo, A. (1990) Evidence for the multistep nature of in vitro human epithelial cell carcinogenesis. *Cancer Res.*, **50** (Suppl.), 5653S–5657S

Rhim, J.S., Thraves, P., Dritschilo, A., Kuettel, M.R. & Lee, M.S. (1993) Radiation-induced neoplastic transformation of human cells. *Scanning Microsc.*, **7**, 209–216

Riballo, E., Critchlow, S.E., Teo, S.H., Doherty, A.J., Priestley, A., Broughton, B., Kysela, B., Beamish, H., Plowman, N., Arlett, C.F., Lehmann, A.R., Jackson, S.P. & Jeggo, P.A.

(1999) Identification of a defect in DNA ligase IV in a radiosensitive leukaemia patient. *Curr. Biol.*, **19**, 699–702

Ribeiro, G.G., Magee, B., Swindell, R., Harris, M. & Banerjee, S.S. (1993) The Christie Hospital breast conservation trial: An update at 8 years from inception. *Clin. Oncol. R. Coll. Radiol.*, **5**, 278–283

Richardson, S., Monfort, C., Green, M., Draper, G. & Muirhead, C. (1995) Spatial variation of natural radiation and childhood leukaemia incidence in Great Britain. *Stat. Med.*, **14**, 2487–2501

Rinchik, E.M., Bell, J.A., Hunsicker, P.R., Friedman, J.M., Jackson, I.J. & Russell, L.B. (1994) Molecular genetics of the brown (p) locus region of mouse chromosome 4. I. Origin and molecular mapping of radiation- and chemical-induced lethal brown deletions. *Genetics*, **137**, 845–854

Rio, P.G., Pernin, D., Bay, J.-O., Albuisson, E., Kwiatkowski, F., De Latour, M., Bernard-Gallon, D.J. & Bignon, Y.-J.. (1998) Loss of heterozygosity of *BRCA1*, *BRCA2* and *ATM* genes in sporadic invasive ductal breast carcinoma. *Int. J. Oncol.*, **13**, 849–853

Robinette, C.D., Jablon, S. & Preston, D.L. (1985) *Mortality of Nuclear Weapons Test Participants*, Washington DC, National Academy Press, pp. 1–47

Roman, E., Doyle, P., Maconochie, N., Davies, G., Smith, P.G. & Beral, V. (1999) Cancer in children of nuclear industry employees: Report on children under 25 years from nuclear industry family study. *Br. med. J.*, **318**, 1443–1450

Ron, E. (1996) Thyroid cancer. In: Schottenfeld, D. & Fraumeni, J.F., Jr, eds, *Cancer Epidemiology and Prevention*, 2nd Ed., New York, Oxford University Press, pp. 1000–1021

Ron, E. & Modan, B. (1980) Benign and malignant thyroid neoplasms after childhood irradiation for tinea capitis. *J. natl Cancer Inst.*, **65**, 7–11

Ron, E., Kleinerman, R.A., Boice, J.D., Jr, LiVolsi, V.A., Flannery, J.T. & Fraumeni, J.F., Jr (1987) A population based case–control study of thyroid cancer. *J. natl Cancer Inst.*, **79**, 1–12

Ron, E., Modan, B., Boice, J.D., Jr, Alfandary, E., Stovall, M.A., Chetrit, A. & Katz, L. (1988a) Tumors of the brain and nervous system after radiotherapy in childhood. *New Engl. J. Med.*, **319**, 1033–1039

Ron, E., Modan, B. & Boice, J.D., Jr (1988b) Mortality after radiotherapy for ringworm of the scalp. *Am. J. Epidemiol.*, **127**, 713–725

Ron, E., Modan, B., Preston, D., Alfandary, E., Stovall, M. & Boice, J.D., Jr (1989) Thyroid neoplasia following low-dose radiation in childhood. *Radiat. Res.*, **120**, 516–531

Ron, E., Modan, B., Preston, D., Alfandary, E., Stovall, M. & Boice, J.D., Jr (1991) Radiation-induced skin carcinomas of the head and neck. *Radiat. Res.*, **125**, 318–325

Ron, E., Boice, J.D., Jr, Hamburger, S. & Stovall, M. (1994) Mortality following radiation treatment for infertility of hormonal origin or amenorrhea. *Int. J. Epidemiol.*, **23**, 1165–1173

Ron, E., Lubin, J.H., Shore, R.E., Mabuchi, K., Modan, B., Pottern, L.M., Schneider, A.B., Tucker, M.A. & Boice, J.D., Jr (1995) Thyroid cancer after exposure to external radiation: A pooled analysis of seven studies. *Radiat. Res.*, **141**, 259–277

Ron, E., Preston, D.L., Kishikawa, M., Kobuke, T., Iseki, M., Tokuoka, S., Tokunaga, M. & Mabuchi, K. (1998a) Skin tumor risk among atomic-bomb survivors in Japan. *Cancer Causes Control*, **9**, 393–401

Ron, E., Doody, M.M., Becker, D.V., Brill, A.B., Curtis, R.E., Goldman, M.B., Harris, B.S., 3rd, Hoffman, D.A., McConahey, W.M., Maxon, H.R., Preston-Martin, S., Warshauer, M.E., Wong, F.L. & Boice, J.D., Jr (1998b) Cancer mortality following treatment for adult hyperthyroidism. Cooperative Thyrotoxicosis Therapy Follow-up Study Group. *J. Am. med. Assoc.*, **280**, 347–355

Rosen, F.S., Cooper, M.D. & Wedgwood, R.J.P. (1984) The primary immunodeficiencies. *New Eng. J. Med.*, **311**, 300–310

Rosin, M.P. & Ochs, H.D. (1986) In vivo chromosomal instability in ataxia-telangiectasia homozygotes and heterozygotes. *Hum. Genet.*, **74**, 335–340

Rowley, M.J., Leach, D.R., Warner, G.A. & Heller, C.G. (1974) Effects of graded doses of ionizing radiation on the human testis. *Radiat. Res.*, **59**, 665–678

Royce, P.C., MacKay, B.R. & DiSabella, P.M. (1979) Value of postirradiation screening for thyroid nodules. A controlled study of recalled patients. *J. Am. med. Assoc.*, **242**, 2675–2678

Rubin, P. & Casarett, G.W. (1968) *Clinical Radiation Pathology*, Philadelphia, PA, W.B. Saunders

Rudolph, N.S., Nagasawa, H., Little, J.B. & Latt, S.A. (1989) Identification of ataxia telangiectasia heterozygotes by flow cytometric analysis of X-ray damage *Mutat. Res.*, **211**, 19–29

Ruifrok, A.C.C., Mason, K.A., Hunter, N. & Thames, H.D. (1994) Changes in the radiation sensitivity of mouse skin during fractionated and prolonged treatments. *Radiat. Res.*, **139**, 334–343

Russell W.L. (1951) X-ray induced mutations in mice. *Cold Spring Harbor Symp. Quant. Biol.*, **16**, 327–336

Russell W.L. (1962) An augmenting effect of dose fractionation on radiation-induced mutation rate in mice. *Proc. natl Acad. Sci. USA*, **48**, 1724–1727

Russell, W.L. (1977) Mutation frequencies in female mice and the estimation of genetic hazards or radiation in women. *Proc. natl Acad. Sci. USA*, **74**, 3523–3527

Russell, W.L. & Kelly, E.M. (1982) Specific locus mutation frequencies in mouse stem cells spermatogonia at very low radiation doses. *Proc. natl Acad. Sci. USA*, **74**, 539–541

Russell, L.B. & Major, M.H. (1957) Radiation-induced presumed somatic mutations in the house mouse. *Genetics*, **42**, 161–175

Russell, L.B. & Rinchik, E.M. (1993) Structural differences between specific-locus mutations induced by different exposure regimes in mouse spermatogonial stem cells. *Mutat. Res.*, **288**, 187–195

Russo, G., Isobe, M., Gatti, R., Finan, J., Batuman, O., Huebner, K., Nowell, P.C. & Croce, C.M. (1989) Molecular analysis of a t(14;14) translocation in leukemic T-cells of an ataxia telangiectasia patient. *Proc. natl Acad. Sci. USA*, **86**, 602–606

Ryan, P., Lee, M.W., North, B. & McMichael, A.J. (1992) Amalgam fillings, diagnostic dental X-rays and tumours of the brain and meninges. *Eur. J. Cancer*, **28B**, 91–95

Ryberg, M., Lundell, M., Nilsson, B. & Pettersson, F. (1990) Malignant disease after radiation treatment of benign gynaecological disorders. A study of a cohort of metropathia patients. *Acta oncol.*, **29**, 563–567

Saar, K., Chrzanowska, K.H., Stumm, M., Jung, M., Nurnberg, G., Wienker, T.F., Seemanova, E., Wegner, R.D., Reis, A. & Sperling, K. (1997) The gene for the ataxia-telangiectasia variant, Nijmegen breakage syndrome, maps to a 1-cM interval on chromosome 8q21. *Am. J. hum. Genet.*, **60**, 605–610

Sabatier, L., Lebeau, J. & Dutrillaux, B. (1994) Chromosomal instability and alterations of telomeric repeats in irradiated human fibroblasts. *Int. J. Radiat. Biol.*, **66**, 611–613

Sadamoto, S., Suzuki, S., Kamiya, K., Kominami, R., Dohi, K. & Niwa, O. (1994) Radiation induction of germline mutation at a hypervariable mouse minisatellite locus. *Int. J. Radiat. Biol.*, **65**, 549–557

Saddi, V., Curry, J., Nohturfft, A., Kusser, W. & Glickman, B.W. (1996) Increased hprt mutant frequencies in Brazilian children accidentally exposed to ionizing radiation. *Environ. mol. Mutag.*, **28**, 267–275

Sanford, K.K. & Parshad, R. (1990) Detection of cancer-prone individuals using cytogenetic response to X-rays. In: Obe, G. & Natarajan, A.T., eds, *Chromosomal Aberrations: Basic and Applied Aspects*, Berlin, Springer-Verlag, pp. 113–120

Sankaranarayanan, K. (1991) Ionizing radiation and genetic risks. III. Nature of spontaneous and radiation-induced mutations in mammalian in vitro systems and mechanisms of induction of mutations by radiation. *Mutat. Res.*, **258**, 75–97

Sankaranarayanan, K. (1996) Environmental chemical mutagens and genetic risks: Lessons from radiation genetics. *Environ. Mol. Mutag.*, **28**, 65–70

Sasaki, S., Kasuga, T., Sato, F. & Kawashima N. (1978a) Late effects of fetal mice X-irradiated at middle or late intra-uterine stage. *Gann*, **69**, 167–177

Sasaki, S., Kasuga, T., Sato, F. & Kawashima, N. (1978b) Induction of hepatocellular tumor by X-ray irradiation at perinatal stage of mice. *Gann*, **69**, 451–452

Savage, J.R.K. (1976) Classification and relationships of induced chromosomal structural changes. *J. med. Genet.*, **13**, 103–22

Savage, J.R. (1979) Chromosomal aberrations at very low radiation dose rates. *Nature*, **277**, 512–513

Savitsky, K., Sfez, S., Tagle, D.A., Ziv, Y., Sartiel, A., Collins, F.S., Shiloh, Y. & Rotman, G. (1995) The complete sequence of the coding region of the ATM gene reveals similarity to cell cycle regulators in different species. *Hum. mol. Genet.*, **4**, 2025–2032

Savkin, M.N., Titov, A.V. & Lebedev, A.N. (1996) Distribution of individual and collective exposure doses for the population in Belarus in the first year after the Chernobyl accident. *Bulletin of the All-Russian Medical and Dosimetry State Registry*, Issue 7, Moscow, pp. 87–113

Schaaper, R.M., Kunkel, T.A. & Loeb, L.A. (1982) Depurination of DNA as a possible mutagenic pathway for cells. *Basic Life Sci.*, **20**, 199–211

Schmahl, W. (1988) Synergistic induction of tumours in NMRI mice by combined foetal X-irradiation with low doses and ethylnitrosourea administered to juvenile offspring. *Carcinogenesis*, **9**, 1493–1498

Schneider, G. & Burkart, W. (1998) [Health risks of ionizing radiation]. *Radiologe,* **38**, 719–725 (in German)

Schneider, A.B., Shore-Freedman, E., Ryo, U.Y., Bekerman, C., Favus, M. & Pinsky, S. (1985) Radiation-induced tumors of the head and neck following childhood irradiation. Prospective studies. *Medicine (Baltimore)*, **64**, 1–15

Schneider, A.B., Ron, E., Lubin, J., Stovall, M. & Gierlowski, T.C. (1993) Dose–response relationships for radiation-induced thyroid cancer and thyroid nodules: Evidence for the prolonged effects of radiation on the thyroid. *J. clin. Endocrinol. Metab.*, **77**, 362–369

Schofield, P.N. (1998) Impact of genomic imprinting on genomic instability and radiation-induced mutation. *Int. J. Radiat. Biol.*, **74**, 705–710

Schröder, J.H. (1971) Attempt to determine the rate of radiation-induced recessive sex-linked lethal and detrimental mutations in immature germ cells of the house mouse (*Mus musculus*). *Genetics*, **68**, 35–57

Schwartz, J.L., Ashman, C.R., Atcher, R.W., Sedita, B.A., Shadley, J.D., Tang, J., Whitlock, J.L. & Rotmensch, J. (1991) Differential locus sensitivity to mutation induction by ionizing radiations of different LETs in Chinese hamster ovary K1 cells. *Carcinogenesis*, **12**, 1721–1726

Schwarz, K., Hansen-Hagge, T.E., Knobloch, C., Friedrich, W., Kleihauer, E. & Bartram, C.R. (1991) Severe combined immunodeficiency (SCID) in man: B cell-negative (B$^-$) SCID patients exhibit an irregular recombination pattern at the J$_H$ locus. *J. exp. Med.*, **174**, 1039–1048

Scott, D. & Zampetti-Bosseler, F. (1982) Cell cycle dependence of mitotic delay in X-irradiated normal and ataxia-telangiectasia fibroblasts. *Int. J. Radiat. Biol.*, **42**, 679–683

Scott, D., Spreadborough, A.R., Jones, L.A., Roberts, S.A. & Moore, C.J. (1996) Chromosomal radiosensitivity in G2-phase lymphocytes as an indicator of cancer predisposition. *Radiat. Res.*, **145**, 3–16

Scott, D., Barber, J.B.P., Levine, E.L., Burrill, W. & Roberts, S.A. (1998) Radiation-induced micronucleus induction in lymphocytes identifies a high frequency of radiosensitive cases among breast cancer patients: A test for predisposition? *Br. J. Cancer*, **77**, 614–620

Scully, R., Chen, J., Plug, A., Xiao, Y., Weaver, D., Feunteun, J., Ashley, T. & Livingston, D.M. (1997) Association of BRCA1 with Rad51 in mitotic and meiotic cells. *Cell*, **88**, 265–275

Searle, A.G. (1974) Mutation induction in mice. In: Lett, J.T., Adler, H. & Zelle, M.R., eds, *Advances in Radiation Biology*, Vol. 4, New York, Academic Press, pp. 131–207

Searle, A.G. & Beechey, C.V. (1985) A specific locus experiment with mainly dominant visible results (Abstract). *Genet. Res.*, **545**, 224

Searle, A.G. & Beechey, C.V. (1986) The role of dominant visibles in mutagenicity testing. In: Ramel, C., Lambert, B. & Magnusson, J., eds, *Genetic Toxicology of Environmental Chemicals, Part B, Genetic Effects and Applied Mutagenesis*, New York, Alan R. Liss, pp. 511–518

Sedgwick, R.P. & Boder, E. (1991) Ataxia-telangiectasia (208900; 208910; 208920). In: Vinken, P.J., Bruyn, G.W., Klawans, H.L. & Vianney de Jong, J.M.B., eds, *Hereditary Neuropathies and Spinocerebellar Atrophies*, Amsterdam, Elsevier, pp. 347–423

Seemanová, E. (1990) An increased risk for malignant neoplasms in heterozygotes for a syndrome of microcephaly, normal intelligence, growth retardation, remarkable facies, immunodeficiency and chromosomal instability. *Mutat. Res.*, **238**, 321–324

Sega, G.A., Sotomayor, R.E. & Owens, J.G. (1978) A study of unscheduled DNA synthesis induced by X-rays in the germ cells of male mice. *Mutat. Res.*, **49**, 239–257

Selby, P.B. & Selby, P.R. (1977) Gamma-ray-induced dominant mutations that cause skeletal abnormalities in mice. I. Plan, summary of results and discussion. *Mutat. Res.*, **43**, 357–375

Seltser, R. & Sartwell, P.E. (1965) The influence of occupational exposure to radiation on the mortality of American radiologists and other medical specialists. *Am. J. Epidemiol.*, **81**, 2–22

Selvanayagam, C.S., Davis, C.M., Cornforth, M.N. & Ullrich, R.L. (1995) Latent expression of *p53* mutations and radiation-induced mammary cancer. *Cancer Res.*, **55**, 3310–3317

Seymour, C.B., Mothersill, C. & Alper, T. (1986) High yields of lethal mutations in somatic mammalian cells that survive ionizing radiation. *Int. J. Radiat. Biol. Relat. Stud. Phys-Chem. Med.*, **50**, 167–179

Seyschab, H., Schindler, D., Friedl, R., Barbi, G., Boltshauser, E., Fryns, J.P., Hanefeld, F., Korinthenberg, R., Krägeloh-Mann, I., Scheres, J.M., Schinzel, A., Seemanová, E., Tommerup, N. & Hoehn, H. (1992) Simultaneous measurement, using flow cytometry, of radiosensitivity and defective mitogen response in ataxia telangiectasia and related syndromes. *Eur. J. Pediatr.*, **151**, 756–760

Sharan, S.K., Morimatsu, M., Albrecht, U., Lim, D.-K., Regel, E., Dinh, C., Sands, A., Eichele, G., Hasty, P. & Bradley, A. (1997) Embryonic lethality and radiation hypersensitivity mediated by Rad51 in mice lacking *Bcra2*. *Nature*, **386**, 804–810

Shellabarger, C.J., Bond, V.P., Aponte, G.E. & Cronkite, E.P. (1966) Results of fractionation and protraction of total-body radiation on rat mammary neoplasia. *Cancer Res.*, **26**, 509–513

Shellabarger, C.J., Chmelevsky, D. & Kellerer, A.M. (1980) Induction of mammary neoplasms in the Sprague-Dawley rat by 430-keV neutrons and X-rays. *J. natl Cancer Inst.*, **64**, 821–833

Shieh, S.-Y., Ikeda, M., Taya, Y. & Prives, C. (1997) DNA damage-induced phosphorylation of p53 alleviates inhibition by MDM2. *Cell*, **91**, 325–334

Shiloh, Y. (1997) Ataxia-telangiectasia and the Nijmegen breakage syndrome: Related disorders but genes apart. *Annu. Rev. Genet.*, **31**, 635–662

Shiloh, Y., Tabor, E. & Becker, Y. (1982a) The response of ataxia-telangiectasia homozygous skin fibroblasts to neocarzinostatin. *Carcinogenesis*, **3**, 815–820

Shiloh, Y., Tabor, E. & Becker, Y. (1982b) Colony-forming ability of ataxia-telangiectasia skin fibroblasts is an indicator of their early senescence and increased demand for growth factors. *Exp. Cell Res.*, **140**, 191–199

Shiloh, Y., Tabor, E. & Becker, Y. (1983) Abnormal response of ataxia-telangiectasia cells to agents that break the deoxyribose moiety of DNA via a targeted free radical mechanism. *Carcinogenesis*, **4**, 1317–1322

Shiloh, Y., Parshad, R., Sanford, K.K. & Jones, G.M. (1986) Carrier detection in ataxia-telangiectasia (Letter to the Editor). *Lancet*, **i**, 689–690

Shimizu, Y., Kato, H. & Schull, W.J. (1990) Studies of the mortality of A-bomb survivors. 9. Mortality, 1950–1985: Part 2. Cancer mortality based on the recently revised doses (DS86). *Radiat. Res.*, **121**, 120–141

Shimizu, Y., Pierce, D.A., Preston, D.l. & Mabuchi, K. (1999) Studies of the mortality of atomic bomb survivors. Report 12. Part 11. Noncancer mortality 1950–1990. *Radiat. Res.*, **151**, 374–389

Shin, M.K, Russell, L.B. & Tilghman, S.M. (1997) Molecular characterization of four induced alleles at the *Ednrb* locus. *Proc. natl Acad. Sci. USA*, **94**, 13105–13110

Shore, R.E., Albert, R.E. & Pasternack, B.S. (1976) Follow-up study of patients treated by X-ray epilation for tinea capitis; resurvey of post-treatment illness and mortality experience. *Arch. environ. Health*, **31**, 17–24

Shore, R.E., Woodard, E.D., Pasternack, B.S. & Hempelmann, L.H. (1980) Radiation and host factors in human thyroid tumors following thymus irradiation. *Health Phys.*, **38**, 451–465

Shore, R.E., Albert, R.E., Reed, M., Harley, N. & Pasternack, B. (1984) Skin cancer incidence among children irradiated for ringworm of the scalp. *Radiat. Res.*, **100**, 192–204

Shore, R.E., Woodard, E., Hildreth, N., Dvoretsky, P., Hempelmann, L. & Pasternack, B. (1985) Thyroid tumors following thymus irradiation. *J. natl Cancer Inst.*, **74**, 1177–1184

Shore, R.E., Hildreth, N., Woodard, E., Dvoretsky, P., Hempelmann, L. & Pasternack, B. (1986) Breast cancer among women given X-ray therapy for acute postpartum mastitis. *J. natl Cancer Inst.*, **77**, 689–696

Shore, R.E., Hildreth, N., Dvoretsky, P., Andresen, E., Moseson, M. & Pasternack, B. (1993) Thyroid cancer among persons given X-ray treatment in infancy for an enlarged thymus gland. *Am. J. Epidemiol.*, **137**, 1068–1080

Sikpi, M.O., Dry, S.M., Freedman, M.L. & Lurie, A.G. (1992) Mutations caused by gamma-radiation-induced double-strand breaks in a shuttle plasmid replicated in human lymphoblasts. *Int. J. Radiat. Biol.*, **62**, 555–562

Siliciano, J.D., Canman, C.E., Taya, Y., Sakaguchi, K., Appella, E. & Kastan, M.B. (1997) DNA damage induces phosphorylation of the amino terminus of p53. *Genes Dev.*, **11**, 3471–3481

Sinclair, W.K. (1964) X-ray-induced heritable damage (small-colony formation) in cultured mammalian cells. *Radiat. Res.*, **21**, 584–611

Sinclair, W.K. (1998) The linear no-threshold response: Why not linearity? *Med. Phys.* **25**, 285–290

Skandalis, A., da-Cruz, A.D., Curry, J., Nohturfft, A., Curado, M.P. & Glickman, B.W. (1997) Molecular analysis of T-lymphocyte HPRT⁻ mutations in individuals exposed to ionizing radiation in Goiania, Brazil. *Environ. Mol. Mutag.*, **29**, 107–116

Skomedal, H., Helland, Å., Kristensen, G.B., Holm, R. & Børresen-Dale, A.-L. (1999) Allelic imbalance at chromosome region 11q23 in cervical carcinoma. *Eur. J. Cancer*, **35**, 659–663

van Sloun, P.P., Wijnhoven, S.W., Kool, H.J., Slater, R., Weeda, G., Van Zeeland, A.A., Lohman, P.H.M & Vrieling, H. (1998) Determination of spontaneous loss of heterozygosity mutations in *Aprt* heterozygous mice. *Nucl. Acids Res.*, **26**, 4888–4894

Smith, P.G. & Doll, R. (1981) Mortality from cancer and all causes among British radiologists. *Br. J. Radiol.*, **54**, 187–194

Smith, L.E. & Grosovsky, A.J. (1993) Evidence for high-frequency allele loss at the aprt locus in TK6 human lymphoblasts. *Mutat. Res.*, **289**, 245–254

Socolow, E.L., Hashizume, A., Neriishi, S. & Niitani, R. (1963) Thyroid carcinoma in man after exposure to ionizing radiation. A summary of the findings in Hiroshima and Nagasaki. *New Engl. J. Med.*, **268**, 406–410

Southern, E.M. (1975) Detection of specific sequences among DNA fragments separated by gel electrophoresis. *J. mol. Biol.*, **98**, 503–517

Spector, B.D., Filipovich, A.H., Perry, G.S., III & Kersey, J.H. (1982) Epidemiology of cancer in ataxia-telangiectasia. In: Bridges, B.A. & Harnden, D.G., eds, *Ataxia-Telangiectasia—*

A Cellular and Molecular Link between Cancer, Neuropathology and Immune Deficiency, New York, John Wiley & Sons, pp. 103–138

Spengler, R.F., Cook, D.H., Clarke, E.A., Olley, P.M. & Newman, A.M. (1983) Cancer mortality following cardiac catheterization: A preliminary follow-up study on 4,891 irradiated children. *Pediatrics*, **71**, 235–239

Sproston, A.R.M., West, C.M.L. & Hendry, J.H. (1997) Cellular radiosensitivity in human severe-combined-immunodeficiency (SCID) syndromes. *Radiother. Oncol.*, **42**, 53–57

Stacey, M., Thacker, S. & Taylor, A.M. (1989) Cultured skin keratinocytes from both normal individuals and basal cell naevus syndrome patients are more resistant to gamma-rays and UV light compared with cultured skin fibroblasts. *Int. J. Radiat. Biol.*, **56**, 45–58

Stanbridge, E.J. (1990) Human tumor suppressor genes. *Annu. Rev. Genet.*, **24**, 615–657

Stankovic, T., Weber, P., Stewart, G., Bedenham, T., Murray, J., Byrd, P.J., Moss, P.A.H. & Taylor, A.M.R. (1999) Inactivation of ataxia telangiectasia mutated gene in B-cell chronic lymphocytic leukaemia. *Lancet*, **353**, 26–29

Starostik, P., Manshouri, T., O'Brien, S., Freireich, E., Kantarjian, H., Haidar, M., Lerner, S., Keating, M. & Albitar, M. (1998) Deficiency of the ATM protein expression defines an aggressive subgroup of B-cell chronic lymphocytic leukemia. *Cancer Res.*, **58**, 4552–4557

Steiner, M., Burkart, W., Grosche, B., Kaletsch, U. & Michaelis, J. (1998) Trends in infant leukaemia in West Germany in relation to in utero exposure due to the Chernobyl accident. *Radiat. environ. Biophys.*, **37**, 87–93

Stevens, W., Thomas, D.C., Lyon, J.L., Till, J.E., Kerber, R.A., Simon, S.L., Lloyd, R.D., Elghany, N.A. & Preston-Martin, S. (1990) Leukemia in Utah and radioactive fallout from the Nevada test site. A case–control study. *J. Am. med. Assoc.*, **264**, 585–591

Stewart, A., Webb, J. & Hewitt, D. (1958) A survey of childhood malignancies. *Br. med. J.*, **5086**, 1495–1508

Stilgenbauer, S., Schaffner, C., Litterst, A., Liebisch, P., Gilad, S., Bar-Shira, A., James, M.R., Lichter, P. & Dohner, H. (1997) Biallelic mutations in the *ATM* gene in T-prolymphocytic leukemia. *Nature Med.*, **3**, 1155–1159

Stjernfeldt, M., Samuelsson, L. & Ludvigsson, J. (1987) Radiation in dwellings and cancer in children. *Pediatr. Hematol. Oncol.*, **4**, 55–61

Stoppa-Lyonnet, D., Girault, D., LeDeist, F. & Aurias, A. (1992) Unusual T cell clones in a patient with Nijimegen breakage syndrome. *J. med. Genet.*, **29**, 136–137.

Stoppa-Lyonnet, D., Soulier, J., Laugé, A., Dastot, H., Garand, R., Sigaux, F. & Stern, M.-H. (1998) Inactivation of the *ATM* gene in T-cell prolymphocytic leukemias. *Blood*, **91**, 3920–3926

Storer, J.B., Mitchell, T.J. & Fry, R.J.M. (1988) Extrapolation of the relative risk of radiogenic neoplasms across mouse strains and to man. *Radiat. Res.*, **114**, 331–353

Storm, H.H., Iversen, E. & Boice, J.D., Jr (1986) Breast cancer following multiple chest fluoroscopies among tuberculosis patients. A case–control study in Denmark. *Acta radiol. oncol.*, **25**, 233–238

Storm, H.H., Andersson, M., Boice, J.D., Jr, Blettner, M., Stovall, M., Mouridsen, H.T., Dombernowsky, P., Rose, C., Jacobsen, A. & Pedersen, M. (1992) Adjuvant radiotherapy and risk of contralateral breast cancer. *J. natl Cancer Inst.*, **84**, 1245–1250

Stratton, M.R. & Wooster, R. (1996) Hereditary predisposition to breast cancer. *Curr. Opin. Genet. Dev.*, **6**, 93–97

Straub, W., Miller, M., Sanislow, C. & Fishbeck, W. (1982) Radiation and risk for thyroid cancer. Atypical findings of a community thyroid recall program. *Clin. nucl. Med.*, **6**, 272–276

Straume, T., Langlois, R.G., Lucas, J., Jensen, R.H., Bigbee, W.L., Ramalho, A.T. & Brandao-Mello, C.E. (1991) Novel biodosimetry methods applied to victims of the Goiania accident. *Health Phys.*, **60**, 71–76

Stumm, M., Seemanová, E., Gatti, R.A., Sperling, K., Reis, A. & Wagner, R.-D. (1995) The ataxia-telangiectasia-variant genes 1 and 2 show no linkage to the A-T candidate region on chromosome 11q22-23. *Am. J. hum. Genet.*, **57**, 960–962

Su, L.-K., Kinzle, K.W., Vogelstein, B., Preisinger, A.C., Moser, A.R., Luongo, C., Gould, K.A. & Dove, W.F. (1992) Multiple intestinal neoplasia caused by a mutation in the murine homolog of the APC gene. *Science*, **256**, 668–670

Sullivan, K.E., Veksler, E., Lederman, H. & Lees-Miller, S.P. (1997) Cell cycle checkpoints and DNA repair in Nijmegen breakage syndrome. *Clin. Immunol. Immunopathol.*, **82**, 43–48

Suzuki, K. (1997) Multistep nature of X-ray-induced neoplastic transformation in mammalian cells: Genetic alterations and instability. *J. Radiat. Res. Tokyo*, **38**, 55–63

Swift, M., Morrell, D., Massey, R.B. & Chase, C.L. (1991) Incidence of cancer in 161 families affected by ataxia-telangiectasia. *New Engl. J. Med.*, **325**, 1831–1836

Szabo, C.I. & King, M.C. (1995) Inherited breast and ovarian cancer. *Hum. mol. Genet.*, **4**, 1811–1817

Taalman, R.D.F.M., Jaspers, N.G.J., Scheres, J.M.J.C., de Wit, J. & Hustinx, T.W.J. (1983) Hypersensitivity to ionizing radiation, in vitro, in a new chromosomal breakage disorder, the Nijmegen breakage syndrome. *Mutat. Res.*, **112**, 23–32

Taalman, R.D.F.M., Hustinx, T.W.J., Weemaes, C.M.R., Seemanová, E., Schmidt, A., Passarge, E. & Scheres, J.M.J.C. (1989) Further delineation of the Nijmegen breakage syndrome. *Am. J. med. Genet.*, **32**, 425–431

Taghian, A., de Vathaire, F., Terrier, P., Le, M., Auquier, A., Mouriesse, H., Grimaud, E., Sarrazin, D. & Tubiana, M. (1991) Long-term risk of sarcoma following radiation treatment for breast cancer. *Int. J. Radiat. Oncol. Biol. Phys.*, **21**, 361–367

Takeuchi, S., Koike, M., Park, S., Seriu, T., Bartram, C.R., Taub, H.E., Williamson, I.K., Grewal, J., Taguchi, H. & Koeffler, H.P. (1998) The *ATM* gene and susceptibility to childhood T-cell acute lymphoblastic leukaemia. *Br. J. Haematol.*, **103**, 536–568

Tao, Z.-F. & Wei, L.X. (1986) An epidemiological investigation of mutational diseases in the high background radiation area of Yangjiang, China. *J. Radiat. Res.*, **27**, 141–150

Taylor, L.S. (1981) The development of radiation protection standards (1925–1940). *Health Phys.*, **41**, 227–232

Taylor, A.M.R. & Butterworth, S.V. (1986) Clonal evolution of T-cell chronic lymphocytic leukaemia in a patient with ataxia telangiectasia. *Int. J. Cancer*, **37**, 511–516

Taylor, A.M.R., Harnden, D.G., Arlett, C.F., Harcourt, S.A., Lehmann, A.R., Stevens, S. & Bridges, B.A. (1975) Ataxia-telangiectasia: A human mutation with abnormal radiation sensitivity. *Nature*, **4**, 427–429

Taylor, A.M., Metcalfe, J.R., Oxford, J.M. & Harnden, D.G. (1976) Is chromatid-type damage in ataxia-telangiectasia after irradiation at G_0 a consequence of defective repair? *Nature*, **260**, 441–443

Taylor, A.M.R., Lowe, P.A., Stacey, M., Thick, J., Campbell, L., Beatty, D., Biggs, P. & Formstone, C.J. (1992) Development of T-cell leukaemia in an ataxia telangiectasia patient following clonal selection in t(X;14)-containing lymphocytes. *Leukemia*, **6**, 961–966

Taylor, A.M.R., Metcalfe, J.A., Thick, J. & Mak, Y.-F. (1996) Leukemia and lymphoma in ataxia-telangiectasia. *Blood*, **87**, 423–438

Terzaghi, M. & Little, J.B. (1976) X-radiation-induced transformation in a C3H mouse embryo-derived cell line. *Cancer Res.*, **36**, 1367–74

Thacker, J. (1992) Radiation-induced mutation in mammalian cells at low doses and dose rates. *Adv. Radiat. Biol.*, **16**, 77–124

Thacker, J., Stephens, M.A. & Stretch, A. (1978) Mutation to ouabain-resistance in Chinese hamster cells: Induction by ethyl methanesulphonate and lack of induction by ionising radiation. *Mutat. Res.*, **51**, 255–270

Thames, H.D. & Hendry, J.H. (1987) *Fractionation in Radiotherapy*, London, Taylor & Francis

Thomas, D., Darby, S., Fagnani, F., Hubert, P., Vaeth, M. & Weiss, K. (1992) Definition and estimation of lifetime detriment from radiation exposures: Principles and methods. *Health Phys.*, **63**, 259–272

Thomas, D.B., Rosenblatt, K., Jimenez, L.M., McTiernan, A., Stalsberg, H., Stemhagen, A., Thompson, W.D., McCrea Curnen, M.G., Satariano, W., Austin, D.F., Greenberg, R.S., Key, C., Kolonel, L.N. & West, D.W. (1994) Ionizing radiation and breast cancer in men (United States). *Cancer Causes Control*, **5**, 9–14

Thompson, D.E., Mabuchi, K., Ron, E., Soda, M., Tokunaga, M., Ochikubo, S., Sugimoto, S., Ikeda, T., Terasaki, M., Izumi, S. & Preston, D.L. (1994) Cancer incidence in atomic bomb survivors. Part II: Solid tumors, 1958–1987. *Radiat. Res.*, **137** (Suppl. 2), S17–S67

Tibbetts, R.S., Brumbaugh, K.M., Williams, J.M., Sarkaria, J.N., Cliby, W.A., Shieh, S-Y., Taya, Y., Prives, C. & Abraham, R.T. (1999) A role for ATR in the DNA damage-induced phosphorylation of p53. *Genes Dev.*, **13**, 152–157

Tinkey, P.T., Lembo, T.M., Evans, G.R., Cundiff, J.H., Gray, K.N. & Price, R.E. (1998) Post-irradiation sarcomas in Sprague-Dawley rats. *Radiat. Res.*, **149**, 401–404

Tirmarche, M., Rannou, A., Mollie, A. & Sauve, A. (1988) Epidemiological study of regional cancer mortality in France and natural radiation. *Radiat. Prot. Dosim.*, **24**, 479–482

Tokarskaya, Z.B., Okladnikova, N.D., Belyaeva, Z.D. & Drozhko, E.G. (1997) Multifactorial analysis of lung cancer dose–response relationships for workers at the Mayak nuclear enterprise. *Health Phys.*, **73**, 899–905

Tokunaga, M., Land, C.E., Tokuoka, S., Nishimori, I., Soda, M. & Akiba, S. (1994) Incidence of female breast cancer among atomic bomb survivors, 1950–1985. *Radiat. Res.*, **138**, 209–223

Tomonaga, M., Matsuo, T., Carter, R.L., Bennett, J.M., Kuriyama, K., Imanaka, F., Kusumi, S., Mabuchi, K., Kuramoto, A., Kamada, N., Ichimaru, M., Pisciotta, A.V. & Finch, S.C. (1991) *Differential Effects of Atomic Bomb Irradiation in Inducing Major Leukemia Types: Analysis of Open-city Cases including the Life Span Study Cohort Based upon Updated Diagnostic Systems and the Dosimetry System 1986 (DS86)* (RERF TR 9-91), Hiroshima, Radiation Effects Research Foundation

Trapeznikov, A.V., Pozolotina, V.N., Chebotina, M.Y., Chukanov, V.N., Trapeznikova, V.N., Kulikov, N.V., Nielsen, S.P. & Aarkrog, A. (1993) Radioactive contamination of the Techa river; the Urals. *Health Phys.*, **65**, 481–488

Travis, E.L. (1987) Relative radiosensitivity of the human lung. *Adv. Radiat. Biol.*, **12**, 205–238

Travis, L.B., Curtis, R.E., Stovall, M., Holowaty, E.J., Van Leeuwen, F.E., Glimelius, B., Lynch, C.F., Hagenbeek, A., Li, C.-Y., Banks, P.M., Gospodarowicz, M.K., Adami, J., Wacholder, S., Inskip, P.D., Tucker, M.A. & Boice, J.D., Jr (1994) Risk of leukemia following treatment for non-Hodgkin's lymphoma. *J. natl Cancer Inst.*, **86**, 1450–1457

Travis, L.B., Curtis, R.E., Glimelius, B., Holowaty, E.J., Van Leeuwen, F.E., Lynch, C.F., Hagenbeek, A., Stovall, M., Banks, P.M., Adami, J., Gospodarowicz, M.K., Wacholder, S., Inskip, P.D., Tucker, M.A. & Boice, J.D., Jr (1995) Bladder and kidney cancer following cyclophosphamide therapy for non-Hodgkin's lymphoma. *J. natl Cancer Inst.*, **87**, 524–530

Travis, L.B., Curtis, R.E., Storm, H., Hall, P., Holowaty, E., Van Leeuwen, F.E., Kohler, B.A., Pukkala, E., Lynch, C.F., Andersson, M., Bergfeldt, K., Clarke, E.A., Wiklund, T., Stoter, G., Gospodarowicz, M, Sturgeon, J., Fraumeni, J.F., Jr & Boice, J.D., Jr (1997) Risk of second malignant neoplasms among long-term survivors of testicular cancer. *J. natl Cancer Inst.*, **89**, 1429–1439

Travis, L.B., Holowaty, E., Bergfeldt, K., Lynch, C.F., Kohler, B.A., Wiklund, T., Curtis, R.E., Hall, P., Andersson, M., Pukkala, E., Sturgeon, J. & Stovall, M. (1999) Risk of leukemia after platinum-based chemotherapy for ovarian cancer. *New Eng. J. Med.*, **340**, 351–357

Tsyb, A.F., Stepanenko, V.F., Pitkevich, V.A., Ispenkov, E.A., Sevan'kaev, A.V., Orlov, M., Dmitriev, E.V., Sarapul'tsev, I.A., Zhigareva, T.L. & Prokof'ev, O.N. (1990) [Around the Semipalatinsk proving grounds: The radioecological situation and the population radiation doses in Semipalatinsk Province (based on data from the report of the Interdepartmental Commission.] *Med. Radiol. Mosk.*, **35**, 3–11 (in Russian)

Tucker, M.A., Meadows, A.T., Boice, J.D., Jr, Hoover, R.N. & Fraumeni, J.F., Jr (1984) Cancer risk following treatment of childhood cancer. In: Boice, J.D., Jr & Fraumeni, J.F., Jr, eds, *Radiation Carcinogenesis: Epidemiology and Biological Significance*, New York, Raven Press, pp. 211–224

Tucker, M.A., D'Angio, G.J., Boice, J.D., Jr, Strong, L.C., Li, F.P., Stovall, M., Stone, B.J., Green, D.M., Lombardi, F., Newton, W., Hoover, R.N. & Fraumeni, J.F., Jr (1987a) Bone sarcomas linked to radiotherapy and chemotherapy in children. *New Engl. J. Med.*, **317**, 588–593

Tucker, M.A., Meadows, A.T., Boice, J.D., Jr, Stovall, M., Oberlin, O., Stone, B.J., Birch, J., Voûte, P.A., Hoover, R.N. & Fraumeni, J.F., Jr for the Late Effects Study Group (1987b) Leukemia after therapy with alkylating agents for childhood cancer. *J. natl Cancer Inst.*, **78**, 459–464

Tucker, M.A., Jones, P.H.M., Boice, J.D., Jr, Robison, L.L., Stone, B.J., Stovall, M., Jenkin, R.D.T., Lubin, J.H., Baum, E.S., Siegel, S.E., Meadows, A.T., Hoover, R.N. & Fraumeni, J.F., Jr for the Late Effects Study Group (1991) Therapeutic radiation at a young age is linked to secondary thyroid cancer. *Cancer Res.*, **51**, 2885–2888

Tucker, M.A., Murray, N., Shaw, E.D., Ettinger, D.S., Mabry, M., Huber, M.H., Feld, R., Shepherd, F.A., Johnson, D.H., Grant, S.T., Aisner, J. & Johnson, B.E. (1997) Second primary cancers related to smoking and treatment of small-cell lung cancer. Lung Cancer Working Cadre. *J. natl Cancer Inst.*, **89**, 1782–1788

Tupler, R., Marseglia, G.L., Stefanini, M., Prosperi, E., Chessa, L., Nardo, T., Marchi, A. & Maraschio, P. (1997) A variant of the Nijmegen breakage syndrome with unusual cytogenetic features and intermediate cellular radiosensitivity. *J. med. Genet.*, **34**, 196–202

Turker, M., Walker, K.A., Jennings, C.D., Mellon, I., Yusufji, A. & Urano, M. (1995) Spontaneous and ionizing radiation induced mutations involve large events when selecting for loss of an autosomal locus. *Mutat. Res.*, **329**, 97–105

Uhrhammer, N., Bay, J., Pernin, D., Rio, P., Grancho, M., Kwiatkowski, F., Gosse-Brun, S., Daver, A. & Bignon, Y. (1998) Loss of heterozygosity at the *ATM* locus in colorectal carcinoma. *Oncol. Rep.*, **6**, 655–658

Ulrich, H. (1946) Incidence of leukemia in radiologists. *New Engl. J. Med.*, **234**, 45–46

Ullrich, R.L. (1980) Effects of split doses of X rays or neutrons on lung tumor formation in RFM mice. *Radiat. Res.*, **83**, 138–145

Ullrich, R.L. (1983) Tumor induction in BALB/c female mice after fission neutron or gamma irradiation. *Radiat. Res.*, **93**, 506–515

Ullrich, R.L. & Ponnaiya, B. (1998) Radiation-induced instability and its relation to radiation carcinogenesis. *Int. J. Radiat. Biol.*, **74**, 747–754

Ullrich, R.L. & Storer, J.B. (1979a) Influence of γ irradiation on the development of neoplastic disease in mice. I. Reticular tissue tumors. *Radiat. Res.*, **80**, 303–316

Ullrich, R.L. & Storer, J.B. (1979b) Influence of γ irradiation on the development of neoplastic disease in mice. II. Solid tumors. *Radiat. Res.*, **80**, 317–324

Ullrich, R.L. & Storer, J.B. (1979c) Influence of γ irradiation on the development of neoplastic disease in mice. III. Dose-rate effects. *Radiat. Res.*, **80**, 325–342

Ullrich, R.L., Jernigan, M.C. & Adams, L.M. (1979) Induction of lung tumors in RFM mice after localized exposures of X rays and neutrons. *Radiat. Res.*, **80**, 464–473

Ullrich, R.L., Jernigan, M.C., Satterfield, L.C. & Bowles, N.D. (1987) Radiation carcinogenesis: Time–dose relationships. *Radiat. Res.*, **111**, 179–184

Ullrich, R.L., Bowles, N.D., Satterfield, L.C. & Davis, C.M. (1996) Strain-dependent suscepti-bility to radiation-induced mammary cancer is a result of differences in epithelial cell sensitivity to transformation. *Radiat. Res.*, **146**, 353–355

UNSCEAR (United Nations Scientific Committee on the Effects of Atomic Radiation) (1972) *Ionizing Radiation Levels and Effects, Vol. 2, Effects*, New York, United Nations

UNSCEAR (United Nations Scientific Committee on the Effects of Atomic Radiation) (1986) *Genetic and Somatic Effects of Ionizing Radiation* (United Nations Sales Publication E.86.IX.9), New York, United Nations

UNSCEAR (United Nations Scientific Committee on the Effects of Atomic Radiation) (1988) *Sources, Effects and Risks of Ionizing Radiation. 1988 Report to the General Assembly with Annexes* (United Nations Sales publication E.88.IX.7), New York, United Nations

UNSCEAR (United Nations Scientific Committee on the Effects of Atomic Radiation) (1993) *Sources and Effects of Ionizing Radiation. 1993 Report to the General Assembly* (United Nations Sales publication E.94.IX.2), New York, United Nations

UNSCEAR (United Nations Scientific Committee on the Effects of Atomic Radiation) (1994) *Sources and Effects of Ionizing Radiation, 1994 Report to the General Assembly with*

Scientific Annexes (United Nations Sales Publication E.94.IX.11), New York, United Nations

Upton, A.C. (1968) Radiation carcinogenesis. In: Busch, H., ed., *Methods in Cancer Research*, Vol. 4, New York, Academic Press, pp. 53–82

Upton, A.C. (1981) Health impact of the Three Mile Island accident. *Ann. N.Y. Acad. Sci.*, **365**, 63–75

Upton, A.C. (1999) The linear–nonthreshold dose–response model: A critical reappraisal. In: NCRP Proceedings No. 21, Bethesda, MD, National Council on Radiation Protection and Measurements, pp. 9–31

Upton, A.C., Randolph, M.L. & Conklin, J.W. (1970) Late effects of fast neutrons and gamma-rays in mice as influenced by the dose rate of irradiation: Induction of neoplasia. *Radiat. Res.*, **41**, 467–491

Urlaub, G. & Chasin, L.A. (1980) Isolation of Chinese hamster cell mutants deficient in dihydrofolate reductase activity. *Proc. natl Acad. Sci. USA*, **77**, 4216–4220

Urquhart, J.D., Black, R.J., Muirhead, M.J., Sharp, L., Maxwell, M., Eden, O.B. & Jones, D.A. (1991) Case–control study of leukaemia and non-Hodgkin's lymphoma in children in Caithness near the Dounreay nuclear installation. *Br. med. J.*, **302**, 687–692

Varon, R., Vissinga, C., Platzer, M., Cerosaletti, K.M., Chrzanowska, K.H., Saar, K., Beckmann, G., Seemanová, E., Cooper, P.R., Nowak, N.J., Stumm, M., Weemaes, C.M.R., Gatti, R.A., Wilson, R.K., Digweed, M., Rosenthal, A., Sperling, K., Concannon, P. & Reis, A. (1998) Nibrin, a novel DNA double-strand break repair protein, is mutated in Nijmegen breakage syndrome. *Cell*, **93**, 467–476

de Vathaire, F., Francois, P., Hill, C., Schweisguth, O., Rodary, C., Sarrazin, D., Oberlin, O., Beurtheret, C., Dutreix, A. & Flamant, R. (1989) Role of radiotherapy and chemotherapy in the risk of second malignant neoplasms after cancer in childhood. *Br. J. Cancer*, **59**, 792–796

de Vathaire, F., Francois, P., Schlumberger, M., Schweisguth, O., Hardiman, C., Grimaud, E., Oberlin, O., Hill, C., Lemerle, J. & Flamant, R. (1992) Epidemiological evidence for a common mechanism for neuroblastoma and differentiated thyroid tumour. *Br. J. Cancer*, **65**, 425–428

de Vathaire, F., Hardiman, C., Shamsaldin, A., Campbell, S., Grimaud, E., Hawkins, M., Raquin, M., Oberlin, O., Diallo, I., Zucker, J.M., Panis, X., Lagrange, J.L., Daly-Schveitzer, N., Lemerle, J., Chavaudra, J., Schlumberger, M. & Bonaiti, C. (1999a) Thyroid carcinomas after irradiation for a first cancer during childhood. *Arch. intern. Med.*, **159**, 2713–2719

de Vathaire, F., Hawkins, M.M., Campbell, S., Oberlin, O., Raquin, M.-A., Schlienger, J.-Y., Shamsaldin, A., Diallo, I., Bell, J., Grimaud, E., Hardiman, C., Lagrange, J.-L., Daly-Schveitzer, N., Panis, X., Zucker, J.-M., Sancho-Garnier, H., Eschwège, F., Chavaudra, J. & Lemerle, J. (1999b) Second malignant neoplasms after a first cancer in childhood: Temporal patten of risk according to the type of treatment. *Br. J. Cancer*, **79**, 1884–1893

Venkateswarlu, D. & Leszczynski, J. (1998) Tautomeric equilibria in 8-oxopurines: Implications for mutagenicity. *J. Comput. Aided Mol. Des.*, **12**, 373–382

Viel, J.-F., Pobel, D. & Carré, A. (1995) Incidence of leukaemia in young people around the La Hague nuclear waste reprocessing plant: A sensitivity analysis. *Stat. Med.*, **14**, 2459–2472

Vincent, R.A., Jr, Sheriden, R.B., III & Huang, P.C. (1975) DNA strained breakage repair in ataxia-telangiectasia fibroblast-like cells. *Mutat. Res.*, **33**, 357–366

Virgilio, L., Isobe, M., Narducci, M.G., Carotenuto, P., Camerini, B., Kurosawa, N., Rushdi, A.-A., Croce, C.M. & Russo, G. (1993) Chromosome walking on the *TCL1* locus involved in T-cell neoplasia. *Proc. natl Acad. Sci. USA*, **90**, 9275–9279

Virgilio. L., Narducci, M.G., Isobe, M., Billips, L.G., Cooper, M.D., Croce, C.M. & Russo, G. (1994) Identification of the *TCL1* gene involved in T-cell malignancies. *Proc. natl Acad. Sci. USA*, **91**, 12530–12534

Virgilio, L., Lazzeri, C., Bichi, R., Nibu, K.-I., Narducci, M.G., Russo, G., Rothstein, J.L. & Croce, C.M. (1998) Deregulated expression of *TCL1* causes T cell leukemia in mice. *Proc. natl Acad. Sci. USA*, **95**, 3885–3889

Vorechovsky, I., Luo, L., Dyer, M.J., Catovsky, D., Amlot, P.L., Yaxley, J.C., Foroni, L., Hammarström, L., Webster, A.D.B. & Yuille, M.A.R. (1997) Clustering of missense mutations in the ataxia-telangiectasia gene in a sporadic T-cell leukaemia. *Nat. Genet.*, **17**, 96–99

Vorobtsova, I.E. & Kitaev, E.M. (1988) Urethane-induced lung adenomas in the first-generation progeny of irradiated male mice. *Carcinogenesis*, **9**, 1931–1934

Vorobtsova, I.E., Aliyakparova, L.M. & Anisimov, V.N. (1993) Promotion of skin tumors by 12-*O*-tetradecanoylphorbol-13-acetate in two generations of descendants of male mice exposed to X-ray irradiation. *Mutat. Res.*, **287**, 207–216

Waghray, M., Al-Sedairy, S., Ozand, P.T. & Hannan, M.A. (1990) Cytogenetic characterization of ataxia telangiectasia (AT) heterozygotes using lymphoblastoid cell lines and chronic γ-irradiation. *Hum. Genet.*, **84**, 532–534

Waha, A., Sturne, C., Kessler, A., Koch, A., Kreyer, E., Fimmers, R., Wiestler, O.D., von Deimling, A., Krebs, D. & Schmutzler, R.K. (1998) Expression of the ATM gene is significantly reduced in sporadic breast carcinomas. *Int. J. Cancer*, **78**, 306–309

Walburg, H.E. & Cosgrove, G.E. (1969) Reticular neoplasms in irradiated and unirradiated germ free mice. In: Mirand, E.A. & Back, N., eds, *Germ-Free Biology*, New York, Plenum, pp. 135–141

Wald, N. (1971) Haematological parameters after acute radiation injury. In: *Manual on Radiation Haematology*, Vienna, International Atomic Energy Agency, pp. 253–264

Walter, S.D., Meigs, J.W. & Heston, J.F. (1986) The relationship of cancer incidence to terrestrial radiation and population density in Connecticut, 1935–1974. *Am. J. Epidemiol.*, **123**, 1–14

Wang, J.-X., Inskip, P.D., Boice, J.D., Jr, Li, B.-X., Zhang, J.-Y. & Fraumeni, J.F., Jr (1990a) Cancer incidence among medical diagnostic X-ray workers in China, 1950 to 1985. *Int. J. Cancer*, **45**, 889–895

Wang, Z., Boice, J.D., Jr, Wei, L., Beebe, G.W., Zha, Y., Kaplan, M.M., Tao, Z., Maxon, H.R., III, Zhang, S., Schneider, A.B., Tan, B., Wesseler, T.A., Chen, D., Ershow, A.G., Kleinerman, R.A., Littlefield, L.G. & Preston, D. (1990b) Thyroid nodularity and chromosome aberrations among women in areas of high background radiation in China. *J. natl Cancer Inst.*, **82**, 478–485

Watanabe, K.K., Kang, H.K. & Dalager, N.A. (1995) Cancer mortality risk among military participants of a 1958 atmospheric nuclear weapons test. *Am. J. public Health*, **85**, 523–527

Watters, D., Khanna, K.K., Beamish, H., Birrell, G., Spring, K., Kedar, P., Gatei, M., Stenzel, D., Hobson, K., Kozlov, S., Zhang, N., Farrell, A., Ramsay, J., Gatti, R. & Lavin, M.F. (1997) Cellular localisation of the ataxia-telangiectasia (ATM) gene products and discrimination between mutated and normal forms. *Oncogene*, **14**, 1911–1921

Weemaes, C.M.R., Hustinx, T.W.J., Scheres, J.M.J.C., van Munster, P.J.J., Bakkeren, J.A.J.M. & Taalman, R.D.F.M. (1981) A new chromosomal instability disorder: The Nijmegen breakage-syndrome. *Acta paediatr. scand.*, **70**, 557–564

Weemaes, C.M.R., Smeets, D.F.C.M. & van der Burgt, C.J.A.M. (1994) Nijmegen breakage syndrome: A progress report. *Int. J. Radiat. Biol.*, **66**, 185–188

Wei, L.-X. & Wang, J.-Z. (1994) Estimate of cancer risk for a large population continuously exposed to higher background radiation in Yangjiang, China. *Chin. med. J.*, **107**, 541–544

Wei, L.-X., Zha, Y.-G., Tao, Z.-F., He, W.-H, Chen, D.-Q. & Yuan, Y.-L. (1990) Epidemiological investigation of radiological effects in high background radiation areas of Yangjiang, China. *J. Radiat. Res.*, **31**, 119–136

Weichselbaum R.R., Nove, J. & Little, J.B. (1978) Deficient recovery from potentially lethal radiation damage in ataxia telangiectasia and xeroderma pigmentosum. *Nature*, **271**, 261–262

Weinberg, C.R., Brown, K.G. & Hoel, D.G. (1987) Altitude, radiation, and mortality from cancer and heart disease. *Radiat. Res.*, **112**, 381–390

Weiss, H.A., Darby, S.C. & Doll, R. (1994) Cancer mortality following X-ray treatment for ankylosing spondylitis. *Int. J. Cancer*, **59**, 327–338

Weiss, H.A., Darby, S.C., Fearn, T. & Doll, R. (1995) Leukemia mortality after X-ray treatment for ankylosing spondylitis. *Radiat. Res.*, **142**, 1–11

Weissenborn, U. & Streffer, C. (1988) Analysis of structural and numerical chromosomal anomalies at the first, second, and third mitosis after irradiation of one-cell mouse embryos with X-rays or neutrons. *Int. J. Radiat. Biol.*, **54**, 381–394

Weissenborn, U. & Streffer, C. (1989) Analysis of structural and numerical chromosomal aberrations at the first and second mitosis after X irradiation of two-cell mouse embryos. *Radiat. Res.*, **117**, 214–220

West, C.M. & Hendry, J.H. (1992) Intrinsic radiosensitivity as a predictor of patient response to radiotherapy. *Br. J. Radiother.*, **Suppl. 24**, 146–152

White, S.C. (1992) 1992 assessment of radiation risk from dental radiograph. *Radiology*, **21**, 118–126

Wiggs, L.D., Johnson, E.R., Cox-DeVore, C.A. & Voelz, G.L. (1994) Mortality through 1990 among white male workers at the Los Alamos National Laboratory: Considering exposures to plutonium and external ionizing radiation. *Health Phys.*, **67**, 577–588

Wijnhoven, S.W., Van Sloun, P.P., Kool, H.J., Weeda, G., Slater, R., Lohman, P.H.M., Van Zeeland, A.A. & Vrieling, H. (1998) Carcinogen-induced loss of heterozygosity at the *Aprt* locus in somatic cells of the mouse. *Proc. natl Acad. Sci. USA*, **95**, 13759–13764

Wilkinson, G.S., Tietjen, G.L., Wiggs, L.D., Galke, W.A., Acquavella, J.F., Reyes, M., Voelz, G.L. & Waxweiler, R.J. (1987) Mortality among plutonium and other radiation workers at a plutonium weapons facility. *Am. J. Epidemiol.*, **125**, 231–250

Winegar, R.A., Lutze, L.H., Hamer, J.D., O'Loughlin, K.G. & Mirsalis, J.C. (1994) Radiation-induced point mutations, deletions and micronuclei in *lacI* transgenic mice. *Mutat. Res.*, **307**, 479–487

Wing, S., Shy, C.M., Wood, J.L., Wolf, S., Cragle, D.L. & Frome, E.L. (1991) Mortality among workers at Oak Ridge National Laboratory: Evidence of radiation effects in follow-up through 1984. *J. Am. med. Assoc.*, **265**, 1397–1402

Wing, S., Richardson, D., Armstrong, D. & Crawford-Brown, D. (1997) A reevaluation of cancer incidence near the Three Mile Island nuclear plant: The collision of evidence and assumptions. *Environ. Health Perspectives*, **105**, 52–57

Wingren, G., Hatschek, T. & Axelson, O. (1993) Determinants of papillary cancer of the thyroid. *Am. J. Epidemiol.*, **138**, 482–491

Wingren, G., Hallquist, A. & Hardell, L. (1997) Diagnostic X-ray exposure and female papillary thyroid cancer: A pooled analysis of two Swedish studies. *Eur. J. Cancer Prev.*, **6**, 550–556

Withers, H.R. (1967) The dose–survival relationship for irradiation of epithelial cells of mouse skin. *Br. J. Radiol.*, **40**, 187–194

Withers, H.R. (1989) Failla Memorial Lecture. Contrarian concepts in the progress of radiotherapy. *Radiat. Res.*, **119**, 395–412

Withers, H.R. & Elkind, M.M. (1970) Microcolony survival assay for cells of mouse intestinal mucosa exposed to radiation. *Int. J. Radiat. Biol.*, **17**, 261–267

Withers, H.R., Hunter, N., Barkley, H.T., Jr & Reid, B.O. (1974) Radiation survival and regeneration characteristics of spermatogenic stem cells of mouse testis. *Radiat. Res.*, **57**, 88–103

Withers, H.R., Peters, L.J. & Kogelnik, H.D. (1980) The pathobiology of late effects of irradiation. In: Meyn, R.E. & Withers, H.R., eds, *Radiation Biology in Cancer Research*, New York, Raven Press, pp. 439–448

Withers, H.R., Mason, K.A. & Thames, H.D., Jr (1986) Late radiation response of kidney assayed by tubule-cell survival. *Br. J. Radiol.*, **59**, 587–595

Wong, F.L., Boice, J.D., Jr, Abramson, D.H., Tarone, R.E., Kleinerman, R.A., Stovall, M., Goldman, M.B., Seddon, J.M., Tarbell, N., Fraumeni, J.F., Jr & Li, F.P. (1997) Cancer incidence after retinoblastoma. Radiation dose and sarcoma risk. *J. Am. med. Assoc.*, **278**, 1262–1267

Worgul, B.V., David, J., Odrich, S., Merriam, G.R., Jr, Medvedovsky, C., Merriam, J.C., Trokel, S.L. & Geard, C.R. (1991) Evidence of genotoxic damage in human cataractous lenses. *Mutagenesis*, **6**, 495–499

Xu, Y., Ashley, T., Brainerd, E.E., Bronson, R.T., Meyn, S.M. & Baltimore, D. (1996) Targeted disruption of *ATM* leads to growth retardation, chromosomal fragmentation during meiosis, immune defects, and thymic lymphoma. *Genes Dev.*, **10**, 2411–2422

Yalow, R.S. (1994) Concerns with low-level ionizing radiation. *Mayo Clin. Proc.*, **69**, 436–440

Yalow, R.S. (1995) Radiation risk and nuclear medicine: An interview with a Nobel Prize winner. *J. nucl. Med.*, **36**, 24N

Yamazaki, V., Wegner, R.-D. & Kirchgessner, C.U. (1998) Characterization of cell cycle checkpoint responses after ionizing radiation in Nijmegen breakage syndrome cells. *Cancer Res.*, **58**, 2316–2322

Yandell, D.W., Dryja, T.P. & Little, J.B. (1990) Molecular genetic analysis of recessive mutations at a heterozygous autosomal locus in human cells. *Mutat Res.*, **229**, 89–102

Yoshimoto, M., Kasumi, F., Fukami, A., Nishi, M., Kajitani, T. & Sakamoto, G. (1985) The influence of family history of cancer, irradiation and anticancer medication (mitomycin C)

on the occurence of multiple primary neoplasms with breast cancer—Statistical analysis by the person–year method. *Jpn. J. clin. Oncol.*, **15**, 191–199

Young, R.W. (1987) Acute radiation syndrome. In: Conklin, J.J. & Walker, R.I., eds, *Military Radiobiology*, New York, Academic Press, pp. 165–190

Yuille, M.A.R., Coignet, L.J.A., Abraham, S.M., Yaqub, F., Luo, L., Matutes, E., Brito-Babapulle, V., Vorechovský, I., Dyer, M.J.S. & Catovsky, D. (1998) *ATM* is usually rearranged in T-cell prolymphocytic leukaemia. *Oncogene*, **16**, 789–796

Zajac-Kaye, M. & Ts'o, P.O. (1984) DNAase I encapsulated in liposomes can induce neoplastic transformation of Syrian hamster embryo cells in culture. *Cell*, **39**, 427–437

Zampetti-Bosseler, F. & Scott, D. (1981) Cell death, chromosome damage and mitotic delay in normal human, ataxia telangiectasia and retinoblastoma fibroblasts after X-irradiation. *Int. J. Radiat. Biol.*, **39**, 547–558

Zaridze, D.G., Arkadieva, M.A., Day, N.E. & Duffy, S.W. (1993) Risk of leukaemia after chemotherapy in a case–control study in Moscow. *Br. J. Cancer*, **67**, 347–350

Zaridze, D.G., Li, N., Men, T. & Duffy, S.W. (1994) Childhood cancer incidence in relation to distance from the former nuclear testing site in Semipalatinsk, Kazakhstan. *Int. J. Cancer*, **59**, 471–475

Zhang, N., Chen, P., Khanna, KK., Scott, S., Gatei, M., Kozlov, S., Watters, D., Spring, K., Yen, T. & Lavin, M.F. (1997) Isolation of full-length ATM cDNA and correction of the ataxia-telangiectasia cellular phenotype. *Proc. natl Acad. Sci. USA*, **94**, 8021–8026

Zhang, N., Chen, P., Gatei, M., Scott, S., Khanna, K.K. & Lavin, M.F. (1998) An anti-sense construct of full-length ATM cDNA imposes a radiosensitive phenotype on normal cells. *Oncogene*, **17**, 811–818

Zippin, C., Bailar, J.C., III, Kohn, H.I., Lum, D. & Eisenberg, H. (1971) Radiation therapy for cervical cancer: Late effects on life span and on leukemia incidence. *Cancer*, **28**, 937–942

Ziv, Y., Bar-Shira, A., Pecker, I., Russell, P., Jorgensen, T.J., Tsarfati, I. & Shiloh, Y. (1997) Recombinant ATM protein complements the cellular A-T phenotype. *Oncogene*, **15**, 159–167

NEUTRONS

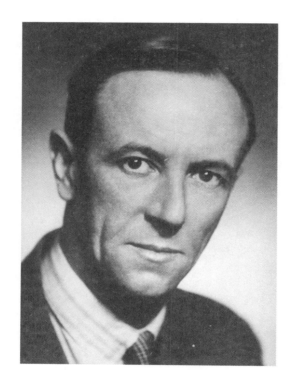

Sir James Chadwick (1891–1974)
Liverpool University, Liverpool, United Kingdom

Sir James received the Nobel Prize in Physics in 1935,
for the discovery of the neutron.

NEUTRONS

1. Exposure Data

Exposure to neutrons can occur from the nuclear fission reactions usually associated with the production of nuclear energy, from cosmic radiation in the natural environment and from sources in which reactions in light target nuclei are used. The main exposures are related to occupation, medical irradiation and cosmic rays.

1.1 Occurrence

The occurrence and characteristics of neutrons are described in detail in the Overall introduction. Neutrons are uncharged particles that interact with the nuclei of atoms, whereas X- and γ-radiation interact primarily with orbital electrons. The spectrum of exposure to neutrons depends on their source, which is ultimately the atomic nucleus. The nuclear constituents are tightly bound, and several million electron volts are required to free a neutron from most nuclei.

Neutrons can be released in several ways, resulting in human exposure. In the interaction of high-energy cosmic radiation with the earth's atmosphere, neutrons are ejected at high energy from the nuclei of molecules in the air. In the fission or fusion of nuclei, nuclear energy is released and many neutrons are produced. Neutrons produced by fusion have more energy (~14 MeV) than those released upon nuclear fission. Fission neutrons (with energy up to several million electron volts) are themselves initiators of the fission event, but their energy must be reduced by collisions with a moderating medium (usually water or graphite) to allow a chain reaction to proceed. Neutrons in the environment of reactors therefore have very little energy. Neutrons produced by nuclear explosions and those that drive breeder reactors have more energy, but not as much as the neutrons resulting from interactions with cosmic radiation. A third way in which neutrons can be released is by collision of charged particles with a lithium or beryllium target, when part of the neutron binding energy in the nucleus of lithium or beryllium is converted into kinetic energy of 14–66 MeV. Radionuclides and ion accelerators that emit α-particles are used to initiate these reactions, and the neutrons emitted are used for radiography and radiotherapy.

The mean free path of neutrons in tissues varies with their energy from a fraction to several tens of centimeters. Since neutrons are uncharged, they do not interact directly with orbital electrons in tissues to produce the ions that initiate the chemical events leading to cell injury. Rather, they induce ionizing events in tissues mainly by elastic collision with the hydrogen nuclei of the tissue molecules; the recoiling nucleus (charged proton) is the source of ionizing events. As about half of the neutron's energy is given to the proton on each collision, the low-energy neutrons provide an internal source of low-energy protons deep within body tissues. The low-energy protons form densely ionizing tracks (high linear energy transfer (LET)) which are efficient in producing biological injury. The ICRP (1991) therefore defined weighting factors for estimating the risks associated with exposure to neutrons which are larger than those for X- or γ-radiation. Neutrons with an energy of about 1 MeV are judged to be the most injurious (see Table 2 of the Overall introduction). After approximately 20–30 collisions with hydrogen, a 1-MeV neutron will come into equilibrium with ambient material and will continue to scatter, both losing and gaining energy in collision until nuclear absorption occurs, usually when hydrogen gives up 2.2-MeV of γ-radiation. Neutrons with > 50 MeV of energy interact mainly with large nuclei (e.g. C, N, O, Ca) in tissue in violent events, producing many low-energy charged particles with a broad distribution of LET (Figure 1; Wilson *et al.*, 1995), and can produce secondaries such as α-particles, protons, deuterons and other neutrons. With increasing energy, the frequency of neutron-induced nuclear disintegration, which produces high-LET α-particles, increases. Exposure to high-energy neutrons is thus quite distinct from exposure to low-energy neutrons, in which only a single recoil proton with LET extending to 100 keV μm^{-1} is formed. The initial LET values of recoil protons are less than about 30 keV μm^{-1} and increase to about 100 keV μm^{-1} as the protons come to a stop. At 100 keV μm^{-1}, the spatial separation of the ionizing events is about 2 nm, comparable to the diameter of the DNA helix, therefore increasing the probability of double-strand breaks in DNA. All neutrons in the course of their interaction with matter generate γ-radiation.

1.2   Relative biological effectiveness

The difference in effectiveness between two radiation qualities, for example, neutrons and γ-radiation, is expressed as the relative biological effectiveness (RBE), which is defined as the ratio of the doses of the two types of radiation that are required to produce the same level of a specified effect. The ratio of the effect of neutrons per unit dose to that of reference low-LET radiation is greater than unity (ICRP, 1984). The reference radiation used has conventionally been X-radiation, but since many experimental and clinical data are derived from studies of the effects of γ-radiation, either X-radiation or γ-radiation can be used as the reference. The effects of X-radiation and γ-radiation at very low doses may, however, be significantly different. While this difference may be important in determining the RBE of stochastic events, it should not be of concern in the case of deterministic effects because of the higher doses required to induce most such effects.

A major disadvantage of RBEs is that they vary not only with radiation quality but also with dose, dose rate and dose fractionation, mainly because these factors affect the response to the reference radiation but only slightly, if at all, the response to neutrons.

Figure 1. Distribution of linear energy transfer produced by a 1-GeV neutron in tissue, and the spectrum of decay of α-particles from ²³⁹Pu for comparison

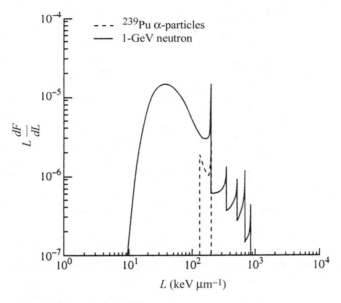

From Wilson *et al.* (1995)

The only singular RBE for any specific effect is the maximum RBE (RBE$_M$ for stochastic effects and RBE$_m$ for deterministic effects). In the case of stochastic effects, the RBE$_M$ is defined as the ratio of the initial and linear slopes of the dose–response curves for the reference radiation and the radiation under study.

RBEs are based on the assumption that the effects of different types or qualities of radiation may differ quantitatively but not qualitatively. Since most deterministic effects depend on cell killing, the assumption that the nature of the induced effect is independent of radiation quality seems justified. In the case of heavy ions, the validity of this assumption has not been proven unequivocally.

The survival curves of cells exposed to neutrons *in vitro* appear to be linear on a semi-logarithmic plot, with little or no evidence of a shoulder and with a steeper curve, reflected in a lower D$_0$ value, than for low-LET radiations (Figure 2; see section 5.1 of the Overall introduction). The slope of the survival curve decreases and the RBE increases with decreasing neutron energy. The effectiveness of the neutrons is maximal at about 400 keV. The lack or the marked reduction of the shoulder of the survival curve reflects a greatly reduced or even completely absent ability to repair sublethal damage after exposure to neutrons (Barendsen, 1990). This lack of repair

Figure 2. Cell survival after exposure to radiation with low and high linear energy transfer (LET) as a function of dose

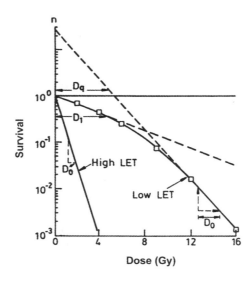

D_1, indicated here for low-LET radiation only, is the dose required to reduce the survival to 37%; n is the extrapolation number; and D_q is the 'quasi-threshold' dose, which, like n, is a measure of the shoulder on the low-LET survival curve. D_0 is the reciprocal of the slope of the linear portion of the curves. Note that the curve for high-LET radiation is steeper than that for low-LET radiation (D_0 is smaller) and that there is a shoulder on the low-LET curve.

results in little or no reduction in effectiveness when the neutron dose is fractionated or when the dose rate is reduced.

The dose–effect relationship of early-responding tissues can be predicted from the responses of the relevant clonogenic cells. There is no apparent difference in the ability of tissues to repopulate after exposure to neutrons, apart from a greater reduction in the number of proliferative cells per unit dose of neutrons than with low-LET radiation. The RBE increases with increasing LET and reaches a maximum, in the case of cell killing and mutagenesis, at LET values of about 100–200 keV μm^{-1}. At higher LET values, the effectiveness decreases. In 1990, a revision of the relationship between the radiation quality factor, which is based on RBEs, and the LET for stochastic effects was introduced which took into account the decrease in effectiveness of radiations with a very high LET. The relationship between RBE and LET for deterministic effects has not been codified explicitly, and the use of quality factors is restricted to stochastic effects. For deterministic effects, the influence of radiation quality is taken into account by using RBEs to adjust the absorbed doses (ICRP, 1990).

RBEs for deterministic effects are derived from the ratios of the threshold doses for neutron and reference radiation or of the doses required to induce a selected level of effect. Since deterministic effects have thresholds by definition, use of the ratio of the threshold doses seems a reasonable approach for determining RBEs. In 1990, however, an ICRP task group introduced the concept of RBE_m, which is comparable to the RBE_M for stochastic effects. The group suggested that singular RBE values for neutrons and other high-LET radiations could be obtained from the linear–quadratic model used to describe the survival curves of the cells responsible for the maintenance of tissues. In the case of deterministic effects, the threshold dose lies on the curved portion of the dose–response curve. Since, in general, deterministic effects result from the killing of a critical number of cells and assuming that the dose–response curve for cell killing can be described by a linear–quadratic model, it is theoretically possible to derive the initial slope of the response. Thus, a RBE_m can be obtained for specific end-points in specific tissues for which there are adequate data on dose–response relationships for different $\alpha{:}\beta$ ratios (see ICRP, 1990, for the method of deriving RBE_m). This approach is, of course, totally dependent on the validity of the linear–quadratic model at low doses at which effects cannot be measured.

The clinical importance of the difference between the effects of neutrons and low-LET radiations on normal tissues was revealed by the high incidence of tissue damage during the early use of neutrons to treat cancer. The effectiveness of fractionated neutrons is underestimated if it is based on the effects of single doses and if the difference in the repair of slowly dividing tissues is not taken into account.

1.3   Exposure

1.3.1   *Natural sources*

The effective dose equivalent rates of cosmic rays are discussed in the Overall introduction (section 4.4.1), in which the rates were evaluated on the basis of measurements with neutron spectrometers, tissue equivalent ion chambers and nuclear emulsion detectors augmented by Monte Carlo calculations. Dose equivalence is derived by summing dose contributions and weighting by LET-dependent quality factors. The ratio of the estimated neutron dose equivalent rate to the total dose equivalent rate according to the parametric atmospheric radiation model is shown for various altitudes in Figure 3. It can be seen that 40–65% of the dose equivalent at ordinary aircraft altitudes is due to neutrons, depending on the latitude and longitude of the flight trajectory. The fraction of neutrons depends on altitude, being nearly negligible at sea level and contributing over half of the exposure at aircraft flight altitudes. The fraction varies little over most of the altitudes at which aircraft operate. Since most commercial flights are at relatively high latitudes, approximately 60% of the dose equivalent is due to neutrons.

Although consistent measurements were made over most geomagnetic latitudes and altitudes during solar cycle 20 which started in October 1964, many of the individual

Figure 3. Fraction of dose equivalent due to neutrons at various altitudes, at minimum solar energy (1965)

$H_{neutron}/H$ at 40 000 ft [~12 000 m]

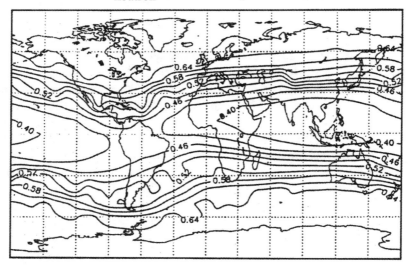

$H_{neutron}/H$ at 50 000 ft [~15 000 m]

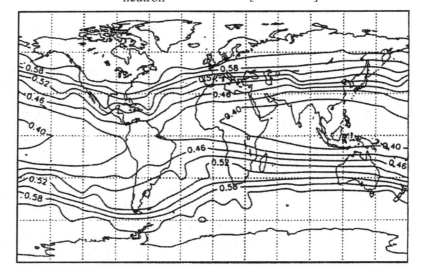

Figure 3 (contd)

Hneutron/H at 65 000 ft [~20 000 m]

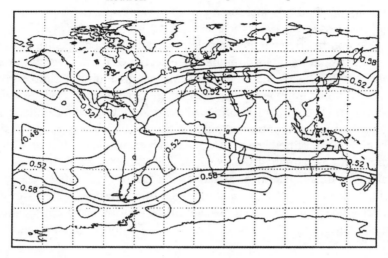

Hneutron/H at 73 000 ft [~22 000 m]

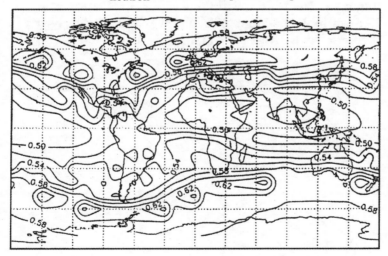

From Wilson *et al.* (1995); H, equivalent dose

components were not resolved because of instrumental limitations at that time. Most of the neutron spectrum therefore depends on theoretical calculations of proton interactions with the atmosphere (Hajnal & Wilson, 1992; National Council on Radiation Protection and Measurements, 1995). Early measurements of the atmospheric neutron spectrum are shown in Figure 4. Hess *et al.* (1961) measured the neutron spectrum in a bismuth fission chamber with a boron fluoride counter, supplemented by a model spectrum. Korff *et al.* (1979) used a liquid scintillator spectrometer (see section 2.1.1 in Overall introduction) sensitive mainly to 1–10-MeV neutrons with analysis assuming a simple power law spectrum. [The Working Group noted that the data of Korff *et al.* (1979) are for a higher altitude than those of Hess *et al.* (1961).] Hewitt *et al.* (1980) used a Bonner sphere set-up (see section 2.1.1 in Overall introduction) at subsonic flight altitudes and analysed the data after assuming a simplified spectral analysis. Their results confirm the importance of high-energy neutrons, although the exact nature of the spectrum remains uncertain owing to limitations of the analytical methods. Nakamura *et al.* (1987) used a Bonner sphere set-up at much lower latitudes and multiplied their results by three for a comparison of spectral shape. Incomplete knowledge of the neutron spectrum thus makes the present estimates uncertain (National Council on Radiation Protection and Measurements, 1995).

Figure 4. Neutron spectra measured at 17.46° N at 23.5 km by Hajnal and Wilson (1992) and that derived theoretically by Hess *et al.* (1961)

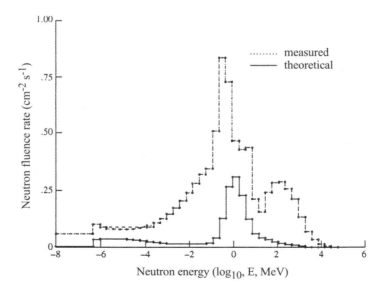

Estimates of dose equivalent rates for exposure to radiation from natural sources are available in a number of publications, but only a few give separate values for the contributions of neutrons. Bagshaw *et al.* (1996) reported that the average rate on long-haul flights from London to Tokyo was 3 μSv h^{-1} for neutrons; an additional 3 μSv h^{-1} for other components gave a total of 6 μSv h^{-1}. Table 1 shows the dose equivalent rates derived with a high-pressure ion chamber and a simplified form of a Bonner sphere, in relation to altitude and latitude (Akatov, 1993). Although the quality of the ionizing dose is not given, it can be seen that the neutron dose equivalent rate represents half or more of the exposure.

Table 1. Atmospheric dose equivalent rates measured on board a Tupolev-144 aeroplane during March–June 1977 (near solar minimum)

Altitude (km)	Latitudes (° N)					
	40–45		46–58		65–72	
	Ionizing (μGy h^{-1})	Neutrons (μSv h^{-1})	Ionizing (μGy h^{-1})	Neutrons (μSv h^{-1})	Ionizing (μGy h^{-1})	Neutrons (μSv h^{-1})
13	2.3	2.6	2.9	4.2	3.5	5.0
14	2.6	3.0	3.2	5.0	4.1	5.9
15	2.8	3.0	3.4	5.4	4.7	6.7
16	2.9	3.2	3.5	5.8	5.2	7.6
17	3.0	3.5	3.7	6.1	–	–
18	3.1	3.4	3.8	5.5	–	–

From Akatov (1993)

In estimating the collective dose equivalent, UNSCEAR (1993) assumed 3×10^9 passenger hours in flight during 1985 and an annual average rate of 2.8 μSv h^{-1} (~1.6 μSv h^{-1} of neutrons) resulting in a collective dose equivalent of 8400 person–Sv (5040 person–Sv of neutrons). By 1997, air travel had grown to 4.3×10^9 passenger hours in flight (ICAO, 1999) leading to a collective dose equivalent of 12 000 person–Sv (7200 person–Sv of neutrons).

1.3.2 *Medical uses*

The medical use of neutrons is limited, as no therapeutic benefit has been noted when compared with conventional radiotherapy; however, neutrons are used to a limited extent in external beam therapy and boron neutron capture therapy.

1.3.3   Nuclear explosions

In the reassessment of the radiation dosimetry associated with the atomic bombings of Hiroshima and Nagasaki, Japan (see Overall introduction, section 4.1.1; Fry & Sinclair, 1987), the estimated dose of neutrons was reduced in both cities, particularly in Hiroshima, where the new value was only 10% of the previously estimated level. The neutron doses were now so small (only 1–2% of the total dose in Hiroshima and less in Nagasaki) that direct estimates of the risk for cancer associated with exposure to neutrons were no longer reliable. The neutron dosimetry is once again under review and may be revised (National Council on Radiation Protection and Measurements, 1997; Rühm et al., 1998).

1.3.4   Occupational exposure

Occupational exposure to neutrons occurs mainly in the nuclear industry. Compilations have been made of the exposure of nuclear workers in the United Kingdom for the years 1946–88 (Carpenter et al., 1994) and of those in the USA for the years 1970–80 (Environmental Protection Agency, 1984). In the United Kingdom compilation, the upper limit of the neutron component was estimated to be 3% of the total exposure (Table 2). The estimates are uncertain because neutron dosimetry was implemented in fuel processing plants only in 1960, a few workers worked at reactors where there was a significant energetic neutron component for which the dosimetry is inadequate, and there were systematic under- and over-recordings when the dosimetry read-outs were below threshold of detection or the dosimeter was in some way inoperative. The average annual dose equivalent for all workers in the United Kingdom was reduced from 12.5 mSv year^{-1} (neutrons, < 0.4 mSv year^{-1}) in the early 1950s to < 2.5 mSv year^{-1} (neutrons, < 0.1 mSv year^{-1}) in 1985. The average cumulative doses

Table 2. Upper limits of estimated cumulative exposure to neutrons of radiation workers, by last site of employment, United Kingdom, 1946–88

Employer	No. of exposed individuals	Cumulative whole-body dose equivalent (mSv)	Collective dose equivalent (person–Sv)
Atomic Energy Authority	21 344	1.2	26
Atomic Weapons Establishment	9 389	0.3	3.1
British Nuclear Fuels, Sellafield	10 028	4.0	40
Total	40 761	1.7	69.1

From Carpenter et al. (1994)

were highest at the Sellafield nuclear fuel processing plant, where 22 workers had single annual doses > 250 mSv (neutrons, > 7.5 mSv year^{-1}), seven of whom had doses > 500 mSv year^{-1} (neutrons, > 15 mSv year^{-1}).

Occupational exposure to neutrons in the USA in 1980 based on data for 1977–84 are shown in Table 3. It was estimated that such exposure had decreased by a factor of two between 1970 and 1980 due to improved protection (Klement et al., 1972; Environmental Protection Agency, 1984).

Table 3. Estimated exposure to neutrons of radiation workers in the United States, 1980

Employer	No. of exposed individuals	Average annual effective dose equivalent (mSv)	Collective effective dose equivalent (person–Sv)
Department of Energy contractors	25 000[a]	2.6	64
Nuclear power stations	1 100	0.5	0.6
US Navy	12 000	0.24	2.9
Total	38 100	1.8	67.5

From National Council for Radiation Protection and Measurements (1987)
[a] Total number of workers

Staff involved in radiotherapy with neutrons are exposed mainly to γ- and β-rays due to activation of the room and equipment. The dose rates are well below 1 μGy h^{-1} and are not detectable by personal dosimetry (Smathers et al., 1978; Finch & Bonnett, 1992; Howard & Yanch, 1995).

Neutron sources are used to chart progress in the search for gas and oil resources. The exposure of oil-well loggers has been monitored with film (Fujimoto et al., 1985) and nuclear track detectors (Inskip et al., 1991). Canadian workers were exposed to 1–2 mSv year^{-1} (Fujimoto et al., 1985), whereas Chinese workers monitored for three months had very low doses of neutrons, only seven of the 1344 workers having doses above the threshold of detection (0.02 mGy) (Inskip et al., 1991).

The exposure of commercial aircraft crews to neutrons depends not only on the flight route (see section 1.3.1) but also on the number of flight hours, which may be as many as 1000 per year. Hughes and O'Riordan (1993) estimated that long-haul crews are airborne for 600 h year^{-1}, while short-haul crews log only 400 h year^{-1}; they therefore used an average value of 500 h year^{-1}. Bagshaw et al. (1996) estimated that crews who fly both ultra-long-haul and long-haul flights fly for 600 h year^{-1}, while those who fly only ultra-long-haul flights fly for up to 900 h year^{-1}. Oksanen (1998) found that the annual average number of flight hours of cabin crews was 673 h, while that of the technical crew was 578 h, with a range of 293–906 h year^{-1}. Air crews have additional exposure during off-duty flights in returning to a home base, which are estimated to account for 20% of the actual flight hours logged.

Hughes and O'Riordan (1993) estimated an average dose equivalent of 3 mSv year^{-1} (neutrons, ~1.8 mSv year^{-1}) for crews on United Kingdom airlines and 6 mSv year^{-1} (neutrons, ~3.6 mSv year^{-1}) for near-polar flights. Montagne *et al.* (1993) estimated that the average exposure of Air France long-haul pilots was 2–3 mSv year^{-1} (neutrons, ~1.2–1.8 mSv year^{-1}). Wilson *et al.* (1994) estimated that the exposure of domestic crews in Australia in 1982–83 was 1–1.8 mSv year^{-1} (neutrons, ~0.6–1.1 mSv year^{-1}), while crews of international flights received 3.8 mSv year^{-1} (neutrons, ~2.3 mSv year^{-1}). Preston (1985) proposed an average dose equivalent of 9.2 µSv h^{-1} (neutrons, ~5.5 µSv h^{-1}) in British Airways operation of the Concorde in 1979, with a maximum observed rate of 38.1 µSv h^{-1} (neutrons, ~23 µSv h^{-1}). The average exposure of the technical crew was 2.8 mSv year^{-1} (neutrons, ~1.7 mSv year^{-1}) and that of the cabin crew was 2.2 mSv year^{-1} (neutrons, ~1.3 mSv year^{-1}). Similar differences (20–30%) between the exposures of personnel on the flight deck and in the cabin were observed by Wilson *et al.* (1994). Differences of up to 20% between aircraft type were also observed.

1.4   Summary

The average effective dose of neutrons received by the world population per year was estimated to be 80 µSv by UNSCEAR (1993). Assuming a 75-year life span, the average lifetime dose would be 6.0 mSv. The highest average lifetime effective dose of neutrons (67.5 mSv) is found in the high-altitude city (3900 m) of La Paz, Bolivia. Table 4 gives the individual and collective lifetime doses for a number of populations. The atomic bombings of Hiroshima and Nagasaki are estimated to have contributed not more than 2% of the total exposure of the survivors, as estimated from the total exposure of 24 000 person–Sv of 86 752 persons and the total exposure of 4 Sv of the 'worst-case' survivors. Insufficient information was available to estimate the individual average exposure of nuclear workers over a working lifetime. The maximal known lifetime exposure of contractors of the Department of Energy in the USA was estimated on the basis of a 50-year career. The collective dose of the world's nuclear workers is based on the assumption that workers in the United Kingdom and the USA represent 20% of such workers. UNSCEAR (1993) estimated that the average total exposure of the world population from air travel was 2 µSv year^{-1}, of which 60% is to neutrons, although the maximal individual exposure due to air travel depends mainly on flight duration. The collective dose for crew members is based on the assumption that there are five crew members for every 100 passengers.

Table 4. Exposure to neutrons of major exposed human populations

Population	Exposure path	Individual lifetime[a] dose (mSv)		Collective dose (person–Sv per year)	Variation
		Average	Maximum		
World (5800 million)	Natural sources (cosmic radiation)	6.0	67.5	4.64×10^5	Large
Tumour therapy	Collateral irradiation of healthy tissue				Highly skewed distribution
Survivors of atomic bombs	Fission neutrons	<5.5	<80.0	<480	Relatively more important at lower exposures (?)
Nuclear workers[b]	Civilian and military nuclear fuel cycle	44.4	130[c]	350[d]	
Aircrews, courriers[e]	Flying at high altitude, cosmic secondary neutrons	30	46	320	Higher on flights over earth poles
Airline passengers	Flying at high altitude, cosmic fusion neutrons	0.09	–	7200	Higher on flights over earth poles

From UNSCEAR (1993)
[a] 75 years
[b] 50-year career
[c] Department of Energy contractors in the USA
[d] Workers in the United Kingdom and the USA assumed to represent 20% of all nuclear workers
[e] 30 years

2. Studies of Cancer in Humans

Until the system for estimating the doses received by the survivors of the atomic bombings in Japan was revised in 1986 (DS86), it was reported consistently that the incidence of cancers after exposure to similar doses was higher among the survivors in Hiroshima than among those in Nagasaki (Kato & Schull, 1982). The bomb dropped on Hiroshima was composed of uranium and that dropped on Nagasaki of plutonium, but it was believed that the design of the two weapons had resulted in greater exposure to neutrons in Hiroshima. For many years, differences in cancer rates and in the frequency of chromosomal aberrations in circulating lymphocytes were attributed to differences in the quality of radiation, and attempts to separate the effects of neutrons and γ-rays were made by comparing the rates in Hiroshima with those in Nagasaki (Committee on the Biological Effects of Ionizing Radiations (BEIR I), 1972). On the basis of these calculations, neutrons were estimated to be about 20 times more carcinogenic than γ-radiation, although it was recognized that a wide range of values was possible.

During the early 1980s, the dosimetry of the radiation from the atomic bombs was reassessed (Fry & Sinclair, 1987; Roesch, 1987a,b). The estimated neutron doses delivered to both cities were now considered to be so small (only 1–2% of the total dose in Hiroshima and less in Nagasaki) that estimates of the risks for cancer associated with exposure to neutrons were not reliable (Jablon, 1993; Little, 1997). The change in the estimates of doses to the Japanese atomic bomb survivors thus meant that there was no longer a useful database of human exposures for estimating the carcinogenic risks of exposure to neutrons.

Some workers in the nuclear industry are occasionally exposed to neutrons, but the number of such workers is too small and the doses are generally too low for any meaningful estimate of risk. In addition, these workers were also exposed to higher doses of γ-radiation. In studies of patients treated with neutrons (Catterall et al., 1975, 1977; Hübener et al., 1989; Richard et al., 1989; Kolker et al., 1990; MacDougall et al., 1990; Silbergeld et al., 1991; Stelzer et al., 1991; Laramore et al., 1993; Russell et al., 1993), the numbers of survivors and those developing second cancers are small, and the dosimetry is very complex (Geraci et al., 1982). Other complicating factors include the killing of cells at the high doses used, scattering of low doses and contaminating exposures to γ-rays. High-energy linear accelerators for medical use produce low levels of neutrons through the photonuclear effect, and a dose of the order of 1 cGy is possible (Hall et al., 1995); however, the dose is again too low—in contrast to the dose used for tumour treatment, of the order of 6000 cGy—to allow quantification of the risk for second cancers attributable to neutrons. Epidemiological studies of air crew, pilots and flight attendants have been initiated because of their exposure to neutrons from cosmic rays during frequent high-altitude flights (Blettner et al., 1998; Boice et al., 1999). The annual exposure of air crew is about 1–2 mSv, which, even after a career of 30 years, is still too low a dose to allow detection, much less quantification, of a cancer excess by epidemiological means. In addition, the dosimetry is complex and this population is also exposed directly to ionizing radiation, making it difficult to evaluate the effects of neutrons.

3. Studies of Cancer in Experimental Animals

Neutrons have been studied in order to compare their carcinogenicity with that of low-LET radiations such as X-radiation and γ-radiation, not only to improve understanding of the risks of exposure to neutrons but also to test biophysical models and their applicability to radiation-induced cancer. This section does not give a comprehensive presentation of all studies in animals. The studies in mice summarized below are those which have provided data on dose–response relationships and on the effects of fractionation and dose rate at low doses of neutrons. The results of experiments in other species provide evidence that the results in mice are not unique.

3.1   Adult animals

3.1.1   *Mouse*

Groups of 21–114 male and 31–197 female non-inbred RF/Un mice, 10 weeks of age, were exposed to 0–9.3 Gy of whole-body irradiation with 1-MeV or 5-MeV neutrons [source and γ-radiation component not specified] at dose rates of 0.04–114 mGy day^{-1} and 0.00003–850 mGy min^{-1}. The animals were allowed to die naturally or were killed when moribund, at which time all animals were necropsied. Only selected lesions were examined histopathologically, as needed, to confirm diagnosis. In the control group of 301 unirradiated females and 115 unirradiated males, neoplasms occurred in about 64% of females and 47% of males. The incidence of myeloid leukaemia was markedly increased by acute exposure, passing through a maximum at 2 Gy and declining at higher doses (Table 5). Chronic irradiation at up to 5.7 Gy also enhanced the incidence, but this declined after exposure to 9.3 Gy. The incidence of reticulum-cell neoplasms, in contrast to those of myeloid leukaemia and thymic lymphoma, decreased with the increased doses delivered at a high rate. Of the unirradiated control mice, 11–14% had pulmonary tumours (adenomas); in treated mice, however, the incidences decreased with increasing dose. The incidence of ovarian tumours (granulosa-cell tumours, luteomas, tubular adenomas and haemangiomas) was statistically significantly increased ($p < 0.05$) only at the lowest dose of 16 mGy at a rate of 0.00003 mGy min^{-1} [statistical method not specified]. The incidences of solid tumours other than of the lung and ovary were increased in the irradiated animals, but the numbers were reported to be insufficient to establish a quantitative dose–effect relationship. The relative biological effectiveness (RBE; see section 1.2) for the induction of myeloid leukaemia was 16 with daily and chronic exposure as

Table 5. Time to death and incidences of tumours in various organs of RF/Un mice exposed to fast neutrons

Mean accumulated dose (Gy)	Average dose rate (mGy min⁻¹)	No. of mice	Mean age at death (days)	Myeloid leukaemia (%)	Thymic lymphoma (%)	Ovarian tumours (%)	Pulmonary tumours (%)	Other solid tumours (%)
Females								
0	–	301	582	3	12	2	11	3
0.016	0.00003	111	584	5	11	19	15	4
0.12	0.00021	97	549	8	11	2	10	1
0.15	0.0015	79	558	6	9	4	13	2
0.16	0.00022	99	566	7	7	4	11	3
0.16	0.0007	117	558	3	8	5	14	4
0.27	0.0004	129	549	4	12	1	12	2
0.28	0.033	50	533	4	8	0	12	2
0.30	0.0062	100	544	8	11	4	15	4
0.31	0.0012	148	578	4	11	2	17	4
0.33	0.0043	90	522	8	19	4	4	3
0.68	0.0037	60	523	7	10	9	17	0
0.75	0.0034	120	471	9	21	2	12	7
0.94	0.0062	197	464	12	19	3	14	4
0.96	0.0099	49	509	5	27	14	5	5
0.98	0.033	85	464	15	20	5	7	4
1.69	0.0033	123	489	14	12	6	17	4
2.10	0.0185	50	451	15	41	4	7	2
2.11	0.0099	49	370	8	39	2	8	0
2.39	0.0275	58	324	20	25	2	4	0
2.91	0.0171	49	431	9	40	2	13	4
3.90	0.0098	120	398	17	35	1	10	3
4.61	0.0207	186	301	12	45	2	6	2
5.70	0.0185	50	363	23	25	0	16	0
9.30	0.083	50	189	2	20	0	2	0

Table 5 (contd)

Mean accumulated dose (Gy)	Average dose rate (mGy min⁻¹)	No. of mice	Mean age at death (days)	Myeloid leukaemia (%)	Thymic lymphoma (%)	Ovarian tumours (%)	Pulmonary tumours (%)	Other solid tumours (%)
Females (contd)								
2.03	850	31	382	20	23	10	0	0
2.60	850	60	304	16	10	7	4	0
3.60	850	98	360	10	23	8	4	2
4.43	850	82	342	9	16	7	2	1
Males								
0	–	115	548	3	1		14	2
0.17	0.0012	77	561	8	1		17	1
0.29	0.0029	69	482	17	1		17	1
1.20	0.0243	21	502	29	5		19	5
1.30	850	27	460	33	7		11	0
1.72	850	48	436	34	11		11	2
2.22	850	114	428	38	4		7	1
2.70	850	103	413	30	5		8	3
3.32	850	79	408	23	9		13	4

From Upton *et al.* (1970)

compared with acute exposure (Upton *et al.*, 1970). [The Working Group noted that the tumour incidences were not analysed for competing causes of death. Since a large fraction of the irradiated mice died early from myeloid leukaemia, such an analysis for solid tumours is essential.]

A total of 3265 female RFM/Un mice, 12 weeks of age, received whole-body irradiation with neutrons at doses of 0.048, 0.096, 0.192, 0.24, 0.47, 0.94 or 1.88 Gy at rates of 50 or 250 mGy min^{-1} or 10 mGy day^{-1}. A reactor was used to deliver the high dose rate, and the low dose rate was produced from a 1.1-mg ^{252}Cf source surrounded by a depleted ^{238}U sphere (Storer *et al.*, 1979). The ratios of neutrons:γ-rays were 7:1 for the reactor and 3:1 for the ^{252}Cf source. A control group of 648 mice was available. The animals were followed for life, and tumours were diagnosed histologically. A positive dose–response relationship for thymic lymphoma was observed at all doses up to 1.0 Gy at both dose rates; at the highest dose, the low dose rate was more effective (Table 6). At low doses, a weak dependence on rate was observed. Increased incidences of thymic lymphoma, lung adenoma and endocrine tumours were seen at doses as low as 0.24 Gy. The highest dose of radiation at the low rate (10 mGy day^{-1}) appeared to induce thymic lymphomas more efficiently than irradiation at the high dose rate (250 mGy min^{-1}). The incidence of ovarian tumours was lower at all doses given at the low rate than at the high rate. After exposure to doses of 0.24–0.47 Gy, the RBE for thymic lymphoma was 3–4 in relation to acute exposure to ^{137}Cs γ-rays, and the induction of mammary tumours also appeared to be more sensitive to neutrons; however, no apparent effect of dose or dose rate was reported over the dose range used. Because of the relatively large carcinogenic effect, the authors concluded that the γ-radiation component had little or no effect on the dose–response relationship observed (Ullrich *et al.*, 1976).

The dose–response relationships for the induction of lung tumours were studied in 592 female RFM/Un mice, 10–12 weeks of age, given thoracic exposure to 0.05–1.5 Gy of fission neutrons at a rate of 50–250 mGy min^{-1} and compared with 88 controls. When the mice were killed nine months after irradiation, the relationship between the number of lung tumours per mouse and doses up to 0.25 Gy was linear, or a threshold model with a linear response above the threshold was reported. The RBE increased with decreasing dose from 25 at 0.25 Gy to 40 at 0.10 Gy in relation to acute exposure to X-rays (Ullrich *et al.*, 1979). In another study (Ullrich, 1980), mice of the same strain were irradiated with 0, 0.1, 0.15, 0.2, 0.5, 1.0 or 1.5 Gy as either single doses or two equal doses separated by 24-h or 30-day intervals. The animals were observed until nine months of age. Dose fractionation had no effect on lung tumour induction at any dose.

In a study with female BALB/c/AnNBd mice, 296 control and 3258 irradiated mice, 12 weeks of age, received whole-body exposure to fission spectrum neutrons at doses of 0, 0.048, 0.096, 0.192, 0.24, 0.47, 0. 94 or 1.88 Gy at a dose rate of 50 or 250 mGy min^{-1} or 10 mGy day^{-1}. The animals were observed for life, and the induced tumours were examined histologically. The tumours that were most sensitive to induction by neutrons

Table 6. Incidences of neoplasms in female RFM/Un mice after neutron irradiation at various doses and rates

Dose rate	Type of neoplasm	Incidence (%)				
		0	0.048 Gy	0.096 Gy	0.192 Gy	0.47 Gy
50 mGy min^{-1}	Thymic lymphoma	7.3	11	11	20	33
	Lung adenoma	24	10	24	30	46
	Endocrine tumours	7.0	5.2	11	50	54
		0	0.24 Gy	0.47 Gy	0.94 Gy	1.88 Gy
250 mGy min^{-1}	Thymic lymphoma	4.6	24	30	40	39
	Reticulum-cell sarcoma	62	53	53	52	31
	Myeloid leukaemia	0	0.56	5.3	1.3	0.62
	Other leukaemias	6.4	6.9	7.5	7.7	9.6
	Lung adenoma	31	42	45	53	16
	Ovarian tumours	0	20	25	52	39
	Pituitary tumours	3.9	7.9	29	21	16
	Harderian gland tumours	0	13	28	35	6.3
	Uterine tumours	1.3	11	25	27	19
	Mammary tumours	2.6	8.0	8.4	10	3.9
	Other solid tumours	3.9	14	24	20	26
10 mGy day^{-1}	Thymic lymphoma	–	18	25	43	63
	Reticulum-cell sarcoma	–	64	58	48	45
	Myeloid leukaemia	–	0	2.4	0.27	0.26
	Other leukaemias	–	4.4	2.9	3.1	4.2
	Lung adenoma	–	48	48	53	32
	Ovarian tumours	–	2.3	8.7	22	24
	Pituitary tumours	–	11	11	19	2.5
	Harderian gland tumours	–	11	20	25	4.5
	Uterine tumours	–	4.8	17	21	18
	Mammary tumours	–	7.3	7.6	5.4	8.9
	Other solid tumours	–	21	14	21	12

From Ullrich *et al.* (1976)

were malignant lung adenocarcinomas, mammary adenocarcinomas and ovarian tumours, and increases in the incidences of these three types of tumours were observed after exposure to doses of neutrons as low as 50–100 mGy at a high dose rate (Table 7; Ullrich *et al.*, 1977).

Groups of 140–182 female BALB/c/AnNBd mice, 12 weeks of age, received a single whole-body exposure to 0.025, 0.05, 0.10, 0.20, 0.50 or 2.0 Gy of fission neutrons at a dose rate of 50–250 mGy min^{-1}. The animals were studied for life, and tumours were examined histologically. A group of 263 controls was available. The ovary was very sensitive to the induction of tumours (granulosa-cell tumours, luteomas

Table 7. Incidences of leukaemias and solid tumours in neutron-irradiated female BALB/c mice

Dose rate	Dose (Gy)	Thymic lymphoma (%)	Reticulum-cell sarcoma (%)	Lung adenoma (%)	Lung adenocarcinoma (%)	Mammary tumours (%)	Ovarian tumours (%)
Control	0	1.1 ± 0.6	41 ± 4.1	26 ± 4.5	13 ± 3.4	7 ± 1.6	6 ± 2.1
50 mGy min⁻¹	0.048	1.0 ± 0.9	39 ± 6.6	11 ± 5.4	27 ± 4.8	7 ± 2.6	7 ± 4.1
	0.096	2.1 ± 1.4	32 ± 6.5	13 ± 6.2	39 ± 5.1	25 ± 4.5	11 ± 4.6
	0.192	2.2 ± 1.6	30 ± 5.8	17 ± 4.9	19 ± 5.1	18 ± 5.0	20 ± 4.9
	0.47	2.8 ± 1.7	27 ± 4.6	28 ± 4.6	22 ± 4.7	17 ± 5.6	49 ± 4.0
250 mGy min⁻¹	0.24	1.8 ± 0.8	29 ± 4.6	25 ± 4.5	19 ± 4.8	17 ± 2.4	37 ± 4.6
	0.47	2.4 ± 0.7	32 ± 6.4	27 ± 5.4	23 ± 5.1	19 ± 3.7	57 ± 5.4
	0.94	4.1 ± 1.3	26 ± 5.4	30 ± 4.9	19 ± 5.7	17 ± 3.9	62 ± 3.5
	1.88	4.5 ± 1.2	21 ± 3.6	23 ± 3.3	13 ± 5.2	15 ± 5.4	39 ± 5.5
10 mGy day⁻¹	0.24	2.1 ± 1.2	38 ± 4.5	28 ± 5.1	13 ± 4.6	14 ± 2.9	7 ± 2.9
	0.47	2.3 ± 0.9	36 ± 4.8	23 ± 5.1	27 ± 5.7	17 ± 3.7	10 ± 3.7
	0.94	2.9 ± 1.0	36 ± 4.1	22 ± 4.0	32 ± 5.5	19 ± 3.8	19 ± 4.2
	1.88	6.1 ± 1.6	28 ± 6.2	13 ± 2.6	43 ± 5.7	45 ± 5.3	21 ± 5.1

From Ullrich et al. (1977); incidences are means ± SE.

and tubular adenomas), the incidence increasing from 2% in controls to 76% after exposure to 0.50 Gy; at 2.0 Gy, the incidence was 56%. For mammary adenocarcinomas, a linear dose–response relationship was reported up to a dose of 0.50 Gy, from 8% in controls to 25%. For lung adenocarcinomas, a convex upward curve was seen over the dose range 0–0.50 Gy. In the dose range 0.1–0.2 Gy, the dose–response curve for the induction of lung and mammary tumours appeared to 'bend over'. The percentage incidences of lung and mammary adenocarcinomas and ovarian tumours are given in Table 8 (Ullrich, 1983).

Table 8. Incidences of solid tumours in female BALB/c mice after fission neutron irradiation

Dose (Gy)	No. of animals	Lung adenocarcinoma (%)	Mammary adenocarcinoma (%)	Ovarian tumours (%)
0	263	15 ± 2.4	8 ± 1.7	2 ± 1.0
0.025	140	17 ± 3.7	11 ± 2.9	3 ± 1.4
0.05	160	21 ± 4.3	17 ± 3.8	7 ± 2.1
0.10	160	18 ± 4.0	18 ± 4.2	10 ± 2.6
0.20	167	$30. \pm 6.1$	20 ± 4.7	16 ± 3.7
0.50	182	37 ± 6.9	25 ± 5.5	76 ± 3.0
2.0	182	27 ± 6.1	8 ± 3.2	56 ± 3.8

From Ullrich (1983); incidences are means $\pm$ SE.

In the same model, the effects of dose rate and of dose fractionation on the carcinogenic effects of fission spectrum neutrons were examined for doses of 0, 0.025, 0.05, 0.10, 0.20 or 0.50 Gy in 263 controls and 140–191 animals in the various irradiated groups. Whole-body irradiation was given as a single dose or split at 24-h or 30-day intervals at dose rates of 10–250 mGy min^{-1}, depending on the total dose. The incidence of ovarian tumours was not altered by fractionation, but lowering the dose rate reduced the incidence of ovarian tumours and enhanced the frequency of mammary tumours at doses as low as 0.025 Gy (Ullrich, 1984).

A total of 1814 male RFM/Un mice, 10 weeks of age, were exposed by whole-body irradiation to 0.05, 0.1, 0.2, 0.4 or 0.8 Gy of fission neutrons at a rate of 0.25 Gy min^{-1}. The radiation facility was the same as that used in previous studies. A group of 602 controls was available. The lifetime incidence of myeloid leukaemia was increased in a dose-related manner from 0.8 ± 0.4 in controls to 2.1 ± 0.5 at 0.05 Gy, 2.6 ± 0.7 at 0.1 Gy, 4.8 ± 1.3 at 0.2 Gy, 7.5 ± 2.2 at 0.4 Gy and $14.9 \pm 3.8\%$ at 0.8 Gy. In comparison with acute ^{137}Cs γ-radiation, the RBE for myeloid leukaemia was 2.8 (Ullrich & Preston, 1987).

Radiation-induced late somatic effects and the shapes of the dose–response curves after graded doses of 1.5-MeV fission neutrons at 0.17, 0.36, 0.71, 1.07, 1.43, 1.79 or

2.14 Gy were reported in 360 male BC3F$_1$ [(C57BL/Cne × C3H/HeCne) F$_1$] mice, three months of age, after whole-body irradiation. The γ-ray component represented about 12.5% of the total dose. A control group of 561 male mice was available. A significant decrease in the mean life span was observed at 0.36 Gy and with increasing doses from 1.07 to 2.14 Gy ($p < 0.001$, Student's t test). Myeloid leukaemia, malignant lymphoma and solid tumours including cancers of the lung, liver and soft tissues were observed. A significant increase in the incidence of myeloid leukaemia was reported at doses of 0.71 to 1.79 Gy ($p < 0.001$, χ^2 test) when compared with controls (0%). A significant decrease in the incidence of malignant lymphoma was observed after exposure to 1.43–2.14 Gy. The incidences of solid tumours were significantly ($p < 0.05$) increased even at doses of 0.36–1.79 Gy when compared with controls (31%). The incidence of myeloid leukaemia fit a curvilinear model, and the RBE at the lowest dose of 0.17 Gy was about 4 with reference to an acute dose of 250-kVp X-rays (Covelli *et al.*, 1989).

The thoraxes of 474 male and 464 female SAS/4 albino outbred mice, three months of age, were exposed locally to 0.10, 0.25, 0.5, 0.75, 1, 2, 3 or 4 Gy of fast neutrons (mean energy, 7.5 MeV, with 3% γ-rays, beryllium target) at a rate of 1.06 Gy min^{-1}; the rest of the body was shielded. At the time of irradiation, the mice were anaesthetized with 57 mg (kg bw)$^{-1}$ sodium pentobarbitone. A group of 219 male and 210 female controls was available. After 12 months of irradiation, the animals were necropsied. Histologically, the lung tumours appeared to be a mixture of benign encapsulated adenomas and malignant invasive adenocarcinomas. The dose–response curve for animals of each sex was 'bell shaped' and steeply linear up to 1 Gy, peaked between 1 and 3 Gy and sharply declined at 4 Gy. In females, the incidences of lung tumours were 9% at 0 Gy (control) and 17.5, 24.1, 25.5, 27.9, 30.5, 33.9, 29.5 and 15.5% at the respective doses; in males, the percentage incidences were 16.5 (controls), 28.3, 32.7, 27.6, 29.1, 41.5, 42.2, 44.9 and 20.0%, respectively. The RBE for doses < 1 Gy of neutrons in comparison with < 3 Gy of 200-kVp acute X-ray exposure was 7.1 for females and 4.5 for males (Coggle, 1988).

Groups of 60 female (C57BL/6N × C3H/He) F$_1$ (B6C3F$_1$) mice, seven to eight weeks of age, were exposed by whole-body irradiation to a dose of 0.27 Gy at 0.059 mGy min^{-1} or 2.7 Gy at 0.53 mGy min^{-1} from ^{252}Cf fission neutrons (mean energy, 2.13 MeV; 35% γ-ray contamination). A group of 60 age-matched females was used as controls. The carcinogenic effects were examined 750 days after irradiation by gross observation and histopathologically. Both doses induced significantly higher incidences of neoplasms in the ovary, pituitary gland, Harderian gland, liver, mammary gland and reticulum cells (at 2.7 Gy only) and of lipoma (at 0.27 Gy only) (χ^2 test). No RBE was reported. There was no significant increase in the incidences of tumours in the lung, uterus and vagina, adrenal gland, soft tissue, bone, pancreas, stomach or thyroid gland, or of haemangiosarcoma or leukaemia after exposure to 0.27 or 2.7 Gy. More frequent development of multiple tumours was reported in the neutron-irradiated animals in comparison with animals exposed to γ-rays (^{60}Co, ^{137}Cs) (Seyama et al., 1991).

In a study of the influences of strain and sex on the development of tumours, 190 male and 151 female B6C3F$_1$ hybrid (C57BL × C3H), 65 male and 60 female C3B6F$_1$, 117 male and 112 female C57BL/6N and 156 male and 139 female C3H/HeN mice, six weeks of age, were exposed by whole-body irradiation to 0 (control), 0.125, 0.5 or 2 Gy of ^{252}Cf neutrons at a rate of 6–8 mGy min^{-1} (mean energy, 2.13 MeV; γ-ray component, 35%) and were observed up to 13 months of age. Tumours were identified histopathologically. The total tumour incidence was high in C3H/HeN, moderate in B6C3F$_1$ and C3B6F$_1$ and low in C57BL/6N mice (Table 9) because of high frequencies of liver tumours in males and ovarian tumours in females. A dose-dependent increase in liver tumours was reported in both males and females of all strains but the increase was greater in males than in females. Ovarian tumours were more frequent in C3H/HeN mice, followed by B6C3F$_1$, C3B6F$_1$ and C57BL/6N. Of the strains and hybrids, B6C3F$_1$, C57BL/6N and C3H/HeN were the most sensitive to low doses around 0.50 Gy (Ito et al., 1992; Takahashi et al., 1992).

In a series of experiments during the period 1971–86, thousands of male and female B6C3F$_1$ mice were exposed by whole-body irradiation to single or fractionated doses of fission neutrons. The effects on survival were reported by Ainsworth et al. (1975), Thomson et al. (1985a,b, 1986) and Thomson and Grahn (1988). In a report on tumour induction, several thousand male and female B6CF$_1$ (C57BL/6 × BALB/c) mice, 110 ± 7 days of age, were exposed to 0–2.4 Gy of fission neutrons, as single doses, 24 equal doses once weekly or 60 equal doses once weekly. The mean energy was 0.85 MeV; 2.5% of the dose was due to γ-radiation and 0.1% was thermal neutrons. A total of 901 age-matched males and 1199 age-matched females were used as controls. All the mice were followed for life, and the tumours were identified histopathologically. Most of those found in both control and irradiated mice were lymphoreticular, vascular and pulmonary tumours. About 85% of the irradiated mice died with or from one or more neoplasms. Dose-dependent increases in the incidence of lymphoreticular, lung, liver, Harderian gland and ovarian tumours were observed. The connective tissues showed less sensitivity to radiation-induced cancers than epithelial tissues, and the latter showed RBE values of 75 or greater with reference to chronic exposure to γ-rays (Grahn et al., 1992).

A total of 742 male BC3F$_1$ mice, three months of age, were exposed to five equal daily fractions of fission neutrons with a mean neutron energy of 4 MeV and a 12% γ-ray component, to yield cumulative doses of 0.025, 0.05, 0.1, 0.17, 0.25, 0.36, 0.535 and 0.71 Gy, given at a rate of 4 mGy min^{-1}. A group of 193 controls was available. The animals were kept for life, and tumours were examined grossly and histopathologically. The incidence of myeloid leukaemia showed a significant positive trend (Peto's test) at doses of 0–0.17 Gy and up to 0.36 Gy. The incidence of epithelial tumours was increased significantly ($p < 0.001$) at doses from 0.17 Gy, those of liver and lung tumours at doses from 0.025 Gy, that of skin tumours from 0.36 Gy and that

Table 9. Strain and sex differences in the incidence of ^{252}Cf neutron-induced tumours in mice

Reference	Dose (Gy)	Strain and sex	Effective no. of mice	Survival rate (%)	Liver tumours (%)	Lymphoma (%)	Adrenal tumours (%)	Ovarian tumours (%)
Ito et al. (1992)		C57BL/6N						
		Male						
	0		23	82	0	0	0	
	0.125		32	100	6.3	9.4	0	
	0.50		31	97	3.2	3.2	0	
	2.0		31	91	9.7	16	3.2	
		Female						
	0		25	89	0	16	0	12
	0.125		30	94	3.3	13	0	20
	0.50		31	97	0	19	3.2	9.7
	2.0		26	81	3.8	15	12	0
		C3H/HeN						
		Male						
	0		43	78	40	2.3	2.3	
	0.125		28	88	61	0	3.6	
	0.50		37	95	70	14	19	
	2.0		48	79	71	6.3	4.2	
		Female						
	0		35	100	11	2.9	0	66
	0.125		29	91	0	0	0	35
	0.50		40	100	18	13	0	94
	2.0		35	79	31	2.9	15	85

Table 9 (contd)

Reference	Dose (Gy)	Strain and sex	Effective no. of mice	Survival rate (%)	Liver tumours (%)	Lymphoma (%)	Adrenal tumours (%)	Ovarian tumours (%)
Ito et al. (1992) (contd)								
		C3B6F₁ Male						
	0		34	100	12	0	0	
	2.0		31	97	55	3.2	0	
		C3B6F₁ Female						
	0		33	97	0	0	0	6.1
	2.0		27	84	19	3.7	30	0
Takahashi et al. (1992)		B6C3F₁ Male				Not studied		
	0		53	96	3.8		0	
	0.03		24	100	13		0	
	0.06		24	100	21		0	
	0.125		30	94	37		3.3	
	0.50		30	94	43		0	
	2.0		29	91	62		0	
		Female						
	0		63	95	3.2		0	4.8
	0.125		29	91	3.4		3.4	28
	0.50		30	94	6.7		6.7	80
	2.0		29	91	28		21	62

of soft-tissue tumours only at the highest dose, 0.71 Gy. The total numbers of solid tumours in the lung, liver, gastrointestinal tract, adrenal gland, kidney, soft tissues, mammary gland, urinary bladder, vascular system, bone, Harderian gland, skin and salivary gland were 33, 41, 25, 28, 24, 24, 26, 20 and 27 at the respective doses. There were no differences in survival or tumour incidence between this study at 4 mGy min⁻¹ (Di Majo *et al.*, 1994) and a previous report (Di Majo *et al.*, 1990) in which dose rates of 50 and 250 mGy min⁻¹ were used. In a subsequent study, it was shown that male CBA/Cne mice were more susceptible to tumour induction than females (Di Majo *et al.*, 1996).

A total of 4689 male and female hybrid B6CF$_1$ (C57BL/6 Bd × BALB/c Bd) mice, 16 weeks of age, were exposed to fission neutrons at doses of 0.06, 0.12, 0.24 or 0.48 Gy in 24 weekly fractions of 0.0025 Gy, 12 fractions of 0.01 Gy every two weeks, six fractions of 0.04 Gy every four weeks or three fractions of 0.16 Gy every eight weeks. A group of 398 male and 396 female controls was available. The animals were observed for life, and tumours were identified histopathologically. The survival and the incidences of most neoplasms increased with dose in the low-dose range (Table 10). Fractionation of the neutron dose did not affect the magnitude of the response at equal total doses (Storer & Fry, 1995).

3.1.2   *Rat*

Most of the studies of the carcinogenicity of neutrons in rats have addressed the effects on the mammary gland (Table 11). The tumour incidence was shown to be influenced by strain and hormonal status (Clifton *et al.*, 1975, 1976a,b; Shellabarger *et al.*, 1978; Jacrot *et al.*, 1979; Shellabarger *et al.*, 1982, 1983). The most comprehensive studies are summarized below.

A total of 312 adult female Sprague-Dawley/ANL rats, two to three months of age, were exposed by whole-body irradiation to single doses of 0 (control), 0.05, 0.10–0.12, 0.18–0.22, 0.35, 0.5, 1.5 or 2.5 Gy of fission neutrons (10–15% γ-ray contamination, see Vogel, 1969). The animals were observed for life, and mammary tumours were examined histologically. At the end of the study, the percentages of rats with mammary tumour were 48, 78, 85, 73, 80, 84, 87 and 76% at the different doses, respectively. Of the 126 mammary tumours in 223 rats irradiated with 0.05–2.5 Gy, 66% were benign (67 fibroadenomas, four fibromas, one fibrolipoma, eight adenofibromas and three cystadenomas), and 34% were malignant (13 sarcomas and 30 carcinomas). The RBE in relation to an acute dose of 250-kVp X-rays was 20–60. In a comparison of partial and whole–body exposures to a dose of 0.35 Gy of neutrons, 28 animals received irradiation of one mammary gland at a mean energy of 540 ± 50 keV and 15 animals were exposed to 0.35 Gy of fission neutrons with a mean energy of about 1 MeV. Palpable mammary tumours (mostly fibroadenomas) developed in 75% of those receiving partial irradiation and 80% of those given whole-body exposure (Vogel & Zaldivar, 1972).

Table 10. Survival and incidences of tumours in various organs of BCF$_1$ mice exposed to single or fractionated doses of fission neutrons

Dose (Gy)	No. of animals	Mean survival (days)	Incidence (%)									
			Lung carci-noma	Reticulum-cell carcinoma	Other lym-phoma and leukaemia	Fibro-sarcoma	Vascular tissue	Liver tumour	Breast carcinoma	Osteo-sarcoma	Ovarian tumour	Other epithelial
Single doses												
Males												
0	398	913	32	17	2.8	29	6.8	8.3	–	–	–	–
0.025	396	888	31	22	2.8	32	6.4	9.7	–	–	–	–
0.05	393	875	28	23	3.2	36	4.9	11	–	–	–	–
0.1	397	870	36	25	2.5	32	5.8	12	–	–	–	–
0.2	398	848	39	24	3.5	49	6.8	13	–	–	–	–
Females												
0	396	938	13	35	12	6.6	6.1	0.51	9.1	0.76	1.3	
0.025	386	943	12	32	9.3	5.7	6.2	1.6	9.0	0.52	2.6	
0.05	389	926	12	39	14	8.3	8.8	1.5	7.4	0.60	2.4	
0.1	391	895	15	41	12	7.6	9.4	2.9	10	0.94	5.7	
0.2	390	866	21	46	13	5.5	7.5	2.8	9.6	1.7	11	
Fractionated doses												
Males												
0	398	913	32	17	2.8	29	6.8	8.3	–	–	–	1.3
24 × 0.0025 = 0.06	193	875	36	20	3.0	36	2.7	5.9	–	–	–	3.6
12 × 0.01 = 0.12	191	825	41	26	11	47	4.5	9.2	–	–	–	4.5
6 × 0.06 = 0.24	196	825	43	3.1	2.8	49	6.0	11	–	–	–	11
3 × 0.16 = 0.48	199	777	60	43	7.5	67	8.5	15	–	–	–	17
Females												
0	396	938	13	35	12	6.6	6.1	0.51	9.1	0.76	1.3	
24 × 0.0025 = 0.06	194	926	17	42	10	7.1	4.4	–	4.9	0.65	1.9	
12 × 0.01 = 0.12	190	894	13	48	15	11	4.8	2.6	8.4	1.4	3.2	
6 × 0.06 = 0.24	192	841	23	56	20	16	14	12	12	0.93	5.0	
3 × 0.16 = 0.48	194	800	33	68	22	11	3.3	11	12	3.3	11	

From Storer & Fry (1995); –, no tumours

Table 11. Mammary tumours in rats and mice after exposure to neutrons

Species and strain	Dose (Gy)	Mean energy (MeV)	No. of animals	No. of animals with tumours	Incidence of tumours (%)	Reference
Sprague-Dawley/ ANL rat	0	1	89	43	48	Vogel & Zaldivar (1972)
	0.05		27	21	78	
	0.10–0.12		34	29	86	
	0.18–0.22		41	30	73	
	0.35		25	20	80	
	0.50		31	26	84	
	1.50		31	27	87	
	2.50		34	26	76	
Fischer rat	0	Not reported	24	2	8	Clifton et al. (1976a)
	0.50		24	17	71	
Sprague-Dawley rat	0	0.43	167	20	12	Shellabarger (1976)
	0.01		182	28	15	
	0.04		89	16	18	
	0.16		68	21	31	
	0.64		45	26	58	
Sprague-Dawley rat	0	14.5	31	2	6.5	Montour et al. (1977)
	0.25		30	0	0	
	0.5		30	6	20	
	0.10		25	6	24	
	0.20		25	6	40	
	0.40		25	17	68	
Sprague-Dawley rat	0	1.2	62	2	3	Vogel (1978)
	0.5 + 0.5		40	6	15	
	0.10		38	10	26	
	0.10 + 0.10		29	15	52	
	0.20		29	10	34	
	0.35 + 0.35		35	22	63	
	0.70		37	20	54	
Sprague-Dawley rat	0	14.8	60	1	1.7	Jacrot et al. (1979)
	0.6		38	4	11	
Wistar/ Furth rat	0	2.0	18	0	0	Yokoro et al. (1980)
	0.48		16	1	6.3	
	0.089		16	0	0	
	0.195		16	0	0	

Table 11 (contd)

Species and strain	Dose (Gy)	Mean energy (MeV)	No. of animals	No. of animals with tumours	Incidence of tumours (%)	Reference
Sprague-Dawley rat	0	0.5	40	Not reported	30	Broerse *et al.* (1987)
	0.02		40		15	
	0.08		40		53	
	0.32		40		63	
	0	15	40		30	
	0.05		40		40	
	0.15		40		65	
	0.50		40		90	
WAG/Rij rat	0	0.5	40		27	
	0.05		40		20	
	0.2		40		33	
	0.8		40		53	
	0	15	40		27	
	0.15		40		35	
	0.50		40		58	
	1.5		40		56	
BN/Bi rat	0	0.5	40		8	
	0.05		40		11	
	0.2		40		19	
	0.8		40		44	
	0	15	40		8	
	0.15		40		22	
	0.5		40		56	
	1.5		40		78	
BALB/c mouse	0	1	263	Not reported	7.9	Ullrich (1983, 1984)
	0.25		140		11	
	0.5		160		17	
	0.10		160		18	
	0.20		167		20	
	0.50		182		25	
	2.00		182		8.4	

Groups of 110 female Sprague-Dawley rats, two months of age, were exposed to single doses of 0.1, 0.2 or 0.7 Gy or to split doses of 0.05 + 0.05, 0.1 + 0.1 and 0.35 + 0.35 Gy at 24-h intervals; 62 rats served as unirradiated controls. The radiation was ^{235}U fission neutrons with a mean energy of 1.2 MeV and a neutron:γ-ray ratio of approximately 7:1. Induction of mammary tumours was examined 11 or 12 months after irradiation [mode of examination not given]. Mammary tumours were reported in 2/62 controls, 10/38 at the single dose of 0.1 Gy and 6/40 given split exposure, in 10/29 at the single dose of 0.2 Gy and 15/29 given split exposure, in 20/37 at the single dose of 0.7 Gy and 22/35 given split exposure. No significant difference was seen in the incidence of mammary tumours with the single and the paired neutron doses (Vogel, 1978).

Groups of 15 and 34 female Long-Evans/Simonsen, 14 and 36 female Sprague-Dawley/Harlan, 15 and 34 female Buffalo/Simonsen, 14 and 36 female Fischer 344/Simonsen and 14 and 36 female Wistar-Lewis/Simonsen rats, two months of age, received whole-body irradiation with a single dose of 0 (control) or 0.5 Gy of fission neutrons (see Vogel, 1969). One year after irradiation, mammary tumours were identified histopathologically. The Long-Evans and Sprague-Dawley strains were the most sensitive, Buffalo and Fischer rats were moderately sensitive, and Wistar-Lewis rats were quite resistant to radiation-induced mammary tumours, the incidences being 56, 56, 29, 26 and 5.5% in exposed rats of the five strains, respectively (Table 12). This result strongly suggested a genetic predisposition in neutron-induced mammary tumorigenesis in rats (Vogel & Turner, 1982).

Groups of 20 (intermediate and high dose) or 40 (control and low dose) female WAG/Rij, BN/BiRij and Sprague-Dawley rats, eight weeks of age, were exposed by whole-body irradiation to single or fractionated doses of monoenergetic neutrons of 0.5, 4 or 15 MeV. In subsequent experiments, the numbers of animals in these groups were increased to 40 and 60, respectively. The animals were observed for life, and tumours were identified by gross and histopathological observation. The three strains developed different types of tumours and showed marked differences in susceptibility for mammary tumorigenesis. The RBE of the 0.5-MeV energy neutrons in relation to acute exposure to 300-kVp X-rays was 15 for the induction of adenocarcinomas and 13 for fibroadenomas in WAG/Rij rats and 7 for the induction of fibroadenomas in Sprague-Dawley rats (Broerse et al., 1986, 1987). [The Working Group noted that the numbers of animals in each group were not clearly stated.]

A total of 135 female Sprague-Dawley rats, 35–40 days of age, were exposed to doses of 0.025, 0.05, 0.1, 0.2 or 0.4 Gy of 14.5-MeV energy neutrons produced by a 35-MeV deuteron beam. A group of 31 controls was available. Mammary tumours were identified histopathologically as adenocarcinoma, fibroadenoma (including adenofibroma) and fibrosarcoma. By 11 months after exposure, 2/31 unirradiated rats had developed single fibroadenomas, whereas 42 mammary tumours were reported in 39/135 irradiated rats. The incidence increased with dose, from 0/30 to 6/30, 6/25, 6/25 and 17/25. Six of the rats that died within 11 months after irradiation had mammary tumours. Three rats died with neoplasms at other sites: lymphocytic type lymphosarcoma (0.4 Gy at seven months), osteogenic sarcoma (0.4 Gy at 11 months) and myxosarcoma (0.25 Gy at 11 months). The RBE increased from 5 at 0.4 Gy to 13.8 at 0.25 Gy, when compared with γ-rays (Montour et al., 1977). [The Working Group noted that the γ-ray source was not described.]

A total of 551 adult female Sprague-Dawley rats were exposed to 0.43-MeV neutrons at doses of 0 (167 controls), 1, 4, 16 or 64 mGy and the incidences of mammary tumours were examined histologically up to the age of 14 months. At the

Table 12. Mammary tumours in five strains of rat after single whole-body exposure to 0.5 Gy of fission neutrons

Strain	No. of rats with mammary tumours/no. of unirradiated rats	No. of rats with mammary tumours/no. of irradiated rats	All mammary tumours (%)	Fibroadenomas and adeno-fibromas (%)	Adeno-carcinomas (%)	Regressed tumours (%)
Long-Evans/Simonsen	0/15	19/34	56	11	5	0
Sprague-Dawley/Harlan	0/14	20/36	56	8	8	1
Buffalo/Simonsen	1/15	10/34	29	7	3	0
Fischer-344/Simonsen	0/15	9/35	26	6	1	0
Wistar-Lewis/Simonsen	0/14	2/36	5.5	0	1	1

From Vogel & Turner (1982)

end of the study, exposure to 1 mGy was found to have induced a higher incidence (15%) of adenocarcinomas and all other tumours than in the controls (12%). The incidences at the other doses were 18% at 4 mGy, 31% at 16 mGy and 58% at 64 mGy. The first tumours appeared five months after exposure to 1 mGy, three months after 4 mGy, four months after 16 mGy and two months after 64 mGy; in controls, the first tumour appeared at eight months. RBEs of about 100 for the low doses and about 8 for the high doses were reported with reference to an acute dose of 250-kVp X-irradiation (Shellabarger, 1976).

The role of prolactin in the induction of mammary tumours after low-dose whole-body irradiation with fission neutrons was examined in groups of 16–18 female Wistar/Furth rats, seven weeks of age, that were exposed to 0 (control), 0.048, 0.089 or 0.195 Gy of neutrons (mean energy, 2.0 Mev) [γ-ray component not specified]. To promote the development and growth of radiation-induced mammary tumours from dormant initiated cells, prolactin-secreting pituitary tumours (MtT.W95) were grafted subcutaneously 25 days after irradiation. In a further experiment, MtT.W95 were grafted only in tumour-free animals 12 months after irradiation. The rats died naturally or were killed when moribund, and mammary tumours were identified histologically as adenocarcinoma or fibroadenoma. Only 1/48 rats developed mammary tumours after neutron irradiation alone, while 20/48 rats developed mammary tumours when MtT.W95 were grafted 25 days after irradiation. The incidences at each dose were 6/16, 5/15 and 9/17, respectively. When MtT.W95 were grafted in tumour-free animals 12 months after irradiation, the incidences were 4/15, 3/15 and 4/15 at the respective doses (Yokoro et al., 1980, 1987).

A total of 767 male and female Sprague-Dawley rats, three months of age, were exposed by whole-body irradiation to fission neutrons at doses of 0.012, 0.02, 0.06, 0.1, 0.3, 0.5 (irradiation period, one day), 1.5, 2.3 (irradiation period, 14 days), 3.9 (irradiation period, 23 days), 5.3 or 8 Gy (irradiation period, 42 days) from a neutron reactor (1.6 MeV; neutron:γ-ray ratio, 3:1) and were observed for the induction of pulmonary neoplasms for life. Tumours were identified histopathologically. The lung tumours included bronchogenic carcinomas, bronchoalveolar carcinomas, lung carcinomas, adenomas and sarcomas. The numbers of animals with lung carcinomas were dose-dependent up to doses of 2.3 Gy, with a reduced mean survival. The numbers of animals with lung carcinoma or adenomas also increased at doses up to 2.3 Gy, but decreased at higher doses. An apparent life-shortening was observed at higher doses (Table 13) (Chmelevsky et al., 1984). [The Working Group noted that no data were given on controls.]

A total of 596 male Sprague-Dawley rats, three months of age, were exposed by whole-body irradiation to fission neutrons at 0.016 (mean of the two doses, 0.012 and 0.02), 0.08 (0.06 and 0.10) or 0.40 (0.32 and 0.49) Gy with a mean energy of 1.6 MeV (neutron:γ-ray ratio, 3:1). The duration of exposure was 20 h at 0.016 Gy and 22 h at the other doses. A group of 579 controls was available. The animals were observed for life. Lung carcinomas (bronchogenic and bronchoalveolar) and lung sarcomas were

Table 13. Pulmonary tumours in Sprague-Dawley rats after exposure to fission neutrons

Reference	Dose (Gy)	Irradiation period	No of animals	No. of animals examined	Mean survival (days)	No. of animals with lung carcinomas			No. of animals with lung sarcomas
						Total	Broncho-genic	Broncho-alveolar	
Chmelevsky et al. (1984)	0		NR	NR	NR	NR	NR	NR	NR
	0.012	1 day	150	148	752	4	3	1	1
	0.02	1 day	150	149	741	2	1	1	–
	0.06	1 day	80	77	679	4	1	3	–
	0.1	1 day	78	75	669	6	5	1	2
	0.3	1 day	75	71	584	9	4	5	2
	0.5	1 day	75	72	525	10	7	3	3
	1.5	14 days	40	94	487	14	5	11	3
	2.3	14 days	60	99	450	18	9	10	1
	3.9	23 days	20	20	390	–	–	–	–
	5.3	42 days	19	19	340	4	2	3	1
	8	42 days	20	20	240	2	1		–
Lafuma et al. (1989)	0		586	579	754	5	4	1	1
	0.012	20 h	150	149	757	4	3	1	3
	0.02	20 h	150	149	742	2	1	1	2
	0.06	22 h	80	77	679	4	1	3	–
	0.10	22 h	78	75	669	6	5	1	–
	0.32	22 h	75	72	583	9	4	5	2
	0.49	22 h	75	74	522	10	7	3	2

NR, not reported

identified by gross and histological examination. As shown in Table 13, increased incidences of animals with bronchogenic or bronchoalveolar carcinomas were observed. The RBE was 30–40 at the dose of 0.1 Gy and > 50 at the dose of 0.016 Gy in relation to acute ^{60}Co γ-irradiation (Lafuma *et al.*, 1989).

A group of 114 female Wistar rats, three to four months of age, were irradiated locally in the region of the liver with 0.2 Gy of neutrons at 14-day intervals for up to two years, for a total of 50 fractions and a total dose of 10 Gy and were observed for life. A group of 114 controls was available. The first liver tumour appeared one year after the beginning of irradiation. At the end of the study, 45 irradiated animals had liver tumours. Of the 83 liver tumours that were classified histologically, 14 were hepatocellular adenomas, 18 were hepatocellular carcinomas, 28 were bile-duct adenomas, nine were bile-duct carcinomas, one was a haemangioma and five were haemangiosarcomas; eight animals had Kupffer-cell sarcomas (Spiethoff *et al.*, 1992).

3.1.3   *Rabbit*

A total of 20 male and 18 female adult Dutch rabbits, 7–18 months of age, were irradiated ventro-dorsally with doses of 1.8–5.5 Gy of fission neutrons of about 0.7 MeV mean energy at a dose rate of about 23 Gy h^{-1} with γ-ray contamination of about 2.7 Gy h^{-1}. A control group of 17 rabbits was available. The rabbits were kept for life (six to nine years) and were killed when moribund. Full autopsies were carried out, and the tissues were studied histologically. The mean age at death was significantly lower after the doses of 3.7 Gy and 4.1–5.5 Gy (Student's *t* test). Increased incidences of subcutaneous fibrosarcomas were observed, with 0/17 in controls, 4/15 at 1.8 Gy, 10/16 at 3.7 Gy and 5/7 at 4.1–5.5 Gy. Osteosarcomas were found in 0, 1, 2 and 2 rabbits in the respective groups, and basal-cell tumours of the skin were found in 0, 10, 5 and 1 rabbits, respectively. The RBE for neutrons in relation to acute γ-irradiation was estimated to be 3–3.5 (Hulse, 1980).

3.1.4   *Dog*

A total of 46 male beagle dogs, one year of age, were exposed to fast neutrons with a mean energy of 15 MeV in one of three dose-limiting normal tissues, spinal cord, lung and brain. The radiation was given in four fractions per week for five weeks to the spinal cord, for six weeks to the lung or for seven weeks to the brain. A group of 11 controls was available. The animals were observed for life, and tumours were identified grossly and microscopically. No tumours were reported in the unirradiated controls. Nine neoplasms developed within the irradiated fields in seven dogs receiving fast neutrons, comprising a haemangiosarcoma of the heart (10 Gy to the hemithorax region), an oligodendroglioma and a glioblastoma in the left basal nuclei (13.33 Gy to the brain), an osteosarcoma in the subcutis, an adenocarcinoma of the lung and a haemangiosarcoma of the heart (15 Gy to the hemithorax region), a neurofibroma of the cervical nerve (17.5 Gy to the spinal cord), an osteosarcoma of the vertebrae and a myxofibrosarcoma of the subcutis (26.25 Gy to the spinal cord). The incidence of neoplasia was 15%, and the latent period for radiation-induced cancers varied from 1 to 4.5 years (Bradley *et al.*, 1981).

3.1.5   *Rhesus monkey*

Nine rhesus monkeys (*Macaca mulatta*), three years of age, were exposed by whole-body irradiation to neutrons (^{235}U; energy, 1 MeV) at doses of 2.3, 3.5, 3.8, 4.1 or 4.4 Gy at a rate of 0.08 Gy min^{-1} [γ-ray component unspecified]. A few hours after irradiation, the monkeys were grafted intravenously with $2–4 \times 10^8$ autologous bone-marrow cells (in Hank balanced salt solution) per kg bw. A group of 21 monkeys served as unirradiated controls. Between 4 and 10 years after irradiation, seven animals died with various malignant tumours, including glomus tumours in the pelvis, scrotum and subcutis, sarcomas or osteosarcomas in the humerus, osteosarcomas in the calvaria and papillary cystadenocarcinoma of the kidney and cerebral astrocytoma and glioblastoma. Benign tumours (islet-cell adenoma, subcutis haemangioma and skin fibroma) were also reported. No malignancies were observed in the 21 untreated controls. A RBE of approximately 4 was reported in relation to an acute dose of 300-kVp X-radiation. The latency for death with neoplastic disease after irradiation with fission neutron was 7 years (Broerse *et al.*, 1981, 1991).

3.1.6   *Relative biological effectiveness*

As shown in Table 14, neutrons were generally more carcinogenic than X-rays and γ-rays. Additional studies not described in the text are included in the Table.

3.2   **Prenatal exposure**

Mouse: Groups of pregnant female BC3F$_1$ [(C57BL/Cne × C3H/HeCne) F$_1$] mice were exposed to 0, 0.09, 0.27, 0.45 or 0.62 Gy of fission neutrons (mean energy, about 0.4 MeV; γ-ray contamination, about 12% of the total dose; minimum and maximum fast neutron dose rates, about 0.049 and 0.248 Gy min^{-1}) on day 17 of gestation and were allowed to deliver their offspring, which were observed for life. Liver tumours were examined histologically. A total of 379 offspring were necropsied. The incidences of liver adenomas and carcinomas were increased to 11, 31, 29 and 52% with the respective neutron doses but decreased to 18% after exposure to the highest dose of 0.62 Gy (Table 15). An RBE of 28 at 0.09 Gy was reported in relation to an acute dose of 250-kVp X-radiation (Di Majo *et al.*, 1990; Covelli *et al.*, 1991a,b).

Table 14. Relative biological effectiveness (RBE) of neutrons for various end-points, in relation to dose and energy

Species	Strain	Effect	Dose (Gy)	Energy (MeV)	RBE	Reference
Mouse	RF/Un	Myeloid leukaemia	0.001	1 and 5	1.8	Upton et al. (1970)
		Thymic lymphoma	0.001	1 and 5	3.3	Ullrich et al. (1979)
	RFM	Lung tumour	0.25	NR	25	
		Lung tumour	0.10		40	
	BALB/c	Lung adenocarcinoma	0.001	NR	19	Ullrich (1983)
		Mammary tumour	0.001		33	
	CBA/H	Myeloid leukaemia	0.001	NR	13	Mole (1984)
	B6C3F$_1$	Lymphoreticular tumour	0.001	~0.85	2–5	Thomson et al. (1985b)
		Lung tumour	0.001		23–24	
		Decreased survival	0.001		15	
	RFM	Myeloid leukaemia	0.001	NR	2.8	Ullrich & Preston (1987)
	BC3F$_1$	Decreased survival	0.01	1.5	12	Covelli et al. (1988)
	SAS/4	Lung tumour (male)	< 1	7.5	4.5	Coggle (1988)
		Lung tumour (female)	< 1	7.5	7.4	
	BC3F$_1$	Liver tumour[a]	0.09	0.4	28	Di Majo et al. (1990)
		Liver tumour[b]	0.17	0.4	13	
	B6C3F$_1$	Liver tumour (male)	0–2.0	2.13	15	Takahashi et al. (1992)
		Liver tumour (female)	0–2.0	2.13	2.5	
	CBA/Cne	Decreased survival (male)	0–0.4	0.4	24	Di Majo et al. (1996)
		Decreased survival (female)	0–0.4	0.4	8.6	
		Harderian gland tumour (male)	0–0.4	0.4	20	
		Harderian gland tumour (female)	0–0.4	0.4	9.5	
		Malignant lymphoma (male)	0–0.4	0.4	11	
		Myeloid leukaemia (male)	0–0.4	0.4	2.3	
	C57BL/Cnb	Malignant tumour	0.125–1	3.1	5-8	Maisin et al. (1996)

Table 14 (contd)

Species	Strain	Effect	Dose (Gy)	Energy (MeV)	RBE	Reference
Rat	Sprague-Dawley	Mammary tumour	0.001–0.04	0.43	100	Shellabarger (1976)
		Mammary tumour	0.016–0.064	0.43	8	
	Sprague-Dawley	Mammary tumour	0.4	14.5	5	Montour et al. (1977)
		Mammary tumour	0.025	14.5	14	
	Sprague-Dawley	Mammary fibroadenoma	0.001	2.43	50	Shellabarger et al. (1980)
	ACI	Mammary adenocarcinoma	0.001	2.43	100	Shellabarger et al. (1982)
	WAG/Rij	Mammary adenocarcinoma	0.001	0.5	15	Broerse et al. (1986)
		Mammary fibroadenoma	0.001	0.5	13	
	Sprague-Dawley	Mammary fibroadenoma	0.001	0.5	7	
	Sprague-Dawley	Lung carcinoma	0.016	1.6–2.1	50	Lafuma et al. (1989)
		Lung carcinoma	0.1	1.6–2.1	30–40	
Rabbit	Dutch	All tumours	1.8–5.5	2.5	3–3.5	Hulse (1980)
Rhesus monkey		All tumours	2–4	1	4	Broerse et al. (1981)

NR, not reported
[a] Irradiation on day 17 of gestation
[b] Irradiation at three months of age

**Table 15. Incidences of liver tumours in male BC3F$_1$
mice exposed *in utero* to a whole-body dose of fission
neutrons**

Dose (Gy)	No. of mice autopsied	No. of mice with tumours		Incidence (%)
		Adenoma	Carcinoma	
0	230	24	2	11
0.09	49	15	0	31
0.27	42	9	3	29
0.45	25	10	3	52
0.62	33	5	1	18

From Di Majo *et al.* (1990)

3.3   Parental exposure

Mouse: Groups of male C3H mice, seven weeks of age, were exposed by whole-body irradiation to neutrons (^{252}Cf; mean energy, 2.13 MeV) at total doses of 0, 0.5, 1 or 2 Gy and were mated two weeks or three months later with unexposed C57BL females. On day 18 of gestation, some pregnant mice were killed to detect dominant lethal mutations. The incidence of dominant lethal mutations increased in a dose-dependent manner only after postmeiotic exposure, at two weeks. The other pregnant mice were allowed to deliver, and a total of 387 offspring were killed at the age of 14.5 months. Although tumours were found in various organs, only the incidence of liver tumours correlated with exposure to ^{252}Cf radiation, and these tumours were examined histologically. As shown in Table 16, the numbers of liver tumours per male offspring of male mice exposed to 0.50 or 1 Gy ^{252}Cf at either the postmeiotic or the spermato-gonial stage were significantly higher than those in unirradiated controls. No increase in the incidence of liver tumours was observed in female offspring. The offspring of male parents irradiated with 2 Gy two weeks before mating did not survive more than two days after birth (Takahashi *et al.*, 1992; Watanabe *et al.*, 1996).

4.   Other Data Relevant to an Evaluation of Carcinogenicity and its Mechanisms

4.1   Transmission and absorption in biological tissues

The interaction of neutrons with biological material cannot be discussed outside the context of ionizing radiation in general, and the reader is referred to the Overall introduction for a fuller discussion. Neutrons with the lowest energy distribution, in

Table 16. Incidences of liver tumours in F₁ offspring of male C3H mice exposed to ²⁵²Cf neutrons and mated with unexposed C57BL mice two weeks or three months after irradiation

Paternal dose (Gy)	Sex of offspring	Two weeks (postmeiotic)		Three months (spermatogonial)	
		No. of mice	Liver tumours (%)	No. of mice	Liver tumours (%)
0	Male	31	3.2	33	9.1
0.5		44	43.2*	20	30.0
1		39	15.4	22	22.9
2		0		19	5.3
0	Female	30	3.3		
0.5		58	1.7	18	5.6
1		35	0	24	0
2		0		14	0

From Takahashi *et al*. (1992); Watanabe *et al*. (1996); *$p < 0.01$

thermal equilibrium with their surroundings, are called 'thermal neutrons' and typically have an energy < 0.5 eV. Neutrons with energies between 0.5 and 100 eV are known as 'epithermal', or 'resonance' neutrons. Neutrons with energies up to about 500 keV are usually considered 'intermediate' in energy, and neutrons above 500 keV are called 'fast'. Most neutrons emerging from a fission reaction are fast, but in a reactor their energies are slowed down (moderated) to thermal energies to allow a chain reaction to proceed. The neutron energy spectrum outside a reactor is typically dominated by intermediate energy neutrons. The distribution of energy from neutrons in tissue is different from that from X- or γ-radiation. At low doses, only a small fraction of cells in a tissue is traversed. For example, 1 cGy of 1-MeV neutrons will traverse about one in 20 cells, whereas low-LET radiation may give rise to five traversals per cell (see Overall introduction, section 3.1).

Techniques for measuring exposure to neutrons are described in the Overall introduction (section 2.1.1).

4.2 Adverse effects other than cancer

Less information is available about the deterministic effects in humans of neutron radiation than of low-LET radiation because fewer patients are treated with neutrons than with low-LET radiation. Although there was a neutron component present in the radiation released by the nuclear explosion at Hiroshima, the effects of neutrons alone are difficult to separate out accurately. The information about the biological effects of neutrons is derived from studies of patients treated with neutrons of various energies and from experimental studies with animals exposed to neutrons of similar energies and to fission neutrons (for reviews see UNSCEAR, 1982; ICRP, 1990, 1991; Engels & Wambersie, 1998).

4.2.1 *Modifying factors*

A characteristic property of neutrons is that their effects are modified considerably less by dose rate, dose fractionation, oxygenation and cell cycle stage than are the effects of low-LET radiations.

(*a*)   *Dose rate and fractionation*

In the case of dose rate and fractionation, the difference between neutrons and low-LET radiation can be attributed to the difference in the capability of the exposed cells to repair the damage induced by the different radiation qualities. With increasing LET, the size of the shoulder on the survival curve decreases and the slope increases. The characteristic reappearance of a shoulder, which is observed with fractionated exposure to low-LET radiation, is either much less pronounced or absent with neutrons. The reduction in repair appears to become maximal as the LET approaches 100 keV μm^{-1}.

(*b*)   *Effect of oxygen*

In general, cells and tissues are more radiosensitive when exposed to low-LET radiation in the presence of oxygen than under hypoxic conditions. The 'oxygen enhancement ratio' is the ratio of the doses required to produce a given level of a specific effect in the presence and absence of oxygen. The ratio for photons is in the range of 2.5–3.0. With increasing LET values above 60 keV μm^{-1}, the oxygen enhancement ratio for survival of human kidney cells decreases until it becomes 1 at LETs of about 180 keV μm^{-1} and higher. It was the low oxygen enhancement ratio that encouraged use of neutrons in cancer therapy (Field & Hornsey, 1979).

(*c*)   *Cell cycle*

Radiosensitivity varies with the age of a cell, with maximum resistance to cell killing late in S phase. The variation in radiosensitivity is less for neutrons than for low-LET radiation. In synchronized Chinese hamster cells exposed to neutrons, the D_0 for S-phase cells was about 25% higher than that for cells in G_1, whereas with X-radiation the difference was nearly 90% (Sinclair, 1968). In clonogenic cells of the jejunal crypt, the variation in cell survival throughout the cycle was about 30% greater with γ-radiation than with 50-MeV neutrons (Withers *et al.*, 1974).

4.2.2   *Effects in normal tissues*

There is considerable sparing of tissues after exposure to low-LET radiation because they can recover from sublethal damage; markedly less sparing is seen with exposure to neutrons. Since exposure frequently involves a number of relatively small dose fractions, the RBE for damage to tissues may be relatively high. Furthermore, slow repair may occur in slowly dividing or late-responding tissues after low-LET but not after high-LET radiation. Table 17 shows the RBE_m values (see section 1.2), calculated on the basis of the linear–quadratic model, for a number of representative end-points in tissues. The RBE_m values are higher and the $\alpha{:}\beta$ ratios are lower for the late-responding tissues than for the early-responding tissues, which have more rapid cell renewal. In reviewing their experience of the radiosensitivity of tissues in patients undergoing neutron radiotherapy, Laramore and Austin-Seymour (1992) stressed the steepness of the dose–response curves for the induction of damage to normal tissue, which renders the therapeutic window rather narrow.

(*a*)   Skin

The responses of mouse skin to high- and low-LET radiations are qualitatively similar, as are the time courses of the effects. The influence of the neutron energy is reflected in the RBE, which is about 7–8 for 2–3-MeV neutrons and about 3–5 for 15–25-MeV neutrons (Denekamp *et al.*, 1984). The RBE for late effects (3.2–3.4) is greater than that for early effects in pig skin exposed to γ-rays or 50-MeV (Be) neutrons (Withers *et al.*, 1977).

(*b*)   Gastrointestinal tract

(i)   Oesophagus

Death within 8–40 days due to either obstruction or perforation of the oesophagus can occur in mice exposed to high doses of neutrons to the thorax. Geraci *et al.* (1976) reported an RBE of 1.9 for 8-MeV neutrons generated by bombarding a beryllium source with 22-MeV deuterons. Phillips *et al.* (1974) obtained an RBE of 4 with 15-MeV monoenergetic neutrons.

(ii)   Small intestine

The murine crypt microcolony assay (Withers & Elkind, 1970) has been used to determine the RBE of single and fractionated doses of neutrons. Gueulette *et al.* (1996) reported RBE values for single doses of fast neutrons used for therapy at seven facilities in five countries, determined from the doses of each neutron source that resulted in 20 crypt microcolonies per circumference of the small intestine relative to the dose of ^{60}Co γ-radiation that caused the same effect. The RBEs were 1.5–2.2. Withers *et al.* (1993) reported RBE values in mice of 3.2–4.6 for neutrons produced by cyclotrons with deuteron energies of 16, 22, 35 and 50 MeV. Composite survival curves for crypt clonogenic cells after exposure to single doses were constructed from

Table 17. Maximum values of relative biological effectiveness (RBE$_m$) for tissue damage induced by fast neutrons and α:β ratios of the dose–response relationships for reference radiation (X- or γ-rays)

Tissue	End-point	Species	Neutron energy (MeV)	α:β (Gy) photons	RBE$_m$	Reference
Skin	Moist desquamation	Human	7.5	10.0	4.5	Field & Hornsey (1979)
Haematopoeitic system	LD$_{50}$ at 30 days	Mouse	14.0	5.0	2.0	Broerse & Barendsen (1973)
Respiratory system	LD$_{50}$ at > 30 days	Mouse	7.5	3.0	6.8	Field & Hornsey (1979)
Central nervous system	Late effects	Rat	14.0	3.0	7.2	Van der Kogel (1985)
Kidney	Late effects	Mouse	7.5	2.2	8.6	Joiner & Johns (1988)

data obtained with multiple fractions, and RBEs were calculated from the ratio of the α values for each neutron energy and γ-radiation. These ratios were considered to be RBE_m values. The RBE increased with decreasing neutron energy, which is consistent with the results of other studies (Hall *et al.*, 1979; see ICRP, 1990).

(c)   Haematopoietic system

The effects of neutrons and comparisons of their effectiveness with that of low-LET radiation have been determined from survival curves for progenitor cells, such as colony forming cells in the haematopoietic system, or from dose–response relationships for lethality expressed as LD_{50} at 30 days. Broerse *et al.* (1978) determined an RBE of about 2.0 for the occurrence of bone-marrow syndrome in rhesus monkeys exposed to fission neutrons. In studies of the effects of neutrons and mixed-field radiation in large animals in the 1950s and 1960s (see Alpen, 1991 for review), the RBE for fast neutrons, based on the LD_{50} at 30 days in dogs and goats, was about 1.0. In contrast, the RBEs for lethality in small rodents were about 2.0–2.5. Two factors are important: the characteristic effects of radiation are less affected by body mass in small animals than in large animals, and the RBE of neutrons for lethality is based on damage to the gut in rodents whereas the bone-marrow syndrome predominates in large animals such as dogs.

Accidental exposures and the atomic bombing of Hiroshima exposed humans to a mixture of fission neutrons and γ-radiation. The effect of mixed radiation on the haematopoietic syndrome has been studied in dogs (MacVittie *et al.*, 1991) in which the RBE for the LD_{50} at 30 days was about 1.7 on the basis of midline doses of ^{60}Co γ-radiation relative to mixed neutron and γ-radiation, the neutrons having an average energy of 0.85 MeV. The RBE based on the D_0 for granulocyte–macrophage colony-forming cells harvested from rib and pelvic bone-marrow aspirates 24 h after exposure of the dogs was reported to be about 2.

In a study of the survival of canine bone-marrow progenitor cells after exposure *in vitro* to ^{60}Co γ-radiation and fission neutrons (mean energy, 0.85 MeV), the D_0 values were about 77 cGy and 28 cGy, respectively, giving an RBE of about 2.8. The higher RBE of fission neutrons is consistent with neutron energy-dependence and with the RBE values of 1–2 reported for higher neutron energies. The RBE values for effects on the haematopoietic system are generally lower than those for solid tissues, which is consistent with the relatively small amounts of sublethal damage and repair in bone-marrow cells exposed to γ-radiation. The D_0 of the survival curve after γ-irradiation of bone-marrow progenitor cells isolated from dogs exposed *in vivo* to 7.0 cGy of γ-rays per day for 500 or 1000 days was reported to be significantly higher (2–2.5-fold) than that of cells from unirradiated dogs, whereas the increase in radioresistance to neutrons was much smaller. The mechanism of the acquired resistance is not known (Seed & Kaspar, 1991).

The determination of RBEs in deep tissues of large animals, including humans, requires accurate estimation of the doses of neutrons and of the reference radiation at the target tissue. In the experiment of MacVittie *et al.* (1991), the neutron:γ-radiation ratio was 5.4:1 in air but 1.7:1 at midline. The absorbed dose to the bone marrow and the resultant change in the neutron:γ ratio are not known. Inhomogeneity of the dose to the bone marrow is a confounding factor.

The effects of single and fractionated doses and low dose rates of fission neutrons on the survival of colony-forming units in the bone marrow were studied in B6CF$_1$ mice. The RBE was 2.6 for inactivation by a single dose but somewhat higher for fractionated doses. When mice were exposed to 0.96 Gy of neutrons or 2.47 Gy of γ-radiation in nine fractions, the populations of colony-forming units in femur cells had not returned to control levels by three months, but this sustained depression of progenitor cells contrasted with the number of circulating leukocytes, which was maintained at a normal level by some compensatory mechanism (Ainsworth *et al.*, 1989).

(d)   Central nervous system

The brain is considered to be relatively radioresistant, but damage to normal tissue has been a limiting factor in the treatment of brain tumours with neutron radiotherapy. In a small number of patients treated with 15.6 Gy of 16-MeV neutrons, severe injury and progressive dementia occurred. When the contaminating γ-radiation dose was included, the total dose was about 17.6 Gy. Damage to the vasculature was thought to account for lesions in normal brain tissue. A neutron dose of about 13 Gy can cause changes such as cerebral oedema (UNSCEAR, 1982).

Van der Kogel *et al.* (1982) described a so-called early type of damage that takes about five to six months to develop after exposure to low-LET radiation. The target is the glial cells responsible for myelinization. Late injury to the vasculature develops within two to five years after single doses of low-LET radiation. Similar lesions and particularly the earlier type of damage occur after neutron irradiation. RBE$_m$ values of about 5–7 have been estimated for 7.5-MeV and 14-MeV neutrons (Van der Kogel, 1985), and values of 6–10 were determined for degeneration of the white matter (White & Hornsey, 1980; Hornsey *et al.*, 1981).

(e)   Reproductive system

The effects of neutrons on the testis and in particular on the survival of type B spermatogonia, a highly radiosensitive cell type, have been reported. D$_0$ values of about 28 cGy for γ-radiation and 4–9 cGy for neutrons were observed (Hornsey *et al.*, 1977). Loss of testicular weight as a function of the dose of high-LET radiation and the survival of various types of spermatogonia have been used to assess the effects of neutrons (for references to individual studies see UNSCEAR, 1982; ICRP, 1990).

The effectiveness of 1-MeV, 2.3-MeV and 5.6-MeV fast neutrons in killing type B spermatogonia in mice was determined by scoring the number of preleptotene spermatocytes 48 h after the start of irradiation, because the surviving type B spermatogonia would have developed to this stage at that time. A decrease in the number of spermatocytes was considered to indicate accurately the loss of spermatogonia to the spermatogenesis process. D_0 values were determined from the loss of spermatogonia as a function of neutron and X-radiation dose. The survival curves were exponential. The RBE_m values were 5.7 for fission neutrons of 1.0 MeV mean energy and 4.6 and 3.0 for the 2.5-MeV and 5.6-MeV neutrons, respectively (Gasinska *et al.*, 1987).

(*f*)　*Renal system*

Stewart *et al.* (1984) used local irradiation of the kidney in mice to determine RBE values for changes in urine output, isotope clearance and haematocrit induced by single and multiple fractions of 3-MeV neutrons. The repair capacity of the kidney was very limited: the RBE for a single dose of about 6 Gy was approximately 2.4 and increased to 4.5–5.1 with eight fractions of about 1 Gy of neutron radiation.

(*g*)　*Respiratory system*

Damage to the lung induced by neutron radiation occurs both early, described as pneumonitis, and late after exposure, in the form of fibrosis. In contrast to most other tissues, the lung does not show significant differences in the RBE values for early and late effects. The RBE values based on the LD_{50} 60–180 days after exposure of mice to 7.5-MeV neutrons were reported to be 1.5 after single doses and about 3.4 after 15 fractions (Hornsey *et al.*, 1975). Parkins *et al.* (1985) studied the effects of irradiation of the mouse thorax with up to 20 fractions of 3-MeV neutrons or 240-kVp X-radiation on relative breathing rate and found an RBE_m value of about 7.

(*h*)　*Ocular lens*

The effects of neutrons on the lens in humans and experimental animals were reviewed by Medvedovsky and Worgul (1991), who reported that neutron-induced changes in the lens are indistinguishable from those produced by low-LET radiation, but neutrons are quantitatively more effective, the incidence being higher and the latent period shorter per unit dose. Reduction of the dose rate has little or no influence on the effectiveness of neutrons to induce cataracts.

The induction and development of lens opacities depend on how much of the total volume of the lens is irradiated and on the dose, the age at exposure and the radiation quality. The effectiveness of neutrons depends on their energy, the most effective energy being ≤ 1 MeV. The induction of various types of lenticular lesions has been used to assess the effect of radiation for the purposes of radiation protection, in order to prevent the induction of cataracts.

(i)　*Cataracts in humans*

Some of the physicists involved in testing the cyclotron developed cataracts (Abelson & Kruger, 1949). Although the doses were not measured precisely, it was estimated that the lens opacities occurred as a result of exposure to < 1 Gy of mixed γ- and neutron radiation. If this estimate is correct, the threshold dose was one-half to one-fifth that estimated for γ-radiation alone, which would indicate an appreciable RBE for the neutron component.

Data on the induction of cataracts in humans by high-LET radiation come from two sources. Roth *et al.* (1976) reported on the incidence of cataracts in patients treated with 7.5-MeV neutrons and found slight, permanent loss of vision in patients exposed to a total dose of 2.2 Gy in 12 fractions, with an RBE estimated to be about 2.5. The second source of information on the effects of neutrons on the eye is studies of the survivors of the atomic bombings, who have been examined for over three decades. The estimated threshold doses to the eye were reported to be 0.06 Gy (95% CI, 0–0.16) of neutrons and 0.73 Gy (95% CI, 0–1.39) of γ-rays, and the RBE was calculated to be approximately 32 (95% CI, 12–89) (Otake & Schull, 1990). Concern has been raised about errors in the dosimetry for this population in general but about the neutron component of the radiation released during the nuclear explosion over Hiroshima in particular (see section 1.3.3). The risk for cataract per unit dose was studied in persons who reported epilation after the atomic bombing and in those with no epilation, in two studies. The authors of one study attributed the difference between the two groups of survivors to a 48% random error in the dose estimates (Neriishi *et al.*, 1995), while the others concluded that it was not possible to decide whether the differences in the frequency of cataracts was due to differences in individual radio-sensitivity or to random errors in the dose estimate (Otake *et al.*, 1996). Because of these uncertainties, the data for experimental animals are important.

(ii)   *Cataracts in experimental animals*

Bateman *et al.* (1972) reported high RBE values for radiation-induced lens opacities in mice on the basis of the presence of flecks and other minor changes, which also occurred in unirradiated mice but at later ages. Neutrons thus shortened the latency to the appearance of these lesions. Data for 430-keV neutrons suggested that the relationship of the RBE to the neutron dose (D_n) in grays could be described as:

$$RBE = 4 \sqrt{1+1.5/D_n} \ .$$

At the lowest dose, the RBE was about 100.

Di Paola *et al.* (1978), using similar techniques, obtained RBE values of 9–21 with decreasing doses of 14-MeV neutrons from 0.38 to 0.01 Gy.

Despite differences in the methods of scoring lenticular opacities, Worgul *et al.* (1996) noted a reasonable degree of agreement in the results for neutron-induced cataracts in most species. They suggested that the RBE for cataractogenesis increases from < 10 at doses ≥ 1 Gy to > 100 at doses ≤ 10 mGy. The commonly used RBE of 20 is not consistent with their results for very low doses, because at a neutron dose of 2 mGy the RBE could be estimated to exceed 250. There is no evidence that the RBE for clinically significant cataracts in humans reaches such high values.

It has become possible to detect very small radiation-induced lesions in the lens, and the estimates of threshold dose have become thresholds of detection. For the purposes of radiation protection, it is the threshold dose for clinically significant opacities (some loss of vision) that is important. Fortunately, the treatment of cataracts has become so effective that the impact of radiation-induced cataracts has been reduced greatly. The experimental data for the induction of lenticular lesions by radiation are some of the best available for examining the relationship between RBE and dose and for testing the validity and consistency of models of the action of radiation. Lesions in the ocular lens can be assessed quantitatively at much lower doses of radiation than is the case for most, if not all, other tissues.

4.3   Radiation-sensitivity disorders

High-LET ionizing radiation kills mammalian cells more efficiently per unit dose than does X-radiation or γ-radiation (Cox *et al.*, 1977a,b; Barendsen, 1985; Goodhead, 1988). Studies of the relationship between the RBE of various forms of radiation and energy deposition in cells can provide additional insight into the mechanisms of the early events in carcinogenesis, such as DNA damage and mutations. It is of interest, therefore, to consider the response to neutron radiation of cells in persons with syndromes such as ataxia telangiectasia, who are known to be sensitive to X-radiation and γ-radiation.

Hypersensitivity to low-LET ionizing radiation is a common characteristic of cells from patients with the chromosomal breakage syndrome ataxia telangiectasia (Taylor *et al.*, 1975; Chen *et al.*, 1978; Cox *et al.*, 1978; see the monograph on 'X-radiation and γ-radiation', section 4.3.1). Cells from such patients have also been reported to be more sensitive than control cells to high-LET radiation, but the difference in sensitivity decreased as the LET of the radiation increased (Cox, 1982). Other characteristics of cells from patients with this syndrome include reduced inhibition of DNA synthesis after exposure to γ-radiation (Edwards & Taylor, 1980; Houldsworth & Lavin, 1980; Ford & Lavin, 1981) or to X-radiation (Painter & Young, 1980; De Wit *et al.*, 1981) and greater and more prolonged accumulation of cells in the G_2 phase of the cell cycle after irradiation (Imray & Kidson, 1983; Ford *et al.*, 1984; Bates & Lavin, 1989).

Exposure of control lymphoblastoid cell lines and cell lines from patients with ataxia telangiectasia to neutrons of a mean energy of 1.7 MeV affects cell survival and the incorporation of [³H]thymidine into DNA. In addition, neutrons influence the progression of cells through the cell cycle. While high-LET radiation was considerably more effective in killing cells from the patients than from controls, the relative sensitivity of the two cell types was variable in the case of low-LET radiation. While fibroblasts from patients with ataxia telangiectasia were hypersensitive to X-radiation and γ-radiation, their radiosensitivity to α-particles was comparable to that of control cells (Lücke-Huhle *et al.*, 1982). In a later study, Lücke-Huhle (1994) failed to observe increased killing by densely ionizing α-particles of cells from these patients when compared with control cells, indicating that the RBE for inactivation of cells from patients with ataxia telangiectasia is much less dependent on ionization density than that of control cells, for which it reaches a maximum of approximately 4 at a LET value of 100 keV μm⁻¹ (Cox *et al.*, 1977a,b). In fibroblasts from these patients, the maximum RBE was ≤ 2 at 100 keV μm⁻¹ (Cox, 1982). These data suggest that the lesions induced in DNA by high-LET radiation are inefficiently repaired in both cell types and the two can be distinguished only on the basis of DNA damage induced by low-LET radiation, which is readily repairable in controls. In a study with two lymphoblastoid cell lines from patients with ataxia telangiectasia, fast neutrons (mean energy, 1.7 MeV) were considerably more effective than γ-rays in inducing cell death. Fast neutrons inhibited DNA synthesis to the same extent in cells from patients with this syndrome as in those from controls (radioresistant DNA synthesis), but the long-term delay in G$_2$/M phase was greater in the cells from the patients, as was observed after γ-irradiation (Bates & Lavin, 1989). Thus, a correlation between G$_2$/M delay and cell killing was seen in these lymphoblastoid cells, regardless of the LET value of the radiation (Houldsworth *et al.*, 1991); this was not the case with fibroblasts from these patients (Lücke-Huhle *et al.*, 1982).

In keeping with the data on the survival of fibroblasts, marked differences in the rejoining kinetics of γ-radiation-induced double-strand breaks in DNA were found between control cells and those from patients with ataxia telangiectasia, but similar kinetics of rejoining of these breaks was observed after exposure to ²⁴¹Am α-particles (Coquerelle *et al.*, 1987). When the production of micronuclei was determined in lymphocytes from such patients after irradiation, the increase over that in control cells was less pronounced after exposure to neutrons than after exposure to γ-rays (Vral *et al.*, 1996).

4.4   Genetic and related effects

4.4.1   *Humans*

Chromosomal aberrations were examined in lymphocytes from eight men aged 24–56 who were exposed during a criticality accident to mixed γ-radiation and fission neutrons at doses estimated to range from 0.23 to 3.65 Gy. The neutrons contributed about 26% of the total dose. Five of the men received doses that were estimated to exceed 2.3 Gy, and the three others received lower doses. The blood samples were drawn about 2.5 years after the irradiation; blood from five unirradiated subjects was used as a control. Only chromatid-type aberrations were found in the controls. In the subjects exposed to the higher doses, the frequency of aneuploid cells was 7–23%, and gross aberrations, such as rings, dicentrics and minutes, were found in 2–20% of the cells. The men who received doses of 0.23–0.69 Gy also had abnormalities but at a much lower frequency (Bender & Gooch, 1962). Analysis of blood samples from the same persons 3.5 years after exposure showed that they still had chromosomal aberra-tions but in most cases at a somewhat lower frequency (Bender & Gooch, 1963).

Chromosomal aberrations in peripheral blood cells were scored in a study of 17 patients who received tumour therapy with 14-meV neutrons at a rate of about

0.2 Gy min⁻¹ with a distance of 80 cm between the source and the skin. Treatment consisted either of daily doses of 0.65–0.80 Gy or of 12 exposures of 1.3 Gy in three fractions per week. The doses of contaminating γ-rays were 5–15% depending on the field size and the depth of the tumour. The intercellular distribution of dicentric chromosomes showed predominantly overdispersion. A positive correlation was found for dicentrics with a total skin dose of 0.8–15.6 Gy, and for total chromosome-type damage (dicentrics, centric rings and excess acentrics). The authors concluded that there was a significant correlation with therapeutic dose, despite the complex influences of biological and physical factors on the aberration yield (Schmid *et al.*, 1980).

[The reports summarized below became available after the meeting of the Working Group, although members of the Group were aware of the existence of some of these publications. In view of their importance for the evaluation, they are included in the monograph for completeness.

[The men studied by Bender and Gooch (1962, 1963) were further examined 7 (Goh, 1968), 8 and 10.5 (Goh, 1975) and 16 and 17 years (Littlefield & Joiner, 1978) after the accident. At 16–17 years, six of the men still had residual chromosomal aberrations; three men who had received the high doses had the highest frequency, and the two who had been exposed to the highest dose had around 10% aberrant cells.

[In a criticality accident in 1965 in Mol, Belgium, a man received doses to the bone marrow estimated to be 500 cGy of γ-radiation and 50 cGy of neutrons. Only 24 mitoses good enough for analysis were obtained. The aberrations included deletions, translocations, dicentrics and rings; some cells had two or even three dicentrics. On the basis of results available at the time on cells exposed *in vitro*, the total dose (mean homogeneous equivalent dose) corresponding in effect to low-LET radiation was estimated to be 470–500 cGy, in good agreement with the physical estimates (Jammet *et al.*, 1980).

[An accident in Vinca, Yugoslavia, in 1958 resulted in the exposure of six persons to neutrons and γ-radiation. More than 50% of the dose was estimated to be neutrons, and the doses were estimated to be 165–227 cGy of neutrons and 158–209 cGy of γ-rays. Five years after the accident, the frequency of structural aberrations in the peripheral lymphocytes was 8–28% (Pendic & Djordjevic, 1968). Nineteen years after the accident, the frequency of aberrations in four men had declined somewhat to 10–22% (Pendic *et al.*, 1980).

[The persistence of chromosomal aberrations in patients who received fractionated neutron therapy (average bone-marrow dose, < 100 to > 1000 cGy) to tumours located at various sites was evaluated recently (Littlefield *et al.*, 2000). Neutron-induced dicentrics and rings disappeared from the peripheral circulation within the first three years after exposure, while translocations persisted for more than 17 years.]

4.4.2 *Experimental systems*

(a) *Mutations* in vivo

(i) *Germ-cell mutations*

Visible dominant mutations: In mice, the spontaneous rate for visible dominant mutations is approximately 8×10^{-6} per gamete per generation. Exposure to fission neutrons (mean energy, 0.7 MeV) gave rise to a spermatogonial mutation rate of 25.5×10^{-5} per gamete per Gy (Batchelor *et al.*, 1966).

Dominant lethal mutations: When male mice were exposed to fission neutrons four to five weeks before mating with untreated females (postgonial stage), the rate of dominant lethal mutations was approximately 25×10^{-2} per gamete per Gy (Grahn *et al.*, 1979). When males were irradiated in the stem-cell stage, no effect of dose rate was observed after single or weekly exposures to neutrons, both of which gave a dominant lethal mutation rate of 40×10^{-3} per gamete per Gy (Grahn *et al.*, 1979).

Experimental evidence of the nature of radiosensitive targets in immature (resting) mouse oocytes led to new experimental designs that permitted measurement of radiation-induced genetic damage in these cells. Such damage has been detected after exposure to monoenergetic 0.43-MeV neutrons, and the genetic sensitivity of the immature oocytes has been compared with that of maturing oocytes. Recoil protons from 0.43-MeV neutrons produce short ionization tracks (mean, 2.6 μm) and can therefore deposit energy in the DNA without simultaneously traversing and damaging the hypersensitive plasma membrane. With these neutrons, dose–response relationships were obtained for both chromosomal aberrations and dominant lethal mutations in oocytes from females irradiated 8–12 weeks earlier, when the oocytes were immature. The intrinsic mutational sensitivity of immature mouse oocytes appeared to be similar to that of maturing oocytes (Straume *et al.*, 1991).

Recessive visible mutations: In male mice, irradiation of post-spermatogonial stages with neutrons at doses of up to 1 Gy resulted in recessive visible mutation rates of $100–150 \times 10^{-6}$ per locus per Gy, with no effect of dose rate (Russell, 1965). In female mice, a rate of 145×10^{-6} per locus per Gy was reported for this type of mutation after single doses of fission neutrons (0.3, 0.6 and 1.2 Gy) (Russell, 1972).

Specific locus mutations: One system for studying mutation induction in mice comprises a series of 12 genes, most of which affect coat colour, six or seven of which are usually tested as a group (Cattanach, 1971). Neutrons show an inverse dose-rate effect, low dose rates of high doses being much more effective. In contrast to spermatogonia, oocytes are difficult to analyse for mutations (Batchelor *et al.*, 1969). A complicating factor is the time of conception after irradiation: with neutrons at low dose rates, mutations could be recovered in litters conceived within seven weeks of irradiation, but later litters had no mutations (Russell 1967).

Comparison of the effects of high-LET and low-LET radiation: Male $B6CF_1$ mice were exposed to once-weekly doses of either fission neutrons or ^{60}Co γ-radiation for up to one year and mated periodically to screen for the induction of dominant lethal mutations. The doses of neutrons were 0.0013–0.027 Gy week^{-1} and those of γ-radiation were 0.05–0.32 Gy week^{-1}. Data on both pre- and postimplantation fetal deaths were obtained. Age- and time-dependent factors made no consistent, significant contribution to the mutation rate; such factors could include changes in radiosensitivity and in spontaneous rates and any cumulative damage to the stem-cell population. Direct comparison of these data with data for males exposed to single doses confirmed that weekly neutron irradiation was significantly more effective than single doses in inducing postimplantation fetal losses, whereas single doses of γ-rays were more effective than the same dose divided into weekly fractions. The RBE of neutrons increased from 5 to 12 for single and weekly doses. The rates of preimplantation loss, although significant, were not considered to be a sensitive measure of genetic injury at the low doses used (Grahn *et al.*, 1986).

Young adult male B6CF$_1$ mice were exposed to single whole-body doses of fission neutrons or ^{60}Co γ-radiation. Post-spermatogonial dominant lethal mutations, the incidence of reciprocal chromosomal translocations in spermatogonia, the incidence of abnormal epididymal sperm four to six weeks after exposure, and testicular weight loss three to six weeks after exposure were measured. The responses to neutron doses of 0.01–0.4 Gy and γ-radiation doses of 0.23–1.45 Gy were analysed in detail, although more limited data from a fourfold higher dose range were integrated into the analysis. Significant effects were seen at 0.01 and 0.025 Gy of neutrons, consistent with extrapolation from higher doses, with the exception of dominant lethal mutations, which occurred in significant excess of expectation. The dose–response relationships were linear or linear–quadratic, depending on the end-point, radiation quality and dose range. For translocation frequencies, the D^2 term in the linear–quadratic dose–response function (see section 5, Overall introduction) was negative for neutron and positive for γ-ray irradiations. The RBE values for testicular weight loss and abnormal sperm were between 5 and 6 over the full dose range and were between 7 and 9 at lower doses (< 0.1 Gy) for translocations. The RBE values for postimplantation loss and total dominant lethal rates were 5–6 at doses > 0.1 Gy and 10–14 at doses < 0.1 Gy. The values for preimplantation loss were between 15 and 25 at doses > 0.1 Gy and possibly higher < 0.1 Gy. The authors suggested that the unusual results at the lower doses may be explained by variation in cell sensitivity, cell selection, probability of neutron traversal per cell, variance of magnitude of the energy deposition events, dose rate and DNA repair (Grahn *et al.*, 1984).

Male mice heterozygous for the Rb(11.13)4Bnr translocation were irradiated for 14.5 min with either 0.15 Gy of fission neutrons or 0.6 Gy of X-rays. These mice are known to show high levels of spontaneous autosomal non-disjunction (20–30%) after anaphase I. The effects of the irradiation on this process were determined in air-dried preparations of primary and secondary spermatocytes. The induced effects were studied at intervals of 2 and 3 h after the start of the irradiation and assessed by scoring: univalents in primary spermatocytes; deletions, aneuploid chromosome counts and precocious centromere separation in secondary spermatocytes; and chromatid gaps and breaks in both cell types. The two types of radiation induced comparable levels of chromosomal damage. The RBE value for neutrons relative to X-rays was calculated to be 5.4 for the meiosis I stage and 3.3 for the meiosis II stage. According to the authors, the significantly higher incidence of cells showing damage at meiosis II than at diakinesis/ meiosis I does not indicate a difference in radiation sensitivity, but is the consequence of the different chromosomal processes taking place during the time between irradiation and fixation (Nijhoff & de Boer, 1980).

(ii)   *Somatic mutations*

Hprt: Mutation induction was measured at the *Hprt* locus in splenic lymphocytes of B6CF$_1$ mice 56 days after whole-body irradiation with fission-spectrum neutrons. Lymphocytes were cultured for 12–16 days in the presence of 5×10^4 feeder cells (syngeneic lymphocytes irradiated with 50 Gy γ-radiation). Animals were exposed to either single doses of neutrons (1.5 Gy) or fractionated doses delivered over two weeks (0.25 Gy × 6; total, 1.5 Gy). The frequency of *Hprt* mutant induction by the single 1.5-Gy dose was $5.98 \pm 1.51 \times 10^{-5}$ (SE). Multiple doses of neutrons (total, 1.5 Gy) gave rise to a mutation frequency of $8.71 \pm 5.39 \times 10^{-5}$ (SE) (Kataoka *et al.*, 1993).

Oncogenes: Point mutations at codon 12 of the K-*Ras* oncogene were analysed by an 'enriched' polymerase chain reaction method in 25-year-old paraffin-embedded samples of normal lung tissue and lung adenocarcinoma tissue from mice that had been exposed to radiation. Significantly more K-*Ras* codon-12 mutations (100%) were observed in normal lung tissue from mice exposed 24 times to once-weekly neutron radiation than in normal lung tissue from sham-irradiated mice (50%; $p < 0.05$). Lung adenocarcinomas from these irradiated mice also had a significantly higher frequency of point mutations in codon 12 of K-*Ras* than lung adenocarcinomas from mice exposed to γ-radiation once a week for 24 or 60 weeks (50%), but the higher frequency was not significantly different from that in spontaneous lung adenocarcinomas from mice (75%; $p > 0.05$). Sequencing of two of the mutants revealed a K-*Ras* 13(Asp) point mutation (Zhang & Woloschak, 1998). [The Working Group noted that it cannot be concluded that the codon-12 mutations were induced by the radiation or arose in clones initially transformed by the radiation.]

N-*Ras* mutations were examined in DNA samples extracted from the spleens of CBA/Ca mice that had developed myeloid leukaemia after exposure to radiations of various qualities. Seventeen cases of myeloid leukaemia comprising five cases of neutron-induced and 12 cases of photon (three γ-radiation and nine X-radiation)-induced myeloid leukaemia were included, with 12 DNA samples from the bone-marrow cells of control mice. Mobility shifts revealed by polymerase chain reaction and single-strand conformational polymorphism indicated mutations only in exon II of the N-*Ras* gene. Such mutations were more prevalent in samples from mice exposed to fast neutrons. Silent point mutations, i.e. base transitions at the third base of codons 57, 62 or 70, were present only in mice that had developed myeloid leukaemia after exposure to fast neutrons. The higher frequency of N-*Ras* mutations in neutron-induced myeloid leukaemia suggested that fast neutrons are more effective in inducing genomic instability at the N-*Ras* region of the genome. More importantly, N-*Ras* mutations appear not to be the initiating event in radiation leukaemogenesis. This conclusion was supported by the finding of N-*ras* mutations only in mice with an overt leukaemic phenotype and not in animals with minimal tissue infiltration of leukaemic cells, suggesting that the disease may be present before the N-*Ras* mutations (Rithidech *et al.*, 1996).

A protocol was developed to induce thymic lymphomas in RF/J mice efficiently by a single acute dose of neutron radiation. Activated *Ras* genes were detected in 4 of 24 of the tumours analysed. One of the tumours contained a K-*Ras* gene activated by a point mutation in codon 146. Activating *Ras* mutations at position 146 have not previously been detected in any known human or animal tumour. The spectrum of *Ras* mutations detected in neutron radiation-induced thymic lymphomas was different from that seen in thymic lymphomas induced by γ-radiation in the same strain of mice (Sloan *et al.*, 1990). A novel K-*ras* mutation in codon 146 was also found in thymic lymphomas induced by neutrons (Corominas *et al.*, 1991).

(iii)   *Cytogenetic effects*

Sister chromatid exchanges were scored in bone-marrow cells from three-month-old rats as a function of time after exposure to 2 Gy of whole-body radiation with 1-MeV fission neutrons. This dose reduced the mean survival time to 445 days after irradiation and induced more than one tumour per animal; by 200 days after irradiation, all of the animals bore tumours at autopsy, but the bone-marrow was not a significant target for tumour induction. In controls, the mean number of sister chromatid exchanges per cell remained constant from 3 to 24 months of age (2.38 per cell; SD, 0.21), but irradiation induced two distinct increases in the frequency: the first occurred during the days following exposure and the second between days 150 and 240. Thereafter, the values levelled off at 3.37 per cell (SD, 0.39) until day 650. Between the two increases (i.e. days 15–150), the number of sister chromatid exchanges dropped to control values. Analysis of the distribution per cell showed that the changes were not confined to a particular cell population. These results suggest that, in irradiated rats, the second increase in sister chromatid exchange coincides with tumour growth, whereas the first increase may be due to DNA damage that is rapidly repaired (Poncy *et al.*, 1988).

A modified mouse splenocyte culture system was standardized and used to evaluate the induction of micronuclei and chromosomal aberrations for the purposes of biological dosimetry after exposure to X-radiation and fission neutrons *in vivo* and/or *in vitro*. After irradiation with 1-MeV fission neutrons *in vivo* and culturing of mouse splenocytes, linear dose–response curves were obtained for the induction of micronuclei and chromosomal aberrations. The lethal effects of neutrons were shown to be significantly greater than those of a similar dose of X-radiation. The RBE was 6–8 in a dose range of 0.25–3 Gy for radiation-induced asymmetrical exchanges (dicentrics and rings) and about 8 for micronuclei in a dose range of 0.25–2 Gy (Darroudi *et al.*, 1992).

The induction of reciprocal translocations in rhesus monkey stem-cell spermatogonia was studied by analysing primary spermatocytes at metaphase. The animals were exposed to 1 Gy of γ-radiation at dose rates of 140 or 0.2 mGy min⁻¹ or to 0.25 Gy of 2-MeV neutrons at 36 mGy min⁻¹. Reduction of the dose rate from 140 to 0.2 mGy min⁻¹ did not lower the frequency of recovered translocations from 0.43% induced by the γ-radiation. The RBE for neutrons in relation to X-radiation was 2.1, which is clearly lower than the value of 4 obtained for mice (Van Buul, 1989).

(*b*)   *Cellular systems*

(i)   *DNA damage*

Radiolysis of water results in numerous products; the most reactive and the most damaging to DNA is the •OH radical. This radical either abstracts •H from deoxyribose and bases or reacts with the bases of all nucleotides. Consequential to these reactions, conformational changes occur in DNA, which lead to the generation of lesions. These lesions include single- and double-strand breaks and modifications of deoxyribose and bases (some of these are alkali-labile sites that are revealed as single-strand breaks after alkaline treatment), intrastrand and interstrand cross-links and DNA–protein cross-links (Burns & Sims, 1981). The RBE of neutrons (in relation to γ-radiation) for generation of these lesions is often higher than 2.5, but there is no qualitative difference in the results of exposure to these types of radiation.

Irradiation of pBR322 plasmid DNA in solution with neutrons or γ-radiation resulted in half the yield of single-strand breaks and a 1.5-times higher yield of double-strand breaks with neutrons as compared with γ-rays (Spotheim-Maurizot *et al.*, 1990, 1996). Scavenging of •OH radicals with ethanol inhibited all neutron-induced single-strand breaks but only 85% of the double-strand breaks, whereas with γ-irradiation the formation of both single- and double-strand breaks was completely inhibited. The results suggest at least three different origins for neutron-induced double-strand breaks. The occurrence of around 30% of these breaks can be explained by a radical transfer mechanism, as proposed by Siddiqi and Bothe (1987), for γ-radiation. In this model, a radical site is transferred from a sugar moiety of the cleaved strand to the complementary intact strand, which occurs with a probability of about 6%. Around 55% of neutron-induced double-strand breaks may be due to the non-random distribution of radicals in high-density tracks of the secondary particles of neutrons, which results in a simultaneous attack of the two strands by •OH radicals. The first two processes are both •OH-mediated and are therefore sensitive to ethanol. The direct effect of fast neutrons and their secondaries (recoil protons, α-particles and recoil nuclei) can account for the remaining 15% of double-strand breaks, which are not inhibited by scavengers (Spotheim-Maurizot *et al.*, 1990). Consistent with this view, Pogozelski *et al.* (1999) found that the decrease in yields of strand breaks in plasmid pBR322 with increasing •OH scavenging capacities was not as pronounced for fission neutrons as for γ-rays. In contrast, damage to restriction fragments or oligo-deoxyribonucleotides induced by fission neutrons can be almost completely suppressed by thiols (Savoye *et al.*, 1997; Swenberg *et al.*, 1997).

In an 80-base-pair DNA fragment exposed to fast neutrons, the probability of strand breakage at a given nucleotide site was not determined by the nature of the nucleotide but by its flanking sequence. The sequence-dependence is due to variations in the accessibility of the H4′ and H5′ atoms. Fitting the experimental results with the calculated reaction probabilities suggested that a C4′-centred radical develops into a strand break three times more efficiently than a C5′-centred radical, and that half of the breaks occur via the 4′ path and half via the 5′ path (Sy *et al.*, 1997).

DNA lesions induced by fast neutrons in L5178Y mouse lymphoma cells were classified into three types on the basis of their repair profiles: rapidly repaired breaks (half-time, 3–5 min), slowly repaired breaks (70 min) and unrepairable breaks. The rates of repair of the first two types of break were almost the same as those of corresponding damage induced by low-LET radiation. Neutrons induced less rapidly repaired damage, a nearly equal amount of slowly repaired damage and more unrepairable damage when compared with equal doses of γ-radiation or X-radiation (Sakai *et al.*, 1987).

The induction and repair of breaks was studied by alkaline elution (Kohn & Grimek-Ewig, 1973) of DNA from Chinese hamster V79 and human P3 epithelial teratocarcinoma cells after exposure to fission-spectrum neutrons (mean energy, 0.85 MeV) and ^{60}Co γ-radiation in the biological dose range. The fission-spectrum neutrons induced fewer direct single-strand breaks per gray of absorbed dose than γ-radiation (Peak *et al.*, 1989). Measurements of cell survival had already indicated incomplete recovery of the cells after exposure to neutrons (Hill *et al.*, 1988). Whereas most single-strand breaks caused by exposure to fission-spectrum neutrons can be rapidly repaired by both hamster and human cell lines, a small but statistically significant fraction (about 10%) of the single-strand breaks induced by exposure to 6 Gy of neutrons was refractory to repair. In contrast, all measurable single-strand DNA breaks induced by 3 Gy of γ-radiation were rapidly repaired (Peak *et al.*, 1989).

Neutron irradiation has been reported to cause single-strand breaks, with RBEs varying from 0.3 to nearly 2 in assays with various cellular and extracellular systems and neutron energies (see, e.g. Van der Schans *et al.*, 1983; Prise *et al.*, 1987; Vaughan *et al.*, 1991). The RBEs for double-strand break induction by neutrons are usually about 1, although higher values have been reported. The breaks differ from those induced by γ-rays mainly in the fact that they are less readily repaired, as described below.

Monolayers of L-929 mouse fibroblasts were irradiated with fast neutrons or 250-kVp X-rays and treated simultaneously with dinitrophenol to prevent the DNA strands from rejoining; single-strand breaks induced in DNA were measured by the alkaline sucrose sedimentation method. The RBE for single-strand breaks was about 1.6, which is essentially the same as that measured from cell survival (Moss *et al.*, 1976).

The effects on cellular viability and the kinetics of induction and repair of DNA strand breaks in HeLa cells were examined after exposure to a thermal neutron beam and compared with those after γ-irradiation. The survival curve had no initial shoulder. The RBEs of the neutron radiation were 2.2 for cell killing (ratio of D_0 values), 1.8 and 0.9 for single-strand breaks measured by alkaline sedimentation and alkaline elution, respectively, and 2.6 for double-strand breaks, determined by neutral elution (Bradley & Kohn, 1979). No difference was observed between thermal neutrons and γ-rays in respect of the repair kinetics of single- and double-strand breaks. It was suggested that the effect of the intracellular nuclear reaction, $^{14}N(n,p)^{14}C$, is mainly responsible for the high RBE values observed (Maki *et al.*, 1986).

The effects of 2.3-MeV (mean energy) neutrons and 250-kVp X-rays on cell survival and DNA double-strand break induction and repair (measured by neutral elution) were investigated in Chinese hamster V79 cells. The lethal effects of neutrons were shown to be significantly greater than those of a similar dose of X-rays (RBE, 3.55 at 10% survival), but the RBE for double-strand break induction, in a dose range of 10–50 Gy, was 1. Radiation-dependent differences were found in the pattern of repair. A fast and a slow repair component were seen in both cases, but the former was reduced after neutron irradiation. Since the amount of slow repair was similar in the two cases, proportionally more unrejoined breaks were seen after exposure to neutrons. The results were similar when the elutions were conducted at pH 9.6 and pH 7.2 (Fox & McNally, 1988).

DNA double-strand break induction and rejoining, measured by field-inversion gel electrophoresis, were compared by cell survival in mutant (XR-V15B) and wild-type parental (V79B) hamster cell lines after low-dose neutron and X-irradiation. Neutrons did not induce more double-strand breaks than X-rays. Even with low doses of neutrons, a visible increase was found in the formation of a smaller subset of DNA fragments, which arise only after very high doses of X-rays. In both cell lines, double-strand breaks induced by neutrons were rejoined more slowly than those induced by X-radiation. At long repair times (4 and 17 h), there were no significant differences between neutrons and X-rays in the fractions of unrejoined double-strand breaks. The authors proposed that neutron-induced double-strand breaks have a higher probability of becoming lethal because they are more likely to be misrepaired during the slow stage of rejoining (Kysela *et al.*, 1993).

Irradiation of viable CHO AA8 cells on ice with 4–25 Gy of either ^{60}Co γ-radiation or d(20 MeV)Be neutrons (mean energy, 7.5 MeV) produced similar resistance to rewinding of nuclear DNA supercoils after treatment with ethidium bromide. The recovery from the effects of 12 Gy of either radiation was also similar, leaving no detectable residual damage. The discrepancy between these data and the reduced ability of neutrons to produce DNA breaks, as defined by the alkaline elution assay, is explained by the discontinuous deposition of energy associated with neutron irradiation. A microdosimetric analysis suggested that neutron radiation interacts with DNA at sites that are on average 5–10 times further apart than those that interact with γ-radiation. The long DNA sequences that result from neutron irradiation are consequently eluted inefficiently during alkaline elution, giving a reported RBE of approximately 0.3. Restrictions in the rewinding of individual supercoils are not dependent on the inter-ionization distance and thus give rise to an RBE of approximately 1. Furthermore, the complete removal of DNA damage, as measured by this technique, supports the hypothesis that the toxicity of neutrons is associated with incorrect, not incomplete, rejoining of the DNA molecule (Vaughan *et al.*, 1991).

The relative sensitivity of Chinese hamster ovary cells to fast neutrons and γ-rays was studied with a panel of mutants characterized by defects in the nucleotide excision repair pathway. These could be further subdivided into mutants that were defective in nucleotide excision repair alone, in base excision repair alone, in DNA-dependent protein kinase-mediated DNA double-strand break repair or in the distinct but overlapping pathway for the repair of DNA cross-links. None of the mutants defective in nucleotide excision repair showed different sensitivities to fast neutrons and γ-radiation. In contrast, deficiency in the base excision repair pathway resulted in significant primary sensitization to both types of radiation (2.0-fold to γ-radiation and 1.8-fold to neutrons). Deficiency in the double-strand break repair pathway mediated by DNA-protein kinase resulted in marked but again similar primary sensitization to γ-radiation (4.2-fold) and neutrons (5.1-fold). Thus, none of the repair pathways examined showed a preferential role in the repair of damage induced by low-LET and intermediate-LET radiations; this resulted in an essentially consistent RBE of approximately 2 in the cell lines studied (Britten & Murray, 1997).

(ii)   *Chromosomal aberrations*

Many studies have been performed of radiation-induced chromosomal aberrations in mammalian cells—often human lymphocytes. Comparisons of the effects of radiation have often been based on the number of dicentric chromosomes induced, although premature chromosome condensation is also an end-point for comparison. The RBEs of neutron irradiation have been determined for dicentrics or for dicentrics plus centric rings in human lymphocytes isolated from peripheral blood exposed to neutrons with different energies (Table 18). Analysis of dicentrics revealed RBE values of 5, 6 and 14 for neutrons of mean energy 21, 14 and 6.5 MeV, respectively, produced on a beryllium target [^{9}Be(d,n)^{10}B] (Fabry *et al.*, 1985).

The yield of chromatid-type aberrations induced by either fission neutrons or X-radiation can be potentiated by post-irradiation treatment with hydroxyurea and caffeine when the cells are irradiated in G_2; however, the frequencies of neutron-induced chromatid-type aberrations are not potentiated by treatment with cytosine arabinoside, except at the highest dose used. In contrast, chromatid aberrations induced by X-radiation were strongly potentiated by cytosine arabinoside. These results indicate that

Table 18. Relative biological effectiveness (RBE) of neutrons for chromosome-type dicentrics (or dicentrics plus centric rings) induced in human peripheral lymphocytes irradiated *in vitro* (reference radiation, ^{60}Co γ-rays; constant dose rate, 0.5 Gy min^{-1}; Lloyd et al., 1975)

Source	Neutron energy (MeV)	Absorbed dose rate (Gy min^{-1})	Sampling time	RBE for 2.0–0.02 aberrations per cell	RBE$_m$	Reference
d, T						
Japan	~ 14.1	–	–	1.2–5.9[a]	14.5	Sasaki (1971)
Germany	~ 15.0 (γ < 4%)	0.12	48 h	1.1–3.6	9.0	Bauchinger et al. (1975)
Glasgow, Scotland	~ 14.7 (γ ~ 7.5%)	0.30	48 h	1.7–6.6	16.7	Lloyd et al. (1976)
Harwell, England	~ 14.9 (γ ~ 3%)	0.25	48 h (O_2)	2.2–6.6	16.2	Prosser & Stimpson (1981)
			(N_2)	1.2–2.1	4.3	
^{3}H(α,n)^{4}He						
Russian Federation (NG–150M)	14.7 (γ < 10%)	0.36–1.85	50–52 h	1.7–3.8	9.0	Sevan'kaev et al. (1979a,b)
d, Be						
Harwell, England (VEC)	~ 20	~ 0.50	52–72 h (with BrdU)	1.4–11.3	29.2	Barjaktarovic & Savage (1980)
Hammersmith, England (cyclotron)	~ 7.6 (γ < 10%)	0.30	48 h	2.1–11.9	30.4	Lloyd et al. (1976)
Louvain, Belgium (cyclotron)	~ 6.2 (γ low)	0.05	48–53 h	1.0–8.3	21.5	Biola et al. (1974)
Japan	~ 2.03	–	–	2.2–17.4[a]	43.3	Sasaki (1971)
Li/Be						
Russian Federation (KG-2.5 accelerator)	~ 0.04 (γ < 7%)	0.01	50–52 h	2.4–6.8	16.5	Sevan'kaev et al. (1979a,b)
	~ 0.09 (γ < 4%)	0.03		1.1–10.8	28.0	

Table 18 (contd)

Source	Neutron energy (MeV)	Absorbed dose rate (Gy min⁻¹)	Sampling time	RBE for 2.0–0.02 aberrations per cell	RBE$_m$	Reference
Fission						
France (CEA/Crac)	Max, ~ 10 (γ very high + thermal)	–	46–53 h (data corrected for γ)	2.8–22.3	57.4	Biola et al. (1974)
France (CEN/Triton)	Max ~ 10 (γ ~ 30–50%)	0.03–0.07	46–53 (data corrected for γ)	2.7–21.6	55.7	Biola et al. (1974)
France (CEN/Harmonie)	Max ~ 1.5 (γ ~ 5%)	0.12	46–53 h	2.0–16.1	41.3	Biola et al. (1974)
Sofia, Bulgaria (IRT-2000)	Max ~ 3	–	52 h	0.8–6.5	16.9	Todorov et al. (1973)
Aldermaston, England	~ 0.9 (γ < 10%)	0.03	48 h	2.2–18.0	46.4	Lloyd et al. (1976)
Argonne, USA (JANUS)	~ 0.85 (γ ~ 3%)	0.06	48–50 h	2.3–18.3[a]	45.6	Carrano (1975)
Russian Federation (BR-10)	~ 0.85 (γ < 5%)	0.06–2.6	50–52 h	2.8–19.9	51.1	Sevan'kaev et al. (1979a,b)
Harwell, England (BEPO)	~ 0.7 (γ ~ 10%)	0.50	48 h	2.6–20.6	53.2	Lloyd et al. (1976)
Harwell, England (BEPO)	~ 0.7 (γ ~ 10%)	0.50	48–56 h	2.6–21	54.1	Scott et al. (1969)
Harwell, England (GLEEP)	~ 0.7 (γ ~ 15%)	0.0005 0.0011	48–46 h	2.5–20.4 3.1–25.2	52.2 65.0	Scott et al. (1969)
Italy (TAPIRO)	~ 0.4 (γ ~ 10%)	0.002–0.07	48 h	2.6–22.2	57.1	Vulpis et al. (1978)
Russian Federation (BR-10)	~ 0.35 (γ < 5%)	0.04–0.4	50–52 h	4.1–32.6	83.9	Sevan'kaev et al. (1979a,b)
Russian Federation (BR-10)	Thermal (γ < 5%)	0.005	50–52 h	1.3–20.6	53.3	Sevan'kaev et al. (1979a,b)

Table 18 (contd)

Source	Neutron energy (MeV)	Absorbed dose rate (Gy min⁻¹)	Sampling time	RBE for 2.0–0.02 aberrations per cell	RBE$_m$	Reference
National Radiological Protection Board (^{252}Cf)	~ 2.13 MeV	0.12–0.17	48 h	1.8–14.8	38.2	Lloyd et al. (1978)

Adapted from Savage (1982)
[a] Dicentrics plus centric rings

neutrons produce a smaller proportion of lesions, the repair of which can be inhibited by this compound, than X-radiation (Antoccia et al., 1992).

Several radiosensitive Chinese hamster cell lines have been studied to explore the relationship between radiation-induced DNA lesions and chromosomal aberrations. The frequency of radiation-induced aberrations in Xrs mutants, which are deficient in double-strand break repair, was higher than in control cells. In a radiosensitive hamster cell line (V-C4), which has no detectable defect in double-strand break repair, the frequencies of X-radiation-induced aberrations are higher than those found in wild-type V79 cells. After treatment with fission neutrons, however, the frequency of aberrations is similar to that in V79 cells, indicating that V-C4 cells are defective in repair of X-radiation-induced lesions other than double-strand breaks. Apparently, these other lesions may also lead to aberrations (Natarajan et al., 1993).

Chromosomal aberrations were scored in BHK21 C13 Syrian hamster fibroblasts exposed in stationary phase to ^{60}Co γ-rays, 250-kV X-rays, 15-MeV neutrons or neutrons of a mean energy of 2.1 MeV produced from the ^{9}Be(d,n)^{10}B reaction. No detectable difference was seen in the responses to ^{60}Co γ-rays and 250-kV X-rays. The RBE for the production of dicentrics, based on the 'one hit' component of the response, was 5 ± 2 for the 15-MeV neutrons and 12 ± 5 for the 2.1-MeV neutrons (Roberts & Holt, 1985).

Micronucleus formation induced by neutrons has been studied in a number of cell types, including human blood lymphocytes and two-cell mouse embryos exposed in late G_2 phase (Molls et al., 1981; Mill et al., 1996; Vral et al., 1996).

There is now substantial evidence that ionizing radiation can induce genomic instability in the form of chromosomal aberrations which appear several cell generations after irradiation. When the progeny of neutron-irradiated human epithelial MCF-10A cells were examined for chromosomal aberrations 5–40 population doublings after irradiation, an increase in the frequency of chromatid-type gaps and breaks was observed, but no such effect was observed for chromosome-type aberrations. Neutron-irradiated cells showed consistently increased frequencies of aberrations when compared with unirradiated control cells at all times examined, indicating that neutrons can cause chromosomal instability (Ponnaiya et al., 1997).

(iii) *Interchromosomal versus intrachromosomal aberrations*

Many attempts have been made to identify specific biomarkers of radiation as the causal agent of biological effects in cells and tissues. The search has included the examination of chromosomal aberrations for what has been termed a chromosomal 'fingerprint' that would indicate the type of radiation responsible for the aberration. Brenner and Sachs (1994) observed that high-LET radiation, in particular α-particles or fission neutrons, produces a remarkably low ratio of interchromosomal to intrachromosomal aberrations, which is two to three times lower than the ratio recorded after X- or γ-irradiation. The authors proposed use of this ratio as a fingerprint for exposure to high-LET radiation.

The two types of aberration are illustrated in Figure 5. Exchange-type chromosomal aberrations are interchromosomal if the DNA double-strand breaks that are the initial cause of the lesion occur on different chromosomes. If the double-strand breaks are on different arms of the same chromosome, the lesion is intrachromosomal. If the double-strand breaks were random and all the double-strand breaks were equally likely to interact with one another, the ratio F of the interchromosomal to intrachromosomal aberrations would be 90, assuming that all chromosome arms were of equal length. Since chromosome arms are not of equal length and there is an increased probability of interaction between double-strand breaks that are close together, the F value is lower and is indicative of lesions induced by low-LET radiations, such as X- and γ-radiation. High-LET radiations, which are densely ionizing because of the inhomogeneity of the energy deposition, induce double-strand breaks that are even closer than those produced by X- or γ-radiation, increasing the yield of intrachromosomal aberrations and resulting in a smaller F value. On the basis of many reports of the induction of chromosomal aberrations in humans and other experimental data, it was suggested that the F value for densely ionizing radiation was about 6 and that this was significantly lower than the values for X- and γ-radiation and for chemical clastogenic agents. If valid, this approach for determining F ratios would have potential use in epidemio-logical studies, such as those on atomic bomb survivors and persons exposed to radon, in establishing the type of radiation involved (Brenner & Sachs, 1994).

Other authors have both supported (Sasaki *et al.*, 1998) and disputed (Bauchinger & Schmid, 1997, 1998) this hypothesis. The report of a workshop set up to examine the use of F values concluded that: (1) there was some evidence to suggest that ratios of different chromosomal aberrations might be used as a biomarker of exposure to high-LET radiations; (2) there are large interlaboratory differences in F values for the same type of radiation; (3) despite these variations, F values do not depend on dose or LET at doses above 1 Gy; (4) further studies are required to establish if F values can be used to identify a causal relationship between the observed chromosomal aberra-tions and specific exposure to radiation. It was suggested that the ratio of intrachromo-somal intra-arm to interchromosomal aberrations (designated the H ratio) should be examined as a possible fingerprint of exposure to high-LET neutrons (Nakamura *et al.*, 1998).

(iv)   *Gene mutations*

Since mutation of a given gene is a relatively rare event, the majority of systems for studying radiation-induced mutations involve placing an irradiated cell population under selective pressure so that only the mutant cells are able to survive and can be enu-merated. Mutation of genes in a hemizygous (single copy) or heterozygous (two copies but only one active) state is usually studied, to enable measurement. Commonly used mutation systems are based on the loss of enzyme activity, e.g. the enzyme HPRT, which renders cells resistant to the drug 6-thioguanine, the enzyme TK, which confers resistance to trifluorothymidine and the enzyme APRT which confers resistance to

Figure 5. Interchromosomal and intrachromosomal, inter-arm aberrations resulting from ionizing radiations of different quality

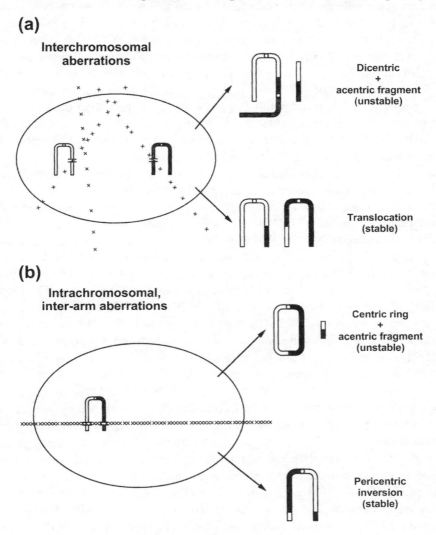

(a)

Interchromosomal aberrations

Dicentric
+
acentric fragment
(unstable)

Translocation
(stable)

(b)

Intrachromosomal, inter-arm aberrations

Centric ring
+
acentric fragment
(unstable)

Pericentric
inversion
(stable)

Adapted from Brenner & Sachs (1994)
Each cross represents an ionization cluster of sufficient localization and multiplicity to produce a double-strand DNA break. Panel **(a)** shows interchromosomal aberrations resulting, in the case shown here, from two independent, sparsely ionizing radiation tracks. This aberration could also result from two double-strand breaks caused by a single radiation track. Panel **(b)** shows intrachromosomal, inter-arm aberrations resulting, in the case shown here, from a single, densely ionizing radiation track.

8-azaadenine and 2-aminopurine (see section 4.4.2 in the monograph on X- and γ-radiation). The *Hprt* gene is located on the X chromosome, while the *Tk* and *Aprt* genes are on autosomes and must therefore be used in a hemi- or heterozygous state.

The effects of the dose rate of high-LET radiation on mouse L5178Y cells were reported (Nakamura & Sawada, 1988) after exposure to ^{252}Cf (2.13-MeV neutrons). At the high dose rate of 1.2 cGy min^{-1}, ^{252}Cf irradiation produced a linear induction of *Hprt* mutants at relatively low doses but showed reduced effectiveness at higher doses. At the lower dose rate of 0.16 cGy min^{-1}, the initial slope for mutant induction (9×10^{-7} per cGy) was approximately the same as that at the higher dose rate, but the induction curve did not appear to 'turn over' at higher doses. Dose-dependent values for the RBE of high-LET radiation in excess of 10 were found for the low-dose rate in a comparison of neutrons from ^{252}Cf with ^{60}Co γ-radiation.

Human B-lymphoblastoid TK6 cells were used to examine the effectiveness of 4.2-MeV (^{230}Pu, Be) neutrons at dose rates of 0.00014–0.04 cGy min^{-1} for up to 20 days. Neutrons at dose rates < 0.0014 cGy min^{-1} were more effective at inducing mutants than were higher dose rates. The RBE of these low dose rates, relative to 100-kV X-rays, can be calculated to be about 10. When TK6 cells were exposed to beams ranging in atomic number from ^{20}Ne to ^{40}Ar over an energy range of 330–670 MeV per atomic mass unit (amu), mutation induction was evaluated for both the *TK* and the *HPRT* loci for a subset of these beams. The results obtained with the ^{20}Ne ions of 425 MeV per amu (LET, 32 keV μm^{-1}) and ^{28}Si ions of 670 MeV per amu (LET, 50 keV μm^{-1}) closely resembled those obtained after brief exposure to (^{230}Pu, Be) neutrons. Alterations in DNA structure within the *TK* locus of mutants induced by neutrons and by ^{40}Ar ions were similar and were dominated by allele loss. Multi-locus deletions inclusive of the c-*erb*A1 locus were common among the *TK*-deficient mutants induced by these densely ionizing radiations (Kronenberg & Little, 1989; Kronenberg, 1991).

A system involving human–hamster hybrid cells was developed by Waldren *et al.* (1979) from a stable hybrid containing the Chinese hamster genome and one copy of the human chromosome 11. The loss of several markers on this chromosome can be determined, and even complete loss of the chromosome is not lethal. This system has been used to measure mutant frequencies after irradiation with neutrons of various energies (0.33–14 MeV), at doses up to 200 cGy. Significant increases in mutant frequency were found at doses as low as 10 cGy, and dose-dependent RBEs of up to 30—for the 0.33-MeV neutrons—were calculated in comparison with ^{137}Cs γ-radiation (Hei *et al.*, 1988).

Fast neutrons produced by proton bombardment of a beryllium target in a cyclotron were used to examine the energy dependence of the induction of mutants at the *Hprt* and *Tk* loci in V79 Chinese hamster cells. The beams of neutrons were produced from protons with 46, 30, 20 and 14 MeV of energy. Gradually increasing cytotoxic and mutagenic effects of the neutrons were noted as the energy decreased. The frequency of induced mutants at the *Tk* gene was higher than at the *Hprt* gene. In a human epithelium teratocarcinoma cell line (P3), the mutation frequency at the *HPRT* locus, as in V79 cells, increased 2.5–4 fold with decreasing neutron energy (Zhu & Hill, 1994; Sharma & Hill, 1996).

A 1-Gy fission neutron dose from a ^{252}Cf source induced a maximal *Hprt* mutation frequency in synchronized L5178Y mouse lymphoma cells when delivered immediately after release from G_2/M block, whereas the maximal response to ^{60}Co γ-radiation was found in G_1 (Tauchi *et al.*, 1993).

The biological effectiveness for mutation induction at the *Hprt* locus in confluent cultures of mouse m5S cells exposed to fission neutrons from ^{252}Cf, relative to γ-radiation, was increased from 4.9 to 7.4 when the dose rate was reduced from 1.8 to 0.12 cGy min^{-1}. The changes in RBE were due mainly to a reduction in the effect of γ-radiation. The authors noted that their observations contrast with reports of proliferating cell cultures and suggested that they could be ascribed to the cell growth conditions used in their experiments (Komatsu *et al.*, 1993).

The toxic and mutagenic effects of X-rays and neutrons were compared in the Chinese hamster ovary cell line K1-BH4 and its transformant, AS52, which lacks the normal *Hprt* gene but instead contains a single autosomally integrated copy of the bacterial equivalent, the *gpt* gene. X-radiation and neutrons appeared to be equitoxic in the two cell lines, but both were 10 times more mutagenic to the *gpt* gene in AS52 cells than to the *Hprt* gene of K1-BH4 cells. The apparent hypermutability of AS52 cells probably results from better recovery of multi-locus deletion mutants in AS52 cells than in K1-BH4 cells, rather than a higher yield of induced mutants (Hsie *et al.*, 1990).

Chinese hamster ovary cells were exposed to thermal neutrons, and the mutation frequency at the *Hprt* locus was determined. The Kyoto University Research Reactor, which produces thermal neutrons with a very low level of contaminating γ-rays and fast neutrons, was used as the source of radiation. The cells were irradiated in the presence or absence of boric acid. Thermal neutron irradiation was 2.5 times as mutagenic as γ-radiation without boron. In the presence of boron, however, thermal neutron radiation was 4.2–4.5 times as mutagenic as γ-radiation. When the mutation frequency was plotted against the surviving fraction, greater mutagenicity was observed in the presence than in the absence of boron, suggesting that the enhancement of thermal neutron-induced mutation with boron is strongly associated with α-particles released by the ^{10}B(n,α)^{7}Li reaction (Kinashi *et al.*, 1997).

(v)   *Cell transformation*

Ionizing radiation of low LET is an effective inducer of cell transformation in various systems (see section 4.4.2 in the monograph on X- and γ-radiation). A large number of studies have also been conducted with neutrons, which are even more effective than X- or γ-rays. The RBE values relative to X- or γ-radiation depend on the energy of the neutrons. Miller *et al.* (1989) examined the effect of low absorbed doses of monoenergetic neutrons with energies of 0.23–13.7 MeV on transformation in asynchronous mouse C3H10T1/2 cells. The dose–response curves were linear or nearly linear for the various neutron energies and curvilinear for the reference X-rays. The RBE values were found to decrease with increasing dose for both cell transformation and survival. The maximal values varied from 13 for 5.9-MeV neutrons to 35 for 0.35-MeV neutrons. Rather lower RBE values were reported in a study with less pure neutron sources (Balcer-Kubiczek & Harrison, 1983): the maximum observed RBE for reactor fission neutrons (with 8–20% γ-ray component) was 3.8, and that for cyclotron neutrons (8% γ-ray component) was 1.2. A subsequent study on fission neutrons at various dose rates gave an RBE for cell transformation of 3 at a high dose rate (0.1 Gy min^{-1}) and 10 at the lowest dose rate studied (0.005 Gy min^{-1}) (Balcer-Kubiczek *et al.*, 1988). In mouse mS5 cells, ^{252}Cf neutrons showed RBE values for cell transformation of 3.3–5.1, depending on the dose rate (1.8–0.12 cGy min^{-1}) (Komatsu *et al.*, 1993).

The claim of Hill *et al.* (1984a,b) that neutron-induced transformation in the C3H10T1/2 system was enhanced by a factor of about 9 at low dose rates triggered much work on dose rates and dose fractionation with respect to the so-called 'inverse dose rate' problem. The effect was confirmed in the same system by several authors (see e.g. Miller *et al.*, 1990) and flatly denied by others (Balcer-Kubiczek *et al.*, 1988, 1991; Saran *et al.*, 1991; Balcer-Kubiczek *et al.*, 1994; Saran *et al.*, 1994). Syrian hamster embryo cells were also reported to show the effect (Jones *et al.*, 1989), and an inverse dose-rate effect of 2.9 was reported for the human hybrid system (HeLa × skin fibroblasts), with fission neutrons of an average energy of 0.85 MeV (Redpath *et al.*, 1990); however, no effect was found in confluent cultures of mouse m5S cells (Komatsu *et al.*, 1993). Several authors reported that the effect is specific to particular sources or energies of neutrons (Elkind, 1991; Miller & Hall, 1991), and there is still some confusion in the area (Masuda, 1994; Brenner *et al.*, 1996). Explanations of the inverse dose-rate effect have involved cell proliferation during irradiation and the postulated existence of a hypersensitive 'window' in the cell cycle (Elkind, 1991).

In experiments with synchronized mouse C3H10T1/2 cells, Miller *et al.* (1995) found that the G$_1$ phase of the cell cycle (4–6 h after mitotic 'shake-off') was the most sensitive to neutron-induced oncogenic transformation, in contrast to what has been observed with X-radiation where the peak was 14–16 h after 'shake-off', reflecting mostly G$_2$ cells. Less variation in the response during the cell cycle was seen for neutrons than for X-rays (Redpath *et al.*, 1995; Pazzaglia *et al.*, 1996).

It is not clear what molecular changes induced by neutrons are responsible for cell transformation. In 5.9-MeV neutron-transformed foci of C3H10T1/2 cells, chromosomal aberrations have been found, but there were no N-*ras* or K-*ras* mutations (Freyer *et al.*, 1996), and it was reported that human keratinocytes transformed by neutrons do not contain mutations in either *RAS* or *p53* (Thraves *et al.*, 1994).

5. Summary of Data Reported and Evaluation

5.1   Exposure data

Exposure to neutrons normally occurs from a mixed irradiation field in which neutrons are a minor component. The exceptions are exposure of patients to neutron radiotherapy beams and exposures of aircraft passengers and crew. In high-altitude cities, neutrons can constitute as much as 25% of cosmic background radiation. A measure of the societal burden is the annual neutron collective dose per year^{-1}. Those values would be 4.6×10^5 person–Sv year^{-1} for the world population exposed at ground level, 350 person–Sv year^{-1} for nuclear workers and 7500 person–Sv year^{-1} for the passengers and crews of aircraft. The individual average lifetime effective dose of neutrons has been estimated to be 6 mSv for the world population exposed at ground level and 30 mSv for aircrews. The maximal lifetime doses of neutrons are estimated to be 68 mSv for the population of the high-altitude city of La Paz, Bolivia, 46 mSv for long-haul pilots and up to 130 mSv for the small proportion of nuclear workers exposed to neutrons.

5.2   Human carcinogenicity data

There are no epidemiological data adequate to evaluate whether neutrons are carcinogenic to humans.

5.3   Animal carcinogenicity data

Neutrons have been tested at various doses and dose rates with wide ranges of mean energy from various sources (reactors, ^{252}Cf, ^{235}U) for carcinogenicity in mice, rats, rabbits, dogs and rhesus monkeys. Fission-spectrum neutrons were used in most of these studies. Neutrons were also tested for carcinogenicity in mice exposed prenatally and in mice after male parental exposure.

In adult animals, the incidences of leukaemia and of ovarian, mammary, lung and liver tumours were increased in a dose-related manner, although the incidence often decreased at high doses. While a γ-ray component was present in the exposure in most studies, it was generally small, and the carcinogenic effects observed could clearly be attributed to the neutrons. Prenatal and parental exposure of mice resulted in increased incidences of liver tumours in the offspring.

In general, there was no apparent reduction in tumour incidence after exposure to low doses at a low dose rate, but enhancement of tumour incidence was often observed with high doses at a low dose rate. In virtually all studies, neutrons were more effective in inducing tumours than were X-radiation or γ-radiation when compared on the basis of absorbed dose.

5.4   Other relevant data

Neutrons are uncharged particles that are penetrating and interact with atomic nuclei, generating densely ionizing charged particles, such as protons, α-particles and nuclear fragments, and sparsely ionizing γ-radiation. The densely ionizing particles produce a spectrum of molecular damage that overlaps with that induced by sparsely ionizing radiation, but they are more effective in causing biological damage because they release more of their energy in clusters of ionizing events, giving rise to more severe local damage.

Comparison of the effects of neutrons with those of X- and γ-radiation is based on the assumption that the effects are the same qualitatively and differ only quantitatively. The assumption is reasonable with regard to deterministic effects because they are, in general, caused by cell killing. Neutrons are more effective than X- and γ-radiation in causing both early and late deterministic effects. The effectiveness of neutrons is dependent on their kinetic energy and decreases with increasing energy up to about 15 MeV. The effects of neutrons are much less dependent on dose rate, fractionation, cell cycle stage and oxygenation than those of X-radiation and γ-radiation. The relative biological effectiveness of neutrons for the induction of deterministic effects is greater than 1 but not as high as those estimated for induction of cancer in experimental animals. For single doses of 1–5-MeV fast neutrons, the relative biological effectiveness values range from 4 to 12, except in the haematopoietic system for which the values are 2–3. The relative biological effectiveness is higher for later-responding tissues than for early-responding tissues.

For individual cells also, neutron energy is an important factor in the stochastic effectiveness of neutrons. The ability of surviving cells to proliferate and increase cell populations does not appear to depend on the quality of radiation; however, because of the greater effectiveness of neutrons per unit dose, the surviving population is smaller and a longer time is required for the proliferation rate to recover. This may be critical in maintenance of the integrity of a tissue.

Cells from patients with ataxia telangiectasia are hypersensitive to cell killing and to induction of micronuclei by fast neutrons, although the degree of hypersensitivity is less pronounced than for sparsely ionizing radiation.

The spectrum of DNA damage from neutrons includes clustered damage of substantial complexity and consequently reduced repairability. Neutrons are comparable to X- and γ-radiation in producing double-strand breaks, but neutron-induced DNA lesions in mammalian cells are less readily repaired than those produced by sparsely ionizing radiation.

Neutrons are very efficient at inducing transformation in rodent and human cellular systems. The relative biological effectiveness of neutrons has been reported to vary from 3 to 35; whether (or under what conditions) the efficiency of neoplastic transformation is greater at low dose rates remains unclear.

Chromosomal aberrations (including rings, dicentrics and acentric fragments) were induced in the circulating lymphocytes of people exposed in an accident involving release of neutrons in a nuclear plant and in the lymphocytes of patients exposed during neutron therapy. In the former study, there was also an increase in the frequency of numerical aberrations. Within the limits of the studies, the effect was found to be dose-dependent.

Gene mutations and chromosomal aberrations are induced in mammalian cells many times more efficiently by neutrons than by the same absorbed dose of X- or γ-radiation. Fission neutrons have been shown to induce germ-line mutations in mice, including visible dominant mutations, dominant lethal mutations, visible recessive mutations and specific locus mutations. When compared with sparsely ionizing radiation on the basis of absorbed dose, fission neutrons are many-fold more effective. Neutrons have been shown to induce *Hprt* mutations in splenic lymphocytes of mice. Point mutations in K-*Ras* and N-*Ras* oncogenes were found in malignant tissue from mice exposed to neutrons, but the mutations cannot be directly ascribed to the exposure. Neutrons have been shown to induce sister chromatid exchange, dicentrics and rings in mice and reciprocal translocations in rhesus monkey stem-cell spermatogonia.

5.5   Evaluation

There is *inadequate evidence* in humans for the carcinogenicity of neutrons.

There is *sufficient evidence* in experimental animals for the carcinogenicity of neutrons.

Overall evaluation

Neutrons are *carcinogenic to humans (Group 1)*.

In making the overall evaluation, the Working Group took into consideration the following:

- When interacting with biological material, fission neutrons generate protons, and the higher-energy neutrons used in therapy generate protons and α-particles. α-Particle-emitting radionuclides (e.g. radon) are known to be human carcinogens. The linear energy transfer of protons overlaps with that of the lower-energy electrons produced by γ-radiation. Neutron interactions also generate γ-radiation, which is a human carcinogen.
- Gross chromosomal aberrations (including rings, dicentrics and acentric fragments) and numerical chromosomal aberrations are induced in the lymphocytes of people exposed to neutrons.
- The spectrum of DNA damage induced by neutrons is similar to that induced by X-radiation but contains relatively more of the serious (i.e. less readily repairable) types.

- Every relevant biological effect of γ- or X-radiation that has been examined has been found to be induced by neutrons.
- Neutrons are several times more effective than X- and γ-radiation in inducing neoplastic cell transformation, mutation *in vitro*, germ-cell mutation *in vivo*, chromosomal aberrations *in vivo* and *in vitro* and cancer in experimental animals.

6.   References

Abelson, P. & Kruger, P.G. (1949) Cyclotron-induced radiation cataracts. *Science*, **110**, 655–657

Ainsworth, E.J., Fry, R.J.M., Brennan, P.C., Stearner, S.P., Rust. J.H. & Williamson, F.S. (1975) Life shortening, neoplasia and systematic injuries in mice after single or fractionated doses of neutron or gamma radiation. In: *Biological and Environmental Effects of Low-level Radiation*, Vol. 1 (WNL 10), Vienna, International Atomic Energy Agency, pp. 77–92

Ainsworth, E.J., Afzal, S.M.J., Crouse, D.A., Hanson, W.R. & Fry, R.J.M. (1989) Tissue responses to low protracted doses of high-LET radiations or photons: Early and late damage relevant to radio-protective countermeasures. *Adv. Space Res.*, **9**, 299–313

Akatov, Y.A. (1993) Some results of dose measurements along civil airways in the USSR. *Radiat. Prot. Dosim.*, **48**, 59–63

Alpen, E.L. (1991) Neutron studies with large animals. *Radiat. Res.*, **128**, S37–S41

Antoccia, A., Palitti, F., Raggi, T., Catena, C. & Tanzarella, C. (1992) The yield of fission neutron-induced chromatid aberrations in G2-stage human lymphocytes: Effect of caffeine, hydroxyurea and cytosine arabinoside post-irradiation. *Int. J. Radiat. Biol.*, **62**, 563–570

Bagshaw, M., Irvine, D. & Davies, D.M. (1996) Exposure to cosmic radiation of British Airways flying crew on ultralonghaul routes. *Occup. environ. Med.*, **53**, 495–498

Balcer-Kubiczek, E.K. & Harrison, G.H. (1983) Oncogenic transformation of C3H/10T1/2 cells by X-rays, fast-fission neutrons, and cyclotron-produced neutrons. *Int. J. Radiat. Biol.*, **44**, 377–386

Balcer-Kubiczek, E.K., Harrison, G.H., Zeman, G.H., Mattson, P.J. & Kunska, A. (1988) Lack of inverse dose-rate effect on fission neutron-induced transformation of C3H/10T1/2 cells. *Int. J. Radiat. Biol.*, **54**, 531–536

Balcer-Kubiczek, E.K., Harrison, G.H. & Hei, T.K. (1991) Neutron dose-rate experiments at the AFRRI nuclear reactor. *Radiat. Res.*, **128**, S65–S70

Balcer-Kubiczek, E.K., Harrison, G.H., Torres, B.A. & McCready, W.A. (1994) Application of the constant exposure time technique to transformation experiments with fission neutrons: Failure to demonstrate dose-rate dependence. *Int. J. Radiat. Biol.*, **65**, 559–569

Barendsen, G.W. (1985) Comparison of transformation, chromosome aberrations, and reproductive death induced in cultured mammalian cells by neutrons of different energies. *Radiat. Res.*, **Suppl. 8**, S158–S164

Barendsen, G.W. (1990) Mechanisms of cell reproductive death and shapes of radiation dose–survival curves of mammalian cells. *Int. J. Radiat. Biol.*, **57**, 485–496

Barjaktarovic, N. & Savage, J.R.K. (1980) R.b.e. for d(42MeV)-Be neutrons based on chromosome-type aberrations induced in human lymphocytes and scored in cells at first division. *Int. J. Radiat. Biol.*, **37**, 667–675

Batchelor, A.L., Phillips, R.J.S. & Searle, A.G. (1966) A comparison of the mutagenic effectiveness of chronic neutron- and gamma irradiation of mouse spermatogonia. *Mutat. Res.*, **3**, 218–229

Batchelor, A.L., Phillips, R.J.S. & Searle, A.G. (1969) The ineffectiveness of chronic irradiation with neutrons and gamma rays in inducing mutations in female mice. *Br. J. Radiol.*, **42**, 448–451

Bateman, J.L., Rossi, H.H., Kellerer, A.M., Robinson, C.V. & Bond, V.P. (1972) Dose-dependence of fast neutron RBE for lens opacification in mice. *Radiat. Res.*, **51**, 381–390

Bates, P.R. & Lavin, M.F. (1989) Comparison of γ-radiation-induced accumulation of ataxia-telangiectasia and control cells in G_2 phase. *Mutat. Res.*, **218**, 165–170

Bauchinger, M. & Schmid, E. (1997) Is there reliable experimental evidence for a chromosomal 'fingerprint' of exposure to densely ionizing radiation? *Radiat. Res.*, **147**, 506–510

Bauchinger, M. & Schmid, E. (1998) LET dependence of yield ratios of radiation-induced intra- and interchromosomal aberrations in human lymphocytes. *Int. J. Radiat. Biol.*, **74**, 17–25

Bauchinger, M., Schmid, E., Rimpl, G. & Kühn, H. (1975) Chromosome aberrations in human lymphocytes after irradiation with 15.0-MeV neutrons *in vitro*. I. Dose–response relation and RBE. *Mutat. Res.*, **27**, 103–109

Bender, M.A. & Gooch, P.C. (1962) Persistent chromosome aberrations in irradiated human subjects. *Radiat. Res.*, **16**, 44–53

Bender, M.A. & Gooch, P.C. (1963) Persistent chromosome aberrations in irradiated human subjects. II. Three and one-half year investigation. *Radiat. Res.*, **18**, 389–396

Biola, M.T., Lego, R., Vacca, G., Ducatez, G., Dacher, J. & Bourguignon, M. (1974) [RBE for various γ/neutron radiations based on induction of chromosomal aberrations in human lymphocytes *in vitro*]. In: *Biological Effects of Neutron Irradiation* (STI/PUB/352), Vienna, International Atomic Energy Agency, pp. 221–236 (in French)

Blettner, M., Grosche, B. & Zeeb, H. (1998) Occupational cancer risk in pilots and flight attendants: Current epidemiological knowledge. *Radiat. environ. Biophys.*, **37**, 75–80

Boice, J.D., Jr, Blettner, M. & Auvinen, A. (2000) *Epidemiologic Studies of Pilots and Aircrew*, NCRP Proceedings 20: *Cosmic Radiation Exposure of Airline Crews, Passengers and Astronauts*, Bethesda, MD, National Council on Radiation Protection and Measurements (in press)

Bradley, M.O. & Kohn, K.W. (1979) X-ray induced DNA double strand break production and repair in mammalian cells as measured by neutral filter elution. *Nucleic Acids Res.*, **7**, 793–804

Bradley, E.W., Zook, B.C., Casarett, G.W., Deye, J.A., Adoff, L.M. & Rogers, C.C. (1981) Neoplasia in fast neutron-irradiated beagles. *J. natl Cancer Inst.*, **67**, 729–738

Brenner, D.J. & Sachs, R.K. (1994) Chromosomal 'fingerprints' of prior exposure to densely ionizing radiation. *Radiat. Res.*, **140**, 134–142

Brenner, D.J., Hahnfeldt, P., Amundson, S.A. & Sachs, R.K. (1996) Interpretation of inverse dose-rate effects for mutagenesis by sparsely ionizing radiation. *Int. J. Radiat. Biol.*, **70**, 447–458

Britten, R.A. & Murray, D. (1997) Constancy of the relative biological effectiveness of 42 MeV (p→Be⁺) neutrons among cell lines with different DNA repair proficiencies. *Radiat. Res.*, **148**, 308–316

Broerse, J.J. & Barendsen, G.W. (1973) Relative biological effectiveness of fast neutrons for effects on normal tissues. *Curr. Top. Radiat. Res. Q.*, **8**, 305–350

Broerse, J.J., van Bekkum, D.W., Hollander, C.F. & Davids, J.A.G. (1978) Mortality of monkeys after exposure to fission neutrons and the effect of autologous bone marrow transplantation. *Int. J. Radiat. Biol.*, **34**, 253–264

Broerse, J.J., Hollander, C.F. & Van Zwieten, M.J. (1981) Tumor induction in rhesus monkeys after total body irradiation with X-rays and fission neutrons. *Int. J. Radiat. Biol.*, **40**, 671–676

Broerse, J.J., Hennen, L.A. & Solleveld, H.A. (1986) Actuarial analysis of the hazard for mammary carcinogenesis in different rat strains after X- and neutron irradiation. *Leukemia Res.*, **10**, 749–754

Broerse, J.J., Hennen, L.A., Klapwijk, W.M. & Solleveld, H.A. (1987) Mammary carcino-genesis in different rat strains after irradiation and hormone administration. *Int. J. Radiat. Biol.*, **51**, 1091–1100

Broerse, J.J., van Bekkum, D.W., Zoetelief, J. & Zurcher, C. (1991) Relative biological effectiveness for neutron carcinogenesis in monkeys and rats. *Radiat. Res.*, **128**, S128–S135

Burns, W.G. & Sims, H.E. (1981) Effect of radiation type in water radiolysis. *J. Chem. Soc. (Faraday Transact.)*, **77**, 2803–2813

Carpenter, L., Higgins, C., Douglas, A., Fraser, P., Beral, V. & Smith, P. (1994) Combined ana-lysis of mortality in three United Kingdom nuclear industry workforces, 1946–1988. *Radiat. Res.*, **138**, 224–238

Carrano, A.V. (1975) Induction of chromosomal aberrations in human lymphocytes by X rays and fission neutrons: Dependence on cell cycle stage. *Radiat. Res.*, **63**, 403–421

Cattanach, B.M. (1971) Specific locus mutation in mice. In: Hollaender, A., ed., *Chemical Mutagens: Principles and Methods for their Detection*, Vol, 2, New York, Plenum Press, pp. 535–540

Catterall, M., Sutherland, I. & Bewley, D.K. (1975) First results of a randomized clinical trial of fast neutrons compared with X or gamma rays in treatment of advanced tumours of the head and neck. *Br. med. J.*, **ii**, 653–656

Catterall, M., Bewley, D.K. & Sutherland, I. (1977) Second report on results of a randomized clinical trial of fast neutrons compared with X or gamma rays in treatment of advanced tumours of head and neck. *Br. med. J.*, **i**, 1642

Chen, P.C., Lavin, M.F., Kidson, C. & Moss, D. (1978) Identification of ataxia telangiectasia heterozygotes, a cancer prone population. *Nature*, **274**, 484–486

Chmelevsky, D., Kellerer, A.M., Lafuma, J., Morin, M. & Masse, R. (1984) Comparison of the induction of pulmonary neoplasms in Sprague-Dwaley rats by fission neutrons and radon daughters. *Radiat. Res.*, **98**, 519–535

Clifton, K.H., Sridharan, B.N. & Douple, E.B. (1975) Brief communication: Mammary carcino-genesis-enhancing effect of adrenalectomy in irradiated rats with pituitary tumor MtT-F4. *J. natl Cancer Inst.*, **55**, 485–487

Clifton, K.H., Sridharan, B.N. & Gould, M.N. (1976a) Risk of mammary oncogenesis from exposure to neutrons or gamma rays, experimental methodology and early findings. In: *Biological and Environmental Effects of Low-level Radiation* (SM-202/211), Vienna, International Atomic Energy Agency, pp. 205–212

Clifton, K.H., Douple, E.B. & Sridharan, B.N. (1976b) Effects of grafts of single anterior pituitary glands on the incidence and type of mammary neoplasm in neutron- or gamma irradiated Fisher female rats. *Cancer Res.*, **36**, 3732–3735

Coggle, J.E. (1988) Lung tumour induction in mice after X-rays and neutrons. *Int. J. Radiat. Biol.*, **53**, 585–598

Committee on the Biological Effects of Ionizing Radiations (BEIR I) (1972) *Health Effects of Exposure to Low Levels of Ionizing Radiation*, Washington DC, National Academy Press

Coquerelle, T.M., Weibezahn, K.F. & Lücke-Huhle, C. (1987) Rejoining of double strand breaks in normal human and ataxia-telangiectasia fibroblasts after exposure to ^{60}Co γ-rays, ^{241}Am α-particles or bleomycin. *Int. J. Radiat. Biol.*, **51**, 209–218

Corominas, M., Sloan, S.R., Leon, J., Kamino, H., Newcomb, E.W. & Pellicer, A. (1991) *ras* activation in human tumors and in animal model systems. *Environ. Health Perspectives*, **93**, 19–25

Covelli, V., Coppola, M., Di Majo, V., Rebessi, S. & Bassani, B. (1988) Tumor induction and life shortening in BC3F$_1$ female mice at low doses of fast neutrons and X-rays. *Radiat. Res.*, **113**, 362–374

Covelli, V., Di Majo, V., Coppola, M. & Rebessi, S. (1989) The dose–response relationships for myeloid leukemia and malignant lymphoma in BC3F$_1$ mice. *Radiat. Res.*, **119**, 553–561

Covelli, V., Coppola, M., Di Majo, V. & Rebessi, S. (1991a) The dose–response relationships for tumor induction after high-LET radiation. *J. Radiat. Res.*, **Suppl. 2**, 110–117

Covelli, V., Di Majo, V., Coppola, M. & Rebessi, S. (1991b) Neutron carcinogenesis in mice: A study of the dose–response curves. *Radiat. Res.*, **128**, S114–S116

Cox, R. (1982) A cellular description of the repair defect in ataxia-telangiectasia. In: Bridges, B.A. & Harnden, D.G., eds, *Ataxia-telangiectasia: A Cellular and Molecular Link between Cancer, Neuropathology, and Immune Deficiency*, London, Wiley, pp. 141–153

Cox, R., Thacker, J., Goodhead, D.T. & Munson, R.J. (1977a) Mutation and inactivation of mammalian cells by various ionising radiations. *Nature*, **267**, 425–427

Cox, R., Thacker, J. & Goodhead, D.T. (1977b) Inactivation and mutation of cultured mammalian cells by aluminium characteristic ultrasoft X-rays. II. Dose–responses of Chinese hamster and human diploid cells to aluminium X-rays and radiations of different LET. *Int. J. Radiat. Biol.*, **31**, 561–576

Cox, R., Hosking, G.P. & Wilson, J. (1978) Ataxia-telangiectasia: Evaluation of radiosensitivity in cultured skin fibroblasts as a diagnostic test. *Arch. Dis. Child.*, **53**, 386–390

Darroudi, F., Farooqi, Z., Benova, D. & Natarajan, A.T. (1992) The mouse splenocyte assay, an in vivo/in vitro system for biological monitoring: Studies with X-rays, fission neutrons and bleomycin. *Mutat. Res.*, **272**, 237–248

De Wit, J., Jaspers, N.G.J. & Bootsma, D. (1981) The rate of DNA synthesis in normal and ataxia-telangiectasia cells after exposure to X-irradiation. *Mutat. Res.*, **80**, 221–226

Denekamp, J., Joiner, M.C. & Maughan, R.L. (1984) Neutron RBEs for mouse skin at low doses per fraction. *Radiat. Res.*, **98**, 317–331

Di Majo, V., Coppola, M., Rebessi, S. & Covelli, V. (1990) Age-related susceptibility of mouse liver to induction of tumors by neutrons. *Radiat. Res.*, **124**, 227–234

Di Majo, V., Coppola, M., Rebessi, S., Saran, A., Pazzaglia, S., Pariset, L. & Covelli, V. (1994) Neutron-induced tumors in BC3F$_1$ mice: Effects of dose fractionation. *Radiat. Res.*, **138**, 252–259

Di Majo, V., Coppola, M., Rebessi, S., Saran, A., Pazzaglia, S., Pariset, L. & Covelli, V. (1996) The influence of sex on life shortening and tumor induction in CBA/Cne mice exposed to X rays or fission neutrons. *Radiat. Res.*, **146**, 81–87

Di Paola, M., Bianchi, M. & Baarli, J. (1978) Lens opacification in mice exposed to 14-MeV neutrons. *Radiat. Res.*, **73**, 340–350

Edwards, M.J. & Taylor, A.M.R. (1980) Unusual levels of (ADP-ribose)$_n$ and DNA synthesis in ataxia telangiectasia cells following γ-ray irradiation. *Nature*, **287**, 745–747

Elkind, M.M. (1991) Physical, biophysical, and cell-biological factors that can contribute to enhanced neoplastic transformation by fission-spectrum neutrons. *Radiat. Res.*, **128**, S47–S52

Engels, H. & Wambersie, A. (1998) Relative biological effectiveness of neutrons for cancer induction and other late effects: A review of radiobiological data. *Recent Results Cancer Res.*, **150**, 54–84

Environmental Protection Agency (1984) *Occupational Exposure to Ionizing Radiation in the United States: A Comprehensive Summary for the Year 1980 and a Summary of Trends for the Years 1960–1985* (EPA 520/1-84-005), Washington DC

Fabry, L., Leonard, A. & Wambersie, A. (1985) Induction of chromosome aberrations in G0 human lymphocytes by low doses of ionizing radiations of different quality. *Radiat. Res.*, **103**, 122–134

Field, S.B. & Hornsey, S. (1979) Aspects of OER and RBE relevant to neutron therapy. *Adv. Radiat. Biol.*, **8**, 1–50

Finch, J. & Bonnett, E. (1992) An investigation of the dose equivalent to radiographers from a high-energy neutron therapy facility. *Br. J. Radiol.*, **65**, 327–333

Ford, M.D. & Lavin, M.F. (1981) Ataxia-telangiectasia: An anomaly in DNA replication after irradiation. *Nucleic Acids Res.*, **9**, 1395–1404

Ford, M.D., Martin, L. & Lavin, M.F. (1984) The effects of ionizing radiation on cell cycle progression in ataxia telangiectasia. *Mutat. Res.*, **125**, 115–122

Fox, J.C. & McNally, N.J. (1988) Cell survival and DNA double-strand break repair following X-ray or neutron irradiation of V79 cells. *Int. J. Radiat. Biol.*, **54**, 1021–1030

Freyer, G.A., Palmer, D.A., Yu, Y., Miller, R.C. & Pandita, T.K. (1996) Neoplastic transformation of mouse C3H10T1/2 cells following exposure to neutrons does not involve mutation of ras gene as analyzed by SSCP and cycle sequencing. *Mutat. Res.*, **357**, 237–244

Fry, R.J. & Sinclair, W.K. (1987) New dosimetry of atomic bomb radiations. *Lancet*, **ii**, 845–848

Fujimoto, K., Wilson, J.A. & Ashmore, J.P. (1985) Radiation exposure risks to nuclear well loggers. *Health Phys.*, **48**, 437–445

Gasinska, A., De Ruiter-Bootsma, A., Davids, J.A.G., Folkard, M. & Fowler, J.F. (1987) Survival of mouse type B spermatogonia for the study of the biological effectiveness of 1 MeV, 2.3 MeV and 5.6 MeV fast neutrons. *Int. J. Radiat. Biol.*, **52**, 237–243

Geraci, J.P., Jackson, K.L., Christensen, G.M., Parker, R.G., Thrower, P.D. & Fox, M. (1976) Single dose fast neutron RBE for pulmonary and esophageal damage in mice. *Radiology*, **120**, 701–703

Geraci, J.P., Jackson, K.L. & Mariano, M.S. (1982) An estimate of the radiation-induced cancer risk from the whole-body stray radiation exposure in neutron radiotherapy. *Eur. J. Cancer clin. Oncol.*, **18**, 1187–1195

Goh, K. (1968) Total-body irradiation and human chromosomes: Cytogenetic studies of the peripheral blood and bone marrow leukocytes seven years after total-body irradiation. *Radiat. Res.*, **35**, 155–170

Goh, K. (1975) Total-body irradiation and human chromosomes. IV. Cytogenetic follow-up studies 8 and 10 1/2 years after total-body irradiation. *Radiat. Res.*, **62**, 364–373

Goodhead, D.T. (1988) Spatial and temporal distribution of energy. *Health. Phys.*, **55**, 231–240

Grahn, D., Frystak, B.H., Lee, C.H., Russell, J.J. & Lindenbaum, A. (1979) Dominant lethal mutations and chromosome aberrations induced in male mice by incorporated ^{239}Pu and by external fission neutron and gamma irradiation. In: *Biological Implications of Radionuclides Released from Nuclear Industries*, Vol. I, Vienna, International Atomic Energy Agency, pp. 163–184

Grahn, D., Carnes, B.A., Farrington, B.H. & Lee, C.H. (1984) Genetic injury in hybrid male mice exposed to low doses of ^{60}Co gamma-rays or fission neutrons. I. Response to single doses. *Mutat. Res.*, **129**, 215–229

Grahn, D., Carnes, B.A. & Farrington, B.H. (1986) Genetic injury in hybrid male mice exposed to low doses of 60Co gamma-rays or fission neutrons. II. Dominant lethal mutation response to long-term weekly exposures. *Mutat. Res.*, **162**, 81–89

Grahn, D., Lombard, L.S. & Carnes, B.A. (1992) The comparative tumorigenic effects of fission neutrons and cobalt-60 gamma rays in B6CF$_1$ mouse. *Radiat. Res.*, **129**, 19–36

Gueulette, J., Beauduin, M., Grégoire, V., Vynckier, S., DeCoster, B.M., Octave-Prignot, M., Wambersie, A., Strijkmans, K., De Schrijver, A., El-Akkad, S., Böhm, L., Slabbert, J.P., Jones, D.T.L., Maughan, R., Onoda, J., Yudelev, M., Porter, A.T., Powers, W.E., Sabattier, R., Breteau, N., Courdi, A., Brassart, N. & Chauvel, P. (1996) RBE variation between fast neutron beams as a function of energy. Intercomparison involving 7 neutrontherapy facilities. *Bull. Cancer Radiother.*, **83** (Suppl. 1), 55S–63S

Hajnal, F. & Wilson, J.W. (1992) High-altitude cosmic ray neutrons: Probable source for the high energy protons at the earth's radiation belts. In: *Proceedings of the 8th Congress of the International Radiation Protection Association*, Montreal, p. 1620

Hall, E.J., Withers, H.R., Geraci, J.P., Meyn, R.E., Rasey, J., Todd, P. & Sheline, G.E. (1979) Radiobiological intercomparisons of fast neutron beams used for therapy in Japan and the United States. *Int. J. Radiat. Oncol. Biol. Phys.*, **5**, 227–233

Hall, E.J., Martin, S.G., Amols, H. & Hei, T.K. (1995) Photoneutrons from medical linear accelerators—Radiobiological measurements and risk estimates. *Int. J. Radiat. Oncol. Biol. Phys.*, **33**, 225–230

Hei, T.K., Hall, E.J. & Waldren, C.A. (1988) Mutation induction and relative biological effectiveness of neutrons in mammalian cells. Experimental observations. *Radiat. Res.*, **115**, 281–291

Hess, W.N., Canfield, E.H. & Lingenfelter, R.E. (1961) Cosmic-ray neutron demography. *J. geophys. Res.*, **66**, 665–667

Hewitt, J.E., Hughes, L., McCaslin, J.B., Smith, A.R., Stephens, L.D., Syvertson, C.A., Thomas, R.H. & Tucker, A.B. (1980) Exposure to cosmic-ray neutrons at commercial jet aircraft altitudes. In: Gessell, T.F. & Lowder, W.M., eds, *Natural Radiation Environment III* (US Department of Energy Report Conf-780422), Springfield, National Technical Information Service, pp. 855–881

Hill, C.K., Han, A. & Elkind, M.M. (1984a) Fission-spectrum neutrons at a low dose rate enhance neoplastic transformation in the linear, low dose region (0–10 cGy). *Int. J. Radiat. Biol.*, **46**, 11–15

Hill, C.K., Han, A. & Elkind, M.M. (1984b) Possible error-prone repair of neoplastic transformation induced by fission-spectrum neutrons. *Br. J. Cancer*, **Suppl**. **6**, 97–101

Hill, C.K., Holland, J., Chang-Liu, C.M., Buess, E.M., Peak, J.G. & Peak, M.J. (1988) Human epithelial teratocarcinoma cells (P3): Radiobiological characterization, DNA damage, and comparison with other rodent and human cell lines. *Radiat. Res.*, **113**, 278–88

Hornsey, S., Kutsutani, Y. & Field, S.B. (1975) Damage to mouse lung with fractionated neutrons and X rays. *Radiology*, **116**, 171–174

Hornsey, S., Myers, R. & Warren, P. (1977) RBE for the two components of weight loss in the mouse testis for fast neutrons relative to X-rays. *Int. J. Radiat. Biol. relat. Stud. Phys. Chem. Med.*, **32**, 297–301

Hornsey, S., Morris, C.C., Myers, R. & White, A. (1981) Relative biological effectiveness for damage to the central nervous system by neutrons. *Int. J. Radiat. Oncol. Biol. Phys.*, **7**, 185–189

Houldsworth, J. & Lavin, M.F. (1980) Effect of ionizing radiation on DNA synthesis in ataxia telangiectasia cells. *Nucleic Acids Res.*, **8**, 3709–3720

Houldsworth, J., Cohen, D., Singh, S. & Lavin, M.F. (1991) The response of ataxia-telangiectasia lymphoblastoid cells to neutron irradiation. *Radiat. Res.*, **125**, 277–282

Howard, W.B. & Yanch, J.C. (1995) Shielding design and dose assessment for accelerator based neutron capture therapy. *Health Phys.*, **68**, 723–730

Hsie, A.W., Xu, Z.D., Yu, Y.J., Sognier, M.A. & Hrelia, P. (1990) Molecular analysis of reactive oxygen-species-induced mammalian gene mutation. *Teratog. Carcinog. Mutag.*, **10**, 115–124

Hübener, K.H., Schwarz, R. & Gleisberg, H. (1989) Neutron therapy of soft tissue sarcomas and status report from the Radiotherapy Department of the Hamburg University Hospital. *Strahlenther. Onkol.*, **165**, 309–310

Hughes, J. S. & O'Riordan, M.C. (1993) *Radiation Exposures of the UK Population—1993 Review* (NRPB-R263), Chilton, Oxfordshire, National Radiation Protection Board

Hulse, E.V. (1980) Tumour incidence and longevity in neutron and gamma-irradiated rabbits, with an assessment of RBE. *Int. J. Radiat. Biol.*, **37**, 633–652

ICAO (International Civil Aviation Authority) (1999) *Annual Civil Aviation Report 1997*. Available at www.icao.org/icao/en/jr/5306 ar3.htm

ICRP (International Commission on Radiological Protection) (1984) *Nonstochastic Effects of Ionizing Radiation* (ICRP Publication 41; Annals of the ICRP 14(3)), Oxford, Pergamon Press

ICRP (International Commission on Radiological Protection) (1990) *RBE for Deterministic Effects* (ICRP Publication 58; Annals of the ICRP 20(4)), Oxford, Pergamon Press

ICRP (International Commission on Radiological Protection) (1991) *1990 Recommendations of the International Commission on Radiological Protection* (ICRP Publication 60; Annals of the ICRP, 21(1-31)), Oxford, Pergamon Press

Imray, F.P. & Kidson, C. (1983) Perturbations of cell-cycle progression in γ-irradiated ataxia telangiectasia and Huntington's disease cells detected by DNA flow cytometric analysis. *Mutat. Res.*, **112**, 369–382

Inskip, P.D., Wang, Z. & Fen, Y. (1991) Suitability of Chinese oil well loggers for an epidemiologic study of the carcinogenic effects of neutrons. *Health Phys.*, **61**, 637–640

Ito, A., Takahashi, T., Watanabe, H., Ogundigie, P.S. & Okamoto T. (1992) Significance of strain and sex differences in the development of ^{252}Cf neutron-induced liver tumors in mice. *Jpn. J. Cancer Res.*, **83**, 1052–1056

Jablon, S. (1993) Neutrons in Hiroshima and uncertainties in cancer risk estimates (Abstract). *Radiat. Res.*, **133**, 130–131

Jacrot, M., Mouriquand, J., Mouriquand., C. & Saez, S. (1979) Mammary carcinogenesis in Sprague-Dawley rats following 3 repeated exposures to 14.8 MeV neutrons and steroid receptor content of these tumor types. *Cancer Lett.*, **8**, 147–153

Jammet, H., Gongora, R., Le Gô, R. & Doloy, M.T. (1980) Clinical and biological comparison of two acute accidental irradiations: Mol (1965) and Brescia (1975). In: Hübner, K.F. & Fry, S.A., eds, *The Medical Basis for Radiation Accident Preparedness*, Amsterdam, Elsevier North Holland, pp. 91–104

Joiner, M.C. & Johns, H. (1988) Renal damage in the mouse: The response to very small doses per fraction. *Radiat. Res.*, **114**, 385–398

Jones, C.A., Sedita, B.A., Hill, C.K. & Elkind, M.M. (1989) Influence of dose rate on the transformation of Syrian hamster embryo cells by fission-spectrum neutrons. In: Baverstock, K.F. & Stather, J.W., eds, *Low Dose Radiation*, London, Taylor & Francis, pp. 539–536

Kataoka, Y., Perrin, J. & Grdina, D.J. (1993) Induction of *hprt* mutations in mice after exposure to fission-spectrum neutrons or ^{60}Co gamma rays. *Radiat. Res.*, **136**, 289–292

Kato, H. & Schull, W.J. (1982) Studies of the mortality of A-bomb survivors. 7. Mortality 1950–1978. Part I. Cancer mortality. *Radiat. Res.*, **90**, 395–432

Kinashi, Y., Masunaga, S., Takagaki, M. & Ono, K. (1997) Mutagenic effects at HPRT locus induced in Chinese hamster ovary cells by thermal neutrons with or without boron compound. *Mutat. Res.*, **377**, 211–215

Klement, A.W., Miller, C.R., Minx, R.P. & Shleien, B., eds (1972) *Estimates of Ionizing Radiation Doses in the United States 1960–2000* (ORP-CSD 72-1), Washington DC, Environmental Protection Agency

Kohn, K.W. & Grimek-Ewig, R.A. (1973) Alkaline elution analysis, a new approach to the study of DNA single-strand interruptions in cells. *Cancer Res.*, **33**, 1849–1853

Kolker, J.D., Halpern, H.J., Krishnasamy, S., Brown, F., Dohrmann, G., Ferguson, L., Hekmatpanah, J., Mullan, J., Wollman, R., Blough, R. & Weichselbaum, R.R. (1990) 'Instant-mix' whole brain photon with neutron boost radiotherapy for malignant gliomas. *Int. J. Radiat. Oncol. Biol. Phys.*, **19**, 409–414

Komatsu, K., Sawada, S., Takeoka, S., Kodama, S. & Okumura, Y. (1993) Dose-rate effects of neutrons and gamma-rays on the induction of mutation and oncogenic transformation in plateau-phase mouse m5S cells. *Int. J. Radiat. Biol.*, **63**, 469–474

Korff, S.A., Mardell, R.B., Merker, M., Light, E.S., Verschell, H.J. & Sandie, W.S. (1979) *Atmospheric Neutrons* (NASA Contractor Report 3126), Washington DC, National Aeronautics and Space Administration

Kronenberg, A. (1991) Perspectives on fast-neutron mutagenesis of human lymphoblastoid cells. *Radiat. Res.*, **128** (Suppl. 1), S87–S93

Kronenberg, A. & Little, J.B. (1989) Molecular characterization of thymidine kinase mutants of human cells induced by densely ionizing radiation. *Mutat. Res.*, **211**, 215–224

Kysela, B.P., Arrand, J.E. & Michael, B.D. (1993) Relative contributions of levels of initial damage and repair of double-strand breaks to the ionizing radiation-sensitive phenotype of the Chinese hamster cell mutant, XR-V15B. Part II. Neutrons. *Int. J. Radiat. Biol.*, **64**, 531–538

Lafuma, J., Chmelevsky, D., Chameaud, J., Morin, M., Masse, R. & Kellerer, A.M. (1989) Lung carcinomas in Sprague-Dawley rats after exposure to low doses of radon daughters, fission neutrons, or γ rays. *Radiat. Res.*, **118**, 230–245

Laramore, G.E. & Austin-Seymour, M.M. (1992) Fast neutron radiotherapy in relation to the radiation sensitivity of human organ systems. *Adv. Radiat. Biol.*, **15**, 153–193

Laramore, G.E., Krall, J.M., Thomas, F.J., Russell, K.J., Maor, M.H., Hendrickson, F.R., Martz, K.L., Griffin, T.W. & Davis, L.W. (1993) Fast neutron radiotherapy for locally advanced prostate cancer. *Am. J. clin. Oncol.*, **16**, 164–167

Little, M.P. (1997) Estimates of neutron relative biological effectiveness derived from the Japanese atomic bomb survivors. *Int. J. Radiat. Biol.*, **72**, 715–726

Littlefield, L.G. & Joiner, E.E. (1978) Cytogenic follow-up studies in six radiation accident victims: 16 and 17 years post-exposure. In: *Late Biological Effects of Ionizing Radiation*, Vol. I, Vienna, International Atomic Energy Agency, pp. 297–308

Littlefield, L.G., McFee, A.F., Sayer, A.M., O'Neill, J.P., Kleinerman, R.A. & Maor, M.H. (2000) Induction and persistence of chromosome aberrations in human lymphocytes exposed to neutrons *in vitro* or *in vivo*: Implications of findings in retrospective biological dosimetry. *Radiat. Prot. Dosim.*, **88**, 59–68

Lloyd, D.C., Purrott, R.J., Dolphin, G.W., Bolton, D., Edwards, A.A. & Corp, M.J. (1975) The relationship between chromosome aberrations and low LET radiation dose to human lymphocytes. *Int. J. Radiat. Biol.*, **28**, 75–90

Lloyd, D.C., Purrott, R.J., Dolphin, G.W. & Edwards, A.A. (1976) Chromosome aberrations induced in human lymphocytes by neutron irradiation. *Int. J. Radiat. Biol.*, **29**, 169–182

Lloyd, D.C., Purrott, R.J., Reeder, E.J., Edwards, A.A. & Dolphin, G.W. (1978) Chromosome aberrations induced in human lymphocytes by radiation from ^{252}Cf. *Int. J. Radiat. Biol.*, **34**, 177–186

Lücke-Huhle, C. (1994) Similarities between human ataxia fibroblasts and murine SCID cells: High sensitivity to γ rays and high frequency of methotrexate-induced DHFR gene amplification, but normal radiosensitivity to densely ionizing α particles. *Radiat. environ. Biophys.*, **33**, 201–210

Lücke-Huhle, C., Comper, W., Hieber, L. & Pech, M. (1982) Comparative study of G2 delay and survival after ^{241}americium-α and ^{60}cobalt-γ irradiation. *Radiat. environ. Biophys.*, **20**, 171–185

MacDougall, R.H., Orr, J.A., Kerr, G.R. & Duncan, W. (1990) Fast neutron treatment for squamous cell carcinoma of the head and neck: Final report of Edinburgh randomised trial. *Br. med. J.*, **301**, 1241–1242

MacVittie, T.J., Monroy, R., Vigneulle, R.M., Zeman, G.H. & Jackson, W.E. (1991) The relative biological effectiveness of mixed fission-neutron–γ radiation on hematopoietic syndrome in the canine: Effect of therapy on survival. *Radiat. Res.*, **128**, S29–S36

Maisin, J.R., Gerber, G.B., Venkerkom, J. & Wambersie, A. (1996) Survival and diseases in C57BL mice exposed to X-rays or 3.1 MeV neutrons at an age of 7 or 21 days. *Radiat. Res.*, **146**, 453–460

Maki, H., Saito, M., Kobayashi, T., Kawai, K. & Akaboshi, M. (1986) Cell inactivation and DNA single- and double-strand breaks in cultured mammalian cells irradiated by a thermal neutron beam. *Int. J. Radiat. Biol. relat. Stud. Phys. Chem. Med.*, **50**, 795–809

Masuda, T. (1994) Radiation-chemical discussion on inverse dose-rate effect observed in radiation-induced strand breaks of plasmid DNA. *J. Radiat. Res. Tokyo*, **35**, 157–167

Medvedovsky, C. & Worgul, B.V. (1991) Neutron effects on the lens. *Radiat. Res.*, **128** (Suppl.), S103–S110

Mill, A.J., Wells, J., Hall, S.C. & Butler, A. (1996) Micronucleus induction in human lymphocytes: Comparative effects of X rays, alpha particles, beta particles and neutrons and implications for biological dosimetry. *Radiat. Res.*, **145**, 575–585

Miller, R.C. & Hall, E.J. (1991) Oncogenic transformation of C3H 10T1/2 cells by acute and protracted exposure to monoenergetic neutrons. *Radiat. Res.*, **128**, S60–S64

Miller, R.C., Geard, C.R., Brenner, D.J., Komatsu, K., Marino, S.A. & Hall, E.J. (1989) Neutron-energy-dependent oncogenic transformation of C3H 10T1/2 mouse cells. *Radiat. Res.*, **117**, 114–127

Miller, R.C., Brenner, D.J., Randers-Pehrson, G., Marino, S.A. & Hall, E.J. (1990) The effects of the temporal distribution of dose on oncogenic transformation by neutrons and charged particles of intermediate LET. *Radiat. Res.*, **124**, S62–S68

Miller, R.C., Geard, C.R., Martin, S.G., Marino, S.A. & Hall, E.J. (1995) Neutron-induced cell cycle-dependent oncogenic transformation of C3H 10T1/2 cells. *Radiat. Res.*, **142**, 270–275

Mole, R.H. (1984) Dose–response relationships. In: Boice, J.D., Jr & Fraumeni, J.F., Jr, eds, *Radiation Carcinogenesis: Epidemiology and Biological Significance*, New York, Raven Press, pp. 403–420

Molls, M., Streffer, C. & Zamboglou, N. (1981) Micronucleus formation in preimplanted mouse embryos cultured in vitro after irradiation with x-rays and neutrons. *Int. J. Radiat. Biol.*, **39**, 307–314

Montagne, C., Donne, J. P., Pelcot, D., Nguyen, V.D., Bouisset, P. & Kerlan, G. (1993) Inflight radiation measurements aboard French airliners. *Radiat. Prot. Dosim.*, **48**, 79–83

Montour, J.L., Hard, R.C., Jr, & Flora, R. (1977) Mammary neoplasia in the rat following high-energy neutron irradiation. *Cancer Res.*, **37**, 2619–2623

Moss, A.J., Jr, Baker, M.L., Prior, R.M., Erichsen, E.A., Nagle, W.A. & Dalrymple, G.V. (1976) Fast neutron and x-ray induced single strand DNA breaks in cultured mammalian cells. *Radiology*, **119**, 459–461

Nakamura, N. & Sawada, S. (1988) Reversed dose-rate effect and RBE of 252-californium radiation in the induction of 6-thioguanine-resistant mutations in mouse L5178Y cells. *Mutat. Res.*, **201**, 65–71

Nakamura, T., Uwamino, Y., Ohkubo, T. & Hara, A. (1987) Altitude variation of cosmic-ray neutrons. *Health Phys.*, **53**, 509–517

Nakamura, N., Tucker, J.D., Bauchinger, M., Littlefield, L.G., Lloyd, D.C., Preston, R.J. Sasaki, M.S., Awa, A.A. & Wolff, S. (1998) F values as cytogenetic fingerprints of prior exposure to different radiation qualities: Prediction, reality and future. *Radiat. Res.*, **150**, 492–494

Natarajan, A.T., Darroudi, F., Jha, A.N., Meijers, M. & Zdzienicka, M.Z. (1993) Ionizing radiation induced DNA lesions which lead to chromosomal aberrations. *Mutat. Res.*, **299**, 297–303

National Council on Radiation Protection and Measurements (1987) *Ionizing Radiation Exposure of the Population of the United States* (NCRP Report No. 93), Bethesda, MD

National Council on Radiation Protection and Measurements (1995) *Radiation Exposure and High-altitude Flight* (NCRP Commentary No. 12), Bethesda, MD

National Council on Radiation Protection and Measurements (1997) *Uncertainties in Fatal Cancer Risk Estimates Used in Radiation Protection* (NCRP Report No. 126), Bethesda, MD

Neriishi, K., Wong, F.L., Nakashima, E., Otake, M., Kodama, K. & Choshi, K. (1995) Relationship between cataracts and epilation in atomic bomb survivors. *Radiat. Res.*, **144**, 107–113

Nijhoff, J.H. & de Boer, P. (1980) Radiation-induced meiotic autosomal non-disjunction in male mice. The effects of low doses of fission neutrons and X-rays in meiosis I and II of a Robertsonian translocation heterozygote. *Mutat. Res.*, **72**, 431–446

Oksanen, P.J. (1998) Estimated individual annual cosmic radiation doses for flight crews. *Aviat. Space Environ. Med.*, **69**, 621–625

Otake, M. & Schull, W.J. (1990) Radiation-related lenticular opacities in Hiroshima and Nagasaki atomic bomb survivors based on the DS86 dosimetry system. *Radiat. Res.*, **121**, 3–13

Otake, M., Neriishi, K. & Schull, W.J. (1996) Cataract in atomic bomb survivors based on a threshold model and the occurrence of severe epilation. *Radiat. Res.*, **146**, 339–348

Painter, R.B. & Young, B.R. (1980) Radiosensitivity in ataxia-telangiectasia: A new explanation. *Proc. natl Acad. Sci. USA*, **77**, 7315–7317

Parkins, C.S., Fowler, J.F., Maughan, R.L. & Roper, M.J. (1985) Repair in mouse lung for up to 20 fractions of X-rays or neutrons. *Br. J. Radiol.*, **58**, 225–241

Pazzaglia, S., Saran, A., Pariset, L., Rebessi, S., Di Majo, V., Coppola, M. & Covelli, V. (1996) Sensitivity of C3H 10T1/2 cells to radiation-induced killing and neoplastic transformation as a function of cell cycle. *Int. J. Radiat. Biol.*, **69**, 57–65

Peak, M.J., Peak, J.G., Carnes, B.A., Liu, C.M. & Hill, C.K. (1989) DNA damage and repair in rodent and human cells after exposure to JANUS fission spectrum neutrons: A minor fraction of single-strand breaks as revealed by alkaline elution is refractory to repair. *Int. J. Radiat. Biol.*, **55**, 761–772

Pendic, B. & Djordjevic, O. (1968) Chromosome aberrations in human subjects five years after whole body irradiation. *Iugoslav. physiol. pharmacol. Acta*, **4**, 231–237

Pendic, B., Barjaktarovic, N. & Kostic, V. (1980) Chromosomal aberrations in persons accidentally irradiated in Vinca 19 years ago. *Radiat. Res.*, **81**, 478–482

Phillips, T.L., Barschall, H.H., Goldberg, E., Fu, K. & Rowe, J. (1974) Comparison of RBE values of 15 MeV neutrons for damage to an experimental tumour and some normal tissues. *Eur. J. Cancer*, **10**, 287–292

Pogozelski, W.K., Xapsos, M.A. & Blakely, W.F. (1999) Quantitative assessment of the contribution of clustered damage to DNA double-strand breaks induced by 60Co gamma rays and fission neutrons. *Radiat. Res.*, **151**, 442–448

Poncy, J.L., Fritsch, P. & Masse, R. (1988) Evolution of sister-chromatid exchanges (SCE) in rat bone marrow cells as a function of time after 2 Gy of whole-body neutron irradiation. *Mutation Res.*, **202**, 45–49

Ponnaiya, B., Cornforth, M.N. & Ullrich, R.L. (1997) Induction of chromosomal instability in human mammary cells by neutrons and gamma rays. *Radiat. Res.*, **147**, 288–294

Preston, F.S. (1985) Eight years' experience of Concorde operations: Medical aspects. *J. R. Soc. Med.*, **78**, 193–196

Prise, K.M., Davies, S. & Michael, B.D. (1987) The relationship between radiation-induced DNA double-strand breaks and cell kill in hamster V79 fibroblasts irradiated with 250 kVp X-rays, 2.3 MeV neutrons or 238Pu alpha-particles. *Int. J. Radiat. Biol.*, **52**, 893–902

Prosser, J.S. & Stimpson, L.D. (1981) The influence of anoxia or oxygenation on the induction of chromosome aberrations in human lymphocytes by 15-MeV neutrons. *Mutat. Res.*, **84**, 365–373

Redpath, J.L., Hill, C.K., Jones, C.A. & Sun, C. (1990) Fission-neutron-induced expression of a tumour-associated antigen in human cell hybrids (HeLa × skin fibroblasts): Evidence for increased expression at low dose rate. *Int. J. Radiat. Biol.*, **58**, 673–680

Redpath, J.L., Antoniono, R.J., Sun, C., Gerstenberg, H.M. & Blakely, W.F. (1995) Late mitosis/early G1 phase and mid-G1 phase are not hypersensitive cell cycle phases for neoplastic transformation of HeLa × skin fibroblast human hybrid cells induced by fission-spectrum neutrons. *Radiat. Res.*, **141**, 37–43

Richard, F., Renard, L. & Wambersie, A. (1989) Neutron therapy of soft tissue sarcoma at Louvain-la-Neuve (interm results 1987). *Strahlenther. Onkol.*, **165**, 306–308

Rithidech, K.N., Dunn, J.J., Gordon, C.R., Cronkite, E.P. & Bond, V.P. (1996) N-ras mutations in radiation-induced murine leukemic cells. *Blood Cells Mol. Dis.*, **22**, 271–280

Roberts, C.J. & Holt, P.D. (1985) Induction of chromosome aberrations and cell killing in Syrian hamster fibroblasts by gamma-rays, X-rays and fast neutrons. *Int. J. Radiat. Biol.*, **48**, 927–942

Roesch, W.C., ed. (1987a) *US–Japan Joint Reassessment of Atomic Bomb Radiation Dosimetry in Hiroshima and Nagasaki,* Vol. 1, Hiroshima, Radiation Effects Research Foundation

Roesch, W.C., ed. (1987b) *US–Japan Joint Reassessment of Atomic Bomb Radiation Dosimetry in Hiroshima and Nagasaki,* Vol. 2, Hiroshima, Radiation Effects Research Foundation

Roth, J., Brown, M., Calterall, M. & Beal, A. (1976) Effects of fast neutrons on the eye. *Br. J. Ophthalmol.*, **60**, 236–244

Rühm, W., Kellerer, A.M., Korschinek, G., Faestermann, T., Knie, K., Rugel, G., Kato, K. & Nolte, E. (1998) The dosimetry system DS86 and the neutron discrepancy in Hiroshima—Historical review, present status, and future options. *Radiat. Environ. Biophys.*, **37**, 293–310

Russell, W.L. (1965) Studies in mammalian radiation genetics. *Nucleonics*, **23**, 53–62

Russell, W.L. (1967) Repair mechanisms in radiation mutation induction in the mouse. In: *Recovery and Repair Mechanisms in Radiobiology* (Brookhaven Symp. Biol. 20), Upton, NY, Brookhaven National Laboratory, pp. 179–189

Russell, W.L. (1972) *The Genetic Effects of Radiation. Peaceful Uses of Atomic Energy* (Fourth International Conference), Vol. 13, Vienna, International Atomic Energy Agency, pp. 487–500

Russell, K.J., Caplan, R.J., Laramore, G.E., Burnison, C.M., Maor, M.H., Taylor, M.E., Zink, S., Davis, L.W. & Griffin, T.W. (1993) Photon versus fast neutron external beam radiotherapy in the treatment of locally advanced prostate cancer: Results of a randomized prospective trial. *Int. J. Radiat. Oncol. Biol. Phys.*, **28**, 47–54

Sakai, N., Suzuki, S., Nakamura, N. & Okada, S. (1987) Induction and subsequent repair of DNA damage by fast neutrons in cultured mammalian cells. *Radiat. Res.*, **110**, 311–320

Saran, A., Pazzaglia, S., Coppola, M., Rebessi, S., Di Majo, V., Garavini, M. & Covelli, V. (1991) Absence of a dose-fractionation effect on neoplastic transformation induced by fission-spectrum neutrons in C3H 10T1/2 cells. *Radiat. Res.*, **126**, 343–348

Saran, A., Pazzaglia, S., Pariset, L., Rebessi, S., Broerse, J.J., Zoetelief, J., Di Majo, V., Coppola, M. & Covelli, V. (1994) Neoplastic transformation of C3H 10T1/2 cells: A study with fractionated doses of monoenergetic neutrons. *Radiat. Res.*, **138**, 246–251

Sasaki, M.S. (1971) Radiation-induced chromosome aberrations in lymphocytes. Possible biological dosimeter in man. In: Sugahara, T. & Hug, O., eds, *Biological Aspects of Radiation Protection*, Tokyo, Igaku Shoin, pp. 81–90

Sasaki, M.S., Takatsuji, T. & Ejima, Y. (1998) The F value cannot be ruled out as a chromosomal fingerprint of radiation quality. *Radiat. Res.*, **150**, 253–258

Savage, J.R.K. (1982) RBE of neutrons for genetic effects. In: Broerse, J.J. & Gerber, G.B., eds, *Radiation Protection. Neutron Carcinogenesis* (EUR 8084 EN). *European Seminar, Rijswijk, NL, 1 April 1982*, Commission of the European Communities

Savoye, C., Swenberg, C., Hugot, S., Sy, D., Sabattier, R., Charlier, M. & Spotheim-Maurizot, M. (1997) Thiol WR-1065 and disulphide WR-33278, two metabolites of the drug ethyol (WR-2721), protect DNA against fast neutron-induced strand breakage. *Int. J. Radiat. Biol.*, **71**, 193–202

Schmid, E., Dresp, J., Bauchinger, M., Franke, H.D., Langendorff, G. & Hess, A. (1980) Radiation-induced chromosome damage in patients after tumour therapy with 14 MeV, DT neutrons. *Int. J. Radiat. Biol.*, **38**, 691–695

Scott, D., Sharpe, H., Batchelor, A.L., Evans, H.J. & Papworth, D.G. (1969) Radiation-induced chromosome damage in human peripheral blood lymphocytes *in vitro*. I. RBE and dose-rate studies with fast neutrons. *Mutat. Res.*, **8**, 367–381

Seed, T.M. & Kaspar, L.V. (1991) Probing altered hematopoietic progenitor cells of pre-leukemic dogs with JANUS fission neutrons. *Radiat. Res.*, **128**, S81–S86

Sevan'kaev, A.V., Zherbin, E.A., Luchnik, N.V., Obaturov, G.M., Kozlov, V.M., Tyatte, E.G. & Kapchigashev, S.P. (1979a) [Cytogenetic effects induced by neutrons in lymphocytes of human peripheral blood *in vitro*. I. Dose-dependence of the effects of neutrons of different energies on various types of chromosome aberrations]. *Genetika*, **15**, 1046–1060 (in Russian)

Sevan'kaev, A.V., Zherbin, E.A., Obaturov, G.M., Kozlov, V.M., Tyatte, E.G. & Kapchigashev, S.P. (1979b) [Cytogenetic effects produced by neutrons in lymphocytes of human peripheral blood *in vitro*. II. Relative biological effectiveness of neutrons of various energies.] *Genetika*, **15**, 1228–1234 (in Russian)

Seyama, T., Yamamoto, O., Kinomura, A. & Yokoro, K. (1991) Carcinogenic effects of tritiated water (HTO) in mice: In comparison to those of neutrons and gamma-rays. *J. Radiat. Res.*, **Suppl. 2**, 132–142

Sharma, S. & Hill, C.K. (1996) Dependence of mutation induction on fast-neutron energy in a human epithelial teratocarcinoma cell line (P3). *Radiat. Res.*, **145**, 331–336

Shellabarger, C.J. (1976) Radiation carcinogenesis, laboratory studies. *Cancer*, **37**, 1090–1096

Shellabarger, C.J., Stone, J.P. & Holtzman, S. (1978) Rat differences in mammary tumor induction with estrogen and neutron radiation. *J. natl Cancer Inst.*, **61**, 1505–1508

Shellabarger, C.J., Chmelevsky, D. & Kellerer, A.M. (1980) Induction of mammary neoplasms in the Sprague-Dawley rat by 430 keV neutrons and X-rays. *J. natl Cancer Inst.*, **64**, 821–833

Shellabarger, C.J., Chmelevsky, D., Kellerer, A.M., Stone, J.P. & Holtzman, S. (1982) Induction of mammary neoplasms in the ACI rat by 430-keV neutrons, X-rays, and diethylstilbestrol. *J. natl Cancer Inst.*, **69**, 1135–1146

Shellabarger, C.J., Stone, J.P. & Holtzman, S. (1983) Effect of interval between neutron radiation and diethylstilbestrol on mammary carcinogenesis in female ACI rats. *Environ. Health Perspectives*, **50**, 227–232

Siddiqi, M.A. & Bothe, E. (1987) Single- and double-strand break formation in DNA irradiated in aqueous solution: Dependence on dose and OH radical scavenger concentration. *Radiat. Res.*, **112**, 449–463

Silbergeld, D.L., Rostomily, R.C. & Alvord, E.C., Jr (1991) The cause of death in patients with glioblastoma is multifactorial: Clinical factors and autopsy findings in 117 cases of supratentorial glioblastoma in adults. *J. Neuro-oncol.*, **10**, 179–185

Sinclair, W.K. (1968) Radiation survival in synchronous and asynchronous Chinese hamster cells *in vitro*. In: *Biophysical Aspects of Radiation Quality* (IAEA STIPUB/171), Vienna, International Atomic Energy Agency, pp. 39–54

Sloan, S.R., Newcomb, E.W. & Pellicer, A. (1990) Neutron radiation can activate K-ras via a point mutation in codon 146 and induces a different spectrum of ras mutations than does gamma radiation. *Mol. Cell Biol.*, **10**, 405–408

Smathers, J.B., Graves, R.G., Sandel, P.S., Almond, P.R., Otte, V.A. & Grant, W.H. (1978) Radiation dose received by TAMVEC neutron therapy staff. *Health Phys.*, **35**, 271–277

Spiethoff, A., Wesch, H., Höver, K.-H. & Wegener, K. (1992) The combined and separate action of neutron radiation and zirconium dioxide on the liver of rats. *Health Phys.*, **63**, 111–118

Spotheim-Maurizot, M., Charlier, M. & Sabattier, R. (1990) DNA radiolysis by fast neutrons. *Int. J. Radiat. Biol.*, **57**, 301–313

Spotheim-Maurizot, M., Savoye, C., Sabattier, R. & Charlier, M. (1996) Comparative study of DNA radiolysis by fast neutrons and γ-rays. *Bull. Cancer Radiother.*, **83** (Suppl.), 27s–31s

Stelzer, K., Griffin, B., Eskridge, J., Eenmaa, J., Mayberg, M., Hummel, S. & Winn, H.R. (1991) Results of neutron radiosurgery for inoperable arteriovenous malformations of the brain. *Med. Dosim.*, **16**, 137–141

Stewart, F.A., Soranson, J., Maughan, R., Alpen, E.L. & Denekamp, J. (1984) The RBE for renal damage after irradiation with 3 MeV neutrons. *Br. J. Radiol.*, **57**, 1009–1021

Storer, J.B. & Fry, R.J.M. (1995) On the shape of neutron dose–effect curves for radiogenic cancers and life shortening in mice. *Radiat. environ. Biophys.*, **34**, 21–27

Storer, J.B., Serrano, L.J., Darden, E.G., Jr, Jernigan, M.C. & Ullrich, R.L. (1979) Life shortening in RFM and BALB/c mice as a function of radiation quality, dose, and dose rate. *Radiat. Res.*, **78**, 122–161

Straume, T., Kwan, T.C., Goldstein, L.S. & Dobson, R.L. (1991) Measurement of neutron-induced genetic damage in mouse immature oocytes. *Mutat. Res.*, **248**, 123–133

Swenberg, C.E., Vaishnav, Y.N., Li, B., Tsao, H., Mao, B. & Geacintov, N.E. (1997) Single-strand breaks in oligodeoxyribonucleotides induced by fission neutrons and gamma-radiation and measured by gel electrophoresis: Protective effects of aminothiols. *J. Radiat. Res. (Tokyo)*, **38**, 241–254

Sy, D., Savoye, C., Begusova, M., Michalik, V., Charlier, M. & Spotheim-Maurizot, M. (1997) Sequence-dependent variations of DNA structure modulate radiation-induced strand breakage. *Int. J. Radiat. Biol.*, **72**, 147–155

Takahashi, T., Watanabe, H., Dohi, K. & Ito, A. (1992) ^{252}Cf relative biological effectiveness and inheritable effects of fission neutrons in mouse liver tumorigenesis. *Cancer Res.*, **52**, 1948–1953

Tauchi, H., Nakamura, N. & Sawada, S. (1993) Cell cycle dependence for the induction of 6-thioguanine-resistant mutations: G2/M stage is distinctively sensitive to ^{252}Cf neutrons but not to ^{60}Co gamma-rays. *Int. J. Radiat. Biol.*, **63**, 475–481

Taylor, A.M.R., Harnden, D.G., Arlett, C.F., Harcourt, S.A., Lehmann, A.R., Stevens, S. & Bridges, B.A. (1975) Ataxia-telangiectasia: A human mutation with abnormal radiation sensitivity. *Nature*, **258**, 427–429

Thomson, J.F. & Grahn, D. (1988) Life shortening in mice exposed to fission neutrons and gamma rays. VII. Effects of 60 once-weekly exposures. *Radiat. Res.*, **115**, 347–360

Thomson, J.F., Williamson, F.S. & Grahn, D. (1985a) Life shortening in mice exposed to fission neutrons and gamma rays. IV. Further studies with fractionated neutron exposures. *Radiat. Res.*, **103**, 77–88

Thomson, J.F., Williamson, F.S. & Grahn, D. (1985b) Life shortening in mice exposed to fission neutrons and gamma rays. V. Further studies with single low doses. *Radiat. Res.*, **104**, 420–428

Thomson, J.F., Williamson, F.S. & Grahn, D. (1986) Life shortening in mice exposed to fission neutrons and gamma rays. VI. Studies with the white-footed mouse *Peromyscus leucopus*. *Radiat. Res.*, **108**, 176–188

Thraves, P.J., Varghese, S., Jung, M., Grdina, D.J., Rhim, J.S. & Dritschilo, A. (1994) Transformation of human epidermal keratinocytes with fission neutrons. *Carcinogenesis*, **15**, 2867–2873

Todorov, S., Bulanova, M., Mileva, M. & Ivanov, B. (1973) Aberrations induced by fission neutrons in human peripheral lymphocytes. *Mutat. Res.*, **17**, 377–383

Ullrich, R.L. (1980) Effects of split doses of X rays or neutrons on lung tumor formation in RFM mice. *Radiat. Res.*, **83**, 138–145

Ullrich, R.L. (1983) Tumor induction in BALB/c female mice after fission neutron or gamma irradiation. *Radiat. Res.*, **93**, 506–515

Ullrich, R.L. (1984) Tumor induction in BALB/c mice after fractionated or protracted exposures to fission-spectrum neutrons. *Radiat. Res.*, **97**, 587–597

Ullrich, R.L. & Preston, R.J. (1987) Myeloid leukemia in male RFM mice following irradiation with fission spectrum neutrons or gamma rays. *Radiat. Res.*, **109**, 165–170

Ullrich, R.L., Jernigan, M.C., Cosgrove, G.E., Satterfield, L.C., Bowlers, N.D. & Storer, J.B (1976) The influence of dose and dose rate on the incidence of neoplastic disease in RFM mice after neutron irradiation. *Radiat. Res.*, **68**, 115–131

Ullrich, R.L., Jernigan, M.C. & Storer, J.B. (1977) Neutron carcinogenesis, dose and dose-rate effects in BALB/c mice. *Radiat. Res.*, **72**, 487–498

Ullrich, R.L., Jernigan, M.C. & Adams, L.M. (1979) Induction of lung tumors in RFM mice after localized exposures to X rays or neutrons. *Radiat. Res.*, **80**, 464–473

UNSCEAR (United Nations Scientific Committee on the Effects of Atomic Radiation) (1982) *Ionizing Radiation: Sources and Biological Effects*, New York, United Nations

UNSCEAR (United Nations Scientific Committee on the Effects of Atomic Radiation) (1993) *Sources and Effects of Ionizing Radiation*, New York, United Nations

Upton, A.C., Randolph, M.L. & Conklin, J.W. (1970) Late effects of fast neutrons and gamma-rays in mice as influenced by the dose rate of irradiation: Induction of neoplasia. *Radiat. Res.*, **41**, 467–491

Van Buul, P.P. (1989) The induction by ionizing radiation of chromosomal aberrations in rhesus monkey pre-meiotic germ cells: Effects of dose rate and radiation quality. *Mutat. Res.*, **225**, 83–89

Van der Kogel, A.J. (1985) Chronic effects of neutrons and charged particles on spinal cord, lung and rectum. *Radiat. Res.*, **104** (Suppl.), S208–S216

Van der Kogel, A.J., Sissingh, H.A. & Zoetelief, J. (1982) Effect of X rays and neutrons on repair and regeneration in the rat spinal cord. *Int, J. Radiat. Oncol. Biol. Phys.*, **8**, 2095–2097

Van der Schans, G.P., Paterson, M.C. & Cross, W.G. (1983) DNA strand break and rejoining in cultured human fibroblasts exposed to fast neutrons or gamma rays. *Int. J. Radiat. Biol.*, **44**, 75–85

Vaughan, A.T.M., Gordon, D.J., Chettle, D.R. & Green, S. (1991) Neutron and cobalt-60 γ irradiation produce similar changes in DNA supercoiling. *Radiat. Res.*, **127**, 19–23

Vogel, H.H., Jr (1969) Mammary gland neoplasms after fission neutron irradiation. *Nature*, **222**, 1279–1281

Vogel, H.H., Jr (1978) *High LET Irradiation of Sprague-Dawley Female Rats and Mammary Neoplasm Induction* (SM 224/233), Vienna, International Atomic Energy Agency, pp. 147–164

Vogel, H.H., Jr & Turner, J.E. (1982) Genetic component in rat mammary carcinogenesis. *Radiat. Res.*, **89**, 264–273

Vogel, H.H., Jr & Zaldivar, R. (1972) Neutron-induced mammary neoplasms in the rat. *Cancer Res.*, **32**, 933–938

Vral, A., Thierens, H. & De Ridder, L. (1996) Micronucleus induction by ^{60}Co γ-rays and fast neutrons in ataxia-telangiectasia lymphocytes. *Int. J. Radiat. Biol.*, **70**, 171–176

Vulpis, N., Tognacci, L. & Scarpa, G. (1978) Chromosome aberrations as a dosimetric technique for fission neutrons over the dose-range 0.2–50 rad. *Int. J. Radiat. Biol.*, **33**, 301–306

Waldren, C., Jones, C. & Puck, T.T. (1979) Measurement of mutagenesis in mammalian cells. *Proc. natl Acad. Sci. USA*, **76**, 1358–1362

Watanabe, H., Takahashi, T., Lee, J.-Y., Ohtaki, M., Roy, G., Ando, Y., Yamada, K., Gotoh, T., Kurisu, K., Fujimoto, N., Satow, Y. & Ito, A. (1996) Influence of paternal ^{252}Cf neutron exposure on abnormal sperm, embryonal lethality, and liver tumorigenesis in the F_1 offspring of mice. *Jpn. J. Cancer Res.*, **87**, 51–57

White, A. & Hornsey, S. (1980) Time dependent repair of radiation damage in the rat spinal cord after X-rays and neutrons. *Eur. J. Cancer.*, **16**, 957–962

Wilson, O.J., Young, B.F. & Richardson, C.K. (1994) Cosmic radiation doses received by Australian commercial flight crews and the implications of ICRP 60. *Health Phys.*, **66**, 493–502

Wilson, J.W., Nealy, J.E., Cucinotta, F.A., Shinn, J.L., Hajnal, F., Reginatto, M. & Goldhagen, P. (1995) *Radiation Safety Aspects of Commercial High-speed Flight Transportation* (NASA TP-3524), Washington DC, National Aeronautics and Space Administration

Withers, H.R. & Elkind, M.M. (1970) Microcolony survival assay for cells of mouse intestinal mucosa exposed to radiation. *Int. J. Radiat. Biol.*, **17**, 261–267

Withers, H.R., Mason, K., Reid, B.O., Dubravsky, N., Barkley, H.T., Jr, Brown, B.W. & Smathers, J.B. (1974) Response of mouse intestine to neutrons and gamma rays in relation to dose fractionation and division cycle. *Cancer*, **34**, 39–47

Withers, H.R., Flow, B.L., Huchton, J.I., Hussey, D.H., Jardine, J.H., Mason, K.A., Raulston, G.L. & Smathers, J.B. (1977) Effect of dose fractionation on early and late-skin responses to γ-rays and neutrons. *Int. J. Radiat. Oncol. Biol. Phys.*, **3**, 227–233

Withers, H.R., Mason, K.A., Taylor, J.M.J., Kim, D.K. & Smathers, J.B. (1993) Dose–survival curves, alpha/beta ratios, RBE values and equal effect per fraction for neutron irradiation of jejunal crypt cells. *Radiat. Res.*, **134**, 295–300

Worgul, B.V., Medvedovsky, C. Huang, Y., Marino, S.A., Randers-Pehrson, G. & Brenner, D.J. (1996) Quantitative assessment of the cataractogenic potential of very low doses of neutrons. *Radiat. Res.*, **145**, 343–349

Yokoro, K., Sumi, C., Ito, A., Hamada, K., Kanda, K. & Kobayashi, T. (1980) Mammary carcinogenic effect of low-dose fission radiation in Wister/Furth rats and its dependency on prolactin. *J. natl Cancer Inst.*, **64**, 1459–1466

Yokoro, K., Niwa, O., Hamada, K., Kamiya, K., Seyama, T. & Inoh A. (1987) Carcinogenic and co-carcinogenic effects of radiation in rat mammary carcinogenesis and mouse T-cell lymphogenesis: A review. *Int. J. Radiat. Biol.*, **51**, 1069–1080

Zhang, Y. & Woloschak, G.E. (1998) Detection of codon 12 point mutations of the K-ras gene from mouse lung adenocarcinoma by 'enriched' PCR. *Int. J. Radiat. Biol.*, **74**, 43–51

Zhu, L.X. & Hill, C.K. (1994) Neutron-energy-dependent mutagenesis in V79 Chinese hamster cells. *Radiat. Res.*, **139**, 300–306

GLOSSARY

GLOSSARY

Absorbed dose: mean energy imparted by *ionizing radiation* to an irradiated medium per unit mass, expressed in *grays* (Gy)

Activity: amount of radioactivity of a *radionuclide* defined as the mean number of decays per unit time

α-particle: two neutrons and two protons bound as a single particle that is emitted from the nucleus of certain radioactive *isotopes* in the process of decay or disintegration; a positively charged particle indistinguishable from the nucleus of a helium atom

α-radiation: α-particles emerging from radioactive atoms

α-rays: stream of α-particles

Ankylosing spondylitis: arthritis of the spine

Background radiation: amount of radiation to which a population is exposed from natural sources, such as *terrestrial radiation* due to naturally occurring *radionuclides* in the soil, *cosmic radiation* originating in outer space and naturally occurring *radionuclides* deposited in the human body

β-particle: charged particle emitted from the nucleus of an atom, with mass and charge equal to those of an *electron*

β-rays: stream of β-particles

Brachytherapy: method of radiation therapy in which an encapsulated source or group of sources is used to deliver *β-* or *γ-radiation* at a distance of a few centimeters, by surface, intracavitary or interstitial application

Bremsstrahlung: secondary *photon* radiation produced by deceleration of charged particles passing through matter

Collective dose: sum of individual doses received over a given time by a specified population from exposure to a specified source of radiation

Collective dose commitment: infinite time integral of the product of the size of a specified population and the per caput *dose rate* to a given organ or tissue for that population

Collective effective dose equivalent: product of the number of exposed individuals and their average *effective dose* equivalent, expressed in person–sieverts

Commited dose equivalent: dose to some specific organ or tissue over 50 years after intake of radioactive material by an individual

Committed effective dose equivalent: *committed dose equivalent* for a given organ multiplied by a *weighting factor*

Cosmic radiation or **cosmic rays**: radiation of very high energy reaching the earth from outer space or produced in the earth's atmosphere by particles from outer space; part of *background radiation*

Criticality: term used in reactor physics to describe the situation in which the number of *neutrons* released by *nuclear fission* is exactly balanced by the number being absorbed (by the fuel and poisons) and escaping the reactor core. A reactor is said to be 'critical' when it achieves a self-sustaining nuclear chain reaction, as when it is operating.

Cumulative dose: total dose resulting from repeated exposure to radiation

Deterministic effect: health effect, the severity of which varies with dose and for which a threshold is believed to exist; e.g. radiation-induced cataract (also called a non-stochastic effect) (see ***Stochastic effect***)

D_0: reciprocal of the final slope of the curve of cell survival as a function of dose, representing cell killing due to multiple events

Dose: a general term denoting the quantity of radiation or energy absorbed

Dose equivalent: quantity that expresses all kinds of radiation on a common scale for calculating the *effective* absorbed *dose*

Dose fractionation: delivery of a given dose of radiation as several smaller doses, separated by intervals of time

Dose protraction: spreading out of a radiation dose over time by continuous delivery at a lower *dose rate*

Dose rate: absorbed dose delivered per unit time

Effective attributable risk (EAR): reduced attributable risk, such as the fraction of total deaths from lung cancer that would be eliminated by reducing exposure to radon

Effective dose: sum of *equivalent doses*, weighted by the appropriate tissue *weighting factors*, in all the tissues and organs of the body

Electromagnetic radiation: travelling wave motion resulting from changing electric or magnetic fields; familiar types range from *X-rays* and *γ-rays* of short wave-length, through the ultraviolet, visible and infrared regions to radar and radio waves of relatively long wavelength

Electron: subatomic charged particle. Negatively charged electrons are parts of stable atoms. Both negatively and positively charged electrons may be expelled from the radioactive atom when it disintegrates (see also *β-particle*).

Electron volt (eV): unit of energy; 1 eV is equivalent to the energy gained by an *electron* in passing through a potential difference of 1 V.

Equivalent dose: obtained by weighting the *absorbed dose* in an organ or tissue by a *weighting factor* that reflects the biological effectiveness of the radiation that produces *ionization* within the tissue

Excess relative risk (ERR): model that describes the risk imposed by exposures as a multiplicative increment to the excess disease risk above the background rate of disease

Fall-out: radioactive debris from a nuclear detonation or other source

Fast neutron: *neutron* with kinetic energy greater than that of its surroundings when released during fission (see ***Thermal neutron***)

Fission product: element or compounds resulting from *nuclear fission*

Flux: term applied to the amount of some types of particle (e.g. *neutrons*, *α-radiation*) or energy (e.g. *photons*, heat) crossing a unit area per unit time; expressed as number of particles or energy per square centimeter per second

γ-radiation or **γ-rays**: short-wavelength *electromagnetic radiation* of nuclear origin; similar to *X-radiation* but emitted at very specific energies characteristic of the decaying atoms

Gray (Gy): unit of absorbed dose of radiation (1 Gy = 1 J kg^{-1})

Half thickness or **half-value layer**: thickness of a specified material that, when introduced into the path of a given beam of radiation, reduces its intensity to one-half of its original value

High-LET radiation (see also ***Linear energy transfer***): heavy, charged particles such as *protons* and *α-particles* that produce dense ionizing events close together on the scale of a cellular nucleus

Ion: atomic particle, atom or chemical radical bearing an electric charge, either negative or positive

Ionization: process by which a neutral atom or molecule acquires a positive or negative charge

Ionization density: number of *ion* pairs per unit volume

Ionization path (track): trail of *ion* pairs produced by *ionizing radiation* in its passage through matter

Ionization radiation: radiation sufficiently energetic to dislodge *electrons* from an atom thereby causing an *ion* pair; includes *X-radiation* and *γ-radiation*, *electrons* (*β-particles*), *α-particles* (helium nuclei) and heavier charged atomic nuclei

Isotope: *nuclide* with same number of *protons* in its nuclei as another nuclide, and hence the same atomic number, but differing in the number of *neutrons* and therefore in the mass number

Kerma (kinetic energy released in matter): unit of exposure that represents the kinetic energy transferred to charged particles per unit mass of irradiated medium when indirectly ionizing (uncharged) particles, such as *photons* or *neutrons*, traverse the medium. If all of the kinetic energy is absorbed 'locally', the kerma is equal to the *absorbed dose*.

Lineal energy: quotient of *e* over *l* where *e* is the energy imparted to the matter in a volume of interest by an energy deposition event and *l* is the mean chord length in that volume

Linear energy transfer (LET): average amount of energy lost per unit of particle track length. Low LET is characteristic of *electrons*, *X-rays* and *γ-rays*; high LET is characteristic of *protons* and *α-particles*.

Linear model (linear dose–effect model): expresses an effect (e.g. mutation or cancer) as a proportional (linear) function of dose.

Linear–quadratic model (linear–quadratic dose–effect model): expresses an effect (e.g. mutation or cancer) as a function of two components, one directly proportional to the dose (linear term) and one proportional to the square of the dose (quadratic term); the linear term predominates at lower doses and the quadratic term at higher doses.

Low-LET radiation: light, charged particles such as *electrons* or *X-rays* and *γ-rays* that produce sparse ionizing events far apart on the scale of a cellular nucleus

Monte Carlo calculation: method for evaluation of a probability distribution by means of random sampling

Neutron: elementary particle that is a constituent of all atomic nuclei except that of normal hydrogen; has no electric charge and a mass only very slightly greater than that of the *proton*. Outside the nucleus, the neutron decays, with a half-life of 12 min, into a *proton*, an *electron* and a neutrino. Upon collision with atomic nuclei, neutrons generate *recoil protons*, which are a source of *high-LET radiation*.

Nuclear fission: splitting of an atomic nucleus into at least two other nuclei and release of a relatively large amount of energy. Two or three *neutrons* are usually released during this type of nuclear transformation.

Nuclear fusion: event in which at least one heavier, more stable nucleus is produced from two lighter, less stable nuclei. Reactions of this type are responsible for enormous releases of energy, such as that of stars.

Nuclear medicine: use of very small amounts of radioactive materials or radio-pharmaceuticals to diagnose and treat disease

Nuclide: species of atom characterized by the constitution of its nucleus and hence by the number of *protons*, the number of *neutrons*, and the energy content

Orbital electron capture: process in which a *proton* of a nucleus is transformed into a *neutron*, by capturing an orbital *electron* accompanied by emission of a neutrino, the captured electron being replaced by one of the other shell electrons causing emission of characteristic radiation

Phantom: anthropomorphic representation of the human body's characteristics in terms of radiation attenuation, physical morphology and geometry; used to calibrate radiation detection systems for measuring radioactive material in the human body

Photon: quantum of *electromagnetic radiation* that has zero rest mass and energy equal to the product of the frequency of the radiation and Planck's constant; generated when a particle with an electric charge changes its momentum, in collisions between nuclei or *electrons* and in the decay of certain atomic nuclei and particles

Proportional counter: radiation instrument in which an electronic detection system receives pulses that are proportional to the number of *ions* formed in a gas-filled tube by *ionizing radiation*

Proton: Stable elementary particle with electric charge equal in magnitude to that of the *electron* but of opposite sign and with mass 1836.12 times greater than that of the electron. The proton is a hydrogen ion (i.e. a normal hydrogen atomic nucleus) and a constituent of all other atomic nuclei.

Radiation shielding (see also *Shielding factor*): reduction of radiation by interposing a shield of absorbing material between any radioactive source and a person, work area or radiation-sensitive device

Radioactivity: property of some *nuclides* of spontaneously emitting particle or *γ-radiation*, emitting *X-radiation* after *orbital electron capture* or undergoing spontaneous *nuclear fission*

Radionuclide: radioactive species of an atom characterized by the constitution of its nucleus; in *nuclear medicine*, an atomic species emitting *ionizing radiation* and capable of existing for a measurable time, so that it may be used to image organs and tissues

Radiosensitivity: relative susceptibility of cells, tissues, organs and organisms to the injurious action of radiation

Recoil: motion imparted to a particle as a result of interaction with radiation or as a result of a nuclear transformation

Recoil proton: product of the elastic collision of a *neutron* with an atomic nucleus; source of *high-LET radiation*

Reference man: person with the anatomical and physiological characteristics of an average individual which is used in calculations of internal dose (also called 'Standard man').

Relative biological effectiveness (RBE): factor used to compare the biological effectiveness of *absorbed* radiation *doses* due to different types of radiation; more specifically, the experimentally determined ratio of an absorbed dose of a radiation in question to that of a reference radiation required to produce an identical biological effect in a particular experimental organism or tissue

Shielding factor: ratio of the detector response at a location behind a shield on which radiation is incident to the detector response at the same location without the presence of the shield; a measure of the effectiveness of the shield

Specific energy: actual energy per unit mass deposited per unit volume in a given event; a stochastic quantity as opposed to the average value over a larger number of instances (i.e. the *absorbed dose*)

Stochastic effect: effect that occurs by chance, generally without a threshold level of dose, whose probability is proportional to the dose and whose severity is independent of the dose. In the context of radiation protection, the main stochastic effects are cancer and genetic effects.

Target volume: (i) volume containing those tissues that are to be irradiated to a specified *absorbed dose* according to a specified time–dose pattern. For curative treatment, the target volume consists of the demonstrated tumour(s), if present, and any other tissue with presumed tumour; (ii) volume of a discrete biological entity (i.e. chromosome strand, bacterium, gene, virus) in which the effect of radiation is primarily seen

Telangiectasia: dilatation of the capillary vessels and very small arteries

Teletherapy: radiation treatment administered from a source at a distance from the body; usually *γ-ray* beams from *radionuclide* sources

Terrestrial radiation: portion of natural *background radiation* that is emitted by naturally occurring radioactive materials, such as uranium, thorium and radon in the earth

Thermal neutron: neutron that has (by collision with other particles) reached an energy state equal to that of its surroundings, typically on the order of 0.025 eV (*electron volts*) (see **Fast neutron**)

Thermoluminescent detector: small device used to measure radiation as the amount of visible light emitted from a crystal in the detector when exposed to *ionizing radiation*

Thermonuclear: adjective referring to the process in which very high temperatures are used to bring about the fusion of light nuclei, such as those of the hydrogen *isotopes* deuterium and tritium, with the accompanying liberation of energy

Threshold dose: minimal *absorbed dose* that will produce a detectable degree of any given effect

Track (see **Ionization path**)

Weighting factor (w_T): multiplier of the *equivalent dose* to an organ or tissue used for radiation protection purposes to account for different sensitivities of different organs and tissues to the induction of *stochastic effects* of radiation

X-radiation or **X-rays**: penetrating *electromagnetic radiation* whose wavelength is shorter than that of visible light; usually produced by bombarding a metallic target with fast *electrons* in a high vacuum; in nuclear reactions, it is customary to refer to *photons* originating in the nucleus as *γ-radiation* and those originating in the extra-nuclear part of the atom as X-radiation. Dose of X-rays is expressed in kVp, the maximum (p for peak) applied voltage (kV) that an X-ray machine can produce.

CUMULATIVE CROSS INDEX TO *IARC MONOGRAPHS ON THE EVALUATION OF CARCINOGENIC RISKS TO HUMANS*

The volume, page and year of publication are given. References to corrigenda are given in parentheses.

A

A-α-C	*40*, 245 (1986); *Suppl. 7*, 56 (1987)
Acetaldehyde	*36*, 101 (1985) (*corr. 42*, 263);
	Suppl. 7, 77 (1987); *71*, 319 (1999)
Acetaldehyde formylmethylhydrazone (*see* Gyromitrin)	
Acetamide	*7*, 197 (1974); *Suppl. 7*, 389 (1987);
	71, 1211 (1999)
Acetaminophen (*see* Paracetamol)	
Acridine orange	*16*, 145 (1978); *Suppl. 7*, 56 (1987)
Acriflavinium chloride	*13*, 31 (1977); *Suppl. 7*, 56 (1987)
Acrolein	*19*, 479 (1979); *36*, 133 (1985);
	Suppl. 7, 78 (1987); *63*, 337 (1995)
	(*corr. 65*, 549)
Acrylamide	*39*, 41 (1986); *Suppl. 7*, 56 (1987);
	60, 389 (1994)
Acrylic acid	*19*, 47 (1979); *Suppl. 7*, 56 (1987);
	71, 1223 (1999)
Acrylic fibres	*19*, 86 (1979); *Suppl. 7*, 56 (1987)
Acrylonitrile	*19*, 73 (1979); *Suppl. 7*, 79 (1987);
	71, 43 (1999)
Acrylonitrile-butadiene-styrene copolymers	*19*, 91 (1979); *Suppl. 7*, 56 (1987)
Actinolite (*see* Asbestos)	
Actinomycin D (*see also* Actinomycins)	*Suppl. 7*, 80 (1987)
Actinomycins	*10*, 29 (1976) (*corr. 42*, 255)
Adriamycin	*10*, 43 (1976); *Suppl. 7*, 82 (1987)
AF-2	*31*, 47 (1983); *Suppl. 7*, 56 (1987)
Aflatoxins	*1*, 145 (1972) (*corr. 42*, 251);
	10, 51 (1976); *Suppl. 7*, 83 (1987);
	56, 245 (1993)
Aflatoxin B₁ (*see* Aflatoxins)	
Aflatoxin B₂ (*see* Aflatoxins)	
Aflatoxin G₁ (*see* Aflatoxins)	
Aflatoxin G₂ (*see* Aflatoxins)	
Aflatoxin M₁ (*see* Aflatoxins)	
Agaritine	*31*, 63 (1983); *Suppl. 7*, 56 (1987)
Alcohol drinking	*44* (1988)
Aldicarb	*53*, 93 (1991)
Aldrin	*5*, 25 (1974); *Suppl. 7*, 88 (1987)
Allyl chloride	*36*, 39 (1985); *Suppl. 7*, 56 (1987);
	71, 1231 (1999)

Allyl isothiocyanate — *36*, 55 (1985); *Suppl. 7*, 56 (1987); *73*, 37 (1999)

Allyl isovalerate — *36*, 69 (1985); *Suppl. 7*, 56 (1987); *71*, 1241 (1999)

Aluminium production — *34*, 37 (1984); *Suppl. 7*, 89 (1987)
Amaranth — *8*, 41 (1975); *Suppl. 7*, 56 (1987)
5-Aminoacenaphthene — *16*, 243 (1978); *Suppl. 7*, 56 (1987)
2-Aminoanthraquinone — *27*, 191 (1982); *Suppl. 7*, 56 (1987)
para-Aminoazobenzene — *8*, 53 (1975); *Suppl. 7*, 390 (1987)
ortho-Aminoazotoluene — *8*, 61 (1975) (*corr. 42*, 254); *Suppl. 7*, 56 (1987)

para-Aminobenzoic acid — *16*, 249 (1978); *Suppl. 7*, 56 (1987)
4-Aminobiphenyl — *1*, 74 (1972) (*corr. 42*, 251); *Suppl. 7*, 91 (1987)

2-Amino-3,4-dimethylimidazo[4,5-*f*]quinoline (*see* MeIQ)
2-Amino-3,8-dimethylimidazo[4,5-*f*]quinoxaline (*see* MeIQx)
3-Amino-1,4-dimethyl-5*H*-pyrido[4,3-*b*]indole (*see* Trp-P-1)
2-Aminodipyrido[1,2-*a*:3′,2′-*d*]imidazole (*see* Glu-P-2)
1-Amino-2-methylanthraquinone — *27*, 199 (1982); *Suppl. 7*, 57 (1987)
2-Amino-3-methylimidazo[4,5-*f*]quinoline (*see* IQ)
2-Amino-6-methyldipyrido[1,2-*a*:3′,2′-*d*]imidazole (*see* Glu-P-1)
2-Amino-1-methyl-6-phenylimidazo[4,5-*b*]pyridine (*see* PhIP)
2-Amino-3-methyl-9*H*-pyrido[2,3-*b*]indole (*see* MeA-α-C)
3-Amino-1-methyl-5*H*-pyrido[4,3-*b*]indole (*see* Trp-P-2)
2-Amino-5-(5-nitro-2-furyl)-1,3,4-thiadiazole — *7*, 143 (1974); *Suppl. 7*, 57 (1987)
2-Amino-4-nitrophenol — *57*, 167 (1993)
2-Amino-5-nitrophenol — *57*, 177 (1993)
4-Amino-2-nitrophenol — *16*, 43 (1978); *Suppl. 7*, 57 (1987)
2-Amino-5-nitrothiazole — *31*, 71 (1983); *Suppl. 7*, 57 (1987)
2-Amino-9*H*-pyrido[2,3-*b*]indole (*see* A-α-C)
11-Aminoundecanoic acid — *39*, 239 (1986); *Suppl. 7*, 57 (1987)
Amitrole — *7*, 31 (1974); *41*, 293 (1986) (*corr. 52*, 513; *Suppl. 7*, 92 (1987)

Ammonium potassium selenide (*see* Selenium and selenium compounds)
Amorphous silica (*see also* Silica) — *42*, 39 (1987); *Suppl. 7*, 341 (1987); *68*, 41 (1997)

Amosite (*see* Asbestos)
Ampicillin — *50*, 153 (1990)
Anabolic steroids (*see* Androgenic (anabolic) steroids)
Anaesthetics, volatile — *11*, 285 (1976); *Suppl. 7*, 93 (1987)
Analgesic mixtures containing phenacetin (*see also* Phenacetin) — *Suppl. 7*, 310 (1987)
Androgenic (anabolic) steroids — *Suppl. 7*, 96 (1987)
Angelicin and some synthetic derivatives (*see also* Angelicins) — *40*, 291 (1986)
Angelicin plus ultraviolet radiation (*see also* Angelicin and some synthetic derivatives) — *Suppl. 7*, 57 (1987)
Angelicins — *Suppl. 7*, 57 (1987)
Aniline — *4*, 27 (1974) (*corr. 42*, 252); *27*, 39 (1982); *Suppl. 7*, 99 (1987)
ortho-Anisidine — *27*, 63 (1982); *Suppl. 7*, 57 (1987); *73*, 49 (1999)

para-Anisidine — *27*, 65 (1982); *Suppl. 7*, 57 (1987)
Anthanthrene — *32*, 95 (1983); *Suppl. 7*, 57 (1987)
Anthophyllite (*see* Asbestos)
Anthracene — *32*, 105 (1983); *Suppl. 7*, 57 (1987)

Benzidine   *1*, 80 (1972); *29*, 149, 391 (1982);
                                                           Suppl. 7, 123 (1987)

Benzidine-based dyes   *Suppl. 7*, 125 (1987)
Benzo[*b*]fluoranthene   *3*, 69 (1973); *32*, 147 (1983);
                                                           Suppl. 7, 58 (1987)

Benzo[*j*]fluoranthene   *3*, 82 (1973); *32*, 155 (1983);
                                                           Suppl. 7, 58 (1987)

Benzo[*k*]fluoranthene   *32*, 163 (1983); *Suppl. 7*, 58 (1987)
Benzo[*ghi*]fluoranthene   *32*, 171 (1983); *Suppl. 7*, 58 (1987)
Benzo[*a*]fluorene   *32*, 177 (1983); *Suppl. 7*, 58 (1987)
Benzo[*b*]fluorene   *32*, 183 (1983); *Suppl. 7*, 58 (1987)
Benzo[*c*]fluorene   *32*, 189 (1983); *Suppl. 7*, 58 (1987)
Benzofuran   *63*, 431 (1995)
Benzo[*ghi*]perylene   *32*, 195 (1983); *Suppl. 7*, 58 (1987)
Benzo[*c*]phenanthrene   *32*, 205 (1983); *Suppl. 7*, 58 (1987)
Benzo[*a*]pyrene   *3*, 91 (1973); *32*, 211 (1983)
                                                           (*corr. 68*, 477); *Suppl. 7*, 58 (1987)
Benzo[*e*]pyrene   *3*, 137 (1973); *32*, 225 (1983);
                                                           Suppl. 7, 58 (1987)

1,4-Benzoquinone (see *para*-Quinone)
1,4-Benzoquinone dioxime   *29*, 185 (1982); *Suppl. 7*, 58 (1987);
                                                           71, 1251 (1999)
Benzotrichloride (*see also* α-Chlorinated toluenes and benzoyl chloride)   *29*, 73 (1982); *Suppl. 7*, 148 (1987);
                                                           71, 453 (1999)
Benzoyl chloride (*see also* α-Chlorinated toluenes and benzoyl chloride)   *29*, 83 (1982) (*corr. 42*, 261);
                                                           Suppl. 7, 126 (1987); *71*, 453 (1999)
Benzoyl peroxide   *36*, 267 (1985); *Suppl. 7*, 58 (1987);
                                                           71, 345 (1999)
Benzyl acetate   *40*, 109 (1986); *Suppl. 7*, 58 (1987);
                                                           71, 1255 (1999)
Benzyl chloride (*see also* α-Chlorinated toluenes and benzoyl chloride)   *11*, 217 (1976) (*corr. 42*, 256); *29*,
                                                           49 (1982); *Suppl. 7*, 148 (1987);
                                                           71, 453 (1999)
Benzyl violet 4B   *16*, 153 (1978); *Suppl. 7*, 58 (1987)
Bertrandite (*see* Beryllium and beryllium compounds)
Beryllium and beryllium compounds   *1*, 17 (1972); *23*, 143 (1980)
                                                           (*corr. 42*, 260); *Suppl. 7*, 127
                                                           (1987); *58*, 41 (1993)

Beryllium acetate (*see* Beryllium and beryllium compounds)
Beryllium acetate, basic (*see* Beryllium and beryllium compounds)
Beryllium-aluminium alloy (*see* Beryllium and beryllium compounds)
Beryllium carbonate (*see* Beryllium and beryllium compounds)
Beryllium chloride (*see* Beryllium and beryllium compounds)
Beryllium-copper alloy (*see* Beryllium and beryllium compounds)
Beryllium-copper-cobalt alloy (*see* Beryllium and beryllium compounds)
Beryllium fluoride (*see* Beryllium and beryllium compounds)
Beryllium hydroxide (*see* Beryllium and beryllium compounds)
Beryllium-nickel alloy (*see* Beryllium and beryllium compounds)
Beryllium oxide (*see* Beryllium and beryllium compounds)
Beryllium phosphate (*see* Beryllium and beryllium compounds)
Beryllium silicate (*see* Beryllium and beryllium compounds)
Beryllium sulfate (*see* Beryllium and beryllium compounds)
Beryl ore (*see* Beryllium and beryllium compounds)
Betel quid   *37*, 141 (1985); *Suppl. 7*, 128 (1987)

C

Cabinet-making (*see* Furniture and cabinet-making)
Cadmium acetate (*see* Cadmium and cadmium compounds)
Cadmium and cadmium compounds

2, 74 (1973); *11*, 39 (1976)
(*corr. 42*, 255); *Suppl. 7*, 139
(1987); *58*, 119 (1993)

Cadmium chloride (*see* Cadmium and cadmium compounds)
Cadmium oxide (*see* Cadmium and cadmium compounds)
Cadmium sulfate (*see* Cadmium and cadmium compounds)
Cadmium sulfide (*see* Cadmium and cadmium compounds)
Caffeic acid

56, 115 (1993)

Caffeine

51, 291 (1991)

Calcium arsenate (*see* Arsenic and arsenic compounds)
Calcium chromate (see Chromium and chromium compounds)
Calcium cyclamate (*see* Cyclamates)
Calcium saccharin (*see* Saccharin)
Cantharidin

10, 79 (1976); *Suppl. 7*, 59 (1987)

Caprolactam

19, 115 (1979) (*corr. 42*, 258);
39, 247 (1986) (*corr. 42*, 264);
Suppl. 7, 390 (1987); *71*, 383
(1999)

Captafol

53, 353 (1991)

Captan

30, 295 (1983); *Suppl. 7*, 59 (1987)

Carbaryl

12, 37 (1976); *Suppl. 7*, 59 (1987)

Carbazole

32, 239 (1983); *Suppl. 7*, 59
(1987); *71*, 1319 (1999)

3-Carbethoxypsoralen

40, 317 (1986); *Suppl. 7*, 59 (1987)

Carbon black

3, 22 (1973); *33*, 35 (1984);
Suppl. 7, 142 (1987); *65*, 149
(1996)

Carbon tetrachloride

1, 53 (1972); *20*, 371 (1979);
Suppl. 7, 143 (1987); *71*, 401
(1999)

Carmoisine

8, 83 (1975); *Suppl. 7*, 59 (1987)

Carpentry and joinery

25, 139 (1981); *Suppl. 7*, 378
(1987)

Carrageenan

10, 181 (1976) (*corr. 42*, 255); *31*,
79 (1983); *Suppl. 7*, 59 (1987)

Catechol

15, 155 (1977); *Suppl. 7*, 59
(1987); *71*, 433 (1999)

CCNU (*see* 1-(2-Chloroethyl)-3-cyclohexyl-1-nitrosourea)
Ceramic fibres (see Man-made mineral fibres)
Chemotherapy, combined, including alkylating agents (*see* MOPP and
        other combined chemotherapy including alkylating agents)
Chloral

63, 245 (1995)

Chloral hydrate

63, 245 (1995)

Chlorambucil

9, 125 (1975); *26*, 115 (1981);
Suppl. 7, 144 (1987)

Chloramphenicol

10, 85 (1976); *Suppl. 7*, 145
(1987); *50*, 169 (1990)

Chlordane (*see also* Chlordane/Heptachlor)

20, 45 (1979) (*corr. 42*, 258)

Chlordane/Heptachlor

Suppl. 7, 146 (1987); *53*, 115
(1991)

Chlorotrianisene (*see also* Nonsteroidal oestrogens)   *21*, 139 (1979); *Suppl. 7*, 280
                                                             (1987)
2-Chloro-1,1,1-trifluoroethane   *41*, 253 (1986); *Suppl. 7*, 60
                                                             (1987); *71*, 1355 (1999)
Chlorozotocin   *50*, 65 (1990)
Cholesterol   *10*, 99 (1976); *31*, 95 (1983);
                                                             Suppl. 7, 161 (1987)

Chromic acetate (*see* Chromium and chromium compounds)
Chromic chloride (*see* Chromium and chromium compounds)
Chromic oxide (*see* Chromium and chromium compounds)
Chromic phosphate (*see* Chromium and chromium compounds)
Chromite ore (*see* Chromium and chromium compounds)
Chromium and chromium compounds (*see also* Implants, surgical)   *2*, 100 (1973); *23*, 205 (1980);
                                                             Suppl. 7, 165 (1987); *49*, 49 (1990)
                                                             (*corr. 51*, 483)

Chromium carbonyl (*see* Chromium and chromium compounds)
Chromium potassium sulfate (*see* Chromium and chromium compounds)
Chromium sulfate (*see* Chromium and chromium compounds)
Chromium trioxide (*see* Chromium and chromium compounds)
Chrysazin (*see* Dantron)
Chrysene   *3*, 159 (1973); *32*, 247 (1983);
                                                             Suppl. 7, 60 (1987)
Chrysoidine   *8*, 91 (1975); *Suppl. 7*, 169 (1987)
Chrysotile (*see* Asbestos)
CI Acid Orange 3   *57*, 121 (1993)
CI Acid Red 114   *57*, 247 (1993)
CI Basic Red 9 (*see also* Magenta)   *57*, 215 (1993)
Ciclosporin   *50*, 77 (1990)
CI Direct Blue 15   *57*, 235 (1993)
CI Disperse Yellow 3 (see Disperse Yellow 3)
Cimetidine   *50*, 235 (1990)
Cinnamyl anthranilate   *16*, 287 (1978); *31*, 133 (1983);
                                                             Suppl. 7, 60 (1987)
CI Pigment Red 3   *57*, 259 (1993)
CI Pigment Red 53:1 (*see* D&C Red No. 9)
Cisplatin (*see also* Etoposide)   *26*, 151 (1981); *Suppl. 7*, 170
                                                             (1987)
Citrinin   *40*, 67 (1986); *Suppl. 7*, 60 (1987)
Citrus Red No. 2   *8*, 101 (1975) (*corr. 42*, 254);
                                                             Suppl. 7, 60 (1987)
Clinoptilolite (*see* Zeolites)
Clofibrate   *24*, 39 (1980); *Suppl. 7*, 171
                                                             (1987); *66*, 391 (1996)
Clomiphene citrate   *21*, 551 (1979); *Suppl. 7*, 172
                                                             (1987)
Clonorchis sinensis (infection with)   *61*, 121 (1994)
Coal dust   *68*, 337 (1997)
Coal gasification   *34*, 65 (1984); *Suppl. 7*, 173 (1987)
Coal-tar pitches (*see also* Coal-tars)   *35*, 83 (1985); *Suppl. 7*, 174 (1987)
Coal-tars   *35*, 83 (1985); *Suppl. 7*, 175 (1987)
Cobalt[III] acetate (*see* Cobalt and cobalt compounds)
Cobalt-aluminium-chromium spinel (*see* Cobalt and cobalt compounds)
Cobalt and cobalt compounds (*see also* Implants, surgical)   *52*, 363 (1991)
Cobalt[II] chloride (*see* Cobalt and cobalt compounds)

DDD (*see* DDT)
DDE (*see* DDT)
DDT   *5*, 83 (1974) (*corr. 42*, 253);
                                                           Suppl. 7, 186 (1987); *53*, 179
                                                           (1991)
Decabromodiphenyl oxide   *48*, 73 (1990); *71*, 1365 (1999)
Deltamethrin   *53*, 251 (1991)
Deoxynivalenol (*see* Toxins derived from *Fusarium graminearum,*
     F. culmorum and *F. crookwellense*)
Diacetylaminoazotoluene   *8*, 113 (1975); *Suppl. 7*, 61 (1987)
N,N'-Diacetylbenzidine   *16*, 293 (1978); *Suppl. 7*, 61 (1987)
Diallate   *12*, 69 (1976); *30*, 235 (1983);
                                                           Suppl. 7, 61 (1987)
2,4-Diaminoanisole   *16*, 51 (1978); *27*, 103 (1982);
                                                           Suppl. 7, 61 (1987)
4,4'-Diaminodiphenyl ether   *16*, 301 (1978); *29*, 203 (1982);
                                                           Suppl. 7, 61 (1987)
1,2-Diamino-4-nitrobenzene   *16*, 63 (1978); *Suppl. 7*, 61 (1987)
1,4-Diamino-2-nitrobenzene   *16*, 73 (1978); *Suppl. 7*, 61 (1987);
                                                           57, 185 (1993)
2,6-Diamino-3-(phenylazo)pyridine (*see* Phenazopyridine hydrochloride)
2,4-Diaminotoluene (*see also* Toluene diisocyanates)   *16*, 83 (1978); *Suppl. 7*, 61 (1987)
2,5-Diaminotoluene (*see also* Toluene diisocyanates)   *16*, 97 (1978); *Suppl. 7*, 61 (1987)
ortho-Dianisidine (*see* 3,3'-Dimethoxybenzidine)
Diatomaceous earth, uncalcined (*see* Amorphous silica)
Diazepam   *13*, 57 (1977*); Suppl. 7*, 189
                                                           (1987); *66*, 37 (1996)
Diazomethane   *7*, 223 (1974); *Suppl. 7*, 61 (1987)
Dibenz[*a,h*]acridine   *3*, 247 (1973); *32*, 277 (1983);
                                                           Suppl. 7, 61 (1987)
Dibenz[*a,j*]acridine   *3*, 254 (1973); *32*, 283 (1983);
                                                           Suppl. 7, 61 (1987)
Dibenz[*a,c*]anthracene   *32*, 289 (1983) (*corr. 42*, 262);
                                                           Suppl. 7, 61 (1987)
Dibenz[*a,h*]anthracene   *3*, 178 (1973) (*corr. 43*, 261);
                                                           32, 299 (1983); *Suppl. 7*, 61 (1987)
Dibenz[*a,j*]anthracene   *32*, 309 (1983); *Suppl. 7*, 61 (1987)
7*H*-Dibenzo[*c,g*]carbazole   *3*, 260 (1973); *32*, 315 (1983);
                                                           Suppl. 7, 61 (1987)
Dibenzodioxins, chlorinated (other than TCDD)
     (*see* Chlorinated dibenzodioxins (other than TCDD))
Dibenzo[*a,e*]fluoranthene   *32*, 321 (1983); *Suppl. 7*, 61 (1987)
Dibenzo[*h,rst*]pentaphene   *3*, 197 (1973); *Suppl. 7*, 62 (1987)
Dibenzo[*a,e*]pyrene   *3*, 201 (1973); *32*, 327 (1983);
                                                           Suppl. 7, 62 (1987)
Dibenzo[*a,h*]pyrene   *3*, 207 (1973); *32*, 331 (1983);
                                                           Suppl. 7, 62 (1987)
Dibenzo[*a,i*]pyrene   *3*, 215 (1973); *32*, 337 (1983);
                                                           Suppl. 7, 62 (1987)
Dibenzo[*a,l*]pyrene   *3*, 224 (1973); *32*, 343 (1983);
                                                           Suppl. 7, 62 (1987)
Dibenzo-*para*-dioxin   *69*, 33 (1997)
Dibromoacetonitrile (*see also* Halogenated acetonitriles) *71*, 1369 (1999)

Diethyl sulfate	*4*, 277 (1974); *Suppl. 7*, 198 (1987); *54*, 213 (1992); *71*, 1405 (1999)
Diglycidyl resorcinol ether	*11*, 125 (1976); *36*, 181 (1985); *Suppl. 7*, 62 (1987); *71*, 1417 (1999)
Dihydrosafrole	*1*, 170 (1972); *10*, 233 (1976) *Suppl. 7*, 62 (1987)
1,8-Dihydroxyanthraquinone (*see* Dantron)	
Dihydroxybenzenes (*see* Catechol; Hydroquinone; Resorcinol)	
Dihydroxymethylfuratrizine	*24*, 77 (1980); *Suppl. 7*, 62 (1987)
Diisopropyl sulfate	*54*, 229 (1992); *71*, 1421 (1999)
Dimethisterone (*see also* Progestins; Sequential oral contraceptives)	*6*, 167 (1974); *21*, 377 (1979)
Dimethoxane	*15*, 177 (1977); *Suppl. 7*, 62 (1987)
3,3′-Dimethoxybenzidine	*4*, 41 (1974); *Suppl. 7*, 198 (1987)
3,3′-Dimethoxybenzidine-4,4′-diisocyanate	*39*, 279 (1986); *Suppl. 7*, 62 (1987)
para-Dimethylaminoazobenzene	*8*, 125 (1975); *Suppl. 7*, 62 (1987)
para-Dimethylaminoazobenzenediazo sodium sulfonate	*8*, 147 (1975); *Suppl. 7*, 62 (1987)
trans-2-[(Dimethylamino)methylimino]-5-[2-(5-nitro-2-furyl)-vinyl]-1,3,4-oxadiazole	*7*, 147 (1974) (*corr. 42*, 253); *Suppl. 7*, 62 (1987)
4,4′-Dimethylangelicin plus ultraviolet radiation (*see also* Angelicin and some synthetic derivatives)	*Suppl. 7*, 57 (1987)
4,5′-Dimethylangelicin plus ultraviolet radiation (*see also* Angelicin and some synthetic derivatives)	*Suppl. 7*, 57 (1987)
2,6-Dimethylaniline	*57*, 323 (1993)
N,N-Dimethylaniline	*57*, 337 (1993)
Dimethylarsinic acid (*see* Arsenic and arsenic compounds)	
3,3′-Dimethylbenzidine	*1*, 87 (1972); *Suppl. 7*, 62 (1987)
Dimethylcarbamoyl chloride	*12*, 77 (1976); *Suppl. 7*, 199 (1987); *71*, 531 (1999)
Dimethylformamide	*47*, 171 (1989); *71*, 545 (1999)
1,1-Dimethylhydrazine	*4*, 137 (1974); *Suppl. 7*, 62 (1987); *71*, 1425 (1999)
1,2-Dimethylhydrazine	*4*, 145 (1974) (*corr. 42*, 253); *Suppl. 7*, 62 (1987); *71*, 947 (1999)
Dimethyl hydrogen phosphite	*48*, 85 (1990); *71*, 1437 (1999)
1,4-Dimethylphenanthrene	*32*, 349 (1983); *Suppl. 7*, 62 (1987)
Dimethyl sulfate	*4*, 271 (1974); *Suppl. 7*, 200 (1987); *71*, 575 (1999)
3,7-Dinitrofluoranthene	*46*, 189 (1989); *65*, 297 (1996)
3,9-Dinitrofluoranthene	*46*, 195 (1989); *65*, 297 (1996)
1,3-Dinitropyrene	*46*, 201 (1989)
1,6-Dinitropyrene	*46*, 215 (1989)
1,8-Dinitropyrene	*33*, 171 (1984); *Suppl. 7*, 63 (1987); *46*, 231 (1989)
Dinitrosopentamethylenetetramine	*11*, 241 (1976); *Suppl. 7*, 63 (1987)
2,4-Dinitrotoluene	*65*, 309 (1996) (*corr. 66*, 485)
2,6-Dinitrotoluene	*65*, 309 (1996) (*corr. 66*, 485)
3,5-Dinitrotoluene	*65*, 309 (1996)
1,4-Dioxane	*11*, 247 (1976); *Suppl. 7*, 201 (1987); *71*, 589 (1999)
2,4′-Diphenyldiamine	*16*, 313 (1978); *Suppl. 7*, 63 (1987)
Direct Black 38 (*see also* Benzidine-based dyes)	*29*, 295 (1982) (*corr. 42*, 261)
Direct Blue 6 (*see also* Benzidine-based dyes)	*29*, 311 (1982)

Ethyl tellurac	*12*, 115 (1976); *Suppl. 7*, 63 (1987)
Ethynodiol diacetate	*6*, 173 (1974); *21*, 387 (1979); *Suppl. 7*, 292 (1987); *72*, 49 (1999)
Eugenol	*36*, 75 (1985); *Suppl. 7*, 63 (1987)
Evans blue	*8*, 151 (1975); *Suppl. 7*, 63 (1987)

F

Fast Green FCF	*16*, 187 (1978); *Suppl. 7*, 63 (1987)
Fenvalerate	*53*, 309 (1991)
Ferbam	*12*, 121 (1976) (*corr. 42*, 256); *Suppl. 7*, 63 (1987)
Ferric oxide	*1*, 29 (1972); *Suppl. 7*, 216 (1987)
Ferrochromium (*see* Chromium and chromium compounds)	
Fluometuron	*30*, 245 (1983); *Suppl. 7*, 63 (1987)
Fluoranthene	*32*, 355 (1983); *Suppl. 7*, 63 (1987)
Fluorene	*32*, 365 (1983); *Suppl. 7*, 63 (1987)
Fluorescent lighting (exposure to) (*see* Ultraviolet radiation)	
Fluorides (inorganic, used in drinking-water)	*27*, 237 (1982); *Suppl. 7*, 208 (1987)
5-Fluorouracil	*26*, 217 (1981); *Suppl. 7*, 210 (1987)
Fluorspar (*see* Fluorides)	
Fluosilicic acid (*see* Fluorides)	
Fluroxene (*see* Anaesthetics, volatile)	
Foreign bodies	*74* (1999)
Formaldehyde	*29*, 345 (1982); *Suppl. 7*, 211 (1987); *62*, 217 (1995) (*corr. 65*, 549; *corr. 66*, 485)
2-(2-Formylhydrazino)-4-(5-nitro-2-furyl)thiazole	*7*, 151 (1974) (*corr. 42*, 253); *Suppl. 7*, 63 (1987)
Frusemide (*see* Furosemide)	
Fuel oils (heating oils)	*45*, 239 (1989) (*corr. 47*, 505)
Fumonisin B₁ (*see* Toxins derived from *Fusarium moniliforme*)	
Fumonisin B₂ (*see* Toxins derived from *Fusarium moniliforme*)	
Furan	*63*, 393 (1995)
Furazolidone	*31*, 141 (1983); *Suppl. 7*, 63 (1987)
Furfural	*63*, 409 (1995)
Furniture and cabinet-making	*25*, 99 (1981); *Suppl. 7*, 380 (1987)
Furosemide	*50*, 277 (1990)
2-(2-Furyl)-3-(5-nitro-2-furyl)acrylamide (*see* AF-2)	
Fusarenon-X (*see* Toxins derived from *Fusarium graminearum*, *F. culmorum* and *F. crookwellense*)	
Fusarenone-X (*see* Toxins derived from *Fusarium graminearum*, *F. culmorum* and *F. crookwellense*)	
Fusarin C (*see* Toxins derived from *Fusarium moniliforme*)	

G

γ-radiation	*75*, 121 (2000)
Gasoline	*45*, 159 (1989) (*corr. 47*, 505)

Hexachloroethane	*20*, 467 (1979); *Suppl. 7*, 64 (1987); *73*, 295 (1999)
Hexachlorophene	*20*, 241 (1979); *Suppl. 7*, 64 (1987)
Hexamethylphosphoramide	*15*, 211 (1977); *Suppl. 7*, 64 (1987); *71*, 1465 (1999)
Hexoestrol (*see also* Nonsteroidal oestrogens)	*Suppl. 7*, 279 (1987)
Hormonal contraceptives, progestogens only	*72*, 339 (1999)
Human herpesvirus 8	*70*, 375 (1997)
Human immunodeficiency viruses	*67*, 31 (1996)
Human papillomaviruses	*64* (1995) (*corr. 66*, 485)
Human T-cell lymphotropic viruses	*67*, 261 (1996)
Hycanthone mesylate	*13*, 91 (1977); *Suppl. 7*, 64 (1987)
Hydralazine	*24*, 85 (1980); *Suppl. 7*, 222 (1987)
Hydrazine	*4*, 127 (1974); *Suppl. 7*, 223 (1987); *71*, 991 (1999)
Hydrochloric acid	*54*, 189 (1992)
Hydrochlorothiazide	*50*, 293 (1990)
Hydrogen peroxide	*36*, 285 (1985); *Suppl. 7*, 64 (1987); *71*, 671 (1999)
Hydroquinone	*15*, 155 (1977); *Suppl. 7*, 64 (1987); *71*, 691 (1999)
4-Hydroxyazobenzene	*8*, 157 (1975); *Suppl. 7*, 64 (1987)
17α-Hydroxyprogesterone caproate (*see also* Progestins)	*21*, 399 (1979) (*corr. 42*, 259)
8-Hydroxyquinoline	*13*, 101 (1977); *Suppl. 7*, 64 (1987)
8-Hydroxysenkirkine	*10*, 265 (1976); *Suppl. 7*, 64 (1987)
Hypochlorite salts	*52*, 159 (1991)

I

Implants, surgical	*74*, 1999
Indeno[1,2,3-*cd*]pyrene	*3*, 229 (1973); *32*, 373 (1983); *Suppl. 7*, 64 (1987)
Inorganic acids (*see* Sulfuric acid and other strong inorganic acids, occupational exposures to mists and vapours from)	
Insecticides, occupational exposures in spraying and application of	*53*, 45 (1991)
Ionizing radiation (*see* Neutrons, γ- and X-radiation)	
IQ	*40*, 261 (1986); *Suppl. 7*, 64 (1987); *56*, 165 (1993)
Iron and steel founding	*34*, 133 (1984); *Suppl. 7*, 224 (1987)
Iron-dextran complex	*2*, 161 (1973); *Suppl. 7*, 226 (1987)
Iron-dextrin complex	*2*, 161 (1973) (*corr. 42*, 252); *Suppl. 7*, 64 (1987)
Iron oxide (*see* Ferric oxide)	
Iron oxide, saccharated (*see* Saccharated iron oxide)	
Iron sorbitol-citric acid complex	*2*, 161 (1973); *Suppl. 7*, 64 (1987)
Isatidine	*10*, 269 (1976); *Suppl. 7*, 65 (1987)
Isoflurane (*see* Anaesthetics, volatile)	
Isoniazid (*see* Isonicotinic acid hydrazide)	
Isonicotinic acid hydrazide	*4*, 159 (1974); *Suppl. 7*, 227 (1987)
Isophosphamide	*26*, 237 (1981); *Suppl. 7*, 65 (1987)
Isoprene	*60*, 215 (1994); *71*, 1015 (1999)

Light Green SF	*16*, 209 (1978); *Suppl. 7*, 65 (1987)
d-Limonene	*56*, 135 (1993); *73*, 307 (1999)
Lindane (*see* Hexachlorocyclohexanes)	
Liver flukes (*see Clonorchis sinensis, Opisthorchis felineus* and *Opisthorchis viverrini*)	
Lumber and sawmill industries (including logging)	*25*, 49 (1981); *Suppl. 7*, 383 (1987)
Luteoskyrin	*10*, 163 (1976); *Suppl. 7*, 65 (1987)
Lynoestrenol	*21*, 407 (1979); *Suppl. 7*, 293 (1987); *72*, 49 (1999)

M

Magenta	*4*, 57 (1974) (*corr. 42*, 252); *Suppl. 7*, 238 (1987); *57*, 215 (1993)
Magenta, manufacture of (*see also* Magenta)	*Suppl. 7*, 238 (1987); *57*, 215 (1993)
Malathion	*30*, 103 (1983); *Suppl. 7*, 65 (1987)
Maleic hydrazide	*4*, 173 (1974) (*corr. 42*, 253); *Suppl. 7*, 65 (1987)
Malonaldehyde	*36*, 163 (1985); *Suppl. 7*, 65 (1987); *71*, 1037 (1999)
Malondialdehyde (*see* Malonaldehyde)	
Maneb	*12*, 137 (1976); *Suppl. 7*, 65 (1987)
Man-made mineral fibres	*43*, 39 (1988)
Mannomustine	*9*, 157 (1975); *Suppl. 7*, 65 (1987)
Mate	*51*, 273 (1991)
MCPA (*see also* Chlorophenoxy herbicides; Chlorophenoxy herbicides, occupational exposures to)	*30*, 255 (1983)
MeA-α-C	*40*, 253 (1986); *Suppl. 7*, 65 (1987)
Medphalan	*9*, 168 (1975); *Suppl. 7*, 65 (1987)
Medroxyprogesterone acetate	*6*, 157 (1974); *21*, 417 (1979) (*corr. 42*, 259); *Suppl. 7*, 289 (1987); *72*, 339 (1999)
Megestrol acetate	*Suppl. 7*, 293 (1987); *72*, 49 (1999)
MeIQ	*40*, 275 (1986); *Suppl. 7*, 65 (1987); *56*, 197 (1993)
MeIQx	*40*, 283 (1986); *Suppl. 7*, 65 (1987) *56*, 211 (1993)
Melamine	*39*, 333 (1986); *Suppl. 7*, 65 (1987); *73*, 329 (1999)
Melphalan	*9*, 167 (1975); *Suppl. 7*, 239 (1987)
6-Mercaptopurine	*26*, 249 (1981); *Suppl. 7*, 240 (1987)
Mercuric chloride (*see* Mercury and mercury compounds)	
Mercury and mercury compounds	*58*, 239 (1993)
Merphalan	*9*, 169 (1975); *Suppl. 7*, 65 (1987)
Mestranol	*6*, 87 (1974); *21*, 257 (1979) (*corr. 42*, 259); *Suppl. 7*, 288 (1987); *72*, 49 (1999)
Metabisulfites (*see* Sulfur dioxide and some sulfites, bisulfites and metabisulfites)	
Metallic mercury (*see* Mercury and mercury compounds)	

Methyl methanesulfonate   *7*, 253 (1974); *Suppl. 7*, 66 (1987);
                                                                       71, 1059 (1999)
2-Methyl-1-nitroanthraquinone   *27*, 205 (1982); *Suppl. 7*, 66 (1987)
N-Methyl-*N*'-nitro-*N*-nitrosoguanidine   *4*, 183 (1974); *Suppl. 7*, 248 (1987)
3-Methylnitrosaminopropionaldehyde [*see* 3-(*N*-Nitrosomethylamino)-
    propionaldehyde]
3-Methylnitrosaminopropionitrile [*see* 3-(*N*-Nitrosomethylamino)-
    propionitrile]
4-(Methylnitrosamino)-4-(3-pyridyl)-1-butanal [*see* 4-(*N*-Nitrosomethyl-
    amino)-4-(3-pyridyl)-1-butanal]
4-(Methylnitrosamino)-1-(3-pyridyl)-1-butanone [*see* 4-(-Nitrosomethyl-
    amino)-1-(3-pyridyl)-1-butanone]
N-Methyl-*N*-nitrosourea   *1*, 125 (1972); *17*, 227 (1978);
                                                                       Suppl. 7, 66 (1987)
N-Methyl-*N*-nitrosourethane   *4*, 211 (1974); *Suppl. 7*, 66 (1987)
N-Methylolacrylamide   *60*, 435 (1994)
Methyl parathion   *30*, 131 (1983); *Suppl. 7*, 392
                                                                       (1987)
1-Methylphenanthrene   *32*, 405 (1983); *Suppl. 7*, 66 (1987)
7-Methylpyrido[3,4-*c*]psoralen   *40*, 349 (1986); *Suppl. 7*, 71 (1987)
Methyl red   *8*, 161 (1975); *Suppl. 7*, 66 (1987)
Methyl selenac (*see also* Selenium and selenium compounds)   *12*, 161 (1976); *Suppl. 7*, 66 (1987)
Methylthiouracil   *7*, 53 (1974); *Suppl. 7*, 66 (1987)
Metronidazole   *13*, 113 (1977); *Suppl. 7*, 250
                                                                       (1987)
Mineral oils   *3*, 30 (1973); *33*, 87 (1984)
                                                                       (*corr. 42*, 262); *Suppl. 7*, 252
                                                                       (1987)
Mirex   *5*, 203 (1974); *20*, 283 (1979)
                                                                       (*corr. 42*, 258); *Suppl. 7*, 66 (1987)
Mists and vapours from sulfuric acid and other strong inorganic acids *54*, 41 (1992)
Mitomycin C   *10*, 171 (1976); *Suppl. 7*, 67 (1987)
MNNG (*see N*-Methyl-*N*'-nitro-*N*-nitrosoguanidine)
MOCA (*see* 4,4'-Methylene bis(2-chloroaniline))
Modacrylic fibres   *19*, 86 (1979); *Suppl. 7*, 67 (1987)
Monocrotaline   *10*, 291 (1976); *Suppl. 7*, 67 (1987)
Monuron   *12*, 167 (1976); *Suppl. 7*, 67
                                                                       (1987); *53*, 467 (1991)
MOPP and other combined chemotherapy including   *Suppl. 7*, 254 (1987)
    alkylating agents
Mordanite (*see* Zeolites)
Morpholine   *47*, 199 (1989); *71*, 1511 (1999)
5-(Morpholinomethyl)-3-[(5-nitrofurfurylidene)amino]-2-   *7*, 161 (1974); *Suppl. 7*, 67 (1987)
    oxazolidinone
Musk ambrette   *65*, 477 (1996)
Musk xylene   *65*, 477 (1996)
Mustard gas   *9*, 181 (1975) (*corr. 42*, 254);
                                                                       Suppl. 7, 259 (1987)
Myleran (*see* 1,4-Butanediol dimethanesulfonate)

N

Oral contraceptives, sequential (*see* Sequential oral contraceptives)

Orange I	*8*, 173 (1975); *Suppl. 7*, 69 (1987)
Orange G	*8*, 181 (1975); *Suppl. 7*, 69 (1987)
Organolead compounds (*see also* Lead and lead compounds)	*Suppl. 7*, 230 (1987)
Oxazepam	*13*, 58 (1977); *Suppl. 7*, 69 (1987); *66*, 115 (1996)
Oxymetholone (*see also* Androgenic (anabolic) steroids)	*13*, 131 (1977)
Oxyphenbutazone	*13*, 185 (1977); *Suppl. 7*, 69 (1987)

P

Paint manufacture and painting (occupational exposures in)	*47*, 329 (1989)
Palygorskite	*42*, 159 (1987); *Suppl. 7*, 117 (1987); *68*, 245 (1997)
Panfuran S (*see also* Dihydroxymethylfuratrizine)	*24*, 77 (1980); *Suppl. 7*, 69 (1987)
Paper manufacture (*see* Pulp and paper manufacture)	
Paracetamol	*50*, 307 (1990); *73*, 401 (1999)
Parasorbic acid	*10*, 199 (1976) (*corr. 42*, 255); *Suppl. 7*, 69 (1987)
Parathion	*30*, 153 (1983); *Suppl. 7*, 69 (1987)
Patulin	*10*, 205 (1976); *40*, 83 (1986); *Suppl. 7*, 69 (1987)
Penicillic acid	*10*, 211 (1976); *Suppl. 7*, 69 (1987)
Pentachloroethane	*41*, 99 (1986); *Suppl. 7*, 69 (1987); *71*, 1519 (1999)
Pentachloronitrobenzene (see Quintozene)	
Pentachlorophenol (*see also* Chlorophenols; Chlorophenols, occupational exposures to; Polychlorophenols and their sodium salts)	*20*, 303 (1979); *53*, 371 (1991)
Permethrin	*53*, 329 (1991)
Perylene	*32*, 411 (1983); *Suppl. 7*, 69 (1987)
Petasitenine	*31*, 207 (1983); *Suppl. 7*, 69 (1987)
Petasites japonicus (*see also* Pyrrolizidine alkaloids)	*10*, 333 (1976)
Petroleum refining (occupational exposures in)	*45*, 39 (1989)
Petroleum solvents	*47*, 43 (1989)
Phenacetin	*13*, 141 (1977); *24*, 135 (1980); *Suppl. 7*, 310 (1987)
Phenanthrene	*32*, 419 (1983); *Suppl. 7*, 69 (1987)
Phenazopyridine hydrochloride	*8*, 117 (1975); *24*, 163 (1980) (*corr. 42*, 260); *Suppl. 7*, 312 (1987)
Phenelzine sulfate	*24*, 175 (1980); *Suppl. 7*, 312 (1987)
Phenicarbazide	*12*, 177 (1976); *Suppl. 7*, 70 (1987)
Phenobarbital	*13*, 157 (1977); *Suppl. 7*, 313 (1987)
Phenol	*47*, 263 (1989) (*corr. 50*, 385); *71*, 749 (1999)
Phenoxyacetic acid herbicides (*see* Chlorophenoxy herbicides)	
Phenoxybenzamine hydrochloride	*9*, 223 (1975); *24*, 185 (1980); *Suppl. 7*, 70 (1987)
Phenylbutazone	*13*, 183 (1977); *Suppl. 7*, 316 (1987)
meta-Phenylenediamine	*16*, 111 (1978); *Suppl. 7*, 70 (1987)

Potassium bromate	40, 207 (1986); Suppl. 7, 70 (1987); 73, 481 (1999)
Potassium chromate (see Chromium and chromium compounds)	
Potassium dichromate (see Chromium and chromium compounds)	
Prazepam	66, 143 (1996)
Prednimustine	50, 115 (1990)
Prednisone	26, 293 (1981); Suppl. 7, 326 (1987)
Printing processes and printing inks	65, 33 (1996)
Procarbazine hydrochloride	26, 311 (1981); Suppl. 7, 327 (1987)
Proflavine salts	24, 195 (1980); Suppl. 7, 70 (1987)
Progesterone (see also Progestins; Combined oral contraceptives)	6, 135 (1974); 21, 491 (1979) (corr. 42, 259)
Progestins (see Progestogens)	
Progestogens	Suppl. 7, 289 (1987); 72, 49, 339, 531 (1999)
Pronetalol hydrochloride	13, 227 (1977) (corr. 42, 256); Suppl. 7, 70 (1987)
1,3-Propane sultone	4, 253 (1974) (corr. 42, 253); Suppl. 7, 70 (1987); 71, 1095 (1999)
Propham	12, 189 (1976); Suppl. 7, 70 (1987)
β-Propiolactone	4, 259 (1974) (corr. 42, 253); Suppl. 7, 70 (1987); 71, 1103 (1999)
n-Propyl carbamate	12, 201 (1976); Suppl. 7, 70 (1987)
Propylene	19, 213 (1979); Suppl. 7, 71 (1987); 60, 161 (1994)
Propyleneimine (see 2-Methylaziridine)	
Propylene oxide	11, 191 (1976); 36, 227 (1985) (corr. 42, 263); Suppl. 7, 328 (1987); 60, 181 (1994)
Propylthiouracil	7, 67 (1974); Suppl. 7, 329 (1987)
Ptaquiloside (see also Bracken fern)	40, 55 (1986); Suppl. 7, 71 (1987)
Pulp and paper manufacture	25, 157 (1981); Suppl. 7, 385 (1987)
Pyrene	32, 431 (1983); Suppl. 7, 71 (1987)
Pyrido[3,4-c]psoralen	40, 349 (1986); Suppl. 7, 71 (1987)
Pyrimethamine	13, 233 (1977); Suppl. 7, 71 (1987)
Pyrrolizidine alkaloids (see Hydroxysenkirkine; Isatidine; Jacobine; Lasiocarpine; Monocrotaline; Retrorsine; Riddelliine; Seneciphylline; Senkirkine)	

Q

Quartz (see Crystalline silica)	
Quercetin (see also Bracken fern)	31, 213 (1983); Suppl. 7, 71 (1987); 73, 497 (1999)
para-Quinone	15, 255 (1977); Suppl. 7, 71 (1987); 71, 1245 (1999)
Quintozene	5, 211 (1974); Suppl. 7, 71 (1987)

and repair)

Silica (*see also* Amorphous silica; Crystalline silica)	*42*, 39 (1987)
Silicone (*see* Implants, surgical)	
Simazine	*53*, 495 (1991); *73*, 625 (1999)
Slagwool (*see* Man-made mineral fibres)	
Sodium arsenate (*see* Arsenic and arsenic compounds)	
Sodium arsenite (*see* Arsenic and arsenic compounds)	
Sodium cacodylate (*see* Arsenic and arsenic compounds)	
Sodium chlorite	*52*, 145 (1991)
Sodium chromate (*see* Chromium and chromium compounds)	
Sodium cyclamate (*see* Cyclamates)	
Sodium dichromate (*see* Chromium and chromium compounds)	
Sodium diethyldithiocarbamate	*12*, 217 (1976); *Suppl. 7*, 71 (1987)
Sodium equilin sulfate (*see* Conjugated oestrogens)	
Sodium fluoride (*see* Fluorides)	
Sodium monofluorophosphate (*see* Fluorides)	
Sodium oestrone sulfate (*see* Conjugated oestrogens)	
Sodium *ortho*-phenylphenate (*see also ortho*-Phenylphenol)	*30*, 329 (1983); *Suppl. 7*, 392 (1987); *73*, 451 (1999)
Sodium saccharin (*see* Saccharin)	
Sodium selenate (*see* Selenium and selenium compounds)	
Sodium selenite (*see* Selenium and selenium compounds)	
Sodium silicofluoride (*see* Fluorides)	
Solar radiation	*55* (1992)
Soots	*3*, 22 (1973); *35*, 219 (1985); *Suppl. 7*, 343 (1987)
Spironolactone	*24*, 259 (1980); *Suppl. 7*, 344 (1987)
Stannous fluoride (*see* Fluorides)	
Steel founding (*see* Iron and steel founding)	
Steel, stainless (*see* Implants, surgical)	
Sterigmatocystin	*1*, 175 (1972); *10*, 245 (1976); *Suppl. 7*, 72 (1987)
Steroidal oestrogens	*Suppl. 7*, 280 (1987)
Streptozotocin	*4*, 221 (1974); *17*, 337 (1978); *Suppl. 7*, 72 (1987)
Strobane® (*see* Terpene polychlorinates)	
Strong-inorganic-acid mists containing sulfuric acid (*see* Mists and vapours from sulfuric acid and other strong inorganic acids)	
Strontium chromate (*see* Chromium and chromium compounds)	
Styrene	*19*, 231 (1979) (*corr. 42*, 258); *Suppl. 7*, 345 (1987); *60*, 233 (1994) (*corr. 65*, 549)
Styrene-acrylonitrile-copolymers	*19*, 97 (1979); *Suppl. 7*, 72 (1987)
Styrene-butadiene copolymers	*19*, 252 (1979); *Suppl. 7*, 72 (1987)
Styrene-7,8-oxide	*11*, 201 (1976); *19*, 275 (1979); *36*, 245 (1985); *Suppl. 7*, 72 (1987); *60*, 321 (1994)
Succinic anhydride	*15*, 265 (1977); *Suppl. 7*, 72 (1987)
Sudan I	*8*, 225 (1975); *Suppl. 7*, 72 (1987)
Sudan II	*8*, 233 (1975); *Suppl. 7*, 72 (1987)
Sudan III	*8*, 241 (1975); *Suppl. 7*, 72 (1987)
Sudan Brown RR	*8*, 249 (1975); *Suppl. 7*, 72 (1987)
Sudan Red 7B	*8*, 253 (1975); *Suppl. 7*, 72 (1987)

U

V

Vat Yellow 4	*48*, 161 (1990)
Vinblastine sulfate	*26*, 349 (1981) (*corr. 42*, 261); *Suppl. 7*, 371 (1987)
Vincristine sulfate	*26*, 365 (1981); *Suppl. 7*, 372 (1987)
Vinyl acetate	*19*, 341 (1979); *39*, 113 (1986); *Suppl. 7*, 73 (1987); *63*, 443 (1995)
Vinyl bromide	*19*, 367 (1979); *39*, 133 (1986); *Suppl. 7*, 73 (1987); *71*, 923 (1999)
Vinyl chloride	*7*, 291 (1974); *19*, 377 (1979) (*corr. 42*, 258*); Suppl. 7*, 373 (1987)
Vinyl chloride-vinyl acetate copolymers	*7*, 311 (1976); *19*, 412 (1979) (*corr. 42*, 258); *Suppl. 7*, 73 (1987)
4-Vinylcyclohexene	*11*, 277 (1976); *39*, 181 (1986) *Suppl. 7*, 73 (1987); *60*, 347 (1994)
4-Vinylcyclohexene diepoxide	*11*, 141 (1976); *Suppl. 7*, 63 (1987); *60*, 361 (1994)
Vinyl fluoride	*39*, 147 (1986); *Suppl. 7*, 73 (1987); *63*, 467 (1995)
Vinylidene chloride	*19*, 439 (1979); *39*, 195 (1986); *Suppl. 7*, 376 (1987); *71*, 1163 (1999)
Vinylidene chloride-vinyl chloride copolymers	*19*, 448 (1979) (*corr. 42*, 258); *Suppl. 7*, 73 (1987)
Vinylidene fluoride	*39*, 227 (1986); *Suppl. 7*, 73 (1987); *71*, 1551 (1999)
N-Vinyl-2-pyrrolidone	*19*, 461 (1979); *Suppl. 7*, 73 (1987); *71*, 1181 (1999)
Vinyl toluene	*60*, 373 (1994)

W

Welding	*49*, 447 (1990) (*corr. 52*, 513)
Wollastonite	*42*, 145 (1987); *Suppl. 7*, 377 (1987); *68*, 283 (1997)
Wood dust	*62*, 35 (1995)
Wood industries	*25* (1981); *Suppl. 7*, 378 (1987)

X

X-radiation	*75*, 121 (2000)
Xylenes	*47*, 125 (1989); *71*, 1189 (1999)
2,4-Xylidine	*16*, 367 (1978); *Suppl. 7*, 74 (1987)
2,5-Xylidine	*16*, 377 (1978); *Suppl. 7*, 74 (1987)
2,6-Xylidine (*see* 2,6-Dimethylaniline)	

List of IARC Monographs on the Evaluation of Carcinogenic Risks to Humans*

Volume 1
Some Inorganic Substances, Chlorinated Hydrocarbons, Aromatic Amines, N-Nitroso Compounds, and Natural Products
1972; 184 pages (out-of-print)

Volume 2
Some Inorganic and Organo-metallic Compounds
1973; 181 pages (out-of-print)

Volume 3
Certain Polycyclic Aromatic Hydrocarbons and Heterocyclic Compounds
1973; 271 pages (out-of-print)

Volume 4
Some Aromatic Amines, Hydra-zine and Related Substances, N-Nitroso Compounds and Miscellaneous Alkylating Agents
1974; 286 pages (out-of-print)

Volume 5
Some Organochlorine Pesticides
1974; 241 pages (out-of-print)

Volume 6
Sex Hormones
1974; 243 pages (out-of-print)

Volume 7
Some Anti-Thyroid and Related Substances, Nitrofurans and Industrial Chemicals
1974; 326 pages (out-of-print)

Volume 8
Some Aromatic Azo Compounds
1975; 357 pages

Volume 9
Some Aziridines, N-, S- and O-Mustards and Selenium
1975; 268 pages

Volume 10
Some Naturally Occurring Substances
1976; 353 pages (out-of-print)

Volume 11
Cadmium, Nickel, Some Epoxides, Miscellaneous Industrial Chemicals and General Considerations on Volatile Anaesthetics
1976; 306 pages (out-of-print)

Volume 12
Some Carbamates, Thio-carbamates and Carbazides
1976; 282 pages (out-of-print)

Volume 13
Some Miscellaneous Pharmaceutical Substances
1977; 255 pages

Volume 14
Asbestos
1977; 106 pages (out-of-print)

Volume 15
Some Fumigants, the Herbicides 2,4-D and 2,4,5-T, Chlorinated Dibenzodioxins and Miscella-neous Industrial Chemicals
1977; 354 pages (out-of-print)

Volume 16
Some Aromatic Amines and Related Nitro Compounds—Hair Dyes, Colouring Agents and Miscellaneous Industrial Chemicals
1978; 400 pages

Volume 17
Some N-Nitroso Compounds
1978; 365 pages

Volume 18
Polychlorinated Biphenyls and Polybrominated Biphenyls
1978; 140 pages (out-of-print)

Volume 19
Some Monomers, Plastics and Synthetic Elastomers, and Acrolein
1979; 513 pages (out-of-print)

Volume 20
Some Halogenated Hydrocarbons
1979; 609 pages (out-of-print)

Volume 21
Sex Hormones (II)
1979; 583 pages

Volume 22
Some Non-Nutritive Sweetening Agents
1980; 208 pages

Volume 23
Some Metals and Metallic Compounds
1980; 438 pages (out-of-print)

Volume 24
Some Pharmaceutical Drugs
1980; 337 pages

Volume 25
Wood, Leather and Some Associated Industries
1981; 412 pages

Volume 26
Some Antineoplastic and Immunosuppressive Agents
1981; 411 pages

Volume 27
Some Aromatic Amines, Anthraquinones and Nitroso Compounds, and Inorganic Fluorides Used in Drinking-water and Dental Preparations
1982; 341 pages

Volume 28
The Rubber Industry
1982; 486 pages

Volume 29
Some Industrial Chemicals and Dyestuffs
1982; 416 pages

Volume 30
Miscellaneous Pesticides
1983; 424 pages

---

*Certain older volumes, marked out-of-print, are still available directly from IARCPress. Further, high-quality photo-copies of all out-of-print volumes may be purchased from University Microfilms International, 300 North Zeeb Road, Ann Arbor, MI 48106-1346, USA (Tel.: 313-761-4700, 800-521-0600).

All IARC publications are available directly from
IARCPress, 150 Cours Albert Thomas, F-69372 Lyon cedex 08, France
(Fax: +33 4 72 73 83 02; E-mail: press@iarc.fr).

IARC Monographs and Technical Reports are also available from the
World Health Organization Distribution and Sales, CH-1211 Geneva 27
(Fax: +41 22 791 4857; E-mail: publications@who.int)
and from WHO Sales Agents worldwide.

IARC Scientific Publications, IARC Handbooks and IARC CancerBases are also available from
Oxford University Press, Walton Street, Oxford, UK OX2 6DP (Fax: +44 1865 267782).